Respiratory Diseases: Contemporary Diagnosis and Treatment

Respiratory Diseases: Contemporary Diagnosis and Treatment

Editor: Stephen Rogers

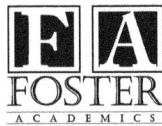

FA
FOSTER
ACADEMICS

www.fosteracademics.com

www.fosteracademics.com

FA
FOSTER
ACADEMICS

Cataloging-in-Publication Data

Respiratory diseases : contemporary diagnosis and treatment / edited by Stephen Rogers.
    p. cm.
Includes bibliographical references and index.
ISBN 978-1-63242-802-8
    1. Respiratory organs--Diseases. 2. Respiratory organs--Diseases--Diagnosis.
3. Respiratory organs--Diseases--Treatment. 4. Respiratory infections. I. Rogers, Stephen.
RC731 .R47 2019
616.2--dc23

Foster Academics,
118-35 Queens Blvd., Suite 400,
Forest Hills, NY 11375, USA

ISBN 978-1-63242-802-8 (Hardback)

Contents

Preface

The diseases related to the organs and tissues involved in gas exchange are called respiratory diseases. They involve the conditions associated with the upper respiratory tract, bronchi, pleura, alveoli, trachea, bronchioles and pleural cavity. Common cold is one of the most common respiratory disease. Other severe respiratory conditions include acute asthma, pneumonia, pulmonary embolism and lung cancer. Pulmonology is the field of medicine dealing with respiratory diseases. Some of the common tests used for diagnosing respiratory diseases include blood tests, chest X-ray, bronchoscopy, ultrasound, computed tomography scan and pulmonary function test. Medications include the intake of antibiotics and leukotriene antagonists, and the inhalation of bronchodilators and steroids. Different approaches, evaluations, methodologies and advanced studies on respiratory diseases have been included in this book. It includes some of the vital pieces of work being conducted across the world, on various topics related to the diagnosis and treatment of respiratory diseases. With state-of-the-art inputs by acclaimed experts of this field, this book targets students and professionals.

This book is the end result of constructive efforts and intensive research done by experts in this field. The aim of this book is to enlighten the readers with recent information in this area of research. The information provided in this profound book would serve as a valuable reference to students and researchers in this field.

At the end, I would like to thank all the authors for devoting their precious time and providing their valuable contribution to this book. I would also like to express my gratitude to my fellow colleagues who encouraged me throughout the process.

Editor

Serum sST2 levels predict severe exacerbation of asthma

Masato Watanabe[*] , Keitaro Nakamoto, Toshiya Inui, Mitsuru Sada, Kojiro Honda, Masaki Tamura, Yukari Ogawa, Takuma Yokoyama, Takeshi Saraya, Daisuke Kurai, Haruyuki Ishii and Hajime Takizawa

Abstract

Background: Neutrophilic inflammation is associated with poorly controlled asthma. Serum levels of sST2, a soluble IL-33 receptor, increase in neutrophilic lung diseases. We hypothesized that high serum sST2 levels in stable asthmatics are a predictor for exacerbation within a short duration.

Methods: This prospective observational study evaluated the serum sST2 levels of 104 asthmatic patients who were treated by a lung disease specialist with follow-ups for 3 months.

Results: High serum sST2 levels (> 18 ng/ml) predicted severe asthma exacerbation within 3 months. Serum sST2 levels correlated positively with asthma severity (treatment step), airway H_2O_2 levels, and serum IL-8 levels. High serum sST2 levels and blood neutrophilia (> 6000 /µl) were independent predictors of exacerbation. We defined a post-hoc exacerbation-risk score combining high serum sST2 level and blood neutrophilia, which stratified patients into four groups. The score predicted exacerbation-risk with an area under curve of 0.91 in the receiver operating characteristic curve analysis. Patients with the highest scores had the most severe phenotype, with 85.7% showing exacerbation, airflow limitation, and corticosteroid-insensitivity.

Conclusions: High serum sST2 levels predicted exacerbation within the general asthmatic population and, when combined with blood neutrophil levels, provided an exacerbation-risk score that was an accurate predictor of exacerbation occurring within 3 months.

Keywords: IL-33, ST2L, Biomarker

Background

Bronchial asthma is a clinical syndrome characterized by chronic airway inflammation, respiratory symptoms, airflow limitation, and bronchial hypersensitivity [1]. Asthma has heterogeneous pathogenic causes and can be classified into different phenotypes [2, 3].

In particular, neutrophilic airway inflammation is found in patients with poorly controlled asthma [4–6]. Neutrophilic asthma is characterized by a high neutrophil count in the sputum (40–76%), along with severe asthma, corticosteroid-insensitivity, chronic airflow obstruction, and acute exacerbation [4, 5, 7–9]. Furthermore, mixed granulocytic (i.e. neutrophilic and eosinophilic) infiltration into the airway causes the greatest disease burden and airflow limitation in asthmatic patients [8, 9]. Patients with

uncontrolled asthma commonly use oral corticosteroid, which may further augment airway neutrophilia. Peripheral blood neutrophilia is another predictor for exacerbation and poor control of asthma [10], which may be related to oral corticosteroids usage. Importantly, the association between neutrophil counts in sputum and peripheral blood is very weak [5]. Combined, these results indicate that asthma related to neutrophilic inflammation can be further classified into subtypes, e.g. airway- or blood-dominance and combined. However, no current serum biomarkers efficiently stratify neutrophil-related asthma into subgroups.

Soluble suppression of tumorigenicity 2 (sST2) is a decoy receptor for interleukin (IL)-33 [11, 12]. IL-33 is released from bronchial epithelial cells and lung blood vessels after exposure to allergic antigens [13] and necrosis [14]. IL-33 causes eosinophilic inflammation and Th2 cytokine production in the lungs [14–17] and is involved

---
* Correspondence: masato@ks.kyorin-u.ac.jp
Department of Respiratory Medicine, Kyorin University School of Medicine, 6-20-3 Sinkawa, Mitaka-city, Tokyo 181-8612, Japan

in arising asthma [17, 18]. In contrast, sST2 is released from bronchial epithelial cells and lung blood vessels by stimulation with proinflammatory cytokines, toll-like receptor (TLR) ligands, and Th2 cytokines [11, 19]. Serum sST2 levels are markedly increased when neutrophilic inflammation is present (i.e. in pneumonia [20], chronic obstructive lung disease [COPD], [21] and sepsis [22]). In patients with atopic asthma, serum sST2 levels are elevated during exacerbation and are associated with the severity of the asthma attack [23]. These indicate that the IL-33/sST2 balance affects granulocyte counts in the airway, and that high serum sST2 levels in asthmatics are associated with exacerbation occurrences.

We hypothesized that high serum sST2 levels in stable asthmatics are a predictor for exacerbation within a short period of time. We also expected that serum sST2 levels would stratify neutrophil-related asthma into subgroups. To address these, we conducted a prospective observational study, in which we recruited 104 asthmatic patients, measured serum sST2 levels, followed-up for 3 months, and evaluated whether serum sST2 levels predicted exacerbation. We also explored the characteristics of patients with high serum sST2 levels, and found that serum sST2 levels and blood neutrophilia were independent predictors of asthma exacerbation. In a post-hoc decision, we defined an asthma exacerbation-risk score based on high serum sST2 levels and blood neutrophilia. Patients that were positive for both were at extremely high exacerbation risk (85.7%), indicating that serum sST2 levels and blood neutrophil counts can classify poorly controlled asthma into clinically relevant subgroups.

Methods
Study design
This was a prospective observational study approved by the institutional review board at Kyorin University (approvals no. 161 and no. 523). All patients gave written informed consent before participating; patients underwent blood tests, lung function tests, and fractional exhaled nitric oxide (FeNO) tests, followed by obtaining exhaled breath condensates (EBC). Afterward, the patients were treated by lung disease specialists in accordance with the guidelines of the Global Initiative for Asthma (GINA) 2015 [24] and were followed-up for 3 months. The primary endpoint was severe exacerbation: defined as worsening asthma that required hospital admission or an emergency room visit.

Patients
We recruited patients with asthma who visited the Department of Respiratory Medicine, Kyorin University Hospital from January 2013 through November 2015. All patients were diagnosed with asthma and assessed for treatment step by a lung disease specialist according

to the criteria of the GINA 2015. No patients had experienced any exacerbation of asthma for at least 4 weeks prior to participating in the study.

Laboratory testing and cytokine measurements
Serum levels of sST2, IL-6, IL-8, IL-33, and IL-5 were quantified using Quantikine ELISA kits (R&D Systems, MN, USA) according to the manufacturer's instructions. EBC was obtained with an RTube (Respiratory Research, TX, USA). Serum and EBC H_2O_2 levels were measured using a d-ROMs test® (WISMERLL, Tokyo, Japan). The FeNO level was measured using a NIOX MINO® device (Aerocrine AB, Solna, Sweden) according to the manufacturer's instructions and the American Thoracic Society-guidelines [25].

Statistics
Normality was assessed using the Shapiro-Wilk test. Data are shown as mean ± SD and median (interquartile range) for parametric and non-parametric data, respectively. For parametric data, two or more groups were compared using the Student's t-test or one-way ANOVA, respectively. For non-parametric data, two or more groups were compared using the Mann-Whitney or Kruskal-Wallis tests, respectively. Categorical data were compared using a Chi-square test or Fisher's Exact test. Multiple comparisons for parametric and non-parametric data were performed using the Dunnett test and the Steel test, respectively. For all correlations, the Spearman's correlation coefficient was used. Using the receiver operating characteristic (ROC) curve analysis, the area under curve (AUC) and cut-off values (determined by the Youden index) were calculated. Hazard ratios were calculated using a Cox-regression analysis. Power analysis was performed with an alpha value of 0.05. Statistical analyses were performed using SPSS statistics version 19.0.0 (IBM, New York, USA), SigmaProt version 11.0 (Systat Software Inc., Illinois, USA), and the free website provided by Osaka University (Osaka, Japan; http://www.gen-info.osa-ka-u.ac.jp/MEPHAS/steel.html).

Results
Characteristics of the patients
A total of 104 asthmatic patients were enrolled. During the three-month follow-up period, 11 patients experienced exacerbation (at-risk), whereas 93 patients did not (stable). Triggers of exacerbation were natural worsening of asthma in 10 patients and infection in one. At-risk patients showed poorer control of asthma, a higher treatment step, higher percentage of oral corticosteroid usage, higher WBC and blood neutrophil counts, lower blood eosinophil counts, higher serum H_2O_2 and IL-6 levels, and lower percentages of predicted vital capacity (%VC) and forced vital capacity (%FVC) than stable patients

(Table 1). Smoking status, serum IgE levels and FeNO did not differ between groups. No patient was treated with biotherapy.

Serum sST2 levels and high-risk exacerbation patients
At-risk patients showed higher serum sST2 levels than stable patients ($p = 0.002$, Fig. 1a). A patient with

Table 1 Patient characteristics

	Stable (N = 93)	At-risk (N = 11)	P-value*†
Age, mean (SD)	52.7 (15.4)	51.7 (19.4)	0.852
Sex, M: F, n (%)	39 (42.0): 54 (58.0)	3 (27.3): 8 (72.7)	0.540
BMI, median (IQR)	22.9 (20.6–26.9)	24.6 (21.8–30.1)	0.089
Smoking, n (%)			
Current-smoker	8 (8.6)	2 (18.2)	0.454
Ex-smoker	27 (29.0)	4 (36.4)	
Never-smoker	58 (62.4)	5 (45.4)	
Asthma control, n (%)			
Well controlled	29 (31.2)	1 (9.1)	**< 0.001**
Partially controlled	51 (54.8)	2 (18.2)	
Uncontrolled	13 (14.0)	8 (72.7)	
Treatment step, n (%)			
1	4 (4.3)	0 (0.0)	**0.008**
2	14 (15.1)	0 (0.0)	
3	20 (21.5)	0 (0.0)	
4	49 (52.7)	7 (63.6)	
5	6 (6.4)	4 (36.4)	
Oral CS use, n (%)	6 (6.5)	4 (36.4)	**0.011**
Laboratory tests			
WBC (/µL), median (IQR)	6300 (5000–7200)	10,500 (6700–12,100)	**< 0.001**
Neutrophil (/µL), median (IQR)	3618 (2745–4772)	8159 (3953–9196)	**< 0.001**
Eosinophil (/µL), median (IQR)	201 (128–334)	79 (32–303)	**0.029**
CRP (mg/dl), median (IQR)	0.1 (0–0.2)	0.1 (0–0.5)	0.208
IgE (IU/ml), median (IQR)	188 (45–533)	185 (12–1539)	0.841
IL-8 (pg/ml), median (IQR)	13.1 (10.6–16.9)	16.0 (9.6–22.6)	0.612
IL-6 (pg/ml), median (IQR)	1.0 (0.5–1.7)	2.4 (1.2–3.7)	**0.035**
Serum H_2O_2 (U.CARR), median (IQR)	336 (302–380)	379 (350–421)	**0.025**
FeNO (ppb), median (IQR)	24 (16–42)	16 (11–99)	0.302
EBC H_2O_2 (U.CARR), median (IQR)	0.5 (0.1–1.0)	0.5 (0.2–0.6)	0.687
Lung function tests			
VC (L), median (IQR)	3.1 (2.5–4.0)	2.8 (2.5–4.0)	0.067
%VC (%), mean (SD)	107.4 (16.1)	94.5 (18.9)	**0.016**
FVC (L), median (IQR)	3.0 (2.5–3.9)	2.5 (1.9–3.6)	0.067
%FVC (%), mean (SD)	98.8 (15.6)	87.4 (18.7)	**0.027**
FEV_1 (L), median (IQR)	2.3 (1.8–2.9)	1.7 (1.3–2.9)	0.104
%FEV_1 (%), mean (SD)	89.6 (19.1)	80.1 (26.1)	0.135
FEV_1/FVC (%), median (IQR)	75.2 (68.4–81)	73.6 (64.3–83.4)	0.958

*P-values for parametric, non-parametric, and categorical data were calculated using the Student's t-test, Mann-Whitney test, and Chi-square test, respectively
†Bold letters, P < 0.05
BMI body mass index, Oral CS oral corticosteroid, WBC white blood cells, FeNO fractional exhaled nitric oxide, EBC exhaled breath condensate, SD standard deviation, IQR interquartile range

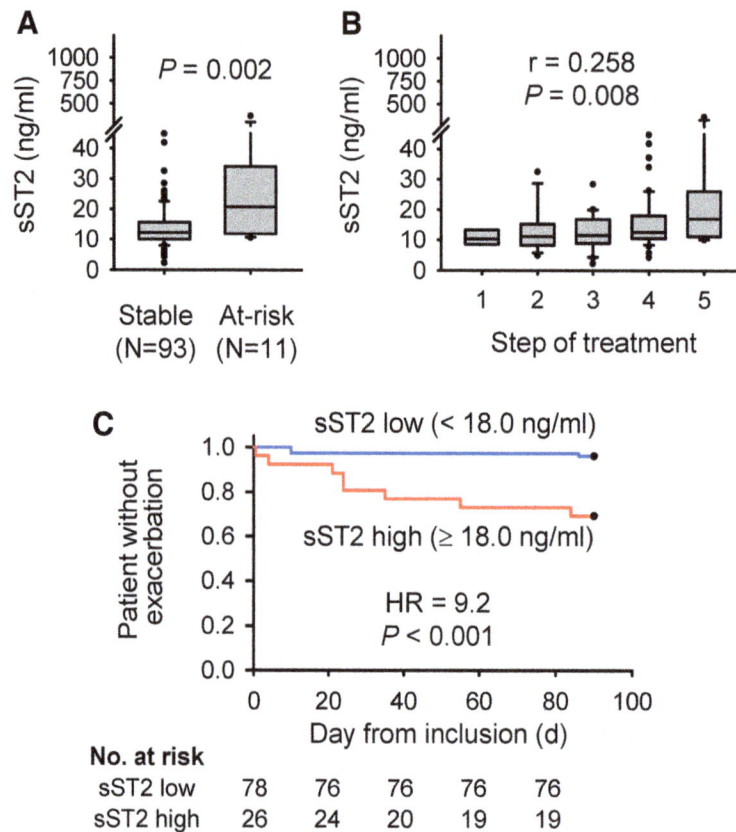

Fig. 1 Serum sST2 levels and asthma exacerbation risk. **a** Serum sST2 levels were higher in patients whose asthma was exacerbated within 3 months (at-risk) than those without exacerbation (stable). **b** Serum sST2 levels correlated positively with the treatment steps defined in the GINA guidelines (2015). **c** Survival analysis comparing durations until exacerbation between patients with high and low serum sST2 levels. **a–c** p-values were calculated using the Mann-Whitney test (**a**), Spearman's rank correlation (**b**), and Cox regression analysis (**c**)

extremely high sST2 levels (364 ng/ml) was exacerbated due to infection within 1 day. Serum sST2 levels correlated positively with treatment step ($r = 0.258$, $p = 0.008$, Fig. 1b). Serum sST2 levels predicted at-risk patients with an AUC (95% CI) of 0.79 (0.63–0.94) in a ROC curve analysis. A cut-off value of 18.0 ng/ml was diagnostic of patients at high risk of exacerbation (sensitivity 0.73, specificity 0.81), with a hazard ratio (95% confidence interval) of 9.2 (2.4–34.7, $P = 0.001$; Fig. 1c). Importantly, a power analysis showed that high serum sST2 levels predicted at-risk patients with a power of 0.983 ($\alpha = 0.05$, $N = 104$, $p < 0.001$), confirming that this study has a sufficient sample size.

These findings demonstrate that serum sST2 levels correlate positively with asthma severity and can diagnose patients at high risk of exacerbation.

Serum sST2 levels and neutrophilic inflammation

To explore the characteristics of patients with high serum sST2 levels, we evaluated the correlation between serum sST2 levels and clinical parameters. Serum sST2 levels correlated positively with serum IL-8 levels and airway oxidative stress levels (EBC H_2O_2) (Table 2). These findings indicate that serum sST2 levels reflect the extent of airway inflammation and systemic chemotaxis activity. On the other hand, blood neutrophil counts correlated positively with serum CRP, IL-6, oxidative stress (H_2O_2) levels, and BMI, and negatively with blood eosinophil (%), serum IgE levels, FeNO levels, and %VC (Table 2). These results suggest that blood neutrophil counts are associated with the extent of systemic inflammation, blood oxidative stress, and obesity, and are strongly associated with neutrophilic inflammation but not eosinophilic or atopic inflammation. Unexpectedly, serum sST2 levels and blood neutrophil counts did not correlate (Table 2). Furthermore, we confirmed that high serum sST2 levels and blood neutrophilia (6000/μl) were independent predictors for asthma exacerbation (Table 3). Importantly, serum sST2 levels were not affected by oral corticosteroid usage, although WBC and blood neutrophil counts were elevated in asthmatics who used regular oral corticosteroid (Additional file 1: Figure S1). We also measured serum IL-5 and IL-33 levels in 40 subjects as preliminary experiments, but the levels were under the detection limit in all 40 subjects.

Table 2 Correlations between serum sST2 levels and clinical parameters

	Serum sST2 level (N = 104)		Blood neutrophil count (N = 104)	
	r	P-value*	r	P-value*
EBC H_2O_2 level[a]	0.281	**0.011**	0.074	0.513
FeNO	0.045	0.653	−0.306	**0.002**
Serum IL-8 level	0.328	**0.001**	0.011	0.915
Serum IL-6 level	0.089	0.370	0.384	**0.001**
Serum CRP level	0.002	0.981	0.305	**0.002**
Serum IgE level	0.046	0.643	−0.241	**0.014**
Serum H_2O_2 level	−0.099	0.318	0.214	**0.029**
BMI	0.185	0.060	0.205	**0.037**
WBC	0.138	0.164	0.901	**< 0.001**
Blood neutrophil count	0.129	0.191	ND	ND
Blood eosinophil count	−0.162	0.100	−0.187	0.057
Blood neutrophil (%)	0.107	0.278	0.794	**< 0.001***
Blood eosinophil (%)	−0.206	**0.036***	− 0.409	**< 0.001***

*Bold letters, $P < 0.05$ calculated using Spearman rank correlation
[a]$N = 81$
R = correlation coefficient, FeNO fractional exhaled nitric oxide, EBC exhaled breath condensate, WBC white blood cell

Taken together, high serum sST2 levels and blood neutrophilia reflect airway and systemic inflammation, respectively, and are independent predictors for asthma exacerbation.

Definition of exacerbation-risk score and the score-based phenotypes

With a post-hoc decision, we defined an exacerbation-risk score for asthma based on serum sST2 levels and blood neutrophil count (Fig. 2a). The exacerbation-risk score predicted asthma worsening with an AUC of 0.91 ($P < 0.001$, Fig. 2b) in the ROC curve analysis. The odds ratios of scores 1 to 3 for predicting exacerbation were 8.4 ($P = 0.109$), 35.5 ($P = 0.014$), and 426 ($P < 0.001$), respectively (Fig. 2c). A survival curve analysis also showed that patients with scores of 2 and 3 were at higher risk of exacerbation than patients with scores of 0 (Fig. 2d). The sensitivities and specificities of each score for predicting exacerbation are shown in Additional file 1: Table S1. Importantly, a power analysis showed that high exacerbation-risk score predicted at-risk patients with a power of 1.000 ($\alpha = 0.05$, $N = 104$, $P < 0.001$), confirming that this study has a sufficient sample size.

Finally, we assessed the characteristics of patients with each score (Table 4). Patients with a score of 3, with both high serum sST2 levels and blood neutrophilia, showed the most severe phenotype. Six out of seven patients (85.7%) experienced exacerbation; their asthma was mostly uncontrolled rather than in intensive treatment (a high treatment step), with airflow limitation and a lower percentage of eosinophil in WBC. Patients with a score of 2, with blood neutrophilia alone, showed a 33.3% exacerbation rate, identical treatment step, and better asthma control compared to patients with a score of 3, and preserved lung function, indicating that they were relatively reactive to corticosteroids. Patients with a score of 1, with high serum sST2 levels alone, showed a 10.5% of exacerbation rate, higher serum IL-8 levels, and a slightly higher treatment step than those with a score of 0. Patients with a score of 0, without serum sST2 level elevation nor blood neutrophilia, were at the lowest exacerbation risk (1.4% exacerbation rate).

Taken together, high serum sST2 levels (greater than 18 ng/ml) are reasonable predictor of exacerbation and, when combined with blood neutrophilia, provided an

Table 3 Multivariate analysis for predicting the risk of asthma exacerbation

	Univariate		Multivariate[a]	
	Hazard ratio (95% CI)	P-value	Hazard ratio (95% CI)	P-value*
High serum sST2 level (> 18 ng/ml)	9.2 (2.4–34.7)	0.001	5.5 (1.4–21.5)	0.015
Blood neutrophilia[b] (> 6000 μl)	26.6 (7.9–100.9)	< 0.001	18.9 (4.8–74.4)	< 0.001

*P-values were calculated using Cox proportional hazard analysis
[a]Correlation coefficients: high serum sST2 level, 1.70; blood neutrophilia, 2.94, respectively
[b]The cut-off value for defining blood neutrophilia was optimized using the receiver operating characteristic curve analysis and calculating the Youden index
CI confidence interval

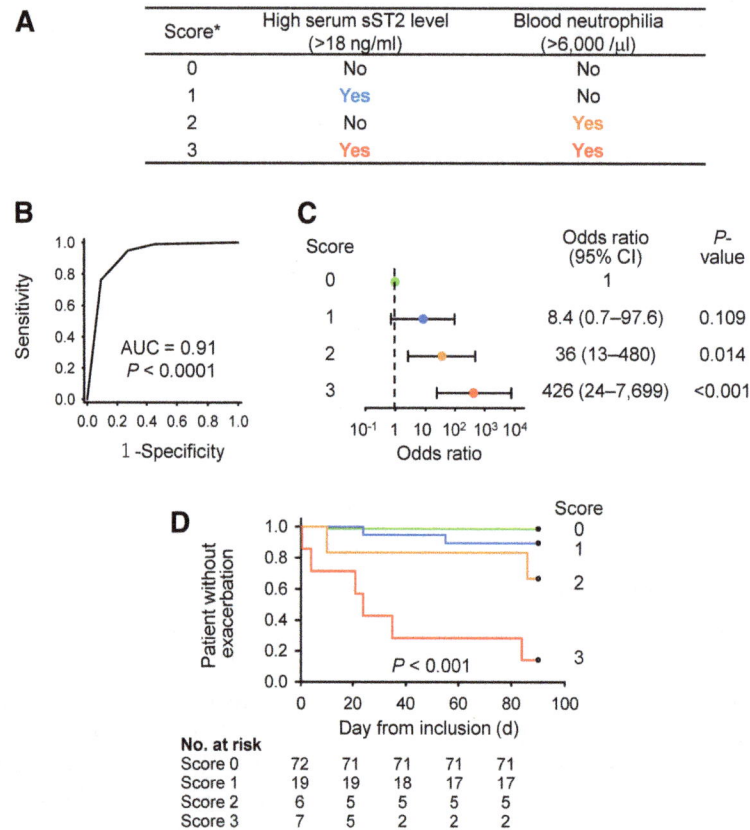

Fig. 2 The exacerbation-risk score and its accuracy. **a** Definition of the exacerbation-risk score. Scores of 1 and 2 were based on the coefficients calculated in Table 3 (high serum sST2 level, 1.70; blood neutrophilia, 2.94) (**b**) The exacerbation-risk score predicted asthma exacerbation with an AUC (95% CI) of 0.91 (0.79–1.02) (P < 0.001) in the ROC curve analysis. **c** Odds ratios predicting exacerbation risk for scores of 1, 2, and 3 as compared with a score of 0. **d** Survival analysis comparing time to exacerbation among patients with scores ranging from 0 to 3. P < 0.05: score 0 vs. 2, score 0 vs. 3, and score 1 vs. 2. (B–D) P-values were calculated using a ROC curve analysis (**b**), Fisher's Exact test (**c**), and Log-Rank test (**d**). CI, confidence interval

exacerbation risk score that is an accurate predictor of exacerbation and which classifies poorly-controlled asthma into subgroups.

Discussion

The present study demonstrated that serum sST2 levels serve as a biomarker for the disease severity of asthma and predicted exacerbation risk within 3 months. Serum sST2 levels reflected the extent of airway oxidative stress and serum chemotaxis activity, whereas peripheral neutrophil counts reflected systemic inflammatory response, blood oxidative stress, and obesity. High serum sST2 levels and peripheral blood neutrophilia independently predicted asthma exacerbation, and a double positive was suggestive of an extremely high risk of worsening asthma, corticosteroid-resistance, and airflow limitation.

High serum sST2 levels serve as biomarker for asthma severity. Oshikawa and colleagues evaluated atopic asthma patients and reported that serum sST2 levels during exacerbation were higher than these at steady state and were associated with asthma severity (i.e. peak

flow volume and arterial blood CO_2 partial pressure) [23]. We assessed asthmatic patients who were recruited irrespective of atopic state and demonstrated that serum sST2 levels at steady state also correlated with disease severity (i.e. treatment step) and that serum sST2 levels greater than 18 ng/ml were a reasonable predictor for exacerbation within 3 months. Taken together, serum sST2 levels in asthmatics correlate with severity at steady state and during exacerbation, and are a reasonable predictor for exacerbation regardless of atopic state.

sST2 is produced in the lungs [11, 19]. Multiple types of human lung cells (i.e. bronchial cells, alveolar cells, and vascular endothelial cells) release sST2 in vitro, which can be enhanced by stimulation with proinflammatory cytokines, lipopolysaccharide, and Th2 cytokines [11, 19]. Serum (or plasma) sST2 levels were elevated in patients with neutrophilic (i.e. bacterial pneumonia [20] and COPD [21]) and eosinophilic (i.e. acute eosinophilic pneumonia [26]) lung disease. Serum sST2 levels correlated with disease severity in pneumonia patients [20]. These suggest that serum sST2 levels reflect the extent

Table 4 Characteristics of patients classified with the exacerbation-risk score

	Exacerbation-risk score				P-value*
	0	1	2	3	
	(N = 72)	(N = 19)	(N = 6)	(N = 7)	
Patients with exacerbation of asthma, n (%)	1 (1.4)	2 (10.5)	2 (33.3)	6 (85.7)	**< 0.001**
Age, mean (SD)	54.1 ± 14.6	56.1 ± 17.3	47.2 ± 20.0	59.7 ± 18.4	0.321
Sex, M: F, n (%)	24 (33.8): 48 (66.7)	13 (68.4): 6 (31.6)	2 (33.3): 4 (66.7)	3 (42.9): 4 (57.1)	0.050
BMI, median (IQR)	22.9 (20.6–27.4)	23.1 (21.5–26.7)	23.1 (19.6–28.6)	27.9 (21.8–30.1)	0.538
Smoking, n (%)					
Current smoker	8 (11.1)	1 (5.3)	0 (0)	1 (28.6)	0.527
Ex-smoker	19 (26.4)	6 (31.6)	4 (66.7)	2 (14.3)	
Never-smoker	45 (62.5)	12 (63.2)	2 (33.3)	4 (57.1)	
Asthma control, n (%)					
Well controlled	20 (27.8)	7 (36.8)	3 (50.0)	0 (0)	**< 0.001**
Partially controlled	42 (58.3)	9 (47.4)	1 (16.7)	1 (14.3)	
Uncontrolled	10 (13.9)	3 (15.8)	2 (33.3)	6 (85.7)	
Treatment step, n (%)					
1	4 (5.5)	0 (0.0)	0 (0.0)	0 (0.0)	**0.005**
2	11 (15.3)	1 (5.3)	1 (16.7)	1 (14.2)	
3	16 (22.2)	4 (21.0)	0 (0.0)	0 (0.0)	
4	39 (54.2)	12 (63.2)	2 (33.3)	3 (42.9)	
5	2 (2.8)	2 (10.5)	3 (50.0)	3 (42.9)	
sST2 (ng/ml), median (IQR)	11.0 (8.8–13.0)	21.1 (18.8–28.4)	11.8 (11.4–14.3)	26.4 (20.8–34.0)	**< 0.001**
WBC (/μL), median (IQR)	6200 (5225–6800)	5900 (4700–7200)	10,250 (9000–12,350)	10,500 (9700–12,100)	**< 0.001**
Neutrophil (/μL), median (IQR)	3496 (2786–4268)	3553 (2248–4650)	6333 (6117–10,381)	8159 (7497–9196)	**< 0.001**
Eosinophil (/μL), median (IQR)	199 (133–335)	201 (45–307)	229 (75–677)	87 (32–303)	0.273
Eosinophil (%), median (IQR)	3.7 (2.1–6.2)	3.4 (0.9–4.9)	2.4 (0.6–7.4)	**1.0 (0.3–2.5) †**	**0.045**
CRP (mg/dl), median (IQR)	0.1 (0–0.2)	0.0 (0–0.)	0.1 (0–0.4)	0.1 (0.1–0.5)	0.195
IgE (IU/ml), median (IQR)	201 (45–684)	236 (104–330)	60 (8–843)	73 (3–2656)	0.432
IL-8 (pg/ml), median (IQR)	13.0 (10.5–15.8)	**21.9 (9.7–31.0) †**	11.7 (7.9–19.8)	16.0 (11.0–25.2)	0.063
IL-6 (pg/ml), median (IQR)	1.0 (0.5–1.8)	0.9 (0.5–1.9)	2.5 (1.2–8.0)	1.8 (0.3–3.7)	0.143
Serum H_2O_2 (U. CARR), median (IQR)	345 (315–401)	322 (294–356)	341 (304–390)	383 (336–390)	0.182
FeNO (ppm), median (IQR)	23.5 (16.0–38.3)	24.0 (15.0–63.0)	19.0 (13.3–49.8)	16.0 (11.0–121.0)	0.892
EBC H_2O_2 (U. CARR) [a]	0.4 (0.0–1.0)	0.5 (0.2–1.1)	0.4 (0.0–0.6)	0.6 (0.3–0.7)	0.751
VC (L), median (IQR)	2.9 (2.5–3.8)	3.7 (2.6–4.4)	3.7 (3.3–3.8)	**2.3 (2.0–2.9) †**	0.079
%VC (%), mean (SD)	106.7 (45.6)	107.9 (19.5)	114.0 (13.0)	**87.3 (14.2) ‡**	**0.014**
FVC (L), median (IQR)	2.9 (2.4–3.7)	3.7 (2.5–4.4)	3.6 (3.2–3.8)	**2.2 (1.8–2.9) †**	0.087
%FVC (%), mean (SD)	98.6 (14.6)	97.1 (15.4)	107.1 (15.4)	**79.4 (12.1) ‡**	**0.009**
FEV_1 (L), median (IQR)	2.3 (1.8–2.7)	2.5 (1.4–3.1)	2.8 (2.0–3.0)	1.6 (1.3–1.9)	0.142
%FEV_1 (%), mean (SD)	90.1 (17.8)	86.5 (23.5)	97.7 (24.3)	**71.1 (22.3) ‡**	0.063
FEV_1/FVC (%), median (IQR)	76.0 (69.2–81.0)	70.3 (67.6–79.8)	79.4 (66.0–82.0)	73.6 (64.0–83.6)	0.550

*P-values for parametric, non-parametric, and categorical data were calculated using a one-way ANOVA test, Kruskal-Wallis test, and Chi-square test, respectively
†$P < 0.05$ vs. a score of 0, calculated using the Steel test
‡$P < 0.05$ vs. a score of 0, calculated using the Dunnett test
*†‡ Bold letters, $P < 0.05$
[a]A total of 81 patients (scores of 0, 1, 2, and 3: N = 56, 17, 4, and 4, respectively) were evaluated
BMI body mass index, *WBC* white blood cells, *FeNO* fractional exhaled nitric oxide, *EBC* exhaled breath condensate, *SD* standard deviation, *IQR* interquartile range

of airway inflammation. In addition, airway H_2O_2 levels correlate with sputum granulocyte (i.e. neutrophil and eosinophil) counts in asthmatic patients [27]. We demonstrated the positive correlation between serum sST2 levels and airway H_2O_2 levels in asthmatics, which also indicated an association between high serum sST2 levels and the presence of airway inflammation. Taken together, serum sST2 levels reflect the extent of neutrophil and/or eosinophil infiltration in lungs.

Neutrophilic inflammation is associated with the development of uncontrolled asthma. Airway neutrophilic inflammation is related to severe asthma; airway mixed-granulocytic infiltration (i.e. both neutrophils and eosinophils) appeared to cause the greatest disease burden in asthmatics [8, 9]. In addition to sputum neutrophilia, peripheral blood neutrophilia was also a risk factor for asthma worsening [10]. However, blood neutrophil counts showed only a low association with sputum neutrophil count [5, 28], suggesting that neutrophilic inflammation-related asthma could be further classified (e.g. into subgroups of airway-dominant, blood-dominant, and mixed neutrophilia). We classified asthmatics into four subtypes using blood neutrophilia (related to systemic inflammation) and high serum sST2 levels (associated with airway inflammation), which provided an accurate predictor for exacerbation (the exacerbation-risk score). These support the concept that neutrophil-related asthma can be further stratified into subgroups that reflect phenotypic severity. Although further investigation regarding the relationship between sputum granulocyte counts (i.e. neutrophil and eosinophil counts) and serum sST2 levels are needed, our observations indicate that sST2 is a potential phenotypic marker for uncontrolled asthma.

IL-33 is related to eosinophilic asthma: it is the nuclear-associated cytokine of IL-1, [29] which is released from allergen-exposed cells [13]. Exogenous administration of IL-33 causes a massive infiltration of eosinophils and Th2 cytokine production [14–16]. In addition, IL-33 stimulates type 2 innate lymphoid cells to produce IL-5 and -13 resulting in eosinophilia and goblet cell hyperplasia, respectively [16]. Genome-wide association studies (GWASs) have demonstrated that *IL-33* and *IL1RL1* (encoding the IL-33 receptor) variants were associated with arising asthma [17, 18] and blood eosinophilia [17]. The *IL-1RL1* variant was also associated with arising neutrophilic asthma whereas the *IL-33* variant was not [17]. Further, some *IL1RL1* variants enhance sST2 production, as demonstrated by human plasma analysis and cell culture experiments [30]. Our data show that high serum sST2 levels are related to low blood eosinophil (%), which was also associated with less airway eosinophilic inflammation [22]. Taken together, an interaction between IL-33, the cell surface, and soluble IL-33 receptors (ST2L and sST2, respectively) regulates the airway granulocyte (i.e. neutrophil

and eosinophil) counts that potentially influence asthma phenotypes.

The sST2/IL-33 axis regulates neutrophilic inflammation in the lungs [29, 31]. In a mouse model of influenza virus infection, IL-33 synthesis increased in the lungs [32]. Similarly, in a mouse COPD exacerbation model caused by influenza virus infection, nasal administration of IL-33 enhanced neutrophil infiltration into lungs, which was attenuated by sST2 administration [33]. IL-33, known as alarmine, [34] is released from necrotized cells [11]. IL-33 is processed by neutrophil elastase from a less-active full-length form to a highly-activated cleaved form [35]. IL-33 restored a decrease in neutrophil chemotaxis that resulted from TLR stimulation [31]. Thus, IL-33 augments neutrophilic airway inflammation in certain situations, such as when viral infections accompany necrotic tissue damage. Importantly, inflamed epithelial cells release an increased amount of sST2 [11, 19]. This attenuates biologically IL-33-induced neutrophilic inflammation and serves clinically as a biomarker for lung inflammation. Taken together, the sST2/IL-33 balance is regulated in the lungs, controlling neutrophilic inflammation and subsequent tissue damage, and serving as a biomarker for airway inflammation.

This study has some limitations. First, it is a relatively small-scale and single-centre study, thus, our findings require further confirmation by a larger study. Second, we did not evaluate sputum cells nor serum IL-33 levels. The relationship among serum sST2 and IL-33 levels, blood neutrophil counts, and asthma phenotypes should also be evaluated with sputum cell counts in future studies. However, our study provides novel diagnostic methods that counter these limitations. Firstly, serum sST2 levels greater than 18 ng/ml were a reasonable predictor for exacerbation within 3 months. Secondly, high serum sST2 levels and blood neutrophilia provided an exacerbation-risk score that can classify neutrophil-related asthma into subgroups where the subgroup with the highest score had an 85.7% exacerbation rate.

Conclusion

High serum sST2 levels predict exacerbation in the general asthmatic population and, when combined with blood neutrophil levels, provide an exacerbation-risk score that is a better predictor of exacerbation than serum sST2 levels alone.

Acknowledgements
We would like to thank all of our colleagues who participated in the study.

Funding
This research was supported in part by the Environmental Restoration and Conservation Agency and by Grants-In-Aid for Scientific Research (KAKENHI; No. 15 K09189).

Authors' contributions
Literature search, study design, figure, data collection, data analysis, data interpretation, and writing: MW. Data collection, data analysis, and data interpretation: KN. Data analysis: KH. Data collection: MS, TI, MT, YO, TY, TS, DK, and HI. Data collection and writing: HT. All authors read and approved the final manuscript.

Competing interests
The authors declare that they have no competing interests.

References
1. Program. NAEaP: Expert panel report 3: guidelines for the diagnosis and Management of Asthma. National Institutes of Health; National Heart, Lung, and Blood Institute; 2007 Publication no 07–4051 2007. https://www.nhlbi.nih.gov/files/docs/guidelines/asthgdln.pdf
2. Wenzel SE. Asthma phenotypes: the evolution from clinical to molecular approaches. Nat Med. 2012;18:716–25.
3. Fajt ML, Wenzel SE. Asthma phenotypes and the use of biologic medications in asthma and allergic disease: the next steps toward personalized care. J Allergy Clin Immunol. 2015;135:299–310. quiz 311
4. Moore WC, Meyers DA, Wenzel SE, Teague WG, Li H, Li X, D'Agostino R Jr, Castro M, Curran-Everett D, Fitzpatrick AM, et al. Identification of asthma phenotypes using cluster analysis in the severe asthma research program. Am J Respir Crit Care Med. 2010;181:315–23.
5. Hastie AT, Moore WC, Li H, Rector BM, Ortega VE, Pascual RM, Peters SP, Meyers DA, Bleecker ER. Biomarker surrogates do not accurately predict sputum eosinophil and neutrophil percentages in asthmatic subjects. J Allergy Clin Immunol. 2013;132:72–80.
6. Fahy JV. Eosinophilic and neutrophilic inflammation in asthma: insights from clinical studies. Proc Am Thorac Soc. 2009;6:256–9.
7. Chung KF. Neutrophilic asthma: a distinct target for treatment? Lancet Respir Med. 2016;4:765–7.
8. Israel E, Reddel HK. Severe and difficult-to-treat asthma in adults. N Engl J Med. 2017;377:965–76.
9. Moore WC, Hastie AT, Li X, Li H, Busse WW, Jarjour NN, Wenzel SE, Peters SP, Meyers DA, Bleecker ER. Sputum neutrophil counts are associated with more severe asthma phenotypes using cluster analysis. J Allergy Clin Immunol. 2014;133:1557–63. e1555
10. Nadif R, Siroux V, Boudier A, le Moual N, Just J, Gormand F, Pison C, Matran R, Pin I. Blood granulocyte patterns as predictors of asthma phenotypes in adults from the EGEA study. Eur Respir J. 2016;48:1040–51.
11. Yagami A, Orihara K, Morita H, Futamura K, Hashimoto N, Matsumoto K, Saito H, Matsuda A. IL-33 mediates inflammatory responses in human lung tissue cells. J Immunol. 2010;185:5743–50.
12. Hayakawa H, Hayakawa M, Kume A, Tominaga S. Soluble ST2 blocks interleukin-33 signaling in allergic airway inflammation. J Biol Chem. 2007;282:26369–80.
13. Hristova M, Habibovic A, Veith C, Janssen-Heininger YM, Dixon AE, Geiszt M, van der Vliet A. Airway epithelial dual oxidase 1 mediates allergen-induced IL-33 secretion and activation of type 2 immune responses. J Allergy Clin Immunol. 2016;137:1545–56. e1511
14. Luthi AU, Cullen SP, McNeela EA, Duriez PJ, Afonina IS, Sheridan C, Brumatti G, Taylor RC, Kersse K, Vandenabeele P, et al. Suppression of interleukin-33 bioactivity through proteolysis by apoptotic caspases. Immunity. 2009;31:84–98.
15. Schmitz J, Owyang A, Oldham E, Song Y, Murphy E, McClanahan TK, Zurawski G, Moshrefi M, Qin J, Li X, et al. IL-33, an interleukin-1-like cytokine that signals via the IL-1 receptor-related protein ST2 and induces T helper type 2-associated cytokines. Immunity. 2005;23:479–90.
16. Bartemes KR, Iijima K, Kobayashi T, Kephart GM, McKenzie AN, Kita H. IL-33-responsive lineage- CD25+ CD44(hi) lymphoid cells mediate innate type 2 immunity and allergic inflammation in the lungs. J Immunol. 2012;188:1503–13.
17. Gudbjartsson DF, Bjornsdottir US, Halapi E, Helgadottir A, Sulem P, Jonsdottir GM, Thorleifsson G, Helgadottir H, Steinthorsdottir V, Stefansson H, et al. Sequence variants affecting eosinophil numbers associate with asthma and myocardial infarction. Nat Genet. 2009;41:342–7.
18. Moffatt MF, Gut IG, Demenais F, Strachan DP, Bouzigon E, Heath S, von Mutius E, Farrall M, Lathrop M, Cookson WO. A large-scale, consortium-based genomewide association study of asthma. N Engl J Med. 2010;363:1211–21.
19. Mildner M, Storka A, Lichtenauer M, Mlitz V, Ghannadan M, Hoetzenecker K, Nickl S, Dome B, Tschachler E, Ankersmit HJ. Primary sources and immunological prerequisites for sST2 secretion in humans. Cardiovasc Res. 2010;87:769–77.
20. Watanabe M, Takizawa H, Tamura M, Nakajima A, Kurai D, Ishii H, Takata S, Nakamoto K, Sohara E, Honda K, et al. Soluble ST2 as a prognostic marker in community-acquired pneumonia. J Inf Secur. 2015;70:474–82.
21. Xia J, Zhao J, Shang J, Li M, Zeng Z, Wang J, Xu Y, Xie J. Increased IL-33 expression in chronic obstructive pulmonary disease. Am J Physiol Lung Cell Mol Physiol. 2015;308:L619–27.
22. Hoogerwerf JJ, Tanck MW, van Zoelen MA, Wittebole X, Laterre PF, van der Poll T. Soluble ST2 plasma concentrations predict mortality in severe sepsis. Intensive Care Med. 2010;36:630–7.
23. Oshikawa K, Kuroiwa K, Tago K, Iwahana H, Yanagisawa K, Ohno S, Tominaga SI, Sugiyama Y. Elevated soluble ST2 protein levels in sera of patients with asthma with an acute exacerbation. Am J Respir Crit Care Med. 2001;164:277–81.
24. Global Strategy for Asthma Management and Prevention (GINA). Global Initiative for Asthma 2015.
25. Dweik RA, Boggs PB, Erzurum SC, Irvin CG, Leigh MW, Lundberg JO, Olin AC, Plummer AL, Taylor DR. An official ATS clinical practice guideline: interpretation of exhaled nitric oxide levels (FENO) for clinical applications. Am J Respir Crit Care Med. 2011;184:602–15.
26. Oshikawa K, Kuroiwa K, Tokunaga T, Kato T, Hagihara SI, Tominaga SI, Sugiyama Y. Acute eosinophilic pneumonia with increased soluble ST2 in serum and bronchoalveolar lavage fluid. Respir Med. 2001;95:532–3.
27. Loukides S, Bouros D, Papatheodorou G, Panagou P, Siafakas NM. The relationships among hydrogen peroxide in expired breath condensate, airway inflammation, and asthma severity. Chest. 2002;121:338–46.
28. Zhang XY, Simpson JL, Powell H, Yang IA, Upham JW, Reynolds PN, Hodge S, James AL, Jenkins C, Peters MJ, et al. Full blood count parameters for the detection of asthma inflammatory phenotypes. Clin Exp Allergy. 2014;44:1137–45.
29. Molofsky AB, Savage AK, Locksley RM. Interleukin-33 in tissue homeostasis, injury, and inflammation. Immunity. 2015;42:1005–19.
30. Ho JE, Chen WY, Chen MH, Larson MG, McCabe EL, Cheng S, Ghorbani A, Coglianese E, Emilsson V, Johnson AD, et al. Common genetic variation at the IL1RL1 locus regulates IL-33/ST2 signaling. J Clin Invest. 2013;123:4208–18.
31. Alves-Filho JC, Sonego F, Souto FO, Freitas A, Verri WA Jr, Auxiliadora-Martins M, Basile-Filho A, McKenzie AN, Xu D, Cunha FQ, Liew FY. Interleukin-33 attenuates sepsis by enhancing neutrophil influx to the site of infection. Nat Med. 2010;16:708–12.
32. Le Goffic R, Arshad MI, Rauch M, L'Helgoualc'h A, Delmas B, Piquet-Pellorce C, Samson M. Infection with influenza virus induces IL-33 in murine lungs. Am J Respir Cell Mol Biol. 2011;45:1125–32.
33. Kearley J, Silver JS, Sanden C, Liu Z, Berlin AA, White N, Mori M, Pham TH, Ward CK, Criner GJ, et al. Cigarette smoke silences innate lymphoid cell function and facilitates an exacerbated type I interleukin-33-dependent response to infection. Immunity. 2015;42:566–79.
34. Pichery M, Mirey E, Mercier P, Lefrancais E, Dujardin A, Ortega N, Girard JP. Endogenous IL-33 is highly expressed in mouse epithelial barrier tissues, lymphoid organs, brain, embryos, and inflamed tissues: in situ analysis using a novel Il-33-LacZ gene trap reporter strain. J Immunol. 2012;188:3488–95.
35. Lefrancais E, Roga S, Gautier V, Gonzalez-de-Peredo A, Monsarrat B, Girard JP, Cayrol C. IL-33 is processed into mature bioactive forms by neutrophil elastase and cathepsin G. Proc Natl Acad Sci U S A. 2012;109:1673–8.

2

IL-32γ attenuates airway fibrosis by modulating the integrin-FAK signaling pathway in fibroblasts

Gyong Hwa Hong[1,2†], So-Young Park[3†], Hyouk-Soo Kwon[2], Bo-Ram Bang[1,2], Jaechun Lee[4], Sang-Yeob Kim[1,5], Chan-Gi Pack[1,5], Soohyun Kim[6], Keun-Ai Moon[1,2], Tae-Bum Kim[2], Hee-Bom Moon[2] and You Sook Cho[2*]

Abstract

Background: Fibrosis in severe asthma often leads to irreversible organ dysfunction. However, the mechanism that regulates fibrosis remains poorly understood. Interleukin (IL)-32 plays a role in several chronic inflammatory diseases, including severe asthma. In this study, we investigated whether IL-32 is involved in fibrosis progression in the lungs.

Methods: Murine models of chronic airway inflammation induced by ovalbumin and *Aspergillus melleus* protease and bleomycin-induced pulmonary fibrosis were employed. We evaluated the degree of tissue fibrosis after treatment with recombinant IL-32γ (rIL-32γ). Expression of fibronectin and α-smooth muscle actin (α-SMA) was examined and the transforming growth factor (TGF)-β-related signaling pathways was evaluated in activated human lung fibroblasts (MRC-5 cells) treated with rIL-32γ.

Results: rIL-32γ significantly attenuated collagen deposition and α-SMA production in both mouse models. rIL-32γ inhibited the production of fibronectin and α-SMA in MRC-5 cells stimulated with TGF-β. Additionally, rIL-32γ suppressed activation of the integrin-FAK-paxillin signaling axis but had no effect on the Smad and non-Smad signaling pathways. rIL-32γ localized outside of MRC-5 cells and inhibited the interaction between integrins and the extracellular matrix without directly binding to intracellular FAK and paxillin.

Conclusions: These results demonstrate that IL-32γ has anti-fibrotic effects and is a novel target for preventing fibrosis.

Keywords: Interleukin-32γ, Asthma, Airway inflammation, Subepithelial fibrosis, Pulmonary fibrosis

Background

Fibrosis, characterized by the accumulation of fibroblasts and excess extracellular matrix, is a common feature of various pathological states in many organs, resulting in dysfunction. Interstitial lung diseases and chronic inflammatory airway diseases of the lungs, such as severe asthma and chronic obstructive pulmonary disease (COPD), lead to sub-bronchial fibrosis and pulmonary fibrosis, both of which result in irreversible structural changes that affect patient survival [1–3]. Because lung fibrosis is mainly a consequence of chronic inflammation, therapeutic strategies have focused on preventing

inflammation by administering immunosuppressive agents or anti-inflammatory drugs, including corticosteroids [4, 5]. However, recent studies have suggested that inflammation alone is not sufficient for inducing fibrosis development. Many studies showed that immunosuppressive therapies do not prevent lung fibrosis [6]. To date, targeting fibrosis itself has been unsuccessful.

Interleukin (IL)-32, initially described as NK4 generated by activated T cells or NK cells [7], is produced by various cells, including epithelial cells, endothelial cells, and macrophages. IL-32 induces the production of several pro-inflammatory mediators, such as tumor necrosis factor (TNF)-α, IL-1β, and IL-6, by activating the nuclear factor-κB and p38 mitogen-activated protein kinase signaling pathways [8, 9]. IL-32 is also involved in several chronic inflammatory diseases, such as rheumatoid arthritis and COPD [10–12]. In addition to its role in

* Correspondence: yscho@amc.seoul.kr
†Gyong Hwa Hong and So-Young Park contributed equally to this work.
2Department of Internal Medicine, Division of Allergy and Clinical Immunology, Asan Medical Center, University of Ulsan College of Medicine, 88 Olympic-ro 43-gil, Songpa-gu, Seoul 138-736, Korea
Full list of author information is available at the end of the article

inflammation, recent studies suggested that IL-32 is involved in liver fibrosis in patients with chronic hepatitis by affecting cytokine induction [13]. Although the precise effects of IL-32 on tissue fibrosis are largely unknown, IL-32 contains an RGD motif, which is known to bind several integrins [14]. Moreover, a 3-dimensional reconstruction model of IL-32 revealed that its structure was highly similar to that of the focal adhesion targeting (FAT) region of focal adhesion kinase (FAK). FAK-related non-kinase, a peptide with a structure similar to the FAT region, inhibits FAK signal transduction [15]. Because the integrin-FAK signaling axis is critical for the development of tissue fibrosis [16, 17], we predicted that IL-32 interrupts the signaling pathway by binding to these molecules, thereby inhibiting FAK activation and alleviating fibrosis.

We hypothesized that IL-32γ modulates fibrosis in chronic airway and lung diseases by disrupting the integrin-FAK signaling pathway. Here, we used murine models of chronic airway inflammation and bleomycin-induced pulmonary fibrosis to examine the role of IL-32γ in fibrosis of the airways and lungs, respectively. We also evaluated the role of IL-32γ in mechanisms underlying fibroblast function.

Methods
Generation of murine models of airway inflammation and pulmonary fibrosis
To generate the bleomycin-induced pulmonary fibrosis model, mice were administered intratracheal injection of bleomycin (1 U/kg body weight) on day 2. To evaluate the effect of IL-32γ treatment, mice were administered 500 ng of human recombinant IL-32γ (rIL-32γ) via intranasal injection on days 1, 2, 14, and 28. In this model, rIL-32γ was injected intranasally; 1 h later, bleomycin was injected intratracheally. Mice were sacrificed at 30 days. To generate the chronic asthma model, wild-type (WT) mice were sensitized by intranasal administration of 22 μg of ovalbumin (OVA) and 8 μg of protease (*Aspergillus melleus* protease; Sigma, St. Louis, MO, USA) twice per week for 8 weeks, as previously described [23]. Mice were sacrificed at 58 days. To evaluate the effect of IL-32γ treatment, mice were treated with 500 ng human recombinant IL-32γ (rIL-32γ) 2 h before each immunization. IL-32γ transgenic (TG) mice on a C57BL/6 background were generated as previously described [18]. The Institutional Animal Care and Use Committee approved all experimental procedures (Animal Utilization Protocol 2014-14-013). Additional details are provided in the Additional file 1.

Histopathologic examination and quantification of tissue fibrosis
Lungs were removed and fixed in 10% neutral-buffered formalin, embedded in paraffin, and sectioned (4 μm). Sections were subjected to Masson's trichrome staining and immunofluorescence staining using several antibodies. To quantify tissue fibrosis, we measured hydroxyproline levels in the tissue. Additionally, quantification graphs were drawn from intensity measurement data using the Image J program (NIH, Bethesda, MD, USA).

Additional details are provided in the Additional file 1.

Cell culture and study design
The human lung fibroblast cell line MRC-5 was purchased from the American Type Culture Collection (Manassas, VA, USA). Mouse embryonic fibroblasts (MEFs) obtained from IL-32γ TG mice were also used. MRC-5 cells were seeded at 2×10^5 cells/well and stimulated with recombinant proteins. Expression of various cellular molecules was measured by *Western* blotting, reverse transcription-PCR, and semi-quantitative PCR. Additional details are provided in the Additional file 1. All in vitro experiments were conducted at least 3 times.

Cell adhesion assay
For crystal violet staining, 96-well culture dishes were coated with collagen (Advanced BioMatrix, Inc., San Diego, CA, USA) and seeded with MRC-5 cells. Plates were incubated for 30, 60, or 180 min. Cells were washed with PBS to remove non-adherent cells, and adhered cells were stained with crystal violet. Additional details are provided in the Additional file 1.

His pull-down assay and immunoprecipitation
His-tagged IL-32γ was incubated with Ni-NTA agarose beads (Qiagen, Hilden, Germany), which were washed with buffer containing imidazole (Sigma). TGF-β-stimulated MRC-5 cells were lysed and centrifuged; the supernatant was incubated with Ni-NTA agarose-bound IL-32γ. Proteins attached to the beads were subjected to immunoblotting. For immunoprecipitation, MRC-5 cells overexpressing flag-tagged IL-32γ were lysed and incubated with protein G Sepharose beads (GE Healthcare, Little Chalfont, UK) coated with an anti-flag antibody. Proteins were electrotransferred for immunoblotting. Additional details are provided in the Additional file 1.

Live cell imaging of IL-32γ
MRC-5 cells were cultured in a μ-Dish 35 mm, High, IbiTreat (Ibidi GmbH, Martinsried, Germany) and treated with Flamma496-labeled IL-32γ. After 10 min, the cells were washed with medium. Fluorescence images were obtained under a Nikon Ti-E inverted I wamicroscope (Tokyo, Japan) equipped with PFS, iXon Ultra 897 EMCCD camera (Andor Technology, Belfast, UK), and excitation and emission filter wheels.

Statistical analysis

All data are reported as the mean ± standard error of mean. Means were compared using the Mann–Whitney test in GraphPad Prism software (version 4.0; GraphPad, Inc., La Jolla, CA, USA). A value of $p < 0.05$ was considered statistically significant.

Results

IL-32γ modulates fibrosis in mouse models of airway inflammation and pulmonary fibrosis

First, histopathological analysis of bleomycin-induced lung fibrosis was conducted to determine the effect of IL-32γ on pulmonary fibrosis. Treatment with rIL-32γ significantly reduced collagen deposition and α-smooth muscle actin (SMA) expression (Fig. 1a and b). Hydroxyproline levels showed a tendency to be lower in the bleomycin-induced fibrosis group treated with rIL-32γ than in the group without rIL-32γ treatment (34.01 ±

7.24 vs. $25.52 ± 3.66$, $p = 0.048$; Fig. 1c). Next, to determine the effect of IL-32γ on airway remodeling in chronic asthma, a murine model of chronic airway inflammation with subepithelial fibrosis was treated with rIL-32γ. Treatment with rIL-32γ reduced peribronchial collagen deposition (Fig. 1d). This was accompanied by reduced expression of α-SMA, a marker of activated fibroblasts, around the bronchi of treated mice (Fig. 1e). Figure 1f is a graph showing quantification of hydroxyproline. Hydroxyproline levels were significantly lower in the chronic asthma model treated with rIL-32γ ($32.35 ± 1.752$ vs. $24.20 ± 1.344$, $P = 0.010$).

rIL-32γ attenuates fibroblast activation

Next, to determine whether IL-32γ affects fibrosis by regulating fibroblast activation, expression of fibronectin and α-SMA was measured in the human fibroblast cell line MRC-5 after treatment with TGF-β in the presence

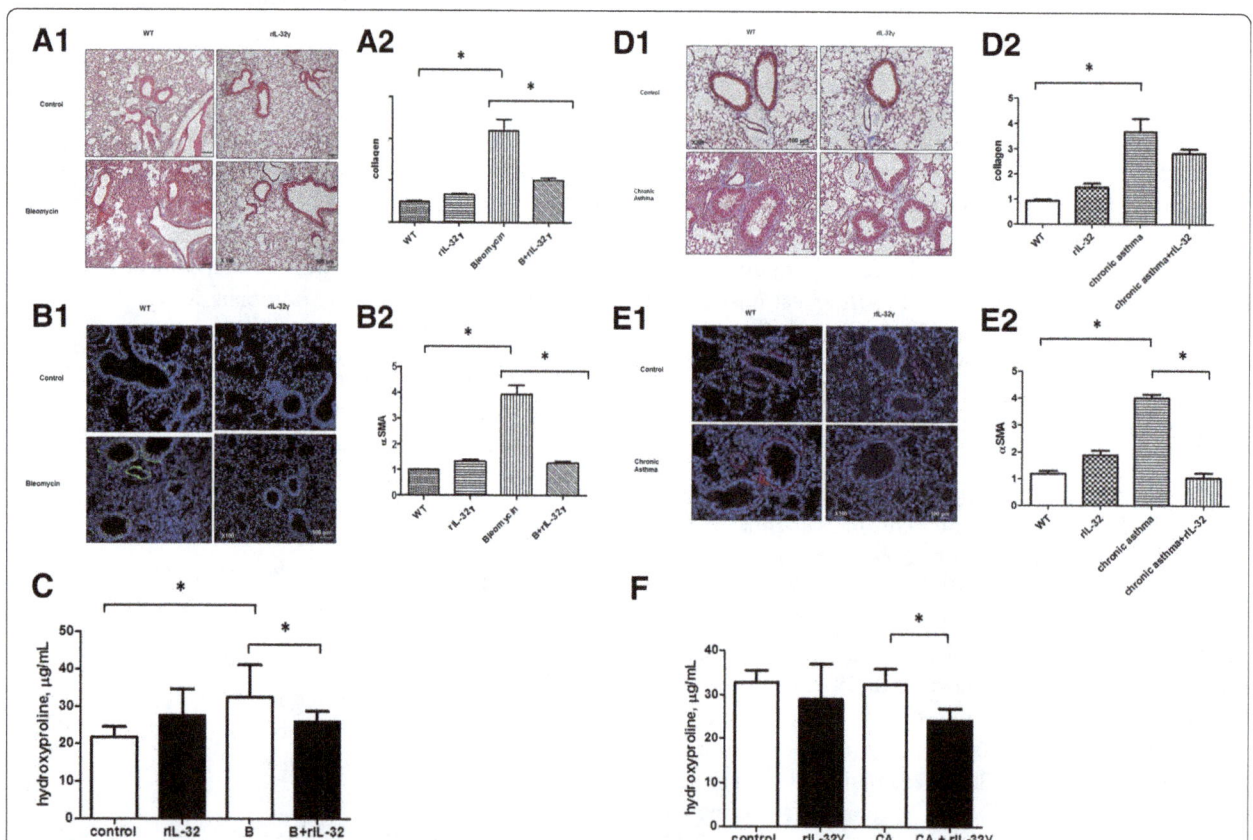

Fig. 1 Human IL-32γ prevents fibrosis in chronic asthma and bleomycin-induced pulmonary fibrosis models. **a** Evaluation of collagen deposits in the lungs of bleomycin-induced mice using Masson's trichrome stain (original magnification: 100×). The quantification graphs of histological analysis in bleomycin-induced fibrosis groups. **b** Immunofluorescence analysis of α-SMA (green) expression in the lungs of bleomycin-induced mice. DAPI staining is blue (original magnification: 100×). **c** Hydroxyproline quantification. In the group with bleomycin-induced fibrosis treated with rIL-32γ ($N = 5$, B ± rIL-32γ), hydroxyproline levels tended to decrease compared to in the non-rIL-32γ-treated bleomycin-induced fibrosis model ($N = 6$, B) ($32.40 ± 3.885$ vs. $26.70 ± 1.287$, $P = 0.166$). **d** Evaluation of collagen deposition in the lungs of chronic asthmatic mice using Masson's trichrome stain (original magnification: × 200). **e** Immunofluorescence analysis of α-SMA (red) expression in the lungs of mice with chronic asthma. DAPI staining is blue (original magnification: × 200). **f** Hydroxyproline quantification graph. Similar results were obtained in each independent experiment, each using five mice per group ($32.35 ± 1.752$ vs. $24.20 ± 1.344$, $P = 0.010$). *$P ≤ 0.05$

or absence of rIL-32γ. Fibronectin expression in rIL-32γ-treated cells was significantly lower than that in untreated cells, whereas α-SMA expression was slightly lower at early time points (Fig. 2a and b). However, overexpression of endogenous intracellular IL-32γ did not noticeably affect the production of fibronectin and α-SMA by MEFs from WT or IL-32γ TG mice (Fig. 2c and Additional file 2: Figure S1). Endogenous IL-32 expression is shown in Fig. 2d.

Anti-fibrotic effect of rIL-32γ occurs independently of TNF-α
Because IL-32 induces the production of TNF-α and vice versa, we next examined whether IL-32γ exerts anti-fibrotic effects by inducing TNF-α expression. First, we found that significant expression of IL-32γ mRNA was induced by TNF-α, although no significant change in TNF-α mRNA expression was observed (see Additional file 3: Figure S2A and B). Similar to IL-32γ, treatment with rTNF-α inhibited the expression of fibronectin and α-SMA in TGF-β-stimulated MRC-5 cells

(Fig. 3a). However, IL-32 was not expressed by rTNF-α under IL-32γ-knockdown conditions (Fig. 3b) and an anti-fibrotic effect of TNF-α was not observed in IL-32γ-knockdown MRC-5 cells (Fig. 3c and Additional file 4: Figure S3A). Additionally, rIL-32γ inhibited fibronectin and α-SMA expression after TNF-α inhibitor treatment (Fig. 3d and Additional file 4: Figure S3B).

rIL-32γ does not appear to be involved in TGF-β-mediated Smad or non-Smad signaling
We next examined the effect of IL-32γ on activation of the Smad pathway, a well-known TGF-β-mediated signaling pathway. There were no significant differences in the expression of Smad signaling molecules (p-Smad 3, smuf2, and TGF-β receptor 1), regardless of rIL-32γ treatment (Fig. 4a). Next, we examined whether the non-Smad pathway plays a role in the anti-fibrotic effects of rIL-32γ. We found no significant differences in

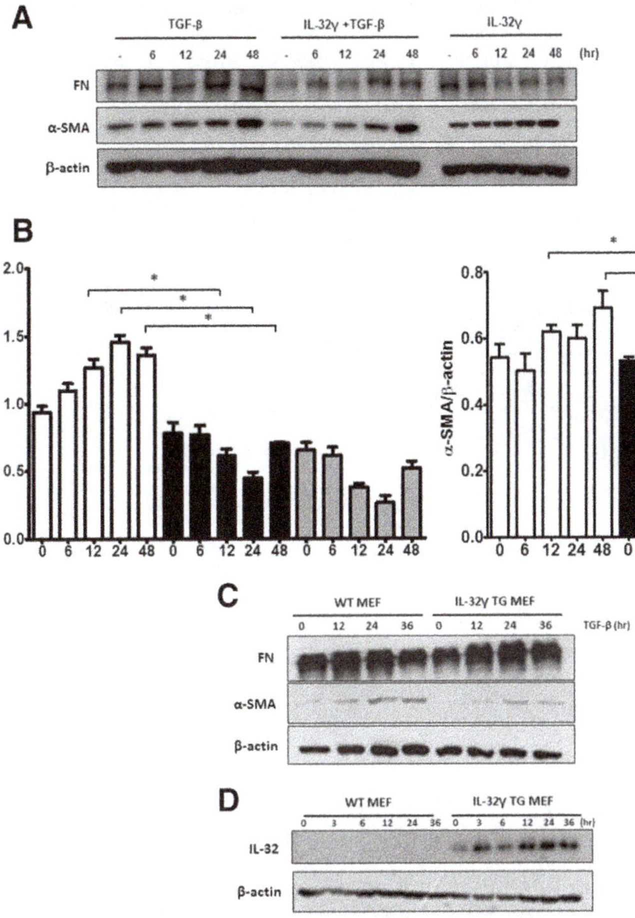

Fig. 2 Exogenous, but not endogenous, IL-32γ attenuates fibroblast activation. Fibronectin and α-SMA expression was detected in rIL-32γ (150 ng/mL)-pretreated MRC-5 cells after TGF-β (5 ng/mL) stimulation. a. Quantification graphs is shown (b). Fibronectin and α-SMA expression are shown in IL-32γ-expressing MEFs after TGF-β (5 ng/mL) stimulation (c). Endogenous IL-32 expression (d). Data are representative of three independent experiments

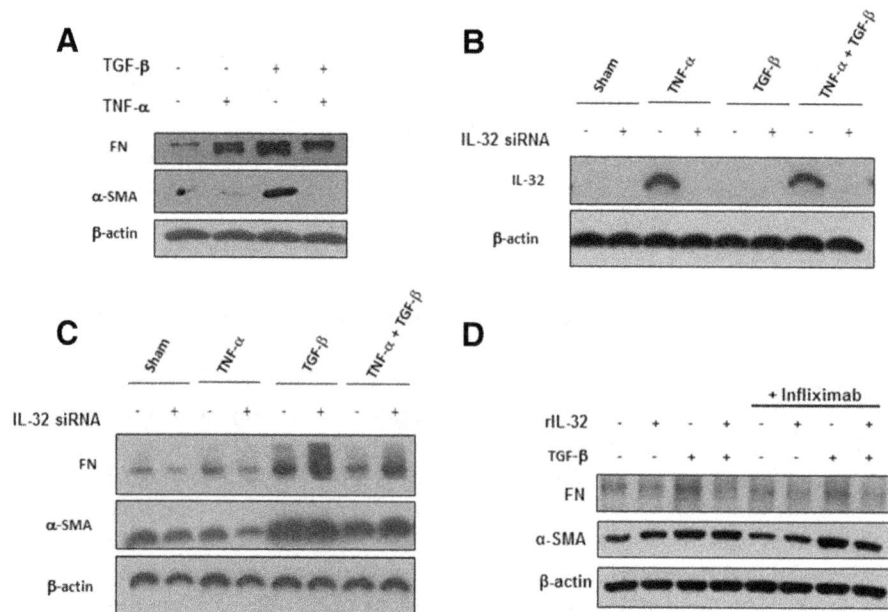

Fig. 3 Anti-fibrotic effects of rIL-32γ are independent of TNF-α. **a** Fibronectin and α-SMA expression in MRC-5 cells after 24 h of stimulation with TNF-α (10 ng/mL) and TGF-β (5 ng/mL). **b** MRC-5 cells were transfected with IL-32 siRNA and then stimulated with TNF-α (10 ng/mL) or TGF-β (5 ng/mL). **c** Fibronectin and α-SMA expression in cell lysates was detected. **d** Infliximab-pretreated MRC-5 cells were stimulated with IL-32γ (150 ng/mL) and TGF-β (5 ng/mL), and fibronectin and α-SMA expression in the cell lysate was detected. Results are representative of two independent experiments, each showing similar results

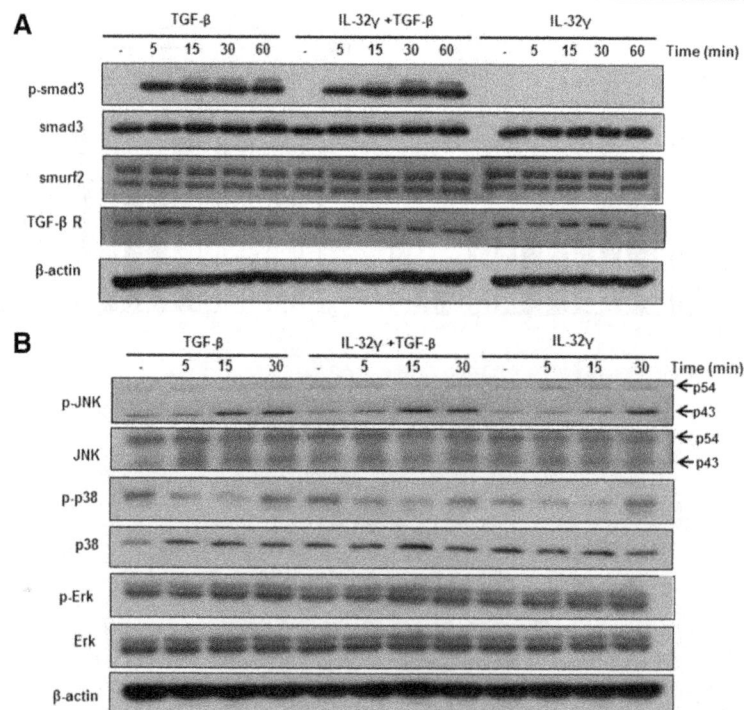

Fig. 4 rIL-32γ has no effect on TGF-β-mediated Smad or non-Smad signaling pathways. MRC-5 wells were stimulated with TGF-β (5 ng/mL) in the presence or absence of rIL-32γ and then harvested at the indicated times. Western blot analysis was performed to examine the expression of proteins in the Smad signaling (**a**) and non-Smad signaling pathways (**b**). Results are representative of three independent experiments

JNK, Erk, and p38 activation between MRC cells treated with rIL-32γ and untreated cells (Fig. 4b).

rIL-32γ inhibits integrin-mediated FAK/paxillin activation

Next, we examined integrin-dependent activation of FAK and paxillin, a critical pathway in fibroblast activation, after treatment with the RGD tripeptide and integrin blocker. RGD peptide inhibited signaling by both FAK and paxillin in MRC-5 cells stimulated with TGF-β (Fig. 5a). Interestingly, rIL-32γ inhibited FAK and paxillin signaling in a manner similar to that of RGD peptide (Fig. 5b).

To investigate how IL-32γ regulates the integrin-FAK-paxillin signaling pathway, we performed a protein-protein binding assay to determine whether IL-32 directly binds to integrin β3, paxillin, or FAK. Both integrin β3 and paxillin were detected in the total cell lysate and flow-through lanes, but no bands were detected in the wash and elution fractions (Fig. 5c). This suggests that these proteins do not directly bind to IL-32γ. Additionally, an anti-flag-IL-32γ antibody did not immunoprecipitate with FAK (Fig. 5d).

rIL-32γ is localized on the cell surface

To determine the mechanism by which rIL-32γ inhibits activation of the FAK/paxillin pathway, we next examined the location of rIL-32γ by live cell imaging for 60 min. rIL-32γ was located outside of MRC-5 cells after 60 min, suggesting that it does not enter cells by endocytosis and is not degraded; therefore, IL-32γ acts extracellularly, at least during the period examined (Fig. 6, see Additional files 5 and 6: Video 1 and 2 in the online Supplement).

rIL-32γ modulates the interaction between integrins and the extracellular matrix

To examine the effect of IL-32γ on integrin signaling, we examined the adhesion of MRC-5 cells to collagen-coated plates in the presence/absence of rIL-32γ. MRC-5 cells adhered to collagen within 30 min in the absence of rIL-32γ; however, the process was impeded in the presence of rIL-32γ (Fig. 7a). Moreover, the number of spindle-shaped MRC-5 cells was much lower in the presence of rIL-32γ, even after 30 min (Fig. 7b). Interestingly, rIL-32γ suppressed integrin/collagen-mediated activation of FAK and paxillin, which is typically induced by cell adhesion to collagen-coated plates in the absence of any other stimulation (Fig. 7c). Finally, we examined the effect of IL-32γ on integrin expression in MRC-5 cells, as TGF-β upregulates integrin expression. Semi-quantitative PCR revealed increased expression of integrin β3 and reduced expression of integrin β8 following TGF-β stimulation. This pattern was not altered by IL-32γ treatment (see Additional file 7: Figure S4).

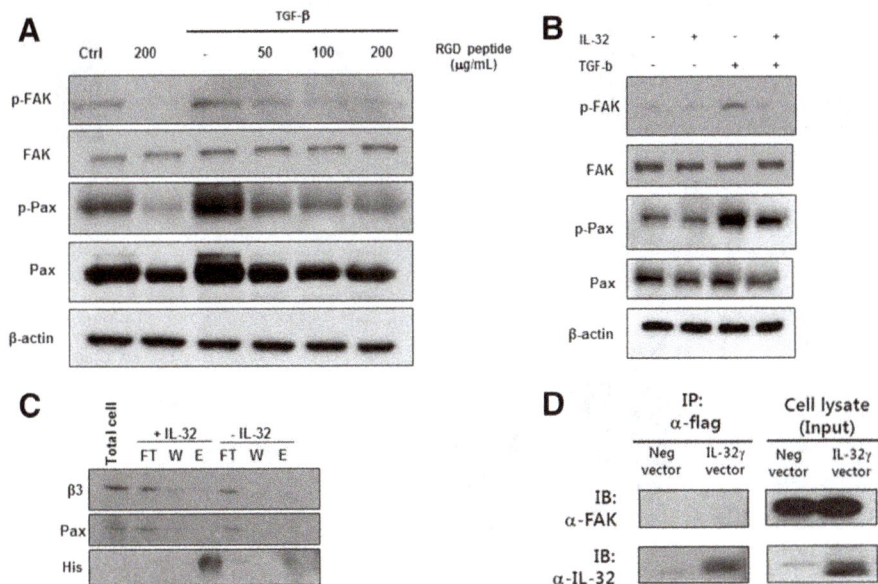

Fig. 5 rIL-32γ inhibits integrin-mediated activation of FAK/paxillin. Phosphorylation of FAK and paxillin was detected in TGF-β (5 ng/mL)-stimulated MRC-5 cells pretreated with an RGD peptide (**a**) or rIL-32γ (**b**). Activated FAK and paxillin were detected after 24 h. Results are representative of three independent experiments. **c** MRC-5 cells were stimulated with TGF-β for 24 h, and His-tagged rIL-32γ was precipitated from cell lysates using Ni-NTA beads. Bound proteins were analyzed by *Western* blotting with antibodies specific for integrin β3, paxillin, and the His-tag. **d** Flag-tagged IL-32γ-overexpressing MRC-5 cells were stimulated with TGF-β and harvested at 24 h. Flag-tagged IL-32γ was then immunoprecipitated from cell lysates using an anti-flag antibody followed by immunoblotting with an anti-FAK antibody. Similar results were obtained from two independent experiments. FT, flow-through; W, wash; E, elution

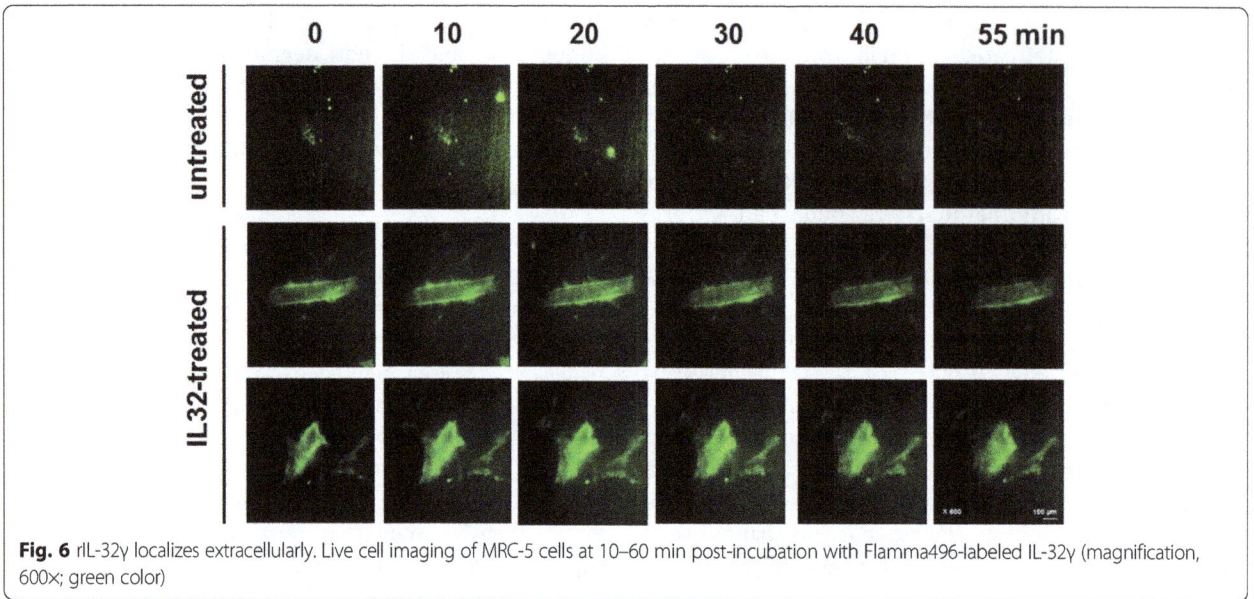

Fig. 6 rIL-32γ localizes extracellularly. Live cell imaging of MRC-5 cells at 10–60 min post-incubation with Flamma496-labeled IL-32γ (magnification, 600×; green color)

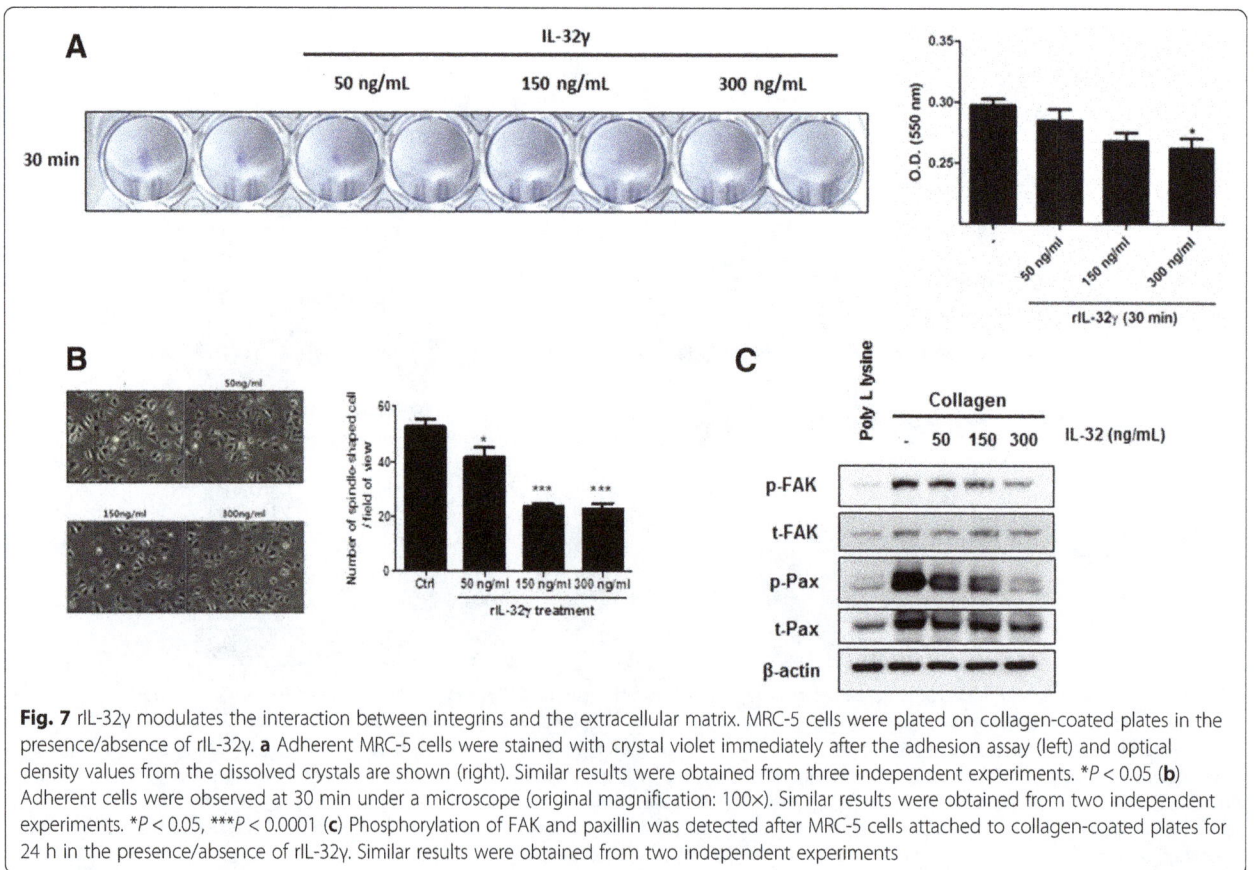

Fig. 7 rIL-32γ modulates the interaction between integrins and the extracellular matrix. MRC-5 cells were plated on collagen-coated plates in the presence/absence of rIL-32γ. **a** Adherent MRC-5 cells were stained with crystal violet immediately after the adhesion assay (left) and optical density values from the dissolved crystals are shown (right). Similar results were obtained from three independent experiments. *$P < 0.05$ (**b**) Adherent cells were observed at 30 min under a microscope (original magnification: 100×). Similar results were obtained from two independent experiments. *$P < 0.05$, ***$P < 0.0001$ (**c**) Phosphorylation of FAK and paxillin was detected after MRC-5 cells attached to collagen-coated plates for 24 h in the presence/absence of rIL-32γ. Similar results were obtained from two independent experiments

Discussion

This study demonstrated the anti-fibrotic effect of IL-32γ both in vitro and in vivo. We showed that rIL-32γ regulates fibroblast activation by modulating the integrin-FAK signaling pathway. Thus, rIL-32γ may be useful for inhibiting tissue fibrosis in the clinical setting.

The mechanism of tissue fibrosis is closely related to that of wound repair, which is a normal healing process in injured tissues. However, dysregulated fibrosis can lead to severe organ dysfunction, which is typically irreversible and has a fatal outcome in many disease states. In the lungs, for example, progressive parenchymal fibrosis is a consequence of serious pulmonary fibrotic diseases such as idiopathic pulmonary fibrosis, leading to high mortality. Additionally, bronchial subepithelial fibrosis can cause irreversible fixed airway obstruction, as observed in chronic inflammatory airway diseases such as chronic severe asthma and COPD, which can become critical if untreated.

Although lung fibrogenesis is thought to result from chronic inflammation, numerous studies have suggested that fibrosis is not completely dependent on inflammatory processes and that anti-inflammatory therapeutic strategies are not always effective. Thus, therapeutic trials have shifted their focus from anti-inflammatory targets to anti-fibrotic targets, as many studies demonstrated that such mechanisms underlie the development of fibrosis [19–22]. However, therapeutic agents that effectively control fibrosis are lacking; therefore, there is an urgent need to identify novel molecules with potent anti-fibrotic activities.

IL-32, previously considered a pro-inflammatory cytokine, is a multifunctional protein with a potential role in lung diseases [12, 23–25]. We previously showed that IL-32γ modulates immune responses by recruiting IL-10-producing monocytic cells in a chronic asthma model [24]. Here, we observed that IL-32γ also exhibits a strong anti-fibrotic effect in a model of sub-bronchial fibrosis. Because chronic inflammation is a major factor driving the progression of fibrosis, its apparent suppressive effect on airway fibrosis may be completely dependent on the anti-inflammatory effects of IL-32γ. Thus, we examined the modulatory effects of IL-32γ in a bleomycin-induced lung injury model, which is considered a prototype of tissue fibrosis but displays lower accumulation of immune cells in the lungs. This is of interest because IL-32γ is a putative immunomodulatory cytokine. The results of the current study suggest that IL-32γ has a novel function in lung fibrosis, as well as anti-inflammatory effects on chronic airway inflammation.

We also used human fibroblasts to further investigate the mechanism underlying the anti-fibrotic effect of IL-32γ, as excessive accumulation of extracellular matrix produced by activated fibroblasts is a major pathological feature in tissue fibrosis, and any possible effects of inflammation in an animal can be excluded. MRC-5 cells were stimulated with TGF-β, which induces fibroblasts to differentiate into fibronectin- and α-SMA-expressing myofibroblasts. We found that IL-32γ effectively inhibited expression of these activation markers upon TGF-β stimulation. Previous studies showed that TNF-α and IL-32γ induce one another. Additionally, TNF-α inhibits the TGF-β-induced Smad signaling pathway [26–29]. Thus, we used cells in which IL-32γ had been silenced and a TNF-α-blocking agent to determine the exact mechanism underlying the suppressive effect of IL-32γ on fibroblast activation. Furthermore, the intracellular pathways linked to the Smad and non-Smad signaling pathways were assessed. We found that the mechanism underlying the role of IL-32γ in fibrogenesis was not dependent on TNF-α expression, nor was it associated with activation of TGF-β downstream of the Smad or non-Smad signaling pathways.

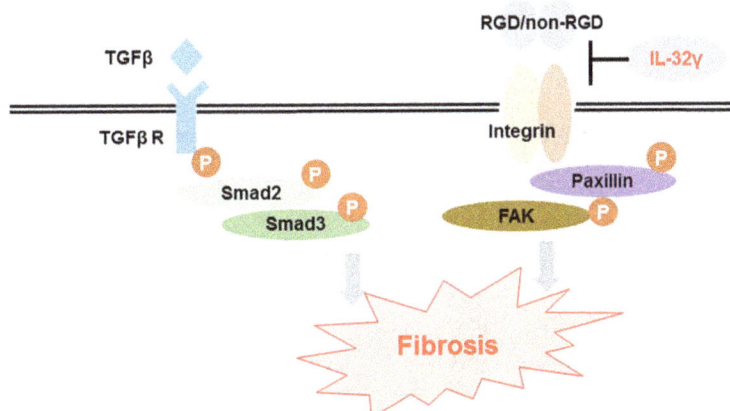

Fig. 8 Suggested role of IL-32γ in the fibrosis pathway. Extracellular IL-32γ suppresses activation of the integrin-FAK-paxillin signaling pathway to exert anti-fibrotic effects but has no effect on the TGF β-Smad signaling pathway

Previous studies indicated that TGF-β-induced fibroblast activation depends on the integrin signaling pathway through FAK/paxillin activation [16, 30–32]. Protein structure modeling suggested that IL-32γ is involved in integrin activation and downstream signaling pathways [14, 33]. In fact, IL-32γ contains an RGD motif that binds to integrins; indeed, several isoforms of IL-32 bind to integrin αVβ3. In addition, IL-32 has a structure resembling the FAT region of FAK (similar to an FAK-inhibitory peptide). However, these studies examined only IL-32α and β, although IL-32γ is considered the most active form [34].

We found that rIL-32γ inhibited the phosphorylation of FAK and paxillin in TGF-β-stimulated fibroblasts without directly binding to these molecules. Based on these results, extracellular rIL-32γ regulates TGF-β-mediated fibroblast activation without entering the cell. Indeed, we observed that rIL-32γ treatment inhibited integrin-mediated cell adhesion, although rIL-32γ remained outside the cell. These results strongly suggest that IL-32γ is involved in the development of tissue fibrosis, likely by disrupting the binding between integrins expressed in the cellular membrane and the extracellular matrix.

No study has fully identified an IL-32-associated pathway in the context of fibrosis, raising the question of whether IL-32 is released by dead cells or via a specific secretory pathway. Notably, in the early phase of several diseases, IL-32 is produced by activated T cells, monocytes, and NK cells and acts as a pro-inflammatory cytokine that stimulates TNF-α, IL-6, and IL-8 production [8, 12, 35, 36]. Because recent studies showed that IL-32 is not secreted [24, 37], IL-32γ released from injured epithelial cells in patients with chronic inflammatory diseases, including those with mycobacterium avium complex pulmonary disease and idiopathic inflammatory bowel disease [22, 37], may play a regulatory role in inflammation or tissue remodeling. For instance, our previous study showed that rIL-32γ suppresses chronic airway inflammation, which is closely associated with airway remodeling [24].

There were some limitations to the current study. First, to obtain more convincing and direct evidence to evaluate our hypothesis, mutations or deletions of the RGD motif of IL-32γ should be used. Second, our results do not clearly define the precise function of intracellular and extracellular IL-32γ. Further studies are necessary to resolve these questions.

In summary, IL-32γ has anti-fibrotic effects likely by blocking the integrin-FAK-paxillin pathway (Fig. 8). Therefore, administration of rIL-32γ may play a pivotal role in modulating both inflammation and fibrosis in patients in which inflammation-related fibrosis pathways are activated.

Conclusions

The present study suggested that IL-32γ prevents tissue damage by regulating fibroblast activation in the chronic stage. The mechanism underlying this modulatory effect may involve disruption of integrin/FAK signaling cascades, without the need for IL-32γ to directly bind molecules involved in these cascades. Thus, IL-32γ is a new candidate for the treatment of lung fibrosis.

Additional files

Additional file 1: Additional methods detail. (DOC 46 kb)

Additional file 2: Figure S1. Extracellular IL-32γ suppresses fibroblast activation. Endogenous IL-32γ did not significantly suppress the expression of fibronectin and α-SMA. (TIF 202 kb)

Additional file 3: Figure S2. IL-32γ mRNA expression was induced by TNF-α. MRC-5 cells were stimulated with each cytokine including LPS (1 μg/mL), Poly I: C (10 μg/mL), TNF-α (10 ng/mL), IL-32γ (150 ng/mL), TGF-β (5 ng/mL), and IL-1β (10 ng/mL). After 24-h stimulation, mRNA level of IL-32γ (A) and TNF-α (B) were measured by quantitative PCR. (TIF 71 kb)

Additional file 4: Figure S3. Anti-fibrotic effect of rIL-32γ is independent of TNF-α. Anti-fibrotic effect of TNF-α was not observed in IL-32γ-knockdown MRC-5 cells (A). rIL-32γ suppressed the expression of fibronectin and α-SMA after TNF-α inhibitor treatment (B). (TIF 96 kb)

Additional file 5: Supplementary video. (MP4 2.42 mb)

Additional file 6: Supplementary video. (MP4 1.98 mb)

Additional file 7: Figure S4. Integrin expression in activated fibroblast is not affected by rIL-32γ. The integrin mRNA levels of α2, αv, β1, β3, β5, β8, and the GAPDH mRNA level were determined by semi-quantitative PCR in MRC-5 after TGF-β or rIL-32γ treatments. (TIF 111 kb)

Abbreviations

COPD: Chronic obstructive pulmonary disease; FAK: Focal adhesion kinase; FAT: Focal adhesion targeting; IL-32: Interleukin 32; MEFs: Mouse embryonic fibroblasts; OVA: Ovalbumin; rIL-32γ: Recombinant interleukin 32 gamma; TG: Transgenic; TGF: Transforming growth factor; TNF: Tumor necrosis factor; WT: Wild-type; α-SMA: Alpha smooth muscle actin

Acknowledgements

We thank Dr. Joon Seo Lim from the Scientific Publications Team at Asan Medical Center for his editorial assistance in preparing this manuscript.

Funding

This work was supported by a National Research Foundation of Korea (NRF) grant, funded by the Korean government (NRF-2013R1A1A2064442).

Authors' contributions

GH Hong designed this study, acquired data, analyzed data, and drafted the manuscript. SY Park designed this study, analyzed data, drafted the manuscript, and revised the manuscript. HS Kwon, J Lee, SY Kim, CG Pack, S Kim, TB Kim, and HB Moon analyzed data and revised the manuscript. KA Moon acquired data and drafted the manuscript. YS Cho designed this study, analyzed data, drafted the manuscript, and revised the manuscript. All authors read and approved the final manuscript. All authors have accountability for all aspects of the work in ensuring that questions related to the accuracy or integrity of any part of the work are appropriately investigated and resolved.

Competing interests

The authors declare that they have no competing interests.

Author details

[1]Asan Institute for Life Science, Seoul, Korea. [2]Department of Internal Medicine, Division of Allergy and Clinical Immunology, Asan Medical Center, University of Ulsan College of Medicine, 88 Olympic-ro 43-gil, Songpa-gu, Seoul 138-736, Korea. [3]Department of Internal medicine, Division of Allergy and Respiratory Medicine, Konkuk University Medical Center, Seoul, Korea. [4]Department of Internal Medicine, Jeju National University School of Medicine, Jeju, Korea. [5]Department of Convergence Medicine, University of Ulsan, Seoul, Korea. [6]Laboratory of Cytokine Immunology, Institute of Biomedical Science and Technology, College of Medicine, Konkuk University, Seoul, Korea.

References

1. Halwani R, Al-Muhsen S, Al-Jahdali H, Hamid Q. Role of transforming growth factor-beta in airway remodeling in asthma. Am J Respir Cell Mol Biol. 2011;44(2):127–33.
2. Murray LA. Commonalities between the pro-fibrotic mechanisms in COPD and IPF. Pulm Pharmacol Ther. 2012;25(4):276–80.
3. Wilson MS, Wynn TA. Pulmonary fibrosis: pathogenesis, etiology and regulation. Mucosal Immunol. 2009;2(2):103–21.
4. Chambers RC. Molecular targets in pulmonary fibrosis. CHEST. 2007;132(4):1311–21.
5. Kreuter M, Bonella F, Wijsenbeek M, Maher TM, Spagnolo P. Pharmacological Treatment of Idiopathic Pulmonary Fibrosis: Current Approaches, Unsolved Issues, and Future Perspectives. Biomed Res Int. 2015;2015:329481.
6. Luzina IG, Todd NW, Iacono AT, Atamas SP. Roles of T lymphocytes in pulmonary fibrosis. J Leukoc Biol. 2008;83(2):237–44.
7. Dahl CA, Schall RP, He HL, Cairns JS. Identification of a novel gene expressed in activated natural killer cells and T cells. J Immunol. 1992;148:597–603.
8. Kim SH, Han SY, Azam T, Yoon DY, Dinarello CA. Interleukin-32: a cytokine and inducer of TNFalpha. Immunity. 2005;22(1):131–42.
9. Netea MG, Azam T, Ferwerda G, Girardin SE, Walsh M, Park JS, Abraham E, Kim JM, Yoon DY, Dinarello CA, Kim SH. IL-32 synergizes with nucleotide oligomerization domain (NOD) 1 and NOD2 ligands for IL-1beta and IL-6 production through a caspase 1-dependent mechanism. Proc Natl Acad Sci U S A. 2005;102(45):16309–14.
10. Dinarello CA, Kim SH. IL-32, a novel cytokine with a possible role in disease. Ann Rheum Dis. 2006;65(Suppl 3):iii61–4.
11. Joosten LA, Netea MG, Kim SH, Yoon DY, Oppers-Walgreen B, Radstake TR, Barrera P, van de Loo FA, Dinarello CA, van den Berg WB. IL-32, a proinflammatory cytokine in rheumatoid arthritis. Proc Natl Acad Sci U S A. 2006;103:3298–303.
12. Calabrese F, Baraldo S, Bazzan E, Lunardi F, Rea F, Maestrelli P, Turato G, Lokar-Oliani K, Papi A, Zuin R, et al. IL-32, a novel proinflammatory cytokine in chronic obstructive pulmonary disease. Am J Respir Crit Care Med. 2008;178(9):894–901.
13. Terasaki Y, Terasaki M, Urushiyama H, Nagasaka S, Takahashi M, Kunugi S, Ishikawa A, Wakamatsu K, Kuwahara N, Miyake K, Fukuda Y. Role of survivin in acute lung injury: epithelial cells of mice and humans. Lab Investig. 2013;93(10):1147–63.
14. Heinhuis B, Koenders MI, van den Berg WB, Netea MG, Dinarello CA, Joosten LA. Interleukin 32 (IL-32) contains a typical alpha-helix bundle structure that resembles focal adhesion targeting region of focal adhesion kinase-1. J Biol Chem. 2012;287(8):5733–43.
15. Nagoshi Y, Yamamoto G, Irie T, Tachikawa T. Expression of FAK-related non-kinase (FRNK) coincides with morphological change in the early stage of cell adhesion. Med Mol Morphol. 2006;39(3):154–60.
16. Thannickal VJLD, White ES, Cui Z, Larios JM, Chacon R, Horowitz JC, Day RM, Thomas PE. Myofibroblast differentiation by TGF-β1 is dependent on cell adhesion and integrin signaling via focal adhesion kinase. J Biol Chem. 2003;278(14):12384–9.
17. Zhang L, Che C, Lin J, Liu K, Li DQ, Zhao G. TLR-mediated induction of proinflammatory cytokine IL-32 in corneal epithelium. Curr Eye Res. 2013;38(6):630–8.
18. Choi JBS, Hong J, Ryoo S, Jhun H, Hong K, Yoon D, Lee S, Her E, Choi W, Kim J, Azam T, Dinarello CA, Kim S. Paradoxical effects of constitutive human IL-32γ in transgenic mice during experimental colitis. Proc Natl Acad Sci U S A. 2010;107(49):21082–6.
19. Royce SG, Cheng V, Samuel CS, Tang ML. The regulation of fibrosis in airway remodeling in asthma. Mol Cell Endocrinol 2012, 351(2):167–175
20. Investigates KG. At the frontiers of lung fibrosis therapy. Nat Biotechnol. 2013;31(9):781–3.
21. Beckett PA, Howarth PH. Pharmacotherapy and airway remodelling in asthma. Thorax. 2003;58(2):163–74.
22. Bai X, Ovrutsky AR, Kartalija M, Chmura K, Kamali A, Honda JR, Oberley-Deegan RE, Dinarello CA, Crapo JD, Chang LY, Chan ED. IL-32 expression in the airway epithelial cells of patients with Mycobacterium avium complex lung disease. Int Immunol. 2011;23(11):679–91.
23. Bang BR, Kwon HS, Kim SH, Yoon SY, Choi JD, Hong GH, Park S, Kim TB, Moon HB, Cho YS. IL-32γ Suppresses Allergic Airway Inflammation in Mouse Models of Asthma. Am J Respir Cell Mol Biol. 2014;50(6):1021–30.
24. Meyer N, Christoph J, Makrinioti H, Indermitte P, Rhyner C, Soyka M, Eiwegger T, Chalubinski M, Wanke K, Fujita H, et al. Inhibition of angiogenesis by IL-32: possible role in asthma. J Allergy Clin Immunol. 2012;129(4):964–73. e967
25. Yamane K, Ihn H, Asano Y, Jinnin M, Tamaki K. Antagnistic effects of TNF-a on TGF-b signaling through downregulation on TGF-b receptor type II in human dermal fibroblast. J Immunol. 2003;171:3855–62.
26. Verrecchia F, Mauviel A. TGF-beta and TNF-alpha : antagonistic cytokines controlling type I collagen gene expression. Cell Signal. 2004;16(8):873–80.
27. Verrecchia F, Pessah M, Atfi A, Mauviel A. Tumor necrosis factor- inhibits transforming growth factor- /Smad signaling in human dermal fibroblasts via AP-1 activation. J Biol Chem. 2000;275(39):30226–31.
28. Franck Verrecchia CT, Erwin F, Wagner EF, Mauviel A. A central role for the JNK pathway in mediating the antagonistic activity of pro-inflammatory cytokines against transforming growth factor beta-driven SMAD3/4-specific gene expression. J Biol Chem. 2003;278(3):1585–93.
29. Mamuya FA, Duncan MK. aV integrins and TGF-beta-induced EMT: a circle of regulation. J Cell Mol Med. 2012;16(3):445–55.
30. Munger JS, Sheppard D. Cross talk among TGF-beta signaling pathways, integrins, and the extracellular matrix. Cold Spring Harb Perspect Biol. 2011;3(11):a005017.
31. Greenberg RS, Bernstein AM, Benezra M, Gelman IH, Taliana L, Masur SK. FAK-dependent regulation of myofibroblast differentiation. FASEB J. 2006;20(7):1006–8.
32. Joosten LA, Heinhuis B, Netea MG, Dinarello CA. Novel insights into the biology of interleukin-32. Cell Mol Life Sci. 2013;70(20):3883–92.
33. Choi JD, Bae SY, Hong JW, Azam T, Dinarello CA, Her E, Choi WS, Kim BK, Lee CK, Yoon DY, et al. Identification of the most active interleukin-32 isoform. Immunology. 2009;126(4):535–42.
34. Kim S. Interleukin-32 in inflammatory autoimmune diseases. Immune Netw. 2014;14(3):123–7.
35. Hong J, Bae S, Kang Y, Yoon D, Bai X, Chan ED, Azam T, Dinarello CA, Lee S, Her E, et al. Suppressing IL-32 in monocytes impairs the induction of the proinflammatory cytokines TNFalpha and IL-1beta. Cytokine. 2010;49(2):171–6.
36. Keswani A, Chustz RT, Suh L, Carter R, Peters AT, Tan BK, Chandra R, Kim SH, Azam T, Dinarello CA, et al. Differential expression of interleukin-32 in chronic rhinosinusitis with and without nasal polyps. Allergy. 2012;67(1):25–32.
37. Shioya M, Nishida A, Yagi Y, Ogawa A, Tsujikawa T, Kim-Mitsuyama S, Takayanagi A, Shimizu N, Fujiyama Y, Andoh A. Epithelial overexpression of interleukin-32alpha in inflammatory bowel disease. Clin Exp Immunol. 2007;149(3):480–6.

3

Smoking is associated with quantifiable differences in the human lung DNA virome and metabolome

Ann C. Gregory[1], Matthew B. Sullivan[1,2], Leopoldo N. Segal[3] and Brian C. Keller[4*]

Abstract

Background: The role of commensal viruses in humans is poorly understood, and the impact of the virome on lung health and smoking-related disease is particularly understudied.

Methods: Genetic material from acellular bronchoalveolar lavage fluid was sequenced to identify and quantify viral members of the lower respiratory tract which were compared against concurrent bronchoalveolar lavage bacterial, metabolite, cytokine and cellular profiles, and clinical data. Twenty smoker and 10 nonsmoker participants with no significant comorbidities were studied.

Results: Viruses that infect bacteria (phages) represented the vast majority of viruses in the lung. Though bacterial communities were statistically indistinguishable across smokers and nonsmokers as observed in previous studies, lung viromes and metabolic profiles were significantly different between groups. Statistical analyses revealed that changes in viral communities correlate most with changes in levels of arachidonic acid and IL-8, both potentially relevant for chronic obstructive pulmonary disease (COPD) pathogenesis based on prior studies.

Conclusions: Our assessment of human lung DNA viral communities reveals that commensal viruses are present in the lower respiratory tract and differ between smokers and nonsmokers. The associations between viral populations and local immune and metabolic tone suggest a significant role for virome-host interaction in smoking related lung disease.

Keywords: Bacteriome, Lung, Virus, Virome, Microbiome, Metabolome, Smoking

Background

Smoking is the leading cause of chronic obstructive pulmonary disease (COPD) and the third highest cause of death globally [1, 2]. Despite the clear associated risk, only a fraction of smokers eventually develop COPD [2, 3]. What causes some smokers, and not others, to develop COPD remains unknown and an area of active research [2–5]. Recent work examining the lung bacteriome of individuals with moderate to severe COPD revealed decreased bacterial diversity compared to nonsmokers [6–11]. As a result, it has been proposed that changes in lung-resident bacterial communities may lead to COPD [4–8]. However, respiratory tract bacterial communities of individuals with mild COPD, "healthy" smokers, and nonsmokers are not significantly different [8, 11–13], suggesting that factors other than commensal bacteria may trigger COPD development.

To date, few studies have examined lung viral communities where the vast majority of viruses have been identified as bacteriophages [14–18]. Phages impact bacterial communities through direct and indirect interactions. Though phage ecological roles are unknown in the lung, their activities are relatively well-documented in the oceans where they regulate bacterial population sizes, diversity, metabolic outputs, and gene flow [19–24]. In humans, phages may stimulate the immune system leading to immune-mediated microbial competition [25], tax the immune system enabling opportunistic infection [26], or work symbiotically at human mucosal surfaces providing a source of additional immunity [27]. Thus,

* Correspondence: Brian.Keller2@osumc.edu
[4]Division of Pulmonary, Critical Care & Sleep Medicine, The Ohio State University College of Medicine, 201 Davis Heart & Lung Research Institute, 473 West 12th Avenue, Columbus, OH 43210, USA
Full list of author information is available at the end of the article

changing lung viral communities could alter the bacteriome leading to dysbiosis and disease progression in pre-affected (e.g., COPD) individuals [6–8]. Here we utilized a historical cohort to explore the impact of smoking on the lung microenvironment with specific focus on the role of double-stranded DNA (dsDNA) viruses. To do this, we applied a quantitative sample-to-sequence dsDNA viral metagenomic processing pipeline [28] that maintains relative abundances between samples and used these data as a baseline to compare and ecologically contextualize lung viromes in relation to lung bacteriomes, metabolomes, and immunologic profiles of "healthy" smokers and nonsmokers.

Methods

Sample collection and processing

Between 2010 and 2013, bronchoalveolar lavage (BAL) fluid was collected from 30 asymptomatic subjects (10 nonsmokers, 14 former smokers, and 6 current smokers) as part of previous studies evaluating the lower airway bacteriome and inflammation [29, 30]. Briefly, bronchoscopy was performed via nasal approach and avoiding suctioning until the scope was positioned for sampling. Sequential BAL was collected from the lingula and right middle lobe, combined, and processed. Metabolites and cytokine numbers were measured as previously described [29, 30], and identified metabolites were reported if present in ≥50% of the samples. Intensity data were mean-centered and divided by the standard deviation using MetaboAnalyst [31]. For in vivo cytokines, 39 cytokines were measured with a Luminex 200IS (Luminext Corp, Austin, TX) using Human Cytokine Panel I (Millipore, Billerica, MA). Data were analyzed with MasterPlex TM QT software (version 1–2, MiraiBio, Inc. Alameda, CA).

16S rRNA gene sequencing

The 16S rRNA gene sequencing dataset collected as part of [30] was analyzed in the context of smoking status. The creation of this dataset has been previously described [30]. Briefly, acellular BAL was obtained after centrifugation at 500 x g for 10 min at 4 °C followed by DNA extraction via ion exchange column (Qiagen). Additionally, DNA was extracted from pre-bronchoscopy saline to determine the level of background microbial contamination. The V4 region of the bacterial 16S rRNA gene was amplified in duplicate reactions, using primer set 515F/806R, which nearly universally amplifies bacterial and archaeal 16S rRNA genes [32, 33]. Each unique barcoded amplicon was generated in pairs of 25 μl reactions with the following reaction conditions: 11 μl Polymerase Chain Reaction (PCR)-grade H2O, 10 μl Hot Master Mix (5 Prime Cat# 2200410), 2 μl of forward and reverse barcoded primer (5 μM) and 2 μl template DNA. Reactions were run on a C1000 Touch Thermal Cycler (Bio-Rad) with the

following cycling conditions: initial denaturing at 94 °C for 3 min followed by 35 cycles of denaturation at 94 °C for 45 s, annealing at 58 °C for 1 min, and extension at 72 °C for 90 s, with a final extension of 10 min at 72 °C. 16S rRNA gene amplicons were sequenced with Illumina MiSeq and analyzed using QIIME. Using this dataset, we normalized absolute operational taxonomic unit (OTU) sequence counts to obtain the relative abundances of the microbiota in each sample. These relative abundances at 97% OTU similarity and each of the 5 higher taxonomic levels (phylum, class, order, family, genus) were tested for univariate associations with clinical variables. The ade4 package in R was used to construct Principal Coordinate Analysis (PCoA) based on weighted UniFrac distances [34, 35].

Shotgun sequencing

DNA extracted from the same acellular BAL samples described above was sheared with a Covaris E210 Focused-ultrasonicator. Libraries were constructed with the NEBNext Ultra DNA Library Prep Kit for Illumina (New England Biolabs, Ipswich, MA) and sequenced with Illumina MiSeq. Reads were QC'd and trimmed using BBDuk (BBtools package) [36], de-duplicated, and aligned to the human genome (95% identity) with BBMap [36]. Following processing, each virome had on average > 1 million reads (Additional file 1: Table S1). Cross-assembly of all 30 viromes using SPAdes [37] assembled no viral contigs > 500 bp. Consequently, to determine if viruses were present in a sample, reads were aligned using Bowtie2 [38] to a custom viral database composed of Viral RefSeq release 78, the VirSorter database [39], 23 core gut phages [36–40], and the crAssphage genome (GenBank Accession #JQ995537). Viruses with reads aligned at ≥95% percent identity [41, 42] to a consecutive 200 bp stretch of the genome were considered present in the lung virome. Median coverage was normalized to decontaminated virome read numbers to determine viral relative abundances. While 16S rRNA data was available from saline control samples from earlier studies [29, 30], insufficient amounts of saline and oral rinse control specimens remained for repeat testing by shotgun sequencing.

Statistics

Ecological diversity statistics were performed using vegan in R [43]. Statistical outliers were evaluated using "pcout" in the mvoutlier package [44]. Bray-Curtis distances were calculated with and without outliers and were statistically ordinated using PCoA; bivariate ellipses were fit to the ordination using "ordiellipse" based on smoking status, race, and gender, and centroids were assessed to be significantly different using the "envfit" functions in vegan. Mantel's tests using a spearman correlation were used to correlate viral Bray-Curtis distances. Differentially abundant viral populations across smokers and nonsmokers were determined with Metastats [45, 46]. For metabolic data, bacterial and viral abundances were vector-fit to the PCoA ("envfit" function). A total of 9999 permutations were used for all vector and centroid fitting, and Mantel's tests were used to further confirm the correlations between changes in metabolic data and changes in bacterial and viral abundances. These vector fittings and Mantel's test p-values were Bonferroni-corrected. To determine if viral pneumotypes existed, the SPIEC-EASI package [47] was applied using the Meinshausen and Bühlmann (MB) method to infer associations between viral populations. A batch file of all bioinformatics parameters and code can be found on iVirus in Cyverse (/iplant/shared/iVirus/Lung_Virome).

Results
Cohort
In a previous study, we explored the association between the lower airway bacteriome and inflammation in healthy, asymptomatic individuals. Utilizing this historical cohort [30], we selected 30 subjects (20 current or former smokers and 10 nonsmokers, Table 1) for which sufficient BAL sample remained for additional virome

analysis to analyze the relationship between smoking and the lower airway microenvironment. As previously described [29], nonsmokers were enrolled from the NYU CTSI-sponsored Healthy Volunteers Bronchoscopy Cohort, characterized by subjects with no significant smoking history, normal spirometry, and absence of pulmonary, cardiovascular, renal, or endocrine disease. Smokers were enrolled from the NYU Early Detection Research Network (EDRN, 5U01CA086137–13), a longitudinal cohort consisting of approximately 2000 subjects with substantial smoking history (43.8 ± 24.3 pack-years). Smoking status was obtained during clinical interview screenings. Smokers and nonsmokers were similar in height, weight and gender distribution, whereas older, white participants were over-represented among smokers. In terms of lung function, smokers and nonsmokers had normal forced vital capacity (FVC), forced expiratory volume in 1 s (FEV_1), and diffusing capacity of the lungs for carbon monoxide (DLCO), whereas smokers had lower mean FEV_1/FVC ratios.

Composition of the lung Virome
DNA was extracted from acellular BAL and sequenced with Illumina MiSeq. Despite removing reads mapping to the human genome at > 95% identity, many contaminating human reads remained. Of the almost 35 million

Table 1 Participant characteristics

Demographics	Smokers (n = 20)	Nonsmokers (n = 10)	Statistical Differences
Age, yr	63.7 (58.5–67.2)	36.2 (28.3–41.9)	p < 0.00001
Gender			p < 0.3980[b]
Male	13 (65%)	8 (80%)	
Female	7 (35%)	2 (20%)	
Height, cm	172.7 (165.1–179.1)	176.5 (173.4–181.6)	p < 0.3125
Weight, kg	79.8 (69.4–91.6)	85.5 (75.1–101.2)	p < 0.6560
Race			p < 0.0037[b]
White	19 (95%)	5 (50%)	
Other	1 (5%)	5 (50%)	
Pulmonary Function Testing[a]			
FVC (% Predicted)	96.9 (90.2–102.8)	96.0 (90.0–103.7)	p < 0.8337
FEV_1 (% Predicted)	94.1 (86.7–104.2)	97.1 (86.2–103.4)	p < 0.9840
FEV_1/FVC	71.7 (69.9–78.4)	83.5 (77.7–84.3)	p < 0.0220
DLCO (% Predicted)	91.0 (79.3–99.0)	94.0 (82.0–98.0)	p < 0.4593
BAL Immune Cell Counts (%)			
Macrophages	90.8 (87.8–94.8)	90.8 (86.0–93.5)	p < 0.9840
Lymphocytes	6.2 (3.9–8.7)	6.6 (5.1–11.5)	p < 0.5552
Neutrophils	1.8 (1.3–2.9)	1.3 (1.2–1.6)	p < 0.1645
Eosinophils	0.3 (0.1–0.6)	0.2 (0.1–0.3)	p < 0.2670

Data is given in counts or median values and interquartile ranges. All comparisons are Mann-Whitney U-test results unless noted. [a]Data based on NHANES predicted values. [b]Chi-squared analysis

reads following human decontamination across all 30 samples, only 9730 reads (0.03% of total reads) mapped to our curated viral database (Additional file 1: Table S1). In total, these reads mapped to 247 different viral populations (Fig. 1). All but one of the viruses detected were found in the Viral RefSeq or VirSorter [39] databases. One virus classified as a core gut virus [40] was detected in the lung of two individuals.

Only three eukaryotic DNA viruses were detected in the acellular BAL samples (Fig. 1). These included human herpesvirus 8, human adenovirus 2, and human papillomavirus type 4. All eukaryotic viruses were present in only one or two subject's lung viromes.

Similar to previous findings [14–17], the majority of lung viruses (> 85% of mean viral community abundances) identified in our study were bacteriophages. The identified phages are predicted to infect a broad array of bacterial phyla based on the hosts of reference viruses in Viral RefSeq and VirSorter [39] with 37% infecting Proteobacteria, 36% Firmicutes, 23% Actinobacteria, 3% Bacteriodetes, 1% Fusobacteria, and < 1% Tenericutes (Additional file 2: Figure S1A). Of the Proteobacteria hosts, the majority included *Neisseria*, *Escherichia*, *Acinetobacter*, and *Burkholderia* (Additional file 2: Figure S1B). Among the Firmicutes and Actinobacteria hosts, the majority belong to a single genus, with 60% from the genus *Streptococcus* and 78% from the genus *Propionibacterium*, respectively (Additional file 2: Figure S1C, D). All of the Bacteriodetes hosts that could be annotated (5 out of 6) belonged to the genus *Prevotella*, while *Leptotrichia* and *Spiroplasma* were the only genera identified from the phyla Fusobacteria and Tenericutes, respectively.

Phage abundances were summed based on host genera across all 30 lung viromes to create the total virome.

Based on percentages of the total virome, *Propionibacterium* phages were the most abundant across the 30 lung viromes, making up 29% of the total viral community (Additional file 3: Figure S2). The next most abundant phages were *Streptococcus*, *Burkholderia*, *Escherichia*, and *Bacillus* phages, each making up > 10% of the mean viral community (Additional file 3: Figure S2). Lastly, phages infecting the genera *Acinetobacter*, *Neisseria*, *Mannheimia*, *Staphylococcus*, *Gardnerella*, and *Shigella* made up > 2% and phages infecting the genera *Bartonella*, *Lactobacillus*, *Methylbacterium*, *Salmonella*, *Streptomyces*, *Prevotella*, *Veillonella*, and *Eubacterium* made up > 1% of total viral community (Additional file 3: Figure S2).

Absence of viral Pneumotypes

Previous work in the human gut identified three distinct microbial enterotypes based on co-occurrence of microbial populations and predominance of specific microbial groups [48]. Using the same samples as used in the current study, we previously identified lower respiratory tract bacterial pneumotypes through hierarchical clustering and PCoA analysis of bacterial communities based on 16S rRNA abundances [29, 30]. Bacterial pneumotypes were present irrespective of smoking status. Similarly, we used hierarchical clustering of viral population abundances to evaluate for viral pneumotypes (Fig. 1; hierarchical clustering of viral communities by individual subject not shown) but found no clear clusters. To further assess if viral pneumotypes were present in our samples, we used SPIEC-EASI which forms a co-occurrence network based on correlations between viral populations (Additional file 4: Figure S3). If distinct viral pneumotypes existed across our samples, we should see clear separation of viral populations into clustered groups. We thus conclude that we could not find distinct viral pneumotypes in our cohort.

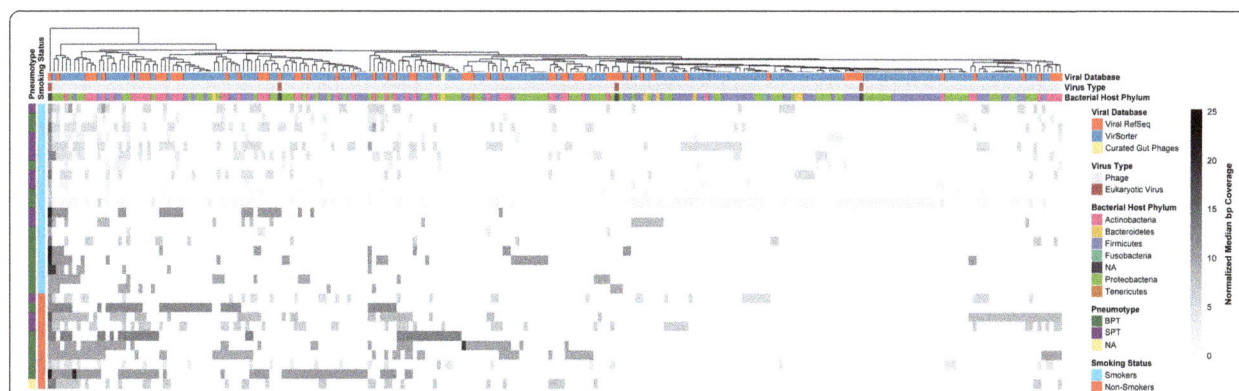

Fig. 1 Identity and relative abundances of viruses in the smoker and nonsmoker lung. Heatmap of relative abundances of the 247 viral populations based on median normalized coverage for each virome. Each row shows the viral community composition of smokers and nonsmokers, also identified by bacterial pneumotype as determined in [26, 27]. Each column represents a distinct viral population coded by host phylum, virus type, and database in which the viral genome can be found. The dendrogram above the heatmap shows hierarchical clustering of viral populations based on abundances across the different viral communities. BPT = background predominant taxa, SPT = supraglottic predominant taxa, NA = not assessed

Lung Virome comparisons between smokers and nonsmokers

We next assessed lung virome composition by smoking status. While a large fraction of the viral populations detected across the 30 samples were shared between smokers and nonsmokers (29%), there were clear differences between abundances of certain phage groups in smoker and nonsmoker viromes. *Prevotella* phages were at least two-fold higher in the smoker virome, whereas in the nonsmoker virome, *Lactobacillus* and *Gardnerella* phages were 10-fold more abundant. Across individuals, statistical analyses of differentially abundant viral populations using Metastats [45, 46], a tool designed to handle sparse counts, revealed similar results. *Prevotella* phages (Metastats: $p = 0.02$) were significantly increased among smokers while *Lactobacillus* and *Gardnerella* phages (Metastats: $p = 0.001$, both) were significantly increased among nonsmokers (Fig. 2). Furthermore, phages infecting *Actinomyces, Aeromonas, Capnocytophaga, Haemophilus, Rodoferax,* and *Xanthomonas* were also increased among smokers, and phages infecting *Enhydrobacter* and *Morganella* were increased among nonsmokers (Metastats: $p < 0.05$).

Some rare viral populations were unique to smoker or nonsmoker total viral communities (Additional file 5: Figure S4). For example, *Actinomyces, Capnocytophaga, Haemophilus* and *Rhodoferax* phages were found only in smokers, and *Enhydrobacter, Enterobacter, Holospora, Morganella,* and *Spiroplasma* phages were found only in nonsmokers. Eukaryotic DNA viruses were only found in the lungs of smokers (Additional file 5: Figure S4).

Ecological comparisons between smokers and nonsmokers

We next examined the lung virome ecology of smokers and nonsmokers. Ecological α diversity measures of richness, biodiversity (Shannon's H), and evenness (Peilou's J) (Fig. 3a) were significantly different (Mann-Whitney U-test; $p < 0.01$) between smoker and nonsmoker viromes with smokers exhibiting lower values in all analyzed metrics. Further, viral community structure (β diversity) was significantly fit by smoking status (Fig. 3b, Bray-Curtis distances, bivariate ellipse fitting (BEF): $r^2 \geq 0.32$, $p \leq 0.02$). Because some effects of smoking are reversible upon cessation, we performed a subgroup analysis of viral communities from current and former smokers and found no significant virome differences (BEF: $p = 1.00$). We also tested whether viral communities could be fit based on their paired bacterial pneumotypes [29, 30] and found no significant association between viral communities and bacterial pneumotypes (BEF: $r^2 \geq 0.17$, $p \leq 0.14$). Finally, we tested if, within smoker and nonsmoker viral communities, there was significant fitting based on their paired bacterial pneumotype and again found no significant fitting (BEF: within smoker: $r^2 \geq 0.12$, $p \leq 0.10$; within nonsmoker: $r^2 \geq 0.34$, $p \leq 0.20$).

Since differences in age and race were noted among the smoker and nonsmoker groups, we tested whether these variables affect the β diversity distribution of the samples. Age was not significantly correlated to Bray-Curtis bacterial and viral community distances (Mantel's test; bacteria: $r = -0.04$, $p < 0.71$; virus: $r = -0.001$, $p < 0.46$). Race also

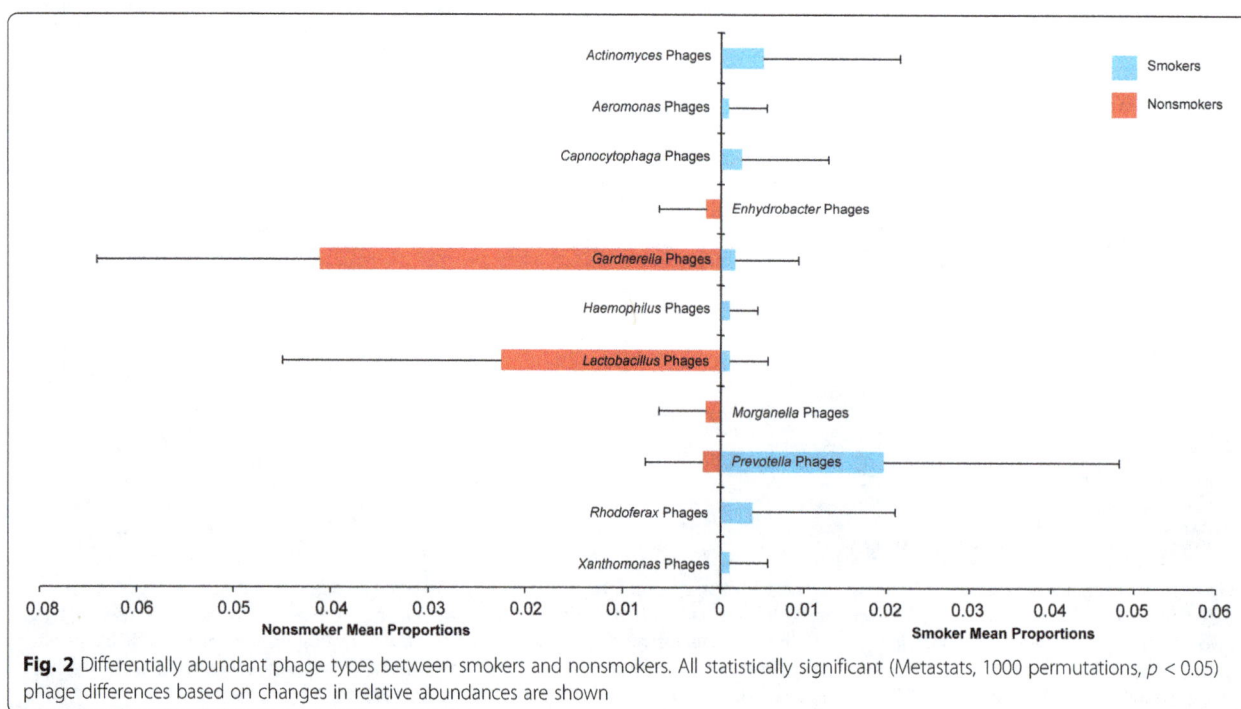

Fig. 2 Differentially abundant phage types between smokers and nonsmokers. All statistically significant (Metastats, 1000 permutations, $p < 0.05$) phage differences based on changes in relative abundances are shown

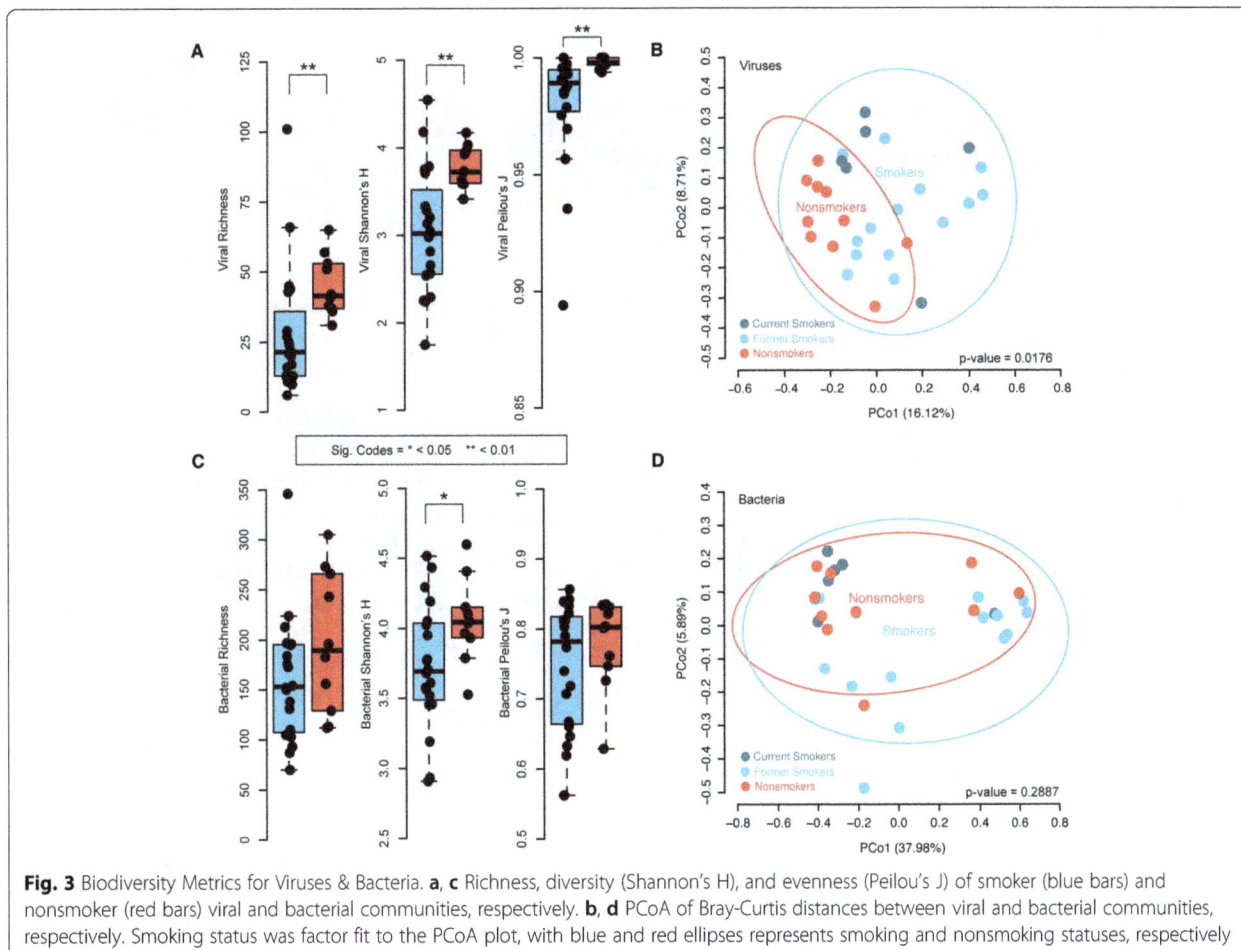

Fig. 3 Biodiversity Metrics for Viruses & Bacteria. **a, c** Richness, diversity (Shannon's H), and evenness (Peilou's J) of smoker (blue bars) and nonsmoker (red bars) viral and bacterial communities, respectively. **b, d** PCoA of Bray-Curtis distances between viral and bacterial communities, respectively. Smoking status was factor fit to the PCoA plot, with blue and red ellipses represents smoking and nonsmoking statuses, respectively

did not significantly explain the variance across all 30 bacterial or viral communities (BEF: bacterial: $r^2 \geq 0.08$, $p \leq 0.74$; viral: $r^2 \geq 0.08$, $p \leq 0.61$ for race).

Previous studies demonstrated changes in the lung bacteriome in moderate to severe COPD [7, 13], but no differences were found in lung bacterial community structure in healthy smokers without COPD compared to nonsmokers [12]. Consistent with this, and in contrast to the lung virome, we found no significant differences in bacterial α diversity (richness, Mann-Whitney U-test, $p < 0.15$; evenness, Peilou's J: Mann-Whitney U-test, $p < 0.50$) and only a slight difference based on Shannon index (Mann-Whitney U-test; $p < 0.05$) (Fig. 3c). Differences in bacterial β diversity were noted, but these differences were not explained by smoking status (Fig. 3d, BEF: $r^2 \geq 0.01$, $p \leq 0.67$). Instead, bacterial communities in our study were previously found to separate based on pneumotypes [29, 30]. Given these results, it was not surprising that bacterial and viral Bray-Curtis distances did not correlate (Mantel's $r = 0.09$, $p < 0.06$).

Low biomass specimens, such as BAL fluid, are at risk of confounding from environmental contamination [49].

To address this, we examined bacteriome differences between pre-bronchoscopy control saline samples from smokers and nonsmokers and found no significant differences (Additional file 6: Figure S5). No *Propionibacterium* bacteria, common reagent and laboratory contaminants, were detectable within the background. In a subgroup of subjects, we previously demonstrated a lack of upper airway carryover into these lower airways specimens (reported in Fig. 2 of [29]).

Metabolic differences between smokers and nonsmokers

To assess the impact of smoking on cellular activities at the functional level, we compared the lung BAL metabolomes of smokers and nonsmokers. In total, we identified 83 distinct metabolites and assessed their abundances across individual smokers and nonsmokers (Fig. 4a). Most metabolites were significantly different between smokers and nonsmokers (Bonferroni corrected Mann-Whitney U-test, $p < 0.05$). These included metabolites involved in multiple metabolic pathways; among the top differences, fatty acid and carboxylic acid metabolites were significantly elevated in smokers.

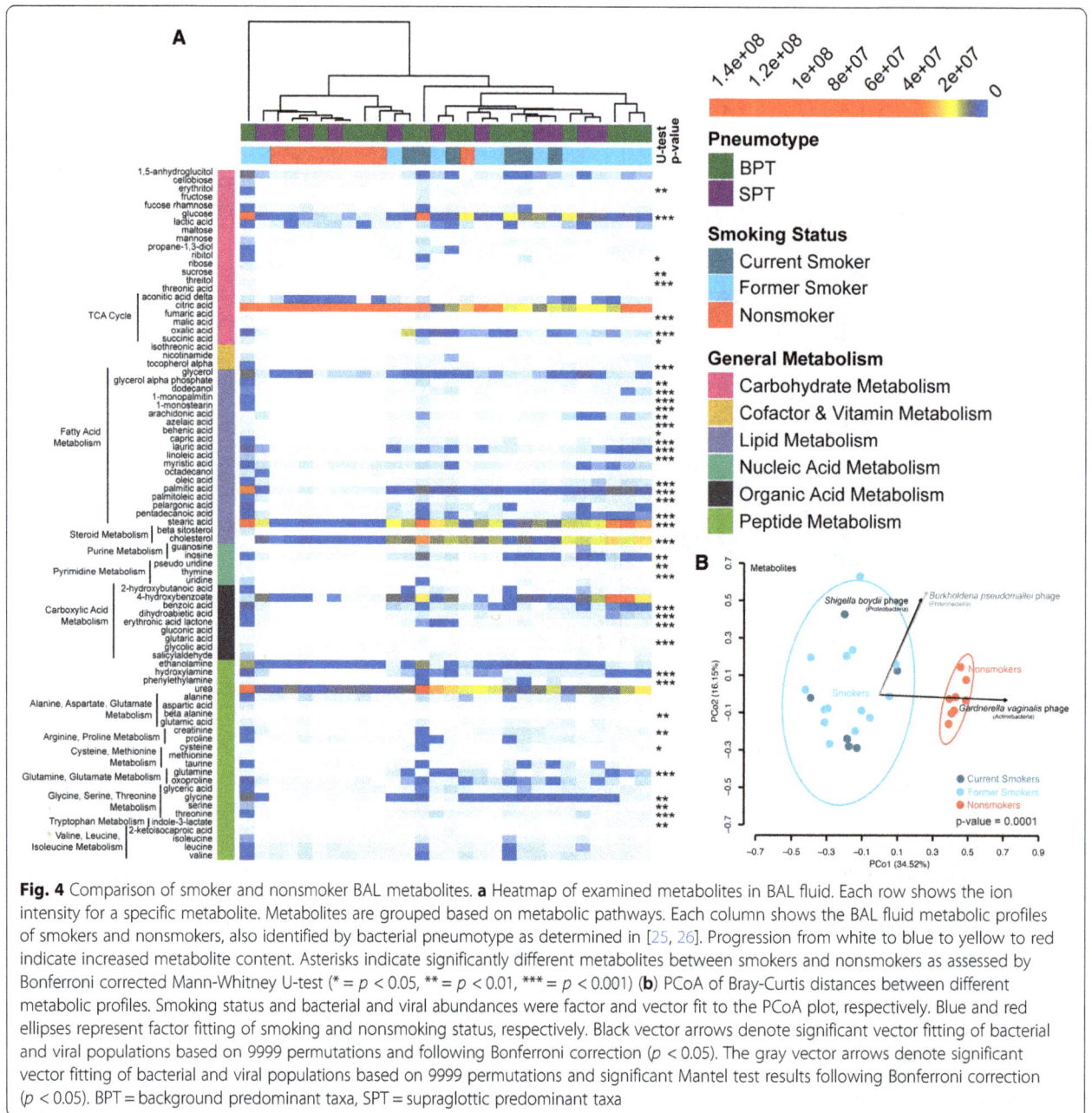

Fig. 4 Comparison of smoker and nonsmoker BAL metabolites. **a** Heatmap of examined metabolites in BAL fluid. Each row shows the ion intensity for a specific metabolite. Metabolites are grouped based on metabolic pathways. Each column shows the BAL fluid metabolic profiles of smokers and nonsmokers, also identified by bacterial pneumotype as determined in [25, 26]. Progression from white to blue to yellow to red indicate increased metabolite content. Asterisks indicate significantly different metabolites between smokers and nonsmokers as assessed by Bonferroni corrected Mann-Whitney U-test (* = $p < 0.05$, ** = $p < 0.01$, *** = $p < 0.001$) (**b**) PCoA of Bray-Curtis distances between different metabolic profiles. Smoking status and bacterial and viral abundances were factor and vector fit to the PCoA plot, respectively. Blue and red ellipses represent factor fitting of smoking and nonsmoking status, respectively. Black vector arrows denote significant vector fitting of bacterial and viral populations based on 9999 permutations and following Bonferroni correction ($p < 0.05$). The gray vector arrows denote significant vector fitting of bacterial and viral populations based on 9999 permutations and significant Mantel test results following Bonferroni correction ($p < 0.05$). BPT = background predominant taxa, SPT = supraglottic predominant taxa

Hierarchical clustering by metabolic profile showed strong clustering of nonsmokers, with nonsmokers having lower metabolite levels than smokers for all metabolites except citric acid. Smoker metabolic profiles also clustered, but with greater variation (Fig. 4a). Metabolic profile Bray-Curtis distances supported the hierarchical clustering and demonstrated significant fitting by smoking status, with low variance among nonsmokers and more variance among smokers (Fig. 4b, BEF: $r^2 \geq 0.56$, $p \leq 0.0001$).

We next evaluated whether distinct bacterial or viral populations may be associated with metabolic profile differences by vector fitting all bacterial and viral abundances to the metabolite Bray-Curtis distances (Fig. 4b). Because PCoA are non-planar, we also ran regressions between Bray-Curtis distances of the bacterial and viral population abundances and the metabolite data converted into Euclidean distances using Mantel's tests. Following Bonferroni correction, three populations emerged as significantly associated with metabolic profile differences (Fig. 4b, $p < 0.05$); all three populations were viruses. Surprisingly, no changes in bacterial abundances were significantly associated with metabolic differences between smokers and nonsmokers. Changes in the abundances of the Proteobacteria phages, *Shigella boydii* phage and *Burkholderia pseudomallei* phage, were associated with a metabolic shift towards smokers, while an Actinobacteria phage, *Gardnerella vaginalis* phage, appeared to influence metabolic differences in nonsmokers.

Associations between viruses and the pulmonary environment

Understanding how viruses and the pulmonary environment impact each other is important for determining the impact of viruses in the lung. We first evaluated what metabolites, immune cells, cytokines, or bacterial populations might be linked to changes in viral community structure. In total, 15 different metabolites, 11 immune cells and cytokines, and 32 different bacterial populations (Fig. 5) correlated with viral community dissimilarity distances (Mantel's test, $p < 0.05$, Mantel's $r > 0.2$). Interestingly, 56% of the bacterial populations correlated with the smoker virome were Proteobacteria, further supporting the role of Proteobacteria and their phages in alterations of host-associated ecosystems [50]. Out of the 26 metabolites, immune cells, and cytokines, arachidonic acid and IL-8 (Fig. 5 top left and top right, respectively) had the highest association with virus community separation based on dissimilarity ($r^2 > 0.3$), and arachidonic acid and IL-8 levels were highest in smokers. No significant

differences in IL-8 or arachidonic acid levels were observed between current and former smokers (Mann-Whitney U-test, IL-8 $p = 0.48$, arachidonic acid $p = 0.13$).

Discussion

In this first study of the effects of smoking on the lung DNA virome, we found that, in contrast to the lung bacteriome, smoking was associated with significant changes in the lung virome and metabolome. Overall, smokers exhibited a contraction of the lung virome, evidenced by lower numbers of viral populations and altered viral ecology. Virome differences between smokers and nonsmokers remained significant even after accounting for age difference between the groups. We hypothesize this altered viral ecology may drive changes in the BAL metabolome between smokers and nonsmokers. Alternatively, changes in the lung metabolic profiles of smokers may lead to downstream effects on the virome, though we consider this less likely as early metabolic changes would presumably also impact bacterial ecology, a link we failed to identify in this study.

Key to our analyses was the ability to quantitatively identify and enumerate viral populations in the lung. While sequence-based 16S rRNA amplification has enabled the rapid quantitative characterization of bacterial

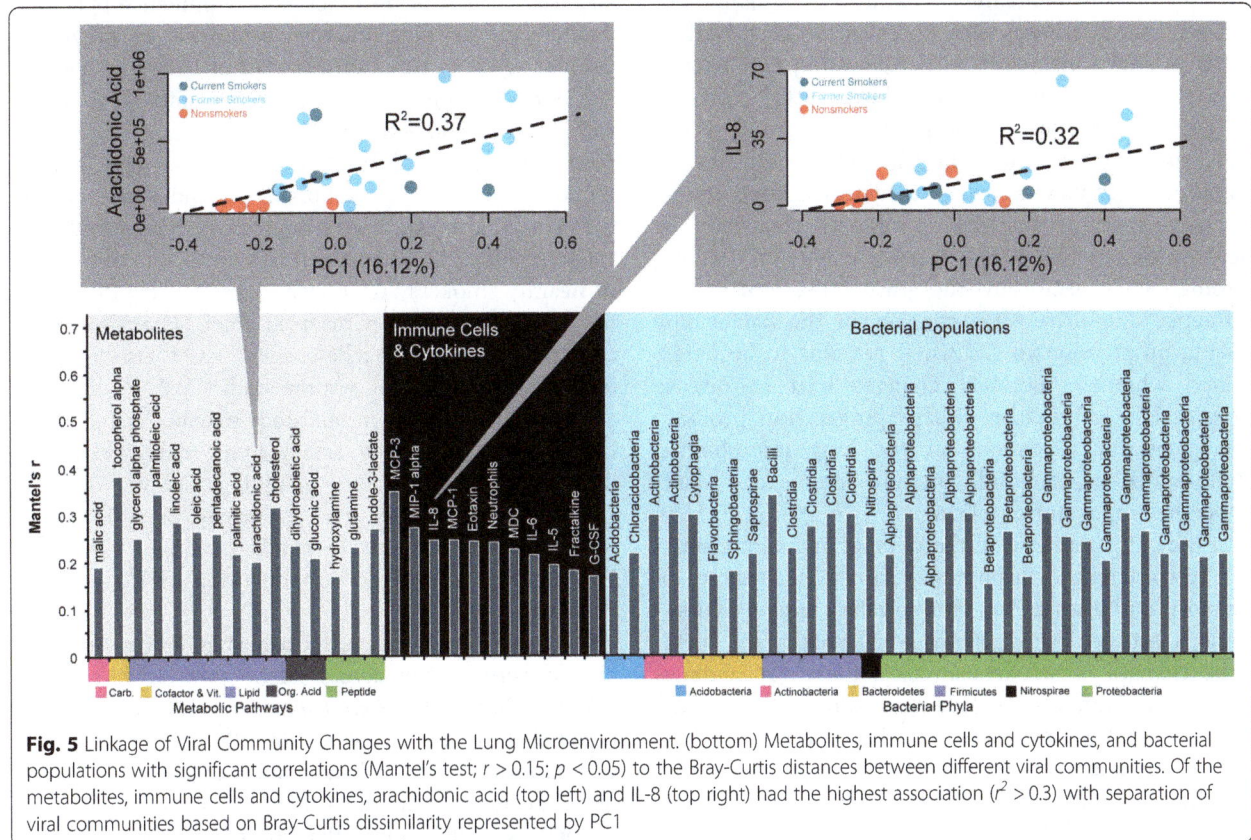

Fig. 5 Linkage of Viral Community Changes with the Lung Microenvironment. (bottom) Metabolites, immune cells and cytokines, and bacterial populations with significant correlations (Mantel's test; $r > 0.15$; $p < 0.05$) to the Bray-Curtis distances between different viral communities. Of the metabolites, immune cells and cytokines, arachidonic acid (top left) and IL-8 (top right) had the highest association ($r^2 > 0.3$) with separation of viral communities based on Bray-Curtis dissimilarity represented by PC1

communities within the lung [51], the identification and enumeration of respiratory viruses has been much slower due to the lack of a single universal viral marker gene and the difficulty in obtaining sufficient viral biomass from airway samples to sequence without amplification. As a result, all lung virome studies to date have used multiple displacement amplification (MDA) to increase viral DNA yield [14–17]. While this amplification step is useful for amplifying single-stranded DNA viruses, it has both systematic and stochastic biases and results in a non-quantitative representation of community members that varies as much as 10,000-fold from the original [52].

Environmental samples often have low biomass and, as a result, low input DNA, especially in aquatic environments. As a result, most research on producing quantitative viral metagenomes has been done with marine samples, which has shown that samples with as low as 100 femtograms of starting DNA are quantitative if MDA is not used [28, 53–55]. Our lung metagenomes were produced using the DNA-to-sequence pipeline used to produce quantitative marine viromes.

It is important to note that in other systems, reduced microbial diversity is associated with dysbiosis [56]. In the lungs of smokers, such dysbiosis might lead to COPD progression. Previous studies demonstrated differences in the bacteriome of patients with advanced COPD compared to healthy controls [7, 13], however no differences were observed between healthy smokers and nonsmokers [12] suggesting that bacterial dysbiosis may not be responsible for COPD disease progression. In contrast, we found that viral diversity was significantly lower in the lungs of healthy smokers, and this viral dysbiosis was associated almost exclusively with changes in phage ecology. We propose that smoking leads to early effects on the lung virome, and specifically the phageome, which may influence and drive later changes in the bacteriome during progression to COPD. It remains to be determined whether microbial changes lead to disease progression or whether disease progression provides the niche for alterations in the lung microbiome. Well-controlled, longitudinal studies are needed to address this important question.

In the gut, alterations in the number and composition of Proteobacteria is hypothesized to be a signature of dysbiosis and disease [50]. Our corollary finding of associations between two Proteobacterial phages and metabolic changes in smokers parallels these gut findings. Given that Proteobacteria changes were not associated with metabolic differences, we hypothesize that increased numbers of Proteobacteria phages may alter metabolic output within their bacterial hosts during infection.

Previously, we described the presence of bacterial pneumotypes in the lungs of healthy volunteers, thought to be related to the degree of silent aspiration of supraglottic taxa. Using these same specimens, we failed to identify unique viral pneumotypes. Nonetheless, the presence of rare viruses such as *Spiroplasma* phage and human herpesvirus 8, appear to enable colonization by new, closely related common virus types and, thus, may be important for establishing viral pneumotypes (Additional file 4: Figure S3) as has been proposed for bacteria [57, 58]. Analyses of more lung viromes are necessary, however, to clarify the existence of, or lack thereof, viral pneumotypes.

Consistent with prior studies [14, 16–18], the vast majority of viruses identified in our lower airway samples were phages. Nonsmoker viromes were enriched with *Lactobacillus* and *Gardnerella* phages while smoker viromes were enriched with *Prevotella* phages. Prior in vitro work has suggested that a byproduct of cigarette smoke induces *Lactobacillus* phages [59]. However, there are about 4000 compounds in cigarette smoke [60], some of which may induce phage while others may suppress phage, though research in this area is lacking. In our study, the majority of smokers were former smokers and therefore, not recently exposed to cigarette smoke. Additionally, we observed an increased relative abundance of *Lactobacillus* phages in the context of the entire DNA virome of nonsmokers. It is possible that bacteria, phages, or host factors may influence phage induction in the lung microenvironment, as previously demonstrated in co-culture studies of lysogenic bacteria and human epithelial cells [61], factors difficult to model with an ex vivo experiment.

Interestingly, we did not observe crAssphage, a virus found ubiquitously in the human gut and vagina and on the skin [62], in our airway samples, nor did we identify single-stranded DNA anelloviruses. In fact, in our cohort of healthy smokers and nonsmokers, we identified very few eukaryotic DNA viruses in total. The absence of crAssphage may be niche-specific, as it also was not identified in other lung virome studies [14–16]. The absence of anelloviruses in our study may be related to the healthy status of our subjects or to differences in sample preparation and sequence analysis compared to other studies. Anelloviruses have primarily been identified in immunocompromised subjects (lung transplant, HIV or deceased organ donors) using MDA-amplified viromes [14, 17].

We did, however, identify high abundances of *Propionibacterium* phage across all 30 lung BAL samples. Notably, *Propionibacterium spp.* bacteria were previously noted in these samples when 16S rRNA gene sequencing was performed with 454 sequencing of the V1-V2 region [29], but not with Illumina MiSeq sequencing of the V4 region [30], indicating that bacteriome comparisons between studies sequencing different regions of the 16S rRNA gene should be made with caution. While the V4 region is excellent at amplifying bacterial and archaeal 16S rRNA genes [32, 33], it has been shown to be less specific for *Propionibacterium spp.* [63]. Our virome data is consistent with the 454 sequencing of V1-V2 [29] which linked *Propionibacterium spp.* to the "background predominant taxa" bacterial pneumotype as suggested by other studies [49]. Due to the low biomass nature of the lower airways and factors associated with BAL collection, the presence of background taxa in these types of samples is inevitable. However, *Propionibacterium spp.* bacteria have been identified in diseased lungs of subjects with bronchiectasis [64] and sarcoidosis [65] as well as in metagenomic studies of lung tissue and extracellular vesicles [9, 66, 67]. In healthy lungs, the data on *Propionibacterium spp.* bacteria in BAL is conflicting [12, 29, 30, 68]. If *Propionibacterium* phage, like *Propionibacterium spp.* bacteria, represent background, it is important to note that these sequences were found in all samples and were not associated with separation of the virome between smokers and nonsmokers.

We note that changes in phageome composition were not reflected in bacteriome changes. There are several potential explanations for this phenomenon. First, it is impossible to know if the viral nucleic acid and bacterial 16S rRNA genes being sequenced represent live or dead microorganisms. Second, viral reference databases, in general, lack robustness, increasing the challenge of properly aligning and assigning taxonomy to short stretches of viral nucleic acid. To improve the likelihood of identifying viral taxa, we combined multiple viral reference databases into a single, custom database. However, the compositional nature of the relative abundance data will be highly impacted by gaps in the reference database used for annotation. Third, phage-bacteria networks are unique to individuals, vary across body sites and are impacted by environmental factors as recently shown in a network-based analytical model by Hannigan et al. [69]. Therefore, it will be important to continue to consider not only the composition of the microbiome (bacteriome, virome, mycobiome), but also the dynamic interactions between those constituents and with the surrounding environment in future studies.

It is still unclear why some smokers progress to COPD while others remain unaffected, though there is evidence that byproducts of lipoxygenation of arachidonic acid, leukotrienes and lipoxins are important for COPD pathogenesis [70]. Recent studies have also implicated IL-8 as an important potential marker of COPD pathogenesis [71, 72]. Interestingly, of all metabolites and cytokines studied, we observed the strongest association between arachidonic acid and IL-8 and changes in the smoker lung virome. Thus, monitoring specific phage

groups or the whole viral community could be important for predicting trends in arachidonic acid and IL-8 and the progression of the smoker lung to COPD. Whether this is a direct interaction or not remains to be determined, but these observations provide a novel pathway of exploration for future studies.

There are several limitations to our study. Statistical power was low in our analyses due to a relatively small sample size. However, due to the invasiveness of the lower airway sampling and cost restraints of our multi-omic approach, particularly in regards to high-throughput next generation sequencing of the virome, we were limited to a cohort of 30 subjects. Nonetheless, our cohort size is in line with current gut virome studies, which do not require an invasive procedure for sample collection. In total, there are 20 gut virome studies with unique datasets [40, 73–91]. Of these studies, the mean number of participants is 35 and the median 20. While smaller than recent lung bacteriome studies, this is the largest study to date to analyze the combined DNA virome, bacteriome and metabolome of BAL fluid. A larger cohort would allow for investigation of the potential role of other important covariates, such as gender, ethnicity, and age, on the lower airway virome. Our study was a cross-sectional analysis of the lower airway microenvironment in smokers and nonsmokers and does not allow for the analysis of trends over time nor the characterization of microbiome changes in relation to COPD progression. Indeed, the lower FEV_1/FVC ratio observed among smokers may be related to early inflammatory airway dysfunction present at a stage where smokers do not meet COPD criteria [72, 92, 93]. Future longitudinal studies are greatly needed to evaluate whether changes in the lower airway virome have an impact on chronic inflammatory airway dysfunction among smokers. We were also limited by availability of historical specimens as we did not have access to matched oral rinse or pre-bronchoscopy saline control samples of sufficient quantity for shotgun sequencing, thereby precluding characterization of the supraglottic or saline virome. Finally, due to technical constraints, we assessed the acellular BAL DNA virome. Shotgun metagenomics sequences all nucleic acid in a sample, and despite the use of acellular BAL to reduce human genomic contamination, the virome sequence space made up only a tiny fraction of all sequences. Further, in low biomass samples, even small increases in host genomic material will quickly swamp low viral signal. Technical advances in BAL virome purification or enrichment, removal of contaminating host and bacterial nucleic acid, and deeper, more affordable sequencing technologies should be a focus moving forward, thereby allowing more detailed analysis of the lung virome.

Conclusions

In summary, our findings provide a foundational glimpse into the ecological interplay between viruses, bacteria, metabolites, and immune cells that likely impact the lung microenvironment and ultimately, perhaps, progression from smoking to COPD. We show that, in contrast to the lung bacteriome, the DNA viromes and metabolomes of smokers and nonsmokers are significantly different. We hypothesize that changes in the metabolic output of Proteobacteria in the lungs driven by their phages could potentially be a biomarker for the smoker metabolic disease state. Further, while we cannot disentangle whether arachidonic acid and IL-8 cause alterations in the lung virome or if virome changes cause increases in arachidonic acid and IL-8, these findings suggest that monitoring the lung virome of smokers may be important for assessing the "tipping point" in transitioning from a healthy lung environment to COPD.

Additional files

Additional file 1: Table S1. Virome library read counts. (DOCX 14 kb)

Additional file 2: Figure S1. Pie charts of host composition of all bacteriophages. **(A)** Relative distribution of bacteriophage host phyla. **(B-D)** Composition of bacteriophage host genera within the Proteobacteria, Firmicutes, and Actinobacteria host phyla, respectively. (DOCX 911 kb)

Additional file 3: Figure S2. Viral community composition of phage by host genera across all virome (overall) and in smokers and nonsmokers. (DOCX 35 kb)

Additional file 4: Figure S3. Viral pneumotype analysis using SPIEC-EASI to examine ecological associations based on abundance profiles. (DOCX 60 kb)

Additional file 5: Figure S4. Venn diagram of the number of viral populations unique to and shared between smokers and nonsmokers. (DOCX 31 kb)

Additional file 6: Figure S5. Comparison of background saline of smokers and nonsmokers. **(A)** PCoA of 16S rRNA gene sequencing data from pre-bronchoscopy control saline samples. **(B)** Heatmap of 16S rRNA OTU abundances (columns) with hierarchical clustering of smoker and nonsmoker pre-bronchoscopy control saline samples (rows). (DOCX 101 kb)

Abbreviations
BAL: Bronchoalveolar lavage; BEF: Bivariate ellipse fitting; BPT: Background predominant taxa; COPD: Chronic obstructive pulmonary disease; DLCO: Diffusing capacity of the lungs for carbon monoxide; DNA: Deoxyribonucleic acid; FEV1: Forced expiratory volume in 1 s; FRC: Functional residual capacity; FVC: Forced vital capacity; HIV: Human immunodeficiency virus; IL-8: Interleukin 8; PCoA: Principal coordinates analyses; RV: Residual volume; SPT: Supraglottic predominant taxa; TLC: Total lung capacity

Acknowledgments
The authors thank Guoyan Zhao and Chandni Desai (Washington University) for bioinformatics assistance and Jessica Hoisington-Lopez (Washington University), Peter Meyn and Adriana Heguy (NYUMC) for sequencing expertise. Sequencing was performed at the Washington University Center for Genome Sciences & Systems Biology and at the NYUMC Genome Technology Center (supported by the Cancer Center Support Grant, P30CA016087).

Funding
T32 AI112542 (to ACG), K23 AI102970 (to LNS), 2 T-32HL007317–36 and T32 HL07317 (to BCK), and a Gordon and Betty Moore Foundation Investigator Award (GBMF#3790 to MBS).

Authors' contributions
LNS and BCK conceived and designed the study. LNS and BCK acquired the data. ACG, MBS, LNS, and BCK analyzed and interpreted the data. ACG, MBS, LNS and BCK drafted or revised the article. ACG, MBS, LNS and BCK approved the final manuscript.

Competing interests
The authors declare that they have no competing interests.

Author details
[1]Department of Microbiology, The Ohio State University, Columbus, OH 43210, USA. [2]Department of Civil, Environmental and Geodetic Engineering, The Ohio State University, Columbus, OH 43210, USA. [3]Division of Pulmonary, Critical Care & Sleep Medicine, New York University School of Medicine, New York, NY 10016, USA. [4]Division of Pulmonary, Critical Care & Sleep Medicine, The Ohio State University College of Medicine, 201 Davis Heart & Lung Research Institute, 473 West 12th Avenue, Columbus, OH 43210, USA.

References
1. Mathers CD, Loncar D. Projections of global mortality and burden of disease from 2002 to 2030. PLoS Med. 2006;3:e442.
2. Mannino DM, Buist AS. Global burden of COPD: risk factors, prevalence, and future trends. Lancet. 2007;370:765–73.
3. Stang P, Lydick E, Silberman C, Kempel A, Keating ET. The prevalence of COPD. Chest. 2000;117:354S–9S.
4. Sze MA, Hogg JC, Sin DD. Bacterial microbiome of lungs in COPD. Int J Chron Obstruct Pulmon Dis. 2014;9:229–38.
5. Dickson RP, Erb-Downward JR, Huffnagle GB. The role of the bacterial microbiome in lung disease. Expert Rev Respir Med. 2013;7:245–57.
6. Sze MA, Dimitriu PA, Suzuki M, McDonough JE, Campbell JD, Brothers JF, Erb-Downward JR, Huffnagle GB, Hayashi S, Elliott WM, et al. Host response to the lung microbiome in chronic obstructive pulmonary disease. Am J Respir Crit Care Med. 2015;192:438–45.
7. Pragman AA, Kim HB, Reilly CS, Wendt C, Isaacson RE. The lung microbiome in moderate and severe chronic obstructive pulmonary disease. PLoS One. 2012;7:e47305.
8. Sze MA, Dimitriu PA, Hayashi S, Elliott WM, McDonough JE, Gosselink JV, Cooper J, Sin DD, Mohn WW, Hogg JC. The lung tissue microbiome in chronic obstructive pulmonary disease. Am J Respir Crit Care Med. 2012;185:1073–80.
9. Kim HJ, Kim YS, Kim KH, Choi JP, Kim YK, Yun S, Sharma L, Dela Cruz CS, Lee JS, Oh YM, et al. The microbiome of the lung and its extracellular vesicles in nonsmokers, healthy smokers and COPD patients. Exp Mol Med. 2017;49:e316.
10. Garcia-Nunez M, Millares L, Pomares X, Ferrari R, Perez-Brocal V, Gallego M, Espasa M, Moya A, Monso E. Severity-related changes of bronchial microbiome in chronic obstructive pulmonary disease. J Clin Microbiol. 2014;52:4217–23.
11. Einarsson GG, Comer DM, McIlreavey L, Parkhill J, Ennis M, Tunney MM, Elborn JS. Community dynamics and the lower airway microbiota in stable chronic obstructive pulmonary disease, smokers and healthy non-smokers. Thorax. 2016;71:795–803.
12. Morris A, Beck JM, Schloss PD, Campbell TB, Crothers K, Curtis JL, Flores SC, Fontenot AP, Ghedin E, Huang L, et al. Comparison of the respiratory microbiome in healthy nonsmokers and smokers. Am J Respir Crit Care Med. 2013;187:1067–75.
13. Erb-Downward JR, Thompson DL, Han MK, Freeman CM, McCloskey L, Schmidt LA, Young VB, Toews GB, Curtis JL, Sundaram B, et al. Analysis of the lung microbiome in the "healthy" smoker and in COPD. PLoS One. 2011;6:e16384.
14. Young JC, Chehoud C, Bittinger K, Bailey A, Diamond JM, Cantu E, Haas AR, Abbas A, Frye L, Christie JD, et al. Viral metagenomics reveal blooms of anelloviruses in the respiratory tract of lung transplant recipients. Am J Transplant. 2015;15:200–9.
15. Willner D, Furlan M, Haynes M, Schmieder R, Angly FE, Silva J, Tammadoni S, Nosrat B, Conrad D, Rohwer F. Metagenomic analysis of respiratory tract DNA viral communities in cystic fibrosis and non-cystic fibrosis individuals. PLoS One. 2009;4:e7370.

16. Willner D, Haynes MR, Furlan M, Hanson N, Kirby B, Lim YW, Rainey PB, Schmieder R, Youle M, Conrad D, Rohwer F. Case studies of the spatial heterogeneity of DNA viruses in the cystic fibrosis lung. Am J Respir Cell Mol Biol. 2012;46:127–31.

17. Abbas AA, Diamond JM, Chehoud C, Chang B, Kotzin JJ, Young JC, Imai I, Haas AR, Cantu E, Lederer DJ, et al. The perioperative lung transplant Virome: torque Teno viruses are elevated in donor lungs and show divergent dynamics in primary graft dysfunction. Am J Transplant. 2016;17(5):1313–24.

18. Elbehery AHA, Feichtmayer J, Singh D, Griebler C, Deng L. The human Virome protein cluster database (HVPC): a human viral metagenomic database for diversity and function annotation. Front Microbiol. 2018;9:1110.

19. Breitbart M. Marine viruses: truth or dare. Annu Rev Mar Sci. 2012;4:425–48.

20. Wilhelm SW, Suttle CA. Viruses and nutrient cycles in the sea. BioScience. 1999;49:781.

21. Fuhrman JA. Marine viruses and their biogeochemical and ecological effects. Nature. 1999;399:541–8.

22. Wommack KEC, R R. Virioplankton: viruses in aquatic ecosystems. Microbiol Mol Biol Rev. 2000;64:69–114.

23. Suttle CA. Marine viruses--major players in the global ecosystem. Nat Rev Microbiol. 2007;5:801–12.

24. Brum JR, Sullivan MB. Rising to the challenge: accelerated pace of discovery transforms marine virology. Nat Rev Microbiol. 2015;13:147–59.

25. Read AF, Taylor LH. The ecology of genetically diverse infections. Science. 2001;292:1099–102.

26. Klainer AS, Beisel WR. Opportunistic infection: a review. Am J Med Sci. 1969; 258:431–56.

27. Barr JJ, Auro R, Furlan M, Whiteson KL, Erb ML, Pogliano J, Stotland A, Wolkowicz R, Cutting AS, Doran KS, et al. Bacteriophage adhering to mucus provide a non-host-derived immunity. Proc Natl Acad Sci U S A. 2013;110:10771–6.

28. Duhaime MB, Deng L, Poulos BT, Sullivan MB. Towards quantitative metagenomics of wild viruses and other ultra-low concentration DNA samples: a rigorous assessment and optimization of the linker amplification method. Environ Microbiol. 2012;14:2526–37.

29. Segal LN, Alekseyenko AV, Clemente JC, Kulkarni R, Wu B, Gao Z, Chen H, Berger KI, Goldring RM, Rom WN, et al. Enrichment of lung microbiome with supraglottic taxa is associated with increased pulmonary inflammation. Microbiome. 2013;1:19.

30. Segal LN, Clemente JC, Tsay J-CJ, Koralov SB, Keller BC, Wu BG, Li Y, Shen N, Ghedin E, Morris A, et al. Enrichment of the lung microbiome with oral taxa is associated with lung inflammation of a Th17 phenotype. Nature Microbiology. 2016;1:16031.

31. Xia J, Sinelnikov IV, Han B, Wishart DS. MetaboAnalyst 3.0--making metabolomics more meaningful. Nucleic Acids Res. 2015;43:W251–7.

32. Caporaso JG, Lauber CL, Walters WA, Berg-Lyons D, Huntley J, Fierer N, Owens SM, Betley J, Fraser L, Bauer M, et al. Ultra-high-throughput microbial community analysis on the Illumina HiSeq and MiSeq platforms. ISME J. 2012;6:1621–4.

33. Walters WA, Caporaso JG, Lauber CL, Berg-Lyons D, Fierer N, Knight R. PrimerProspector: de novo design and taxonomic analysis of barcoded polymerase chain reaction primers. Bioinformatics. 2011;27:1159–61.

34. Dray S, Dufour AB. The ade4 package: implementing the duality diagram for ecologists. J Stat Softw. 2007;22:1–20.

35. Lozupone C, Lladser ME, Knights D, Stombaugh J, Knight R. UniFrac: an effective distance metric for microbial community comparison. ISME J. 2011; 5:169–72.

36. Bushnell B. BBMap. 2015.

37. Bankevich A, Nurk S, Antipov D, Gurevich AA, Dvorkin M, Kulikov AS, Lesin VM, Nikolenko SI, Pham S, Prjibelski AD, et al. SPAdes: a new genome assembly algorithm and its applications to single-cell sequencing. J Comput Biol. 2012;19:455–77.

38. Langmead B, Salzberg SL. Fast gapped-read alignment with bowtie 2. Nat Methods. 2012;9:357–9.

39. Roux S, Enault F, Hurwitz BL, Sullivan MB. VirSorter: mining viral signal from microbial genomic data. PeerJ. 2015;3:e985.

40. Manrique P, Bolduc B, Walk ST, van der Oost J, de Vos WM, Young MJ. Healthy human gut phageome. Proc Natl Acad Sci U S A. 2016;113:10400–5.

41. Brum JR, Ignacio-Espinoza JC, Roux S, Doulcier G, Acinas SG, Alberti A, Chaffron S, Cruaud C, de Vargas C, Gasol JM, et al. Ocean plankton. Patterns and ecological drivers of ocean viral communities. Science. 2015;348:1261498.

42. Gregory AC, Solonenko SA, Ignacio-Espinoza JC, LaButti K, Copeland A, Sudek S, Maitland A, Chittick L, Dos Santos F, Weitz JS, et al. Genomic differentiation among wild cyanophages despite widespread horizontal gene transfer. BMC Genomics. 2016;17:930.

43. Oksanen J, Blanchet G, Friendly M, Kindt R, Legendre P, McGlinn D, Minchin PR, O'Hara RB, Simpson GL, Solymos P, et al. vegan: community ecology package. 2.4–1 ed; 2016.

44. Filzmoser P, Garrett RG, Reimann C. Multivariate outlier detection in exploration geochemistry. Comput Geosci. 2005;31:579–87.

45. White JR, Nagarajan N, Pop M. Statistical methods for detecting differentially abundant features in clinical metagenomic samples. PLoS Comput Biol. 2009;5:e1000352.

46. Schloss PD, Westcott SL, Ryabin T, Hall JR, Hartmann M, Hollister EB, Lesniewski RA, Oakley BB, Parks DH, Robinson CJ, et al. Introducing mothur: open-source, platform-independent, community-supported software for describing and comparing microbial communities. Appl Environ Microbiol. 2009;75:7537–41.

47. Kurtz ZD, Muller CL, Miraldi ER, Littman DR, Blaser MJ, Bonneau RA. Sparse and compositionally robust inference of microbial ecological networks. PLoS Comput Biol. 2015;11:e1004226.

48. Arumugam M, Raes J, Pelletier E, Le Paslier D, Yamada T, Mende DR, Fernandes GR, Tap J, Bruls T, Batto JM, et al. Enterotypes of the human gut microbiome. Nature. 2011;473:174–80.

49. Salter SJ, Cox MJ, Turek EM, Calus ST, Cookson WO, Moffatt MF, Turner P, Parkhill J, Loman NJ, Walker AW. Reagent and laboratory contamination can critically impact sequence-based microbiome analyses. BMC Biol. 2014;12:87.

50. Shin NR, Whon TW, Bae JW. Proteobacteria: microbial signature of dysbiosis in gut microbiota. Trends Biotechnol. 2015;33:496–503.

51. Singleton DR, Furlong MA, Rathbun SL, Whitman WB. Quantitative comparisons of 16S rRNA gene sequence libraries from environmental samples. Appl Environ Microbiol. 2001;67:4374–6.

52. Yilmaz S, Allgaier M, Hugenholtz P. Multiple displacement amplification compromises quantitative analysis of metagenomes. Nat Methods. 2010;7:943–4.

53. Roux S, Solonenko NE, Dang VT, Poulos BT, Schwenck SM, Goldsmith DB, Coleman ML, Breitbart M, Sullivan MB. Towards quantitative viromics for both double-stranded and single-stranded DNA viruses. PeerJ. 2016;4:e2777.

54. Hurwitz BL, Deng L, Poulos BT, Sullivan MB. Evaluation of methods to concentrate and purify ocean virus communities through comparative, replicated metagenomics. Environ Microbiol. 2013;15:1428–40.

55. Solonenko SA, Sullivan MB. Preparation of metagenomic libraries from naturally occurring marine viruses. In: Delong EF, editor. Methods in Enzymology: Microbial community "omics": Metagenomics, metatranscriptomics, and metaproteomics. San Diego: Elsevier; 2013.

56. Lynch SV, Pedersen O. The human intestinal microbiome in health and disease. N Engl J Med. 2016;375:2369–79.

57. Stecher B, Chaffron S, Kappeli R, Hapfelmeier S, Freedrich S, Weber TC, Kirundi J, Suar M, McCoy KD, von Mering C, et al. Like will to like: abundances of closely related species can predict susceptibility to intestinal colonization by pathogenic and commensal bacteria. PLoS Pathog. 2010;6:e1000711.

58. Huang YJ, Erb-Downward JR, Dickson RP, Curtis JL, Huffnagle GB, Han MK. Understanding the role of the microbiome in chronic obstructive pulmonary disease: principles, challenges, and future directions. Transl Res. 2017;179:71–83.

59. Pavlova SI, Tao L. Induction of vaginal lactobacillus phages by the cigarette smoke chemical benzo [a] pyrene diol epoxide. Mutat Res. 2000;466:57–62.

60. Brunnemann KD, Hoffmann D. Analytical studies on tobacco-specific N-nitrosamines in tobacco and tobacco smoke. Crit Rev Toxicol. 1991;21:235–40.

61. Stevens RH, de Moura Martins Lobo Dos Santos C, Zuanazzi D, de Accioly Mattos MB, Ferreira DF, Kachlany SC, Tinoco EM. Prophage induction in lysogenic Aggregatibacter actinomycetemcomitans cells co-cultured with human gingival fibroblasts, and its effect on leukotoxin release. Microb Pathog. 2013; 54:54–59.

62. Dutilh BE, Cassman N, McNair K, Sanchez SE, Silva GG, Boling L, Barr JJ, Speth DR, Seguritan V, Aziz RK, et al. A highly abundant bacteriophage discovered in the unknown sequences of human faecal metagenomes. Nat Commun. 2014;5:4498.

63. Meisel JS, Hannigan GD, Tyldsley AS, SanMiguel AJ, Hodkinson BP, Zheng Q, Grice EA. Skin microbiome surveys are strongly influenced by experimental design. J Invest Dermatol. 2016;136:947–56.

64. Byun MK, Chang J, Kim HJ, Jeong SH. Differences of lung microbiome in patients with clinically stable and exacerbated bronchiectasis. PLoS One. 2017;12:e0183553.

65. Hiramatsu J, Kataoka M, Nakata Y, Okazaki K, Tada S, Tanimoto M, Eishi Y. Propionibacterium acnes DNA detected in bronchoalveolar lavage cells from patients with sarcoidosis. Sarcoidosis Vasc Diffuse Lung Dis. 2003;20: 197–203.

66. Fibla JJ, Brunelli A, Allen MS, Wigle D, Shen R, Nichols F, Deschamps C, Cassivi SD. Microbiology specimens obtained at the time of surgical lung biopsy for interstitial lung disease: clinical yield and cost analysis. Eur J Cardiothorac Surg. 2012;41:36–8.

67. Brown PS, Pope CE, Marsh RL, Qin X, McNamara S, Gibson R, Burns JL, Deutsch G, Hoffman LR. Directly sampling the lung of a young child with cystic fibrosis reveals diverse microbiota. Ann Am Thorac Soc. 2014;11:1049–55.

68. Dickson RP, Erb-Downward JR, Freeman CM, McCloskey L, Falkowski NR, Huffnagle GB, Curtis JL. Bacterial topography of the healthy human lower respiratory tract. MBio. 2017;8

69. Hannigan GD, Duhaime MB, Koutra D, Schloss PD. Biogeography and environmental conditions shape bacteriophage-bacteria networks across the human microbiome. PLoS Comput Biol. 2018;14:e1006099.

70. Jamalkandi SA, Mirzaie M, Jafari M, Mehrani H, Shariati P, Khodabandeh M. Signaling network of lipids as a comprehensive scaffold for omics data integration in sputum of COPD patients. Biochimica Et Biophysica Acta-Molecular and Cell Biology of Lipids. 2015;1851:1383–93.

71. Zhang X, Zheng H, Zhang H, Ma W, Wang F, Liu C, He S. Increased interleukin (IL)-8 and decreased IL-17 production in chronic obstructive pulmonary disease (COPD) provoked by cigarette smoke. Cytokine. 2011;56:717–25.

72. Berger KI, Pradhan DR, Goldring RM, Oppenheimer BW, Rom WN, Segal LN. Distal airway dysfunction identifies pulmonary inflammation in asymptomatic smokers. ERJ Open Res. 2016;2(4):00066–2016.

73. Broecker F, Russo G, Klumpp J, Moelling K. Stable core virome despite variable microbiome after fecal transfer. Gut Microbes. 2017;8:214–20.

74. Chehoud C, Dryga A, Hwang Y, Nagy-Szakal D, Hollister EB, Luna RA, Versalovic J, Kellermayer R, Bushman FD. Transfer of viral communities between human individuals during fecal microbiota transplantation. MBio. 2016;7:e00322.

75. Conceicao-Neto N, Deboutte W, Dierckx T, Machiels K, Wang J, Yinda KC, Maes P, Van Ranst M, Joossens M, Raes J, et al. Low eukaryotic viral richness is associated with faecal microbiota transplantation success in patients with UC. Gut. 2017;67(8):1558–9.

76. Giloteaux L, Hanson MR, Keller BA. A pair of identical twins discordant for Myalgic encephalomyelitis/chronic fatigue syndrome differ in physiological parameters and gut microbiome composition. American Journal of Case Reports. 2016;17:720–9.

77. Kang DW, Adams JB, Gregory AC, Borody T, Chittick L, Fasano A, Khoruts A, Geis E, Maldonado J, McDonough-Means S, et al. Microbiota transfer therapy alters gut ecosystem and improves gastrointestinal and autism symptoms: an open-label study. Microbiome. 2017;5:10.

78. Kramna L, Kolarova K, Oikarinen S, Pursiheimo JP, Ilonen J, Simell O, Knip M, Veijola R, Hyoty H, Cinek O. Gut virome sequencing in children with early islet autoimmunity. Diabetes Care. 2015;38:930–3.

79. Lim ES, Zhou Y, Zhao G, Bauer IK, Droit L, Ndao IM, Warner BB, Tarr PI, Wang D, Holtz LR. Early life dynamics of the human gut virome and bacterial microbiome in infants. Nat Med. 2015;21:1228–34.

80. Ly M, Jones MB, Abeles SR, Santiago-Rodriguez TM, Gao J, Chan IC, Ghose C, Pride DT. Transmission of viruses via our microbiomes. Microbiome. 2016;4:64.

81. Minot S, Grunberg S, Wu GD, Lewis JD, Bushman FD. Hypervariable loci in the human gut virome. Proc Natl Acad Sci U S A. 2012;109:3962–6.

82. Minot S, Sinha R, Chen J, Li H, Keilbaugh SA, Wu GD, Lewis JD, Bushman FD. The human gut virome: inter-individual variation and dynamic response to diet. Genome Res. 2011;21:1616–25.

83. Minot S, Bryson A, Chehoud C, Wu GD, Lewis JD, Bushman FD. Rapid evolution of the human gut virome. Proc Natl Acad Sci U S A. 2013;110: 12450–5.

84. Monaco CL, Gootenberg DB, Zhao G, Handley SA, Ghebremichael MS, Lim ES, Lankowski A, Baldridge MT, Wilen CB, Flagg M, et al. Altered Virome and bacterial microbiome in human immunodeficiency virus-associated acquired immunodeficiency syndrome. Cell Host Microbe. 2016;19:311–22.

85. Norman JM, Handley SA, Baldridge MT, Droit L, Liu CY, Keller BC, Kambal A, Monaco CL, Zhao G, Fleshner P, et al. Disease-specific alterations in the enteric virome in inflammatory bowel disease. Cell. 2015;160:447–60.

86. Perez-Brocal V, Garcia-Lopez R, Vazquez-Castellanos JF, Nos P, Beltran B, Latorre A, Moya A. Study of the viral and microbial communities associated with Crohn's disease: a metagenomic approach. Clin Transl Gastroenterol. 2013;4:e36.

87. Rampelli S, Turroni S, Schnorr SL, Soverini M, Quercia S, Barone M, Castagnetti A, Biagi E, Gallinella G, Brigidi P, Candela M. Characterization of the human DNA gut virome across populations with different subsistence strategies and geographical origin. Environ Microbiol. 2017;19:4728–35.

88. Reyes A, Haynes M, Hanson N, Angly FE, Heath AC, Rohwer F, Gordon JI. Viruses in the faecal microbiota of monozygotic twins and their mothers. Nature. 2010;466:334–8.

89. Reyes A, Blanton LV, Cao S, Zhao G, Manary M, Trehan I, Smith MI, Wang D, Virgin HW, Rohwer F, Gordon JI. Gut DNA viromes of Malawian twins discordant for severe acute malnutrition. Proc Natl Acad Sci U S A. 2015;112: 11941–6.

90. Zhao G, Vatanen T, Droit L, Park A, Kostic AD, Poon TW, Vlamakis H, Siljander H, Harkonen T, Hamalainen AM, et al. Intestinal virome changes precede autoimmunity in type 1 diabetes-susceptible children. Proc Natl Acad Sci U S A. 2017;114:E6166–75.

91. Zuo T, Wong SH, Lam K, Lui R, Cheung K, Tang W, Ching JYL, Chan PKS, Chan MCW, Wu JCY, et al. Bacteriophage transfer during faecal microbiota transplantation in Clostridium difficile infection is associated with treatment outcome. Gut. 2017;67(4):634–43.

92. Martinez CH, Diaz AA, Meldrum C, Curtis JL, Cooper CB, Pirozzi C, Kanner RE, Paine R 3rd, Woodruff PG, Bleecker ER, et al. Age and small airway imaging abnormalities in subjects with and without airflow obstruction in SPIROMICS. Am J Respir Crit Care Med. 2017;195:464–72.

93. Martinez FJ, Han MK, Allinson JP, Barr RG, Boucher RC, Calverley PMA, Celli BR, Christenson SA, Crystal RG, Fageras M, et al. At the root: defining and halting progression of early chronic obstructive pulmonary disease. Am J Respir Crit Care Med. 2018;197:1540–51.

4

Identifying the associated risks of pneumonia in COPD patients: ARCTIC an observational study

Christer Janson[1]* ⓘ, Gunnar Johansson[2], Björn Ställberg[2], Karin Lisspers[2], Petter Olsson[3], Dorothy L. Keininger[4], Milica Uhde[5], Florian S. Gutzwiller[4], Leif Jörgensen[6] and Kjell Larsson[7]

Abstract

Background: Inhaled corticosteroids (ICS) are associated with an increased risk of pneumonia in patients with chronic obstructive pulmonary disease (COPD). Other factors such as severity of airflow limitation and concurrent asthma may further raise the possibility of developing pneumonia. This study assessed the risk of pneumonia associated with ICS in patients with COPD.

Methods: Electronic Medical Record data linked to National Health Registries were collected from COPD patients and matched reference controls in 52 Swedish primary care centers (2000–2014). Levels of ICS treatment (high, low, no ICS) and associated comorbidities were assessed. Patients were categorized by airflow limitation severity.

Results: A total of 6623 patients with COPD and 48,566 controls were analyzed. Patients with COPD had a more than 4-fold increase in pneumonia versus reference controls (hazard ratio [HR] 4.76, 95% confidence interval [CI]: 4.48–5.06). ICS use increased the risk of pneumonia by 20–30% in patients with COPD with forced expiratory volume in 1 s $\geq$ 50% versus patients not using ICS. Asthma was an independent risk factor for pneumonia in the COPD population. Multivariate analysis identified independent predictors of pneumonia in the overall population. The highest risk of pneumonia was associated with high dose ICS (HR 1.41, 95% CI: 1.23–1.62).

Conclusions: Patients with COPD have a greater risk of pneumonia versus reference controls; ICS use and concurrent asthma increased the risk of pneumonia further.

Keywords: Chronic obstructive pulmonary disease, Inhaled corticosteroids, Pneumonia, Sweden, Comorbidities, Asthma

Background

International recommendations for the treatment of patients with chronic obstructive pulmonary disease (COPD) restrict the use of inhaled corticosteroids (ICS) containing treatments in patients at high risk of exacerbation (Global initiative for chronic Obstructive Lung Disease [GOLD] Groups C and D) or patients with asthma-COPD overlap (ACO) [1]. Although ICS-containing treatments are not recommended for patients at low risk of exacerbation (GOLD Groups A and B), they are widely prescribed [2–4]. Until 2015, Swedish national guidelines only recommended the use of ICS in combination with long-acting beta-2 agonists (LABA) for patients with COPD with a forced expiratory volume in 1 s (FEV$_1$) < 50% predicted who were experiencing exacerbations [5]. However, real-world studies indicate that ICS/LABA are often used in Swedish patients with a FEV$_1$ $\geq$ 50% [6].

Associations between ICS use and several adverse effects in patients with COPD were first observed in the TORCH (Towards a Revolution in COPD Health) trial, in particular an increased risk of pneumonia [7], which was most apparent in patients with mild-to-moderate airflow limitation. Further trials demonstrated an association between ICS use and an increased risk of pneumonia [8–12]. Meta-analyses have also confirmed an increase in the risk of pneumonia with ICS use; however,

* Correspondence: christer.janson@medsci.uu.se
[1]Department of Medical Sciences: Respiratory, Allergy and Sleep Research, Uppsala University, Akademiska sjukhuset, 75185 Uppsala, Sweden
Full list of author information is available at the end of the article

no increased risk of mortality from pneumonia was observed [13, 14]. An association between use of ICS and pneumonia has also been found in observational studies using data from electronic medical records (EMRs) and registries, but these studies have largely lacked spirometry data [15, 16].

Asthma is a common comorbidity in COPD and the term "ACO", (patients who have characteristics of both asthma and COPD), has been presented in international recommendations [1, 17]. Notably, several studies found that patients with ACO have more exacerbations and a lower health-related quality of life than patients with COPD alone [18, 19], suggesting that patients who suffer from ACO, are a particularly vulnerable group. To our knowledge, no studies have compared the risk of pneumonia in patients with ACO with COPD only patients.

We analyzed data from a real-world study of Swedish primary care patients with COPD (the ARCTIC observational study) to identify risk factors for pneumonia and determine any relationship with ICS use. Additional aims assessed how airflow limitation severity (measured by FEV_1) and the presence of concurrent asthma affected the risk of pneumonia in patients with COPD. We anticipated that the risk of pneumonia would be higher among patients with COPD taking ICS compared with COPD patients not taking ICS and the reference controls.

Methods
Study design
ARCTIC was a retrospective, observational cohort study of longitudinal patient-level data extracted from the EMRs of Swedish primary care patients. The objectives of the ARCTIC study were to generate evidence to better manage patients with COPD, to foster early diagnosis, and to characterize treatment patterns and associated outcomes. This study was conducted in accordance with the principles of the Declaration of Helsinki and ethical approval was granted by the ethics review board at Uppsala University, Sweden (number: 2014–397).

The general population in Sweden is approximately 10 million [20]. Data were collected from patients with physician-diagnosed COPD and reference patients in 52 primary care centers covering approximately 200,000 patients between the years 2000–2014 using an established software system (Pygargus Customized eXraction Program, CXP 3.0), and included: age, gender, prescriptions (according to the World Health Organization Anatomic Therapeutic Chemical [ATC] codes), disease diagnoses (according to the International Classification of Disease codes [ICD-10 codes]), spirometry measurements (FEV_1 values), laboratory tests, healthcare professional (HCP) visits, and referrals. EMR data were linked by the Swedish National Board of Health and Welfare using

individual patient identification (ID) numbers to National Registry data sources (patient IDs were pseudonymized): (i) the Longitudinal Integration Database for Health Insurance and Labour Market Studies (LISA [21]), which includes socio-demographic data including educational level, marital status and family situation, occupational status, retirement, economic compensation and social benefits; (ii) the National Patient Register [22], which contains data relating to diagnosis (ICD-10 code and associated position), surgery, gender, age, region, hospital visits, specialty visits, hospital admissions and discharges, and medical procedures and surgeries performed in the inpatient and outpatient specialist settings; (iii) the National Prescription register [22], which tracks full details of all dispensed medications (ATC codes), including brand name, prescription date, dose, strength, pack size, specialty of the prescriber and costs associated with the drug prescription; and (iv) the Cause of Death Register [22], which holds information on social security number, home district, sex, date of death and cause of death.

Study subjects
COPD is rare under the age of 40, therefore, patients eligible for inclusion were those aged ≥40 years with lung function measurements and who had received a doctor's diagnosis of COPD (ICD-10 code: J44), and/or asthma (ICD-10 code: J45/J46) in the primary care setting (EMR database) that was then verified as COPD only or COPD and asthma in a hospital setting (according to the National Patient Register). Patients' diagnoses were defined by ICD codes, while lung function was used to assess the degree of airflow limitation based on data collected from EMRs and the National Patient Register. The first patient to receive a COPD diagnosis was in 2000 (index date). An age- and gender-matched reference population was selected from the primary care centers, excluding those who had a diagnosis of COPD and/or asthma. The matching criteria for patients and the reference group included, age, gender and the starting year for the index date. The index date for the reference group was selected as a random date between the start and end of the observation period for the reference patients. To focus exclusively on the effects of ICS, subjects who had taken two or more prescriptions of oral corticosteroids from 2005 to 2014 were excluded. Each COPD patient was matched with a mean of seven reference patients, depending on the size of the age group, to allow for comparisons in the associated risks for pneumonia, with emphasis on ICS use. Patients in the control group were not allowed to take ICS. ICS use was established using the ATC code R03BA from the EMRs and patient registries. The COPD and reference group patients were stratified by the level of ICS exposure after the index

date (high dose: ≥800 μg/day budesonide or equivalent; low dose: < 640 μg/day budesonide or equivalent).

Outcomes

The main outcome of interest was time-to-first pneumonia diagnosis, identified using ICD codes J12–J20. Patients were also categorized by airflow limitation severity: 1) no spirometry data available; 2) $FEV_1 < 50\%$ predicted; and 3) $FEV_1 \geq 50\%$ predicted. These categories were used to stratify results.

Statistical analysis

Data were analyzed concerning wrong personal identifiers and wrong dates, and outliers' analyses were conducted for numeric variables. There was no imputation of missing data; these were reported in the descriptive analysis (the exception being when the day of the month was missing in order to keep the data anonymous, the day of the month was assumed to be the 15th). Patient demographics were described for both patients with COPD and reference controls. Time-to-first pneumonia event analyses were conducted using Cox regression models with 95% confidence intervals (CI) in order to determine the risk of pneumonia associated with varying levels of ICS use, disease states and airflow limitation severity. The statistical reference group for analysis was patients without COPD or asthma who were not taking ICS, except when analyzing the use of ICS, where the reference group included COPD patients not using ICS. The analyses were stratified based on the disease status (asthma with no COPD, asthma and COPD, and COPD with no asthma), level of ICS use (high, low, and no ICS) and the level of airflow limitation severity (no spirometry data available, $FEV_1 < 50\%$ predicted, and $FEV_1 \geq 50\%$ predicted). Finally, risk factors for pneumonia in the COPD group were analyzed in a multivariate model, which included the variables that were statistically associated with pneumonia in the stratified analyses ($p < 0.05$). No immortal time bias was identified in our data. All analyses were performed using SAS version 9.3 or newer (SAS Institute Inc., Cary, NC) statistics software.

A sample size calculation was conducted for the ARCTIC trial before the start of the study, similar to that of another observational matched cohort study in patients with COPD [15]. The power calculation ensured that a sufficiently large sample was obtained to address the study's primary research questions, while also ensuring a large enough sample to address the additional planned sub-analyses. Given the large number of research questions and outcomes of interest, the power calculation was not based on a specific outcome. To achieve a power of 80% to detect a 4% between-group difference at a 5% significance level, 13,800 patients were required.

A target sample size of 15,000 patients with COPD was therefore established before the start of the study.

Results

Patient demographics

From a total of 55,189 patients listed in EMRs with lung function measurements for patients with COPD, 6623 patients with COPD and/or asthma were identified as eligible for inclusion in this study, matched with 48,566 reference controls (Fig. 1). Baseline characteristics for both study populations are presented in Table 1. While the populations were well matched for gender, patients in the COPD population were older than those in the reference population (66 vs. 65 years, $p < 0.0001$) and had significantly higher levels of healthcare utilization, comorbidities and rescue medication use in comparison with the reference controls, all of which were adjusted for in the comparative analyses (Table 1). For example, 38.0% of patients with COPD had cardiovascular disease compared with 20.4% of the reference controls ($p < 0.0001$). The mean FEV_1 in the COPD population was $58.6 \pm 20.1\%$ predicted.

Medication use

Thirty-three percent of patients with COPD were using low dose ICS, while 16% were receiving high dose ICS (Table 1). The majority of patients taking ICS used budesonide (71.5%), whereas only 7.3% used fluticasone propionate (Table 2). Of those patients included in the study, 71.7% had not used oral corticosteroids and 28.3% had collected one prescription.

Pneumonia risk

The diagnosis of pneumonia was collected from primary and secondary care settings. During the follow up (2000–2014), 2324 (35.1%) of COPD patients had at least one episode of pneumonia compared with 5036 (10.4%) in the reference population ($p < 0.0001$). Overall, patients with COPD had a more than 4-fold increase in risk of pneumonia than the reference controls (hazard ratio [HR] 4.76, 95% CI: 4.48–5.06). The risk of pneumonia was higher in men compared with women, both in those with more severe and less severe airflow obstruction ($FEV_1 < 50\%$: HR 1.28, 95% CI: 1.20–1.36; $FEV_1 \geq$ 50%: HR 1.26, 95% CI: 1.19–1.34). Furthermore, for every 1 year increase in age there was a 4% increase in risk of pneumonia (Table 3).

ICS use

COPD was associated with an increased risk of pneumonia irrespective of ICS use (Table 3, Fig. 2). However, ICS use further increased the risk of pneumonia 5-fold among patients with COPD and asthma and in patients with $FEV_1 < 50\%$ or $\geq 50\%$ when the results were

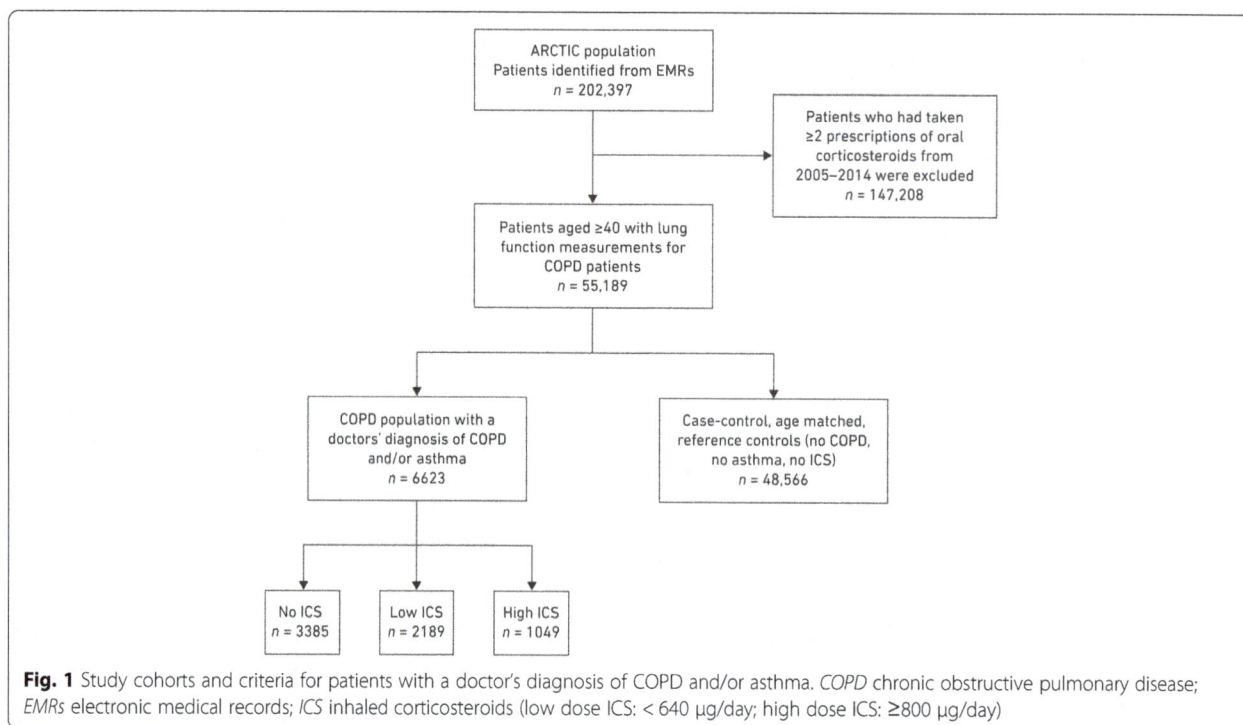

Fig. 1 Study cohorts and criteria for patients with a doctor's diagnosis of COPD and/or asthma. *COPD* chronic obstructive pulmonary disease; *EMRs* electronic medical records; *ICS* inhaled corticosteroids (low dose ICS: < 640 µg/day; high dose ICS: ≥800 µg/day)

stratified by lung function (Table 3). ICS use was associated with a 20–30% increased risk of pneumonia in patients with COPD with $FEV_1 \geq 50\%$ compared with patients who were not using ICS.

Presence of asthma

Overall, patients with concurrent asthma had a higher risk of pneumonia compared with those without asthma (Tables 3 and 4). However, the pattern of risk by ICS use is similar in patients with concurrent asthma and those with COPD alone. For example, in both the low and high dose ICS groups, ICS use was associated with an increased risk of pneumonia (Table 4).

Independent variables associated with pneumonia

A multivariate analysis was carried out to identify independent predictors of pneumonia in patients with COPD. The analysis showed that variables including FEV_1, gender, the use of ICS and presence of asthma were significantly independently associated with an increased risk of a pneumonia event (Table 5). Further, a dose response for ICS was demonstrated, in which the highest risk of pneumonia was associated with the high dose of ICS (high ICS: HR 1.41, 95% CI: 1.23–1.62]; low ICS: HR 1.23, 95% CI: 1.10–1.38]). In addition, no significant association was found between the Charlson Comorbidity Index (CCI) and pneumonia. There was also no significant independent association found between diabetes type II and pneumonia when the CCI was replaced with diabetes type II (HR 0.95, 95% CI: 0.74–1.23).

Discussion

This retrospective real-world study in over 6000 primary care patients with a diagnosis of COPD and/or asthma aged ≥40 years has demonstrated that COPD increases the risk of pneumonia, and that the use of ICS further increases this risk. The presence of concurrent asthma may also be an influential risk factor for pneumonia.

Pneumonia risk and the use of ICS

A higher risk of pneumonia while using ICS has been observed in other randomized clinical trials including the TORCH and Investigating New Standards for Prophylaxis in Reducing Exacerbations (INSPIRE) studies [7, 10, 23, 24]. However, some studies have also demonstrated the opposite effect [25, 26]. In this study, the risk of pneumonia associated with ICS use was lower in comparison with previous reports [16]. This could be related to the low proportion of patients using fluticasone propionate, since previous data suggests its use is associated with a particular increase in the risk of pneumonia. For example, a population-based cohort study showed that patients receiving fluticasone had a higher incidence rate and a higher risk of pneumonia than patients receiving budesonide (12.11 per 100 person-years vs. 10.65 per 100 person-years, adjusted HR 1.13, 95% CI: 1.08–1.20) [27]. An observational study also showed that the rate of serious pneumonia was doubled with fluticasone propionate (rate ratio [RR] 2.01; 95% CI: 1.93–2.10) and increased with the daily dose. In contrast, budesonide was associated with a 17% increase in rate, with no evidence

Table 1 Baseline patient demographics for patients with lung function measurements and reference controls[a] without ICS usage

Variable	COPD with lung function data (N = 6623)	Reference, without ICS usage (N = 48,566)	p-value
Age, mean years ± SD	65.9 ± 10.1	64.5 ± 10.5	< 0.0001
Female, n (%)	3688 (55.7)	26,792 (55.2)	0.4699
Comorbidities below, n (%)			
Asthma, J45	974 (14.7)	0	< 0.0001
Cardiovascular disease, I00-I99	2514 (38.0)	9932 (20.4)	< 0.0001
Hypertensive diseases, I10-I15	1707 (25.8)	5941 (12.2)	< 0.0001
Ischemic heart diseases, I20-I25	584 (8.8)	2052 (4.2)	< 0.0001
Cerebrovascular diseases, I60-I69	213 (3.2)	1182 (2.4)	0.0001
Diabetes Type I, E10	83 (1.2)	757 (1.6)	0.0568
Diabetes Type II, E11 + E13	418 (6.3)	2049 (4.2)	< 0.0001
Hyperlipidemia, E78.5	161 (2.4)	502 (1.0)	< 0.0001
Depression, F32 + F33	456 (6.9)	873 (1.8)	< 0.0001
Osteoporosis, M80 + M81	139 (2.1)	402 (0.8)	< 0.0001
Fractures, S2	356 (5.4)	1968 (4.0)	< 0.0001
Charlson Comorbidity Index value, mean ± SD	1.55 ± 0.8	1.26 ± 0.6	< 0.0001
Health care utilization			
Number of outpatient hospital visits/year in 2 years before index date, mean ± SD	1.53 ± 2.4	1.60 ± 3.7	0.1980
Number of contacts to primary care/year in 2 years before index date, mean ± SD	12.0 ± 16.0	4.14 ± 13.6	< 0.0001
ICS use, n (%)			
No ICS	3385 (51.1)	NA	
Low dose ICS[b]	2189 (33.0)	NA	
High dose ICS[c]	1049 (15.8)	NA	

[a]Patients in the reference control group were excluded if they had a diagnosis of COPD and/or asthma and did not take ICS; [b]Low dose ICS: < 640 µg/day; [c]High dose ICS: ≥800 µg/day
COPD chronic obstructive pulmonary disease, *ICS* inhaled corticosteroids, *NA* not applicable

of a dose response effect [15, 16]. However, evidence for the intra-class differences between ICS compounds in pneumonia risk has been disputed due to the lack of prospective randomized head to head studies [28].

Severity of airflow limitation
Severity of airflow limitation may be an important factor in pneumonia risk, in that patients receiving ICS with

Table 2 Types of inhaled corticosteroids used by the COPD population. Reference patients did not use ICS

Variable	COPD patients with lung function data (N = 6623)[a]
Types of ICS, n (%)	
Budesonide	2317 (71.5)
Fluticasone propionate	236 (7.3)
Budesonide/fluticasone propionate[b]	655 (20.2)
Other	30 (0.9)

[a]No ICS n = 3385; [b]Includes patients that switched from budesonide to fluticasone propionate and fluticasone propionate to budesonide during the study period, as well as a few patients that were using both budesonide and fluticasone propionate at the same time
COPD chronic obstructive pulmonary disease, *ICS* inhaled corticosteroids

severe-to-very severe airflow limitation (i.e. $FEV_1 < 50\%$ predicted), had a higher risk of pneumonia than those with $FEV_1 \geq 50\%$, regardless of ICS dose. This is in accordance with other studies [29]. However, in the 'COPD without asthma' patient group, the association between ICS use and pneumonia was stronger in those with an $FEV_1 \geq 50\%$ predicted (low ICS: HR 1.20; high ICS: HR 1.31, both vs. no ICS use) than in patients with an $FEV_1 < 50\%$ (low ICS: HR 1.06; high ICS HR 0.98, both vs. no ICS use). This result was unexpected and of concern, since these patients were being treated outside the recommendations in Sweden. This finding is not in line with data from the TORCH study [29] and the reason for this is unclear. It could be argued that, although those with severely impaired airflow limitation appear to be at an increased risk of pneumonia, the impact of ICS on the risk in these patients is overestimated, and that patients who require ICS therapy with severely impaired lung function are already predisposed to respiratory tract infections. The results could also represent a survivor effect, in which patients with an

Table 3 Hazard ratio for pneumonia in COPD patients stratified by FEV_1

	$FEV_1 < 50\%$ Hazard ratio (95% CI) (N = 2730)	$FEV_1 \geq 50\%$ Hazard ratio (95% CI) (N = 5547)
Age[a]	1.04 (1.03–1.04)	1.04 (1.04–1.04)
Males[b]	1.28 (1.20–1.36)	1.26 (1.19–1.34)
COPD + asthma compared with reference[c]		
Reference	1	1
No ICS	3.06 (2.35–3.97)	4.61 (3.70–5.75)
Low ICS[d]	6.61 (5.43–8.05)	5.31 (4.57–6.18)
High ICS[e]	6.40 (5.30–7.72)	5.40 (4.56–6.38)
'COPD without asthma' compared with reference[c]		
Reference	1	1
No ICS	4.35 (3.79–4.99)	4.01 (3.58–4.49)
Low ICS	6.15 (5.23–7.24)	4.52 (3.91–5.23)
High ICS	4.91 (3.82–6.31)	4.62 (3.45–6.18)
'COPD without asthma': ICS use compared with no ICS use in the COPD population		
No ICS	1	1
Low ICS	1.06 (0.91–1.25)	1.20 (1.05–1.38)
High ICS	0.98 (0.81–1.17)	1.31 (1.10–1.56)

[a]Increased risk for every one year increase in age; [b]Increased risk for males compared to females; [c]Reference population (n = 48,566); case matched population with no asthma or COPD but with lung function measurements; [d]Low dose ICS: < 640 µg/day; [e]High dose ICS: ≥800 µg/day

CI confidence intervals, *COPD* chronic obstructive pulmonary disease, *FEV_1* forced expiratory volume in 1 s, *ICS* inhaled corticosteroids

$FEV_1 < 50\%$ who may have been at increased risk of pneumonia at higher doses of ICS are no longer alive.

Presence of asthma

In this study, the presence of asthma was an independent risk factor for pneumonia in the COPD population, and was associated with a 13% increase in the risk of pneumonia (HR 1.13, 95% CI: 1.01–1.27). This is consistent with results from previous studies. For example, in a case-control study in four Dutch healthcare centers, a history of asthma was independently associated with an increased risk of community-acquired pneumonia [30]. The study found that asthma was the strongest independent risk factor for pneumonia in both children (odds ratio [OR] 3.57, 95% CI: 1.86–6.88) and young adults

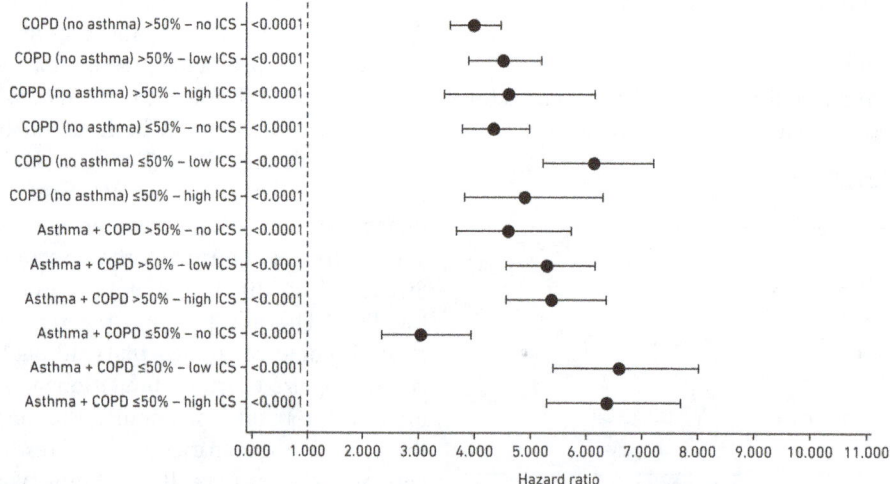

Fig. 2 Forest plot showing the HR for pneumonia in COPD and/or asthma patients versus reference population*. *(No COPD and/or asthma, no ICS). All results were statistically significant, p < 0.0001. HR above 1 is an increased risk of pneumonia. *COPD* chronic obstructive pulmonary disease; *HR* hazard ratio; *ICS* inhaled corticosteroids (low dose ICS: < 640 µg/day; high dose ICS: ≥800 µg/day)

Table 4 Hazard ratio for pneumonia in COPD patients stratified by presence of asthma

	COPD without asthma Hazard ratio (95% CI) (N = 4299)	COPD with asthma Hazard ratio (95% CI) (N = 2324)
Age[a]	1.05 (1.05–1.06)	1.05 (1.05–1.05)
Males[b]	1.19 (1.12–1.27)	1.21 (1.14–1.29)
Reference population[c]	1	1
COPD with no ICS versus ref	3.35 (2.82–3.97)	5.00 (4.56–5.48)
COPD with low ICS[d] versus ref	7.86 (6.96–8.89)	6.36 (5.69–7.11)
COPD with high ICS[e] versus ref	7.08 (6.22–8.04)	4.56 (3.76–5.53)
Within the COPD group: ICS use compared with no ICS use		
No ICS	1	1
Low ICS	1.29 (1.05–1.58)	1.46 (1.28–1.67)
High ICS	1.59 (1.30–1.96)	1.69 (1.37–2.07)

[a]Increased risk for every 1 year increase in age; [b]Increased risk for males compared to females; [c]Reference population = case matched population with no asthma or COPD but with lung function measurements; [d]Low dose ICS: < 640 µg/day; [e]High dose ICS: ≥800 µg/day
CI confidence intervals, COPD chronic obstructive pulmonary disease, ICS inhaled corticosteroids, ref reference

(OR 2.69, 95% CI: 1.23–5.88) [30]. To our knowledge, no previous data on the risk of pneumonia in patients with asthma and COPD are available. However, other studies have identified that patients with COPD and concomitant asthma have more exacerbations and more severe airflow limitation compared with patients with COPD alone [18]. This indicates that patients with both COPD and co-existing asthma are a vulnerable patient group who may require distinct clinical management and surveillance.

Health care utilization and comorbidities
We also found that patients with COPD had significantly higher levels of healthcare utilization and comorbidities than reference controls. Thirty-eight percent of patients had cardiovascular disease and 26% had hypertension.

Table 5 HR for pneumonia in COPD patients only, including FEV$_1$ and comorbidities in a multivariate model

	Hazard ratio (95% CI)	p-value
Age[a]	1.01 (1.00–1.01)	0.06
Male[b]	1.13 (1.03–1.25)	0.01
No ICS	1	
Low ICS[c]	1.23 (1.10–1.38)	0.0003
High ICS[d]	1.41 (1.23–1.62)	< 0.0001
FEV$_1$ < 50%	1.33 (1.21–1.47)	
FEV$_1$ ≥ 50%	1	
No asthma	1	
Asthma	1.13 (1.01–1.27)	0.0310
Charlson Comorbidity index[e]	1.02 (0.96–1.09)	0.4621

[a]Increased risk for every 1 year increase in age; [b]Increased risk for males compared to females; [c]Low dose ICS: < 640 µg/day; [d]High dose ICS: ≥800 µg/day; [e]For each one unit increase in Charlson Comorbidity index
CI confidence intervals, COPD chronic obstructive pulmonary disease, FEV$_1$ forced expiratory volume in 1 s, HR hazard ratio, ICS inhaled corticosteroids

These rates are similar to those reported in other studies [31, 32]. The prevalence of asthma in patients with COPD in this study was higher (15%) compared to the other comorbidities but was low in comparison to other COPD studies, where concomitant asthma was reported in up to 40% of all patients with COPD [33]. In our study, the higher rates of comorbidities in patients with COPD compared to the reference population highlight the importance of a thorough assessment of patients with COPD by physicians and of taking these co-existing conditions into consideration when managing these patients. This will help ensure that delays in COPD diagnosis due to misdiagnosis by HCPs are reduced and that the correct treatment is given. However, further research is needed to understand the full impact of different co-morbidities, including asthma, on COPD outcomes.

Strengths and limitations
This study has a number of strengths. The large sample size of patients with COPD with spirometry data from a primary care setting and real-world study design provides a unique set of data that are reflective of the general patient population. The inclusion of a reference population, several disease states, severity of airflow limitation, concurrent asthma and ICS use (stratified by low, high or no ICS use) are all further strengths of this study, given that only one other cohort study has stratified ICS use [16].

A potential limitation to this study is the retrospective study design, which introduces the potential for bias and confounding due to variables that may not have been accounted for in our analysis. A further limitation was that no investigation into mortality was made. One study demonstrated that mortality rate was approximately 2–6 times higher in patients with COPD compared with the general Swedish population [34]; however, there was no increase in death in those using ICS [35]. There was also no information on smoking or body mass index (BMI). A previous multivariate analysis found that, regardless of treatment, a BMI of < 25 kg/m^2 was a risk factor for pneumonia [24]. We also lacked patient reported outcome data such as the COPD Assessment Test (CAT) and could therefore not use the GOLD A, B, C, D grading system [36]. Furthermore, as the diagnosis of pneumonia was carried out in primary and secondary care, it could be argued that the diagnosis of pneumonia was only accurate in secondary care settings, where chest radiographs and X-rays are used in all patients with suspected pneumonia. Evidence from diagnostic studies also suggests that a diagnosis of pneumonia in general practice is associated with reduced accuracy [37]. Since only Swedish patients were enrolled in this study, the generalizability of results may be limited to patients in other parts of the world. In addition, variability in regional healthcare systems, criteria and practices between and within medical centers make it difficult to compare data [38]. However, we believe our findings have important clinical implications and demonstrate the association between ICS and pneumonia in patients with COPD. As a result, physicians should prescribe ICS judiciously in patients with COPD, particularly taking into account the presence of comorbidities such as asthma.

Clinical implications

Evidence has shown that indacaterol/glycopyrronium, a fixed-dose LABA/long-acting muscarinic antagonist (LAMA) combination, was superior to the ICS/LABA salmeterol/fluticasone in preventing exacerbations and improving patient reported outcomes in patients with COPD with moderate-to-very severe airflow limitation with or without a history of exacerbations [39–41]. Thus, since ICS increases the risk of pneumonia, a LABA/LAMA combination may be an appropriate first choice treatment [39–41]. It is therefore important to understand which patients may benefit from ICS in order to reduce unnecessary exposure of patients to ICS-associated risks. Further studies are needed to determine who should be treated with ICS-containing regimens, focusing on both the benefits and risks, to improve understanding and aid physician decision making.

Conclusion

Despite its limitations, this large-scale primary care study provides important insights into the characteristics of patients with COPD in a real-world setting. We have demonstrated that patients with COPD are at high risk of pneumonia and that the use of ICS and the presence of concomitant asthma are related to a further increase in the risk of pneumonia. Such insights should inform the management of COPD by primary care physicians in order to maximize the chances of positive outcomes among the patients they treat.

Abbreviations

ACO: Asthma-COPD overlap; ATC: Anatomic Therapeutic Chemical; BMI: Body mass index; CI: Confidence intervals; COPD: Chronic obstructive pulmonary disease; EMRs: Electronic medical records; FEV$_1$: Forced expiratory volume in 1 s; GOLD: Global initiative for chronic Obstructive Lung Disease; HCP: Healthcare professionals; HR: Hazard ratio; ICD: International Classification of Disease; ICS: inhaled corticosteroids; ID: Identification; INSPIRE: Investigating New Standards for Prophylaxis in Reducing Exacerbations; LABA: Long-acting beta-2 agonists; LAMA: Long-acting muscarinic antagonist; LISA: Longitudinal Integration Database for Health Insurance and Labour Market Studies; OR: Odds ratio; RR: Rate ratio; TORCH: Towards a Revolution in COPD Health

Acknowledgements

The authors were assisted in the preparation of the manuscript by Laura Brennan, a professional medical writer at CircleScience, an Ashfield Company, part of UDG Healthcare plc.

Funding

Medical writing support was funded by Novartis Pharma AG (Basel, Switzerland).

Authors' contributions

All authors' provided substantial contribution to the design, acquisition of data, analysis and interpretation of data. Authors critically reviewed the manuscript for important intellectual content. All authors read and approved the final version of the manuscript.

Competing interests

Christer Janson has received payments for educational activities from AstraZeneca, Boehringer Ingelheim, Chiesi, Novartis and Teva, and has served on advisory boards arranged by AstraZeneca, Boehringer Ingelheim, Chiesi, GlaxoSmithKline, Novartis and Teva.
Gunnar Johansson has received payments for educational activities from AstraZeneca, Nycomed and Novartis and has served on advisory boards arranged by AstraZeneca, Novartis, Nycomed and Teva.
Björn Ställberg has received honoraria for educational activities and lectures from AstraZeneca, Boehringer Ingelheim, Meda, Novartis and Teva, and has served on advisory boards arranged by AstraZeneca, Novartis, Meda, GlaxoSmithKline, and Boehringer Ingelheim.
Karin Lisspers has received payments for educational activities and lectures from AstraZeneca, GlaxoSmithKline, Meda, MSD, Novartis and Nycomed and has served on advisory boards arranged by Novartis and Meda.
Kjell Larsson has, during the last five years, on one or more occasion served on an advisory board and/or served as speaker and/or participated in education arranged by AstraZeneca, Boehringer Ingelheim, Chiesi, Meda, Orion, Novartis, Teva and Takeda.
Milica Uhde and Leif Jorgensen are employees of IQVIA, who received remuneration in relation to statistical analysis.
Petter Olsson is an employee of Novartis Sverige AB.
Dorothy L Keininger and Florian S. Gutzwiller are employees of Novartis Pharma AG.

Author details
[1]Department of Medical Sciences: Respiratory, Allergy and Sleep Research, Uppsala University, Akademiska sjukhuset, 75185 Uppsala, Sweden. [2]Department of Public Health and Caring Sciences, Family Medicine and Preventive Medicine, Uppsala University, Uppsala, Sweden. [3]Novartis Sverige AB, Täby, Sweden. [4]Novartis, Basel, Switzerland. [5]IQVIA, Stockholm, Sweden. [6]IQVIA, Copenhagen, Denmark. [7]Karolinska Institutet, Solna, Sweden.

References
1. Global Initiative for Chronic Obstructive Lung Disease (GOLD): Global strategy for the diagnosis, management, and prevention of chronic obstructive pulmonary disease. Updated 2017. Available at: http://goldcopd.org/gold-2017-global-strategy-diagnosis-management-prevention-copd/. Last accessed 3 January 2017.
2. Price D, Jones R, Gruffyd-Jones K, Brusselle G, Miravitlles M, Baldwin M, et al. Real-world prescribing patterns among newly diagnosed COPD patients receiving ICS: an analysis of UK patient dataset. Eur Respir J 2014;44(Suppl. 58):P2422 (Abstract).
3. White P, Thornton H, Pinnock H, Georgopoulou S, Booth HP. Overtreatment of COPD with inhaled corticosteroids--implications for safety and costs: cross-sectional observational study. PLoS One. 2013;8:e75221.
4. Miravitlles M, Sicras A, Crespo C, Cuesta M, Brosa M, Galera J, et al. Costs of chronic obstructive pulmonary disease in relation to compliance with guidelines: a study in the primary care setting. Ther Adv Respir Dis. 2013;7: 139–50.
5. Läkemedelverkets Medical Products Agency (Sweden): Läkemedelverkets expert panel. Farmakologisk behandling av kroniskt obstruktiv lungsjukdom (KOL) – behandlingsrekommendationer (In Swedish). 2009:Suppl 2:13–28. Available at: https://lakemedelsverket.se/kol.
6. Lisspers K, Stallberg B, Janson C: Omhändertagande av patienter med kroniskt obstruktiv lungsjukdom (KOL) i Uppsala-Örebroregionen [in Swedish]. 2007. Available at: http://www.praxisstudien.se/texter/KOL-rapport%202007.pdf. Last accessed 4 May 2017.
7. Calverley PM, Anderson JA, Celli B, Ferguson GT, Jenkins C, Jones PW, et al. Salmeterol and fluticasone propionate and survival in chronic obstructive pulmonary disease. N Engl J Med. 2007;356:775–89.
8. Ferguson GT, Anzueto A, Fei R, Emmett A, Knobil K, Kalberg C. Effect of fluticasone propionate/salmeterol (250/50 mg) or salmeterol (50 mg) on COPD exacerbations. Respir Med. 2008;102:1099–108.
9. Anzueto A, Ferguson GT, Feldman G, Chinsky K, Seibert A, Emmett A, et al. Effect of fluticasone propionate/salmeterol (250/50) on COPD exacerbations and impact on patient outcomes. COPD. 2009;6:320–9.
10. Calverley PM, Stockley RA, Seemungal TA, Hagan G, Willits LR, Riley JH, et al. Reported pneumonia in patients with COPD: findings from the INSPIRE study. Chest. 2011;139:505–12.
11. Sharafkhaneh A, Southard JG, Goldman M, Uryniak T, Martin UJ. Effect of budesonide/formoterol pMDI on COPD exacerbations: a double-blind, randomized study. Respir Med. 2012;106:257–68.
12. Dransfield MT, Bourbeau J, Jones PW, Hanania NA, Mahler DA, Vestbo J, et al. Once-daily inhaled fluticasone furoate and vilanterol versus vilanterol only for prevention of exacerbations of COPD: two replicate double-blind, parallel-group, randomised controlled trials. Lancet Respir Med. 2013;1:210–23.
13. Singh S, Amin AV, Loke YK. Long-term use of inhaled corticosteroids and the risk of pneumonia in chronic obstructive pulmonary disease: a meta-analysis. Arch Intern Med. 2009;169:219–29.
14. Festic E, Bansal V, Gupta E, Scanlon PD. Association of inhaled corticosteroids with incident pneumonia and mortality in COPD patients; systematic review and meta-analysis. COPD. 2015;13:312–26.
15. Janson C, Larsson K, Lisspers KH, Stallberg B, Stratelis G, Goike H, et al. Pneumonia and pneumonia related mortality in patients with COPD treated with fixed combinations of inhaled corticosteroid and long acting b_2 agonist: observational matched cohort study (PATHOS). BMJ. 2013;346:f3306.
16. Suissa S, Patenaude V, Lapi F, Ernst P. Inhaled corticosteroids in COPD and the risk of serious pneumonia. Thorax. 2013;68:1029–36.
17. Global initiative for Asthma (GINA). Global strategy for asthma management and Prevention Updated 2017. Available at: https://ginasthma.org/wp-content/uploads/2016/01/wms-GINA-2017-main-report-tracked-changes-for-archive.pdf. Last accessed 4 May 2017.
18. Hardin M, Cho M, McDonald ML, Beaty T, Ramsdell J, Bhatt S, et al. The clinical and genetic features of COPD-asthma overlap syndrome. Eur Respir J. 2014;44:341–50.
19. de Marco R, Marcon A, Rossi A, Anto JM, Cerveri I, Gislason T, et al. Asthma, COPD and overlap syndrome: a longitudinal study in young European adults. Eur Respir J. 2015;46:671–9.
20. Statistics Sweden. Population Statistics. 2017. Available at: https://www.scb.se/BE0101-en. Last accessed: 12th September 2017.
21. Statistics Sweden: Longitudinal integration database for health insurance and labour market studies (LISA by Swedish acronym). 2004. Available at: https://www.scb.se/en/services/guidance-for-researchers-and-universities/vilka-mikrodata-finns/longitudinella-register/longitudinal-integration-database-for-health-insurance-and-labourmarket-studies-lisa/. Last accessed 26 June 2017.
22. Socialstyrelsen. 2017. Available at : http://www.socialstyrelsen.se/register. Last accessed 26 June 2017.
23. Wedzicha JA, Calverley PM, Seemungal TA, Hagan G, Ansari Z, Stockley RA, et al. The prevention of chronic obstructive pulmonary disease exacerbations by salmeterol/fluticasone propionate or tiotropium bromide. Am J Respir Crit Care Med. 2008;177:19–26.
24. Crim C, Calverley PM, Anderson JA, Celli B, Ferguson GT, Jenkins C, et al. Pneumonia risk in COPD patients receiving inhaled corticosteroids alone or in combination: TORCH study results. Eur Respir J. 2009;34:641–7.
25. Welte T, Miravitlles M, Hernandez P, Eriksson G, Peterson S, Polanowski T, et al. Efficacy and tolerability of budesonide/formoterol added to tiotropium in patients with chronic obstructive pulmonary disease. Am J Respir Crit Care Med. 2009;180:741–50.
26. Rennard SI, Tashkin DP, McElhattan J, Goldman M, Ramachandran S, Martin UJ, et al. Efficacy and tolerability of budesonide/formoterol in one hydrofluoroalkane pressurized metered-dose inhaler in patients with chronic obstructive pulmonary disease: results from a 1-year randomized controlled clinical trial. Drugs. 2009;69:549–65.
27. Yang HH, Lai CC, Wang YH, Yang WC, Wang CY, Wang HC, et al. Severe exacerbation and pneumonia in COPD patients treated with fixed combinations of inhaled corticosteroid and long-acting beta2 agonist. Int J Chron Obstruct Pulmon Dis. 2017;12:2477–85.
28. European Medicines Agency (EMA). EMA completes review of inhaled corticosteroids for chronic obstructive pulmonary disease. Review finds no differences between products in risk of pneumonia. Date last updated 29 April 2016. Available at: http://www.ema.europa.eu/ema/index.jsp?curl=pages/news_and_events/news/2016/04/news_detail_002521.jsp&mid=WC0b01ac058004d5c1. Data last accessed 8 January 2018.
29. Jenkins CR, Jones PW, Calverley PM, Celli B, Anderson JA, Ferguson GT, et al. Efficacy of salmeterol/fluticasone propionate by GOLD stage of chronic obstructive pulmonary disease: analysis from the randomised, placebo-controlled TORCH study. Respir Res. 2009;10:59.
30. Teepe J, Grigoryan L, Verheij TJ. Determinants of community-acquired pneumonia in children and young adults in primary care. Eur Respir J. 2010;35:1113–7.
31. Soriano JB, Visick GT, Muellerova H, Payvandi N, Hansell AL. Patterns of comorbidities in newly diagnosed COPD and asthma in primary care. Chest. 2005;128:2099–107.
32. Mannino DM, Thorn D, Swensen A, Holguin F. Prevalence and outcomes of diabetes, hypertension and cardiovascular disease in COPD. Eur Respir J. 2008;32:962–9.
33. Stallberg B, Janson C, Johansson G, Larsson K, Stratelis G, Telg G, et al. Management, morbidity and mortality of COPD during an 11-year period: an observational retrospective epidemiological register study in Sweden (PATHOS). Prim Care Respir J. 2014;23:38–45.
34. Sundh J, Janson C, Lisspers K, Montgomery S, Stallberg B. Clinical COPD questionnaire score (CCQ) and mortality. Int J Chron Obstruct Pulmon Dis. 2012;7:833–42.
35. Joo MJ, Au DH, Fitzgibbon ML, Lee TA. Inhaled corticosteroids and risk of pneumonia in newly diagnosed COPD. Respir Med. 2010;104:246–52.
36. Global Initiative for Chronic Obstructive Lung Disease (GOLD): Global strategy for the diagnosis, management, and prevention of chronic obstructive pulmonary disease. 2018 Report. Available at: http://goldcopd.org/gold-reports/. Last accessed 28 November 2017.
37. Melbye H, Straume B, Aasebo U, Brox J. The diagnosis of adult pneumonia in general practice. The diagnostic value of history, physical examination and some blood tests. Scand J Prim Health Care. 1988;6:111–7.

5

The moderate predictive value of serial serum CRP and PCT levels for the prognosis of hospitalized community-acquired pneumonia

Shuren Guo[1,2], Xiaohuan Mao[3] and Ming Liang[1,2]*

Abstract

Background: To predict the prognosis by observing the dynamic change of C-reactive protein (CRP) and procalcitonin (PCT) for hospitalized community-acquired pneumonia (CAP).

Methods: The data were collected from January to December 2017 from the first affiliated Hospital of Zhengzhou University. Demographic and clinical patient information including age, length of hospital stay and Charlson Comorbidity Index (CCI) were recorded. Blood samples were taken for CRP, PCT, and white blood cell count (WBC). Receiver Operating Characteristic (ROC) curve was used to verify each biomarker's association with the prognosis of pneumonia.

Results: A total of 350 patients were enrolled in the study. The 30-day mortality was 10.86%. Serial serum CRP3, CRP5, PCT3, PCT5 and PCT5c levels were statistically lower in CAP survivors than non-survivors. CRP3c < 0, CRP5c < 0 and PCT5c < 0 were observed with a statistically lower frequency in patients with 30-day mortality and initial treatment failure. The AUC for 30-day mortality for serial CRP levels combined with CRP clearances was 0.85 (95% CI 0.77–0.92), as compared to an AUC of 0.81 (95% CI 0.73–0.9) for serial PCT levels combined with PCT clearances.

Conclusions: Serum serial CRP and PCT levels had moderate predictive value for hospitalized CAP prognosis. The dynamic CRP and PCT changes may potentially be used in the future to predict hospitalized CAP prognosis.

Keywords: Serial serum CRP, PCT, Predictive value, CAP prognosis

Background

Diagnosis of pneumonia in critically ill patients is usually challenging. Signs and symptoms with enormous heterogeneity, such as dyspnea, may be non-diagnostic or atypical, chest X-ray results may be uncertain, also complications may be confounding factors [1–3]. Thus, biomarkers of inflammation or infection, such as procalcitonin (PCT) and C-reactive protein (CRP), have been proposed as a guide in the diagnostic process [4–6]. Elevated serum PCT and CRP were associated with community-acquired pneumonia and ventilator-associated pneumonia (VAP) [5, 7].

CRP is a well-established biomarker in many clinical settings, but has been traditionally considered insufficient as a useful marker in the diagnosis of pneumonia. In fact, all infections, stress reactions, autoimmunity and tumor disease can contribute to the increase in serum CRP values [8].

PCT is a 116-amino acid long precursor of calcitonin, which is produced by the thyroid. In sepsis, macrophages and the monocytic cells of the liver are involved in the synthesis of PCT,which is elevated in sepsis [9, 10]. The degree of induction of PCT correlates with the severity of systemic infection and the presence of organ dysfunction.

Due to multiple confounding factors, several studies have reported controversial results on the role of CRP and PCT in the diagnosis of pneumonia in multiple elderly patients [1, 11, 12]. The importance of serum CRP and PCT

* Correspondence: mingliang@zzu.edu.cn
[1]Department of Clinical Laboratory, The First Affiliated Hospital of Zhengzhou University, East Jianshe Road #1, Zhengzhou, Henan 450002, People's Republic of China
[2]Key Clinical Laboratory of Henan province, Zhengzhou, Henan, People's Republic of China
Full list of author information is available at the end of the article

Table 1 Characteristics of survivors and non-survivors

	All patients (%) n=350	Survivors (%) n=312	Non-Survivors (%) n=38	P value
Age(years)	58.53±19.1	58.59±19.2	58.03±18.9	0.86
Males	204 (58.3)	181(58.0)	23(60.5)	0.7
Comorbidity				
Diabetes Mellitus	30(8.57)	27(8.6)	3(7.8)	0.87
Chronic heart disease	100(28.57)	91(29.1)	9(23.6)	0.48
Chronic liver disease	22(6.29)	20(6.4)	2(5.2)	0.78
Chronic renal disease	47(13.43)	40(12.8)	7(18.4)	0.34
Malignant disease	26(7.43)	24(7.6)	2(5.2)	0.59
History of Shock	17(4.86)	15(4.8)	2(5.2)	0.9
COPD	22(6.29)	18(5.7)	4(10.5)	0.25
Cerebrovascular disease	39(11.14)	35(11.2)	4(10.5)	0.9
Antimicrobial treatment before admission	79(22.6)	70(22.4)	9(23.7)	1
Signs and symptoms				
Cough	268(76.6)	260(83.3)	28(73.6)	0.14
Chest pain	116(33.1)	106(33.9)	10(26.3)	0.34
Expectoration	168(48)	148(47.4)	20(52.6)	0.54
Dyspnea	249(71.1)	221(70.8)	28(73.6)	0.72
Chills	124(35.4)	109(34.9)	15(39.4)	0.58
Headaches	75(21.4)	58(18.5)	17(44.7)	**<0.001**
Myalgia	79(22.6)	71(22.7)	8(21)	0.8
Crackles	114(32.6)	102(32.6)	12(31.5)	0.89
Fever	110(31.4)	96(30.7)	14(36.8)	0.45
Confusion	5(1.4)	1(0.3)	4(10.5)	**<0.001**
CCI class				
0-2	129(36.8)	116(37.1)	13(34.2)	0.7
3-5	180(51.4)	161(51.6)	19(50)	
>5	41(11.7)	35(11.2)	6(15.7)	
CRP1 (mg/L)	65.3±84.7	66.3±85.2	57.1±81.3	0.53
CRP3 (mg/L)	56.4±77.4	50±66.4	109.1±128.4	**<0.001**
CRP3c	556.6±5056.3	575.2±5334.2	401.2±1242.4	0.843
CRP3c<0	223(63.7)	214(68.5)	9(23.6)	**<0.001**
CRP5(mg/L)	44.8±68.5	37.9±61	102.1±96.9	**<0.001**
CRP5c	429.2±3489.6	429.2±3670.1	429.3±1207.6	0.999
CRP5c<0	222(63.4)	213(68.2)	9(23.6)	**<0.001**
PCT1 (ng/mL)	1.8±7.1	1.8±7.3	1.9±5.5	0.96
PCT3 (ng/mL)	1.7±6.3	1.4±4.4	4.1±14.5	**0.012**
PCT3c	791.2±2653.8	793.3±2672.6	774.1±2528.7	0.966
PCT3c<0	174(49.7)	157(50.3)	17(44.7)	0.52
PCT5 (ng/mL)	1.2±3.7	0.8±2	4.3±9.3	**<0.001**
PCT5c	695.3±2463	589.9±2298.2	1555±3454.4	**0.022**
PCT5c<0	179(51.1)	170(54.4)	9(23.6)	**<0.001**
WBC1	10.4±8	10.1±7.2	12.6±12.8	0.081
WBC3	9.5±5	9.2±5	10.8±4.7	0.112

Table 1 Characteristics of survivors and non-survivors *(Continued)*

	All patients (%) n=350	Survivors (%) n=312	Non-Survivors (%) n=38	P value
WBC5	10.5±6.6	10.4±7	10.6±4.7	0.932
CURB class				
0-2	289	256	33	0.46
3-5	61	56	5	

Data are presented as means $\bar{x}$ ±SD, or n (%), CRP, C-reactive protein; CURB-65, confusion, urea > 7 mmol/L, respiratory rate≥30 breaths/min, low blood pressure (systolic<90mm Hg or diastolic≤60 mm Hg) and age≥65 years
PCT procalcitonin, *COPD* Chronic Obstructive Pulmonary Disease, *SD* standard deviation, *WBC* white blood cell, *CRP3c 5c:* CRP clearance on day3, *day5* PCT3c, *5c* PCT clearance on day 3, day 5

levels on diagnosis is well established [5, 7, 13, 14], The mean values of certain cytokines are statistically different from patients with treatment failure vs patients without treatment failure, the wide range of values for particular cytokines make it difficult to use the value of a single patient to predict clinical outcomes. A dynamic approach of assessing biomarkers may provide additional survival information. Markers of the inflammatory response and their kinetics have been studied in the prediction of outcomes in sepsis [15] and VAP [16, 17]. As reported by Huang MY, et al., PCT clearance (PCTc) has been introduced in a previous studies as a tool for monitoring the changes of PCT levels during severe sepsis [18, 19]. Similar to PCTc in the previous study, in our study we introduced CRP clearance (CRPc) to monitor the changes of CRP levels during the treatment of hospitalized CAP. Since PCTc and CRPc measures the relative changes in PCT and CRP to the baseline levels, they are postulated to be a better predictor of prognosis. However, both PCTc and CRPc are not common in clinical practice.

Therefore, the hypothesis of this study is whether CRP and PCT levels and their clearance could serve as prognostic biomarkers for hospitalized CAP patients. The aim of the present study was to evaluate the usefulness of CRP and PCT levels and their clearance as prognostic biomarkers for hospitalized CAP patients.

Methods
Study design and patient population
This was a single-center, prospective observational study. Hospitalized pneumonia patients with a radiological confirmation were recruited. The informed consents were obtained from all subjects or their guardians. The study was approved by ethic committee of Zhengzhou University and met the declaration of Helsinki. Diagnosis of CAP required the presence of at least one respiratory symptom in addition to one auscultatory finding or signs of infection (WBC > 10×10^9/L or < 4×10^9/L cells, shivers, core body temperature > 38.0 °C) and a new infiltrate on chest radiograph. The respiratory symptoms included cough, expectoration, dyspnea, tachypnea, or

Table 2 Univariate and multivariate analysis of biomarkers for 30-day mortality

	Univariate analysis			Multivariate analysis		
	Odds ratio (95% CI)	Estimate	Univariate P-value	Odds ratio (95% CI)	Estimate	Multivariate P-value
CRP1 (mg/L)	0.998(0.994–1.003)	−0.001	0.53			
CRP3 (mg/L)	1.006(1.003–1.01)	0.006	< 0.001	1.013 (1–1.025)	0.012	0.002
CRP3c	0.999(0.999–1)	0	0.845			
CRP3c < 0	1.02(0.991–1.049)	0.019	0.174			
CRP5(mg/L)	1.008(1.004–1.01)	0.008	< 0.001	1.011 (1–1.021)	0.011	0.028
CRP5c	1(0.999–1)	0	0.999			
PCT1 (ng/mL)	1.001(0.955–1.05)	0.001	0.96			
PCT3 (ng/mL)	1.036(0.998–1.07)	0.035	0.06			
PCT3c	0.999(0.999–1)	0	0.966			
PCT5 (ng/mL)	1.21(1.08–1.357)	0.191	< 0.001	1.277 (1.004–1.624)	0.244	0.046
PCT5c	1(0.999–1)	0	0.052			
WBC1	1.025(0.993–1.059)	0.025	0.117			
WBC3	1.061(0.985–1.143)	0.059	0.118			
WBC5	1.004(0.906–1.113)	0.004	0.931			

Table 3 Univariate and multivariate analyses of biomarkers for initial treatment failure

	Initial treatment failure		Univariate Odds ratio(95% CI)	Univariate P-value	Multivariate Odds ratio(95% CI)	Multivariate P-value
	Yes	No				
CRP1 (mg/L)	71±88.7	64±83.9	0.999(0.996-1.003)	0.55	1.008(1.001-1.013)	0.009
CRP3 (mg/L)	89.2±107.6	48.9±66.8	0.995(0.991-0.998)	0.001	0.992(0.985-0.999)	0.035
CRP3c	801.8±3644.9	501±5328.5	1	0.673	1(0.999-1)	0.33
CRP5(mg/L)	79.7±96.3	37.2±58.3	0.993(0.989-0.997)	<0.001	0.996(0.989-1.001)	0.15
CRP5c	682.9±2888.4	371.7±3614.2	1	0.534	1(0.999-1)	0.299
PCT1 (ng/mL)	4.6±13.6	1.2±4.2	0.936(0.892-0.983)	0.009	0.89(0.82-0.965)	0.005
PCT3 (ng/mL)	2.8±11.2	1.4±4.5	0.975(0.941-1.01)	0.163	1.134(1.017-1.263)	0.022
PCT3c	469.1±1972.7	865.2±2784.4	1	0.293	1(0.999-1)	0.403
PCT5 (ng/mL)	2.8±7.3	0.8±2.1	0.868(0.892-0.983)	0.005	0.851(0.751-0.963)	0.01
PCT5c	1013.8±2761.2	622.1±2388.7	1	0.268	1(0.999-1)	0.658

a Variable(s) entered on step 1: CRP1, CRP3, CRP3c, CRP5, CRP5c, PCT1, PCT3, PCT3c, PCT5, PCT5c, and CURB65

pleuritic chest pain [20]. Radiological findings were verified with results of the real-time PCR tests on blood samples and nasopharyngeal swabs. The Clinical severity of the hospitalized CAP was evaluated by the CURB-65 score, which including confusion, urea, respiratory, and blood pressure plus age > 65 years.

Measurement of biomarkers

Followed our study design, WBC counts were measured as a part of routine tests using Beckman-coulter LH750 hematology analyzer. Serum CRP and PCT levels were measured on hospital days 1, 3, and 5 in patients. The blood was drawn in vacuum tube filled with separation gel and centrifuged at 3500 rpm for 5 min, and then CRP and PCT were analyzed by Roche cobas 8000 automatic biochemistry analyzer within 30 min. Concentrations of CRP were determined by an immunoturbidimetric assay. The diagnostic cut-off value of CRP was set by manufacturer at 5 mg/L. PCT (ng/mL) levels were measured by electro chemiluminescence immunoassay with a lower limit of detection of 0.02 ng/ml. CRP and PCT levels measured on day 1, day 3 and day 5 were defined as CRP1 and PCT1, CRP3 and PCT3, CRP5 and PCT5, respectively. PCTc was

calculated based on the previously reported formula [19], (PCTday3/day5-PCTday1)/PCTday1 × 100% = PCT3c /day5c (%). The calculation of CRPc was referred to the PCTc formula. CRPc on day3 and day5 were abbreviated as CRP3c and CRP5c.

The detection of CAP pathogen

Viral RNA or DNA was extracted from the respiratory secretions within 24 h, and was then tested using respiratory virus panel (Shanghai ZJ Bio-Tech Co., Ltd) fast assay to detect influenza A/B virus (lot: RR-0226-02), respiratory syncytial virus (RSV)-A (RR-0160-01) and -B (lot:RR-0160-02), parainfluenzavirus-1, – 2, – 3 and – 4 (lot: RR-0156-01,02,03,04), adenovirus (lot:RD-0195-02), human metapneumovirus (hMPV) (lot: RR-0162-02) in accordance with the manufacturer's instructions.

The autolysin-A (LytA) and wzg (cpsA) genes of *S. pneumoniae* were tested using real-time PCR from blood and swab samples for pneumococcal cases according to the manufacture instructions. *M. pneumoniae* was looked for in blood and nasopharyngeal swabs with nested PCR, as described previously [21]. Routine

Table 4 Correlation of biomarkers characteristics at different time

	PCT1(ng/ml)	PCT3(ng/ml)	PCT5(ng/ml)	PCT3c	PCT5c
CRP1 (mg/L)	R^2=0.35 P=0.0001*				
CRP3 (mg/L)		R^2=0.19 P=0.0001*			
CRP3c				R^2=0.09 P=0.11	
CRP5(mg/L)			R^2=0.21, P=0.0001*		
CRP5c					R^2=0.17 P=0.002*

Correlation is significant at the 0.01 level (2-tailed)
*Pearson Correlation was used to test the correlation between biomarkers

microbiological examinations were also performed at the Microbiology laboratory and included blood culture, sputum culture, and antigenuria.

Statistical analysis and data management

Data were analyzed using SPSS v.17.0 software (SPSS Inc., Chicago, IL, USA) for Windows. Frequency comparison was done using the χ2-test. The two-group comparison for continuous data was done with the Mann-Whitney U-test. We used univariate and multivariate logistic regression analysis to study the association between biomarker levels and outcome adjusting the models for the CAP severity score CURB-65 and age. ROC curves were used to evaluate the sensitivity and specificity of PCT and CRP vs pneumonia prognosis. The areas under the curve (AUC) were reported with its 95% confidence interval (CI). All p-values were two-tailed and were considered significant for $p < 0.05$.

Outcomes

The primary endpoint was 30-day mortality and the secondary endpoint was initial treatment failure. Both endpoints were assessed by seven medical students, blinded to the goal and design of the study, by conducting standardized follow-up interviews by telephone at 30 days after baseline. Initial treatment failure was defined as occurring in patients whose antimicrobial agents were changed by the attending physicians because they were ineffective referring to the CAP guideline in China [22]. Serial changes in PCT, CRP, and WBC were analyzed for their potential to estimate the clinical prognosis/outcome.

Results

Demographics and clinical presentations

Baseline characteristics of survivors and non-survivors were presented in Table 1. This study included a total of 350 patients with a median age of 58.53 years (58.3%

Table 5 Prognostic performance of Biomarkers and CURB-65 in predicting pneumonia prognosis

Variable(s)	AUC	SE	P value	95%CI
CRP1 (mg/L)	0.45	0.05	0.37	0.36-0.55
CRP3 (mg/L)	0.69	0.05	<0.001	0.6-0.8
CRP3c	0.77	0.04	<0.001	0.7-0.85
CRP5(mg/L)	0.76	0.05	<0.001	0.67-0.85
CRP5c	0.81	0.03	<0.001	0.75-0.87
PCT1 (ng/mL)	0.57	0.05	0.11	0.49-0.67
PCT3 (ng/mL)	0.61	0.05	0.02	0.52-0.71
PCT3c	0.57	0.04	0.13	0.49-0.66
PCT5 (ng/mL)	0.73	0.04	<0.001	0.65-0.82
PCT5c	0.65	0.05	<0.001	0.57-0.75
CRP1*PCT1	0.55	0.05	0.36	0.45-0.65
CRP3*CRP3c	0.7	0.05	<0.001	0.6-0.8
CRP5*CRP5c	0.77	0.05	<0.001	0.68-0.86
PCT3*PCT3c	0.65	0.04	<0.001	0.56-0.74
PCT5*PCT5c	0.74	0.04	<0.001	0.66-0.83
CRP3*PCT3	0.7	0.05	<0.001	0.6-0.81
CRP3c*PCT3c	0.76	0.04	<0.001	0.68-0.84
CRP5*PCT5	0.79	0.04	<0.001	0.71-0.87
CRP5c*PCT5c	0.67	0.04	<0.001	0.58-0.76
CRP5*CRP5c*PCT5*PCT5c	0.79	0.04	<0.001	0.71-0.87
CRP3*CRP3c* CRP5*CRP5c	0.85	0.04	<0.001	0.77-0.92
PCT3*PCT3c*PCT5*PCT5c	0.81	0.04	<0.001	0.73-0.9
CRP3*CRP3c* CRP5*CRP5c* PCT3*PCT3c*PCT5*PCT5c	0.81	0.04	<0.001	0.73-0.88
CURB-65	0.53	0.05	0.53	0.44-0.63
CRP3*CRP3c*CRP5*CRP5c*CURB-65	0.77	0.04	<0.001	0.69-0.85
PCT3*PCT3c*PCT5*PCT5c*CURB-65	0.72	0.05	<0.001	0.64-0.81

[a]Under the nonparametric assumption
[b]Null hypothesis: true area = 0.5
[c]ROC receiver operating characteristic, AUC area under the curve, SE standard error, CI confidence interval

males). The 30-day mortality was found in 10.86% (38/ 350) of all patients. Patients had a high burden of comorbidities including chronic heart disease ($n = 100$), chronic liver disease ($n = 22$), chronic renal disease ($n = 47$), malignant disease ($n = 26$), Chronic Obstructive Pulmonary Disease (COPD, $n = 22$) and diabetes ($n = 30$). Cough ($n = 268$, 76.6%) and dyspnea ($n = 249$, 71.1%) were the most frequent symptoms. No significant differences of comorbidities and symptoms were found between survivors and non-survivors. CAP was ascribed to bacteria in 176 (50.29%) patients and to one or more viruses in 115 (32.86%) patients (Additional file 1: Table S1). Serial serum CRP3, CRP5, PCT3, PCT5 and PCT5c levels were statistically lower in CAP survivors than non-survivors (Table 1). CRP3c < 0, CRP5c < 0 and PCT5c < 0 were observed with a statistically lower frequency in patients with 30-day mortality (Table 1).

Statistic analysis for clinical factors and CAP

WBCs, CRP, and PCT levels on hospital days 1, 3, and 5 and their clearance were compared in all groups. The average mean value of these biomarkers comparison is reported in Tables 2, 3 and Additional file 2: Table S2. ANOVA analysis showed that the CAP patients with bacteria pathogens had significantly higher values of CRP and PCT ($P < 0.05$) than those with other causative pathogens (Additional file 2: Table S2).

We used univariate and multivariate logistic regression models to investigate associations between serum biomarker levels and outcome (Table 2). In univariate analysis, no significant association of CRP1 [OR (95% CI): 0.998(0.994–1.003)] and PCT1 levels [OR (95% CI): 1.001(0.955–1.05)] or WBC counts with 30-day mortality was found. Significant predictive ability was found for 30-day mortality with CRP3 [OR (95% CI): 1.006(1.003–1.01)], CRP5 [OR (95% CI): 1.008(1.004–1.01)] and PCT5 [OR (95% CI): 1.21(1.08–1.357)] levels respectively. The significance did not disappear

after adjust for age, sex and CURB-65 in multivariate logistic regression model.

This study did not show that patients with initial treatment failure had significant higher CRP1 levels than others (71 vs 64, $P = 0.55$). On the other hand, patients with initial treatment failure had significantly higher levels of CRP3, CRP5, PCT1, PCT3 and PCT5 than others (Table 3), which indicated that serial measurements of these serum biomarker levels were also useful for predicting whether initial CAP treatment would be successful.

Correlation between PCT and CRP and their clearance

Assessment of correlation between biomarkers was performed by Spearman's rank correlation analysis. Table 4 showed correlations of CRP, PCT and their clearance in the overall population. At baseline, day 3 and day 5, we found significant correlations between PCT and CRP, no correlations were found for PCT3c and CRP3c ($R^2 = 0.09$, $P = 0.11$). However, the maximum correlation coefficient was 0.35, which is smaller than 0.8, indicating the low level of multicollinearity among each biomarker.

Prognostic accuracy of serial values of PCT and CRP

Table 5 showed the ROC curve of each biomarker and each biomarker combined. For the single biomarker, the peak areas under the ROC curve of CRP5c and PCT5 to predict 30-day mortality was 0.81 (95%CI: 0.75–0.87; $P < 0.001$) and 0.73 (95%CI: 0.65–0.82; $P < 0.001$), respectively (Table 5, Fig. 1a, b). The capacity of serial serum biomarkers combined to predict 30-day mortality was higher than only one biomarker or a combination of two of the biomarkers. The AUC for 30-day mortality for serial CRP levels combined with CRP clearances was 0.85 (95% CI 0.77–0.92), as compared to an AUC of 0.81 (95% CI 0.73–0.9) for serial PCT levels combined with PCT clearances. Furthermore, their AUC-ROC did not increase if they were used in combination with CURB65 (Table 5, Fig. 2c, d).

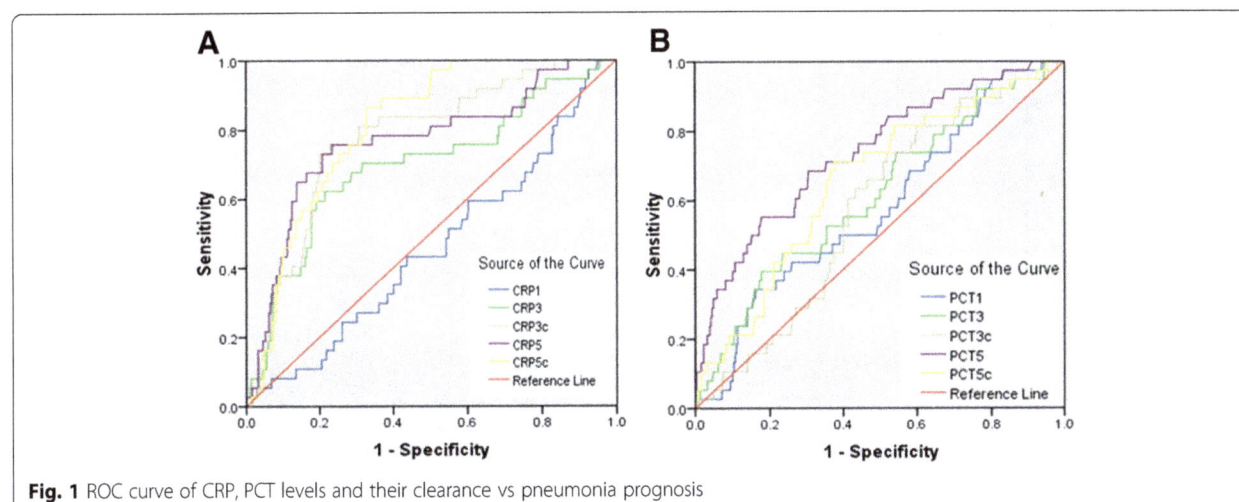

Fig. 1 ROC curve of CRP, PCT levels and their clearance vs pneumonia prognosis

Discussions

In accordance with the current literature, the clinical characteristics of the patients included in this study frequently had a comorbidity of respiratory disorders, diabetes mellitus, congestive heart failure and cancer [23]. So far, most studies focused on the diagnostic performance of serum biomarkers, especially CRP and PCT on the pneumonia diagnosis [1, 5, 7, 11, 24, 25]. Only very few research studied the predictive value of serum biomarkers in the pneumonia outcomes [6, 14, 17, 26–28]. A dynamic approach to biomarkers could capture the progression of disease and might be more effective in evaluating pneumonia prognosis.

In this context, we observed serum CRP and PCT levels measured at different time points after admission. The main findings of this study are threefold. First, circulating CRP and PCT levels were significant different in the pneumonia patients infected with different pathogens. However, there was no significance of the serum CRP1 and PCT1 levels between survivors and non-survivors. This indicated that the initial CRP and PCT levels could not provide useful information to assist with mortality prediction in hospitalized CAP patients, which was consistent with the results from previous studies. Previous studies had showed that simply measuring the initial CRP and PCT levels did not improve clinical score for mortality but

that following the kinetics of PCT did so [6, 29]. However, Akihiro ITO's study found that the initial CRP and PCT levels were significant different between survivors and non-survivors [30]. Furthermore, they found that PCT levels on day3/day1 ≥ 1, CRP levels on day1 ≥ 100 mg/L and CURB-65 ≥ 3 were prognostic variables in CAP. The different basic characteristics of research groups in these studies were the main reasons for the different results. The average age in our study was younger than Akihiro ITO's study (58.53 vs. 73.2), while composition ratio of CURB-65 class was similar (Class 0–2: 82.6 vs. 75.9, Class 3–5: 17.4 vs. 24.1). Similar proportion of CURB-65 in the population aged below and above 65 years old, indicating the more complicate comorbidities or more severe CAP disease in our study which resulting the similar initial CRP and PCT levels between survivors and non-survivors.

Second, consistent with the previous report [6], CRP levels were independent prognostic predictors of CAP clinical outcomes. PCT has been used as a biomarker for initiating or terminating antibiotic therapy in various clinical settings in the previous studies [31, 32]. In this work, we confirmed the predictive role of CRP and PCT in CAP prognosis. Serial serum CRP3, CRP5, PCT3, PCT5 and PCT5c levels were statistically lower in CAP survivors than non-survivors. CRP3c < 0, CRP5c < 0 and PCT5c < 0 were observed with a statistically lower frequency in

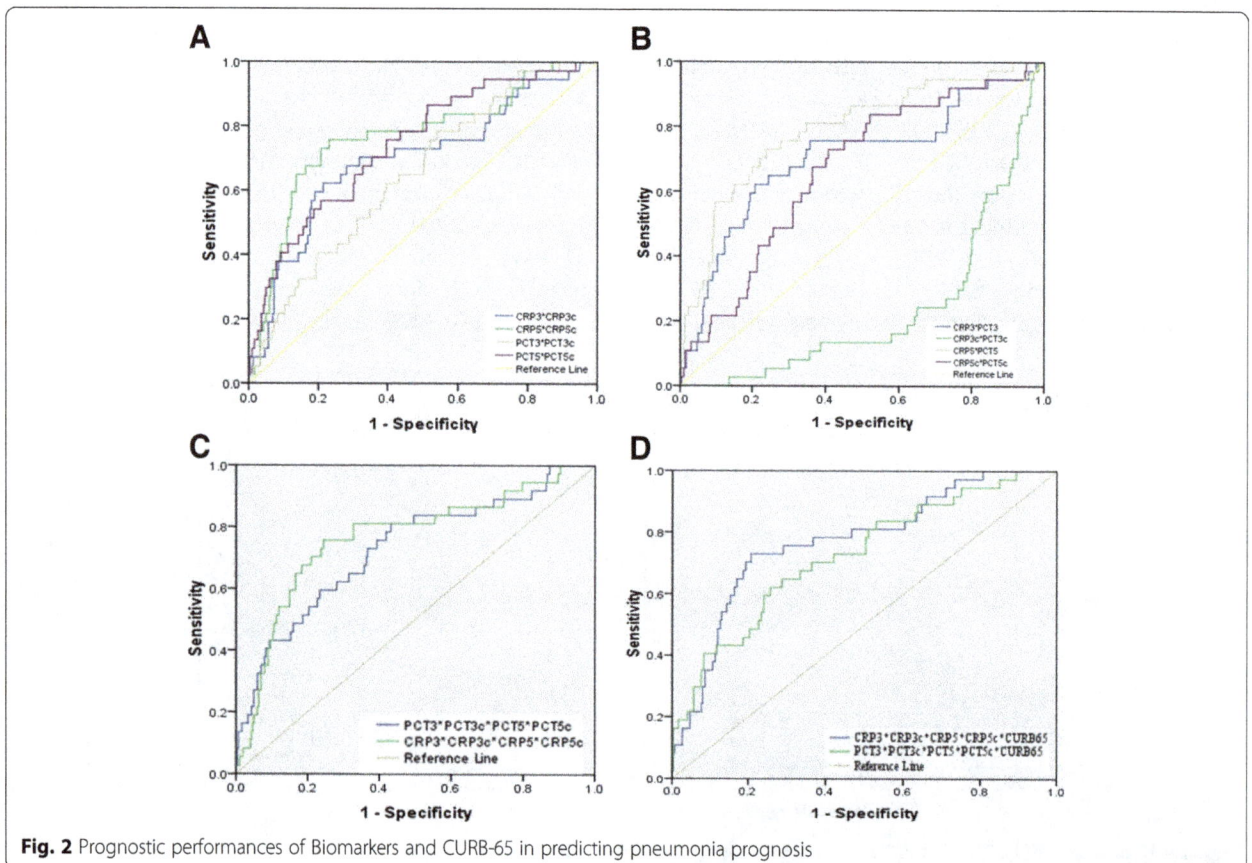

Fig. 2 Prognostic performances of Biomarkers and CURB-65 in predicting pneumonia prognosis

patients with 30-day mortality and initial treatment failure. Significant predictive ability was found for 30-day mortality with CRP3, CRP5 and PCT5 levels.

Third, there was low level of multicollinearity among each biomarker. The capacity of serial serum biomarkers combined to predict 30-day mortality was higher than only one biomarker or a combination of two of the biomarkers. Though the CRP and PCT clearances were not directly associated with the CAP prognosis, when combined with the serum biomarker levels, the increased AUC-ROC indicated the greater prognosis capacity. This was consistent with previous report [33], CRP kinetics can be used to identify ventilator-associated pneumonia patients with poor outcome. This also highlighted the necessary to measure the values of serum biomarkers serially. However, the combination with CURB65 did not increase the predictive AUC-ROC of serum biomarker.

There were some limitations in our study. Firstly, the missing data for laboratory biomarkers in some patients, potential classification bias in the etiologic diagnosis. However, our evaluation has been done in a large study population even excluding missing data. Secondly, since the average age of the patients in our study was near 60 years old, whether these results are generalizable to CAP patients in children or aged greater than 80 years old needs further evaluation. Finally, the objects studied usually combined with other diseases, which might affect the serum CRP and PCT levels. But the complicated diseases were the true status for most hospitalized CAP patients. Thus, further studies with a prospective design are needed to explore the influence of other comorbidity on the biomarkers level and hospitalized CAP prognosis.

Conclusions

This is a large and comprehensive study focused on the predictive value of serum dynamic CRP, PCT levels and their clearance in hospitalized CAP outcomes. The low correlations between the two biomarkers and the only moderate prognostic accuracy calls for a head-to-head trial comparing the ability of both markers to monitor the therapeutic effect and to answer the question which marker is superior in the prognosis prediction

Key messages

The dynamic serum CRP and PCT levels have moderate predictive value on the prognosis of hospitalized CAP.

Abbreviations

AUC: Areas under the curve; CAP: Community-acquired pneumonia; CCI: Charlson Comorbidity Index; CI: Confidence interval; CRP: C-reactive protein; CRPc: CRP clearance; PCT: Procalcitonin; PCTc: PCT clearance; ROC: Receiver operating characteristic; VAP: Ventilator- associated pneumonia; WBC: White blood cell count

Funding
This research received no specific grant from any funding agency in the public, commercial, or not for-profit sectors.

Authors' contributions
SG and XM contributed to designing the study, interpreting data, drafting the manuscript. ML contributed to designing the study, acquisition of and interpreting data and approving the final version of the manuscript. All authors read and approved the final manuscript.

Competing interests
The authors declare that there are no competing interests.

Author details
[1]Department of Clinical Laboratory, The First Affiliated Hospital of Zhengzhou University, East Jianshe Road #1, Zhengzhou, Henan 450002, People's Republic of China. [2]Key Clinical Laboratory of Henan province, Zhengzhou, Henan, People's Republic of China. [3]Department of Clinical Laboratory, Henan Provincial People's Hospital, Henan Province, Zhengzhou 450003, People's Republic of China.

References
1. Nouvenne A, Ticinesi A, Folesani G, Cerundolo N, Prati B, Morelli I, Guida L, Lauretani F, Maggio M, Aloe R, et al. The association of serum procalcitonin and high-sensitivity C-reactive protein with pneumonia in elderly multimorbid patients with respiratory symptoms: retrospective cohort study. BMC Geriatr. 2016;16:16.
2. Gonzalez-Castillo J, Martin-Sanchez FJ, Llinares P, Menendez R, Mujal A, Navas E, Barberan J, Spanish Society of Emergency M, Emergency C, Spanish Society of G, et al. Guidelines for the management of community-acquired pneumonia in the elderly patient. Rev Esp Quimioter. 2014;27:69–86.
3. Faverio P, Aliberti S, Bellelli G, Suigo G, Lonni S, Pesci A, Restrepo MI. The management of community-acquired pneumonia in the elderly. Eur J Intern Med. 2014;25:312–9.
4. Cheng CW, Chien MH, Su SC, Yang SF. New markers in pneumonia. Clin Chim Acta. 2013;419:19–25.
5. Agnello L, Bellia C, Di Gangi M, Lo Sasso B, Calvaruso L, Bivona G, Scazzone C, Dones P, Ciaccio M. Utility of serum procalcitonin and C-reactive protein in severity assessment of community-acquired pneumonia in children. Clin Biochem. 2016;49:47–50.
6. Zhydkov A, Christ-Crain M, Thomann R, Hoess C, Henzen C, Werner Z, Mueller B, Schuetz P. Pro HSG: Utility of procalcitonin, C-reactive protein and white blood cells alone and in combination for the prediction of clinical outcomes in community-acquired pneumonia. Clin Chem Lab Med. 2015; 53:559–66.
7. Habib SF, Mukhtar AM, Abdelreheem HM, Khorshied MM, El Sayed R, Hafez MH, Gouda HM, Ghaith DM, Hasanin AM, Eladawy AS, et al. Diagnostic values of CD64, C-reactive protein and procalcitonin in ventilator-associated pneumonia in adult trauma patients: a pilot study. Clin Chem Lab Med. 2016;54:889–95.
8. Ballou SP, Kushner I. C-reactive protein and the acute phase response. Adv Intern Med. 1992;37:313–36.
9. Cabral L, Afreixo V, Almeida L, Paiva JA. The use of Procalcitonin (PCT) for diagnosis of Sepsis in burn patients: a meta-analysis. PLoS One. 2016;11: e0168475.
10. Yan ST, Sun LC, Jia HB, Gao W, Yang JP, Zhang GQ. Procalcitonin levels in bloodstream infections caused by different sources and species of bacteria. Am J Emerg Med. 2017;35:579–83.

11. Porfyridis I, Georgiadis G, Vogazianos P, Mitis G, Georgiou A. C-reactive protein, procalcitonin, clinical pulmonary infection score, and pneumonia severity scores in nursing home acquired pneumonia. Respir Care. 2014;59: 574–81.

12. Steichen O, Bouvard E, Grateau G, Bailleul S, Capeau J, Lefevre G. Diagnostic value of procalcitonin in acutely hospitalized elderly patients. Eur J Clin Microbiol Infect Dis. 2009;28:1471–6.

13. Meili M, Kutz A, Briel M, Christ-Crain M, Bucher HC, Mueller B, Schuetz P. Infection biomarkers in primary care patients with acute respiratory tract infections-comparison of Procalcitonin and C-reactive protein. BMC Pulm Med. 2016;16:43.

14. Khan F, Owens MB, Restrepo M, Povoa P, Martin-Loeches I. Tools for outcome prediction in patients with community acquired pneumonia. Expert Rev Clin Pharmacol. 2017;10:201–11.

15. Yentis SM, Soni N, Sheldon J. C-reactive protein as an indicator of resolution of sepsis in the intensive care unit. Intensive Care Med. 1995;21:602–5.

16. Luyt CE, Guerin V, Combes A, Trouillet JL, Ayed SB, Bernard M, Gibert C, Chastre J. Procalcitonin kinetics as a prognostic marker of ventilator-associated pneumonia. Am J Respir Crit Care Med. 2005;171:48–53.

17. Abula A, Wang Y, Ma L, Yu X. The application value of the procalcitonin clearance rate on therapeutic effect and prognosis of ventilator associated pneumonia. Zhonghua Wei Zhong Bing Ji Jiu Yi Xue. 2014;26:780–4.

18. Huang MY, Chen CY, Chien JH, Wu KH, Chang YJ, Wu KH, Wu HP. Serum Procalcitonin and Procalcitonin clearance as a prognostic biomarker in patients with severe Sepsis and septic shock. Biomed Res Int. 2016;2016: 1758501.

19. Ruiz-Rodriguez JC, Caballero J, Ruiz-Sanmartin A, Ribas VJ, Perez M, Boveda JL, Rello J. Usefulness of procalcitonin clearance as a prognostic biomarker in septic shock. A prospective pilot study. Med Int. 2012;36:475–80.

20. Woodhead M, Blasi F, Ewig S, Huchon G, Ieven M, Ortqvist A, Schaberg T, Torres A, van der Heijden G, Verheij TJ, et al. Guidelines for the management of adult lower respiratory tract infections. Eur Respir J. 2005; 26:1138–80.

21. Principi N, Esposito S, Blasi F, Allegra L. Mowgli study g: role of mycoplasma pneumoniae and chlamydia pneumoniae in children with community-acquired lower respiratory tract infections. Clin Infect Dis. 2001;32:1281–9.

22. Cao B, Huang Y, She DY, Cheng QJ, Fan H, Tian XL, Xu JF, Zhang J, Chen Y, Shen N, et al. Diagnosis and treatment of community-acquired pneumonia in adults: 2016 clinical practice guidelines by the Chinese thoracic society, Chinese Medical Association. Clin Respir J. 2018;12:1320–60.

23. Fine MJ, Auble TE, Yealy DM, Hanusa BH, Weissfeld LA, Singer DE, Coley CM, Marrie TJ, Kapoor WN. A prediction rule to identify low-risk patients with community-acquired pneumonia. N Engl J Med. 1997;336:243–50.

24. Le Bel J, Hausfater P, Chenevier-Gobeaux C, Blanc FX, Benjoar M, Ficko C, Ray P, Choquet C, Duval X, Claessens YE. Group Es: diagnostic accuracy of C-reactive protein and procalcitonin in suspected community-acquired pneumonia adults visiting emergency department and having a systematic thoracic CT scan. Crit Care. 2015;19:366.

25. Colak A, Yilmaz C, Toprak B, Aktogu S. Procalcitonin and CRP as biomarkers in discrimination of community-acquired pneumonia and exacerbation of COPD. J Med Biochem. 2017;36:122–6.

26. Ugajin M, Yamaki K, Hirasawa N, Yagi T. Predictive values of semi-quantitative procalcitonin test and common biomarkers for the clinical outcomes of community-acquired pneumonia. Respir Care. 2014;59:564–73.

27. Fernandez JF, Sibila O, Restrepo MI. Predicting ICU admission in community-acquired pneumonia: clinical scores and biomarkers. Expert Rev Clin Pharmacol. 2012;5:445–58.

28. Kim MW, Lim JY, Oh SH. Mortality prediction using serum biomarkers and various clinical risk scales in community-acquired pneumonia. Scand J Clin Lab Invest. 2017;77:486–92.

29. Schuetz P, Suter-Widmer I, Chaudri A, Christ-Crain M, Zimmerli W, Mueller B. Prognostic value of procalcitonin in community-acquired pneumonia. Eur Respir J. 2011;37:384–92.

30. Ito A, Ishida T, Tachibana H, Ito Y, Takaiwa T. Serial procalcitonin levels for predicting prognosis in community-acquired pneumonia. Respirology. 2016; 21:1459–64.

31. Bouadma L, Luyt CE, Tubach F, Cracco C, Alvarez A, Schwebel C, Schortgen F, Lasocki S, Veber B, Dehoux M, et al. Use of procalcitonin to reduce patients' exposure to antibiotics in intensive care units (PRORATA trial): a multicentre randomised controlled trial. Lancet. 2010;375:463–74.

32. Mokart D, Leone M. Procalcitonin in intensive care units: the PRORATA trial. Lancet. 2010;375:1605. author reply 1606-1607

33. Povoa P, Martin-Loeches I, Ramirez P, Bos LD, Esperatti M, Silvestre J, Gili G, Goma G, Berlanga E, Espasa M, et al. Biomarkers kinetics in the assessment of ventilator-associated pneumonia response to antibiotics - results from the BioVAP study. J Crit Care. 2017;41:91–7.

6

A biomarker basing on radiomics for the prediction of overall survival in non–small cell lung cancer patients

Bo He[1†], Wei Zhao[2†], Jiang-Yuan Pi[3], Dan Han[1], Yuan-Ming Jiang[1], Zhen-Guang Zhang[1] and Wei Zhao[1*]

Abstract

Background: This study aimed at predicting the survival status on non-small cell lung cancer patients with the phenotypic radiomics features obtained from the CT images.

Methods: A total of 186 patients' CT images were used for feature extraction via Pyradiomics. The minority group was balanced via SMOTE method. The final dataset was randomized into training set ($n = 223$) and validation set ($n = 75$) with the ratio of 3:1. Multiple random forest models were trained applying hyperparameters grid search with 10-fold cross-validation using precision or recall as evaluation standard. Then a decision threshold was searched on the selected model. The final model was evaluated through ROC curve and prediction accuracy.

Results: From those segmented images of 186 patients, 1218 features were obtained via feature extraction. The preferred model was selected with recall as evaluation standard and the optimal decision threshold was set 0.56. The model had a prediction accuracy of 89.33% and the AUC score was 0.9296.

Conclusion: A hyperparameters tuning random forest classifier had greater performance in predicting the survival status of non-small cell lung cancer patients, which could be taken for an automated classifier promising to stratify patients.

Keywords: Non-small cell lung cancer, Radiomics, CT, Random forest, Survival status

Background

Lung cancer, one of the highest risky cancers, is the leading cause of cancer death with a high mortality rate of 82.3% in 5 years after diagnosis (National Cancer Institute). [Noone AM, Howlader N, Krapcho M, et al. SEER Cancer Statistics Review, 1975–2015, https://seer.cancer.gov/csr/1975_2015/] Non-small cell lung cancer is a subtype lung cancer, which accounts for 85% among lung cancers [1]. The 5-year survival rate decreases dramatically as the cancer entering advanced, from 40% for stage I to only 1% for stage IV [2, 3]. It was reported that CT texture analysis could be helpful to further classification of treatment as it provided information on the intratumor

heterogeneity [4] which might be the reason for disparate outcomes of patients. Thibaud P. Coroller and etc. used 7 radiomic features to predict pathological response after chemoradiation [5].

In the past 10 years, medical digital image analysis has grown dramatically as advancement of the pattern recognition tools and increase of the data collection. Radiomics offers unlimited imaging biomarkers which are promising to help cancer detection, prognosis and prediction of treatment response [6, 7]. With the high-throughput computing, it's possible to quickly extract various quantitative features from digital images such as MRI and CT. Since cancers are more likely to be temporal and spatial heterogeneous, the use of biopsy might be limited. Furthermore, medical digital imaging could give a whole picture of the tumor shape, texture and volume, and it is also a noninvasive way to get comprehensive tumor information [8]. Some researches indicated that there was a relationship between radiomic features and tumor grades, histology,

* Correspondence: kyyyzhaowei@vip.km169.net

[†]Bo He and Wei Zhao contributed equally to this work.

[1]Department of Medical Imaging, the First Affiliated Hospital of Kunming Medical University, No.295 Xichang Road, Kunming 650032, Yunnan, China

Full list of author information is available at the end of the article

metabolism, and patient survival and clinical outcomes [9–11]. Kitty Huang et al. also found high risk CT features were significantly associated with local recurrence [12]. Chintan et al. studied the prognostic characteristics of radiomic features between lung cancer and head & neck cancer and found association among 11–13 features and prognosis, histology and stage [13]. Jiangdian et al. investigated the prognostic and predictive ability of phenotypic CT features in non-small cell lung cancer patients and reported an overall clinical stage prediction accuracy of 80.33% [14]. Those previous studies have shown that medical image analysis has a promising ability in improving cancer diagnosis, detection, prognostic prediction on oncology [8].

With those antecedent studies, radiomics displayed its hopeful and cost-effective potential in the area of precision oncology. Even though there have been already numerous researches on the prediction of cancer diagnosis or stage classification, most of them used default parameter or manual selection which might not efficient enough. Most of the time default parameters could give us great result, but the ability of the model would be maximized by parameters optimization when we conduct the training stage [15]. This study intended to construct an automatic grid search [16] hyper-parameters tuning classifier to make detections on the survival status of non-small cell lung cancer patients based on the radiomics features. The dataset was randomized into training set and validation set. A random forest classifier with hyperparameters tuning was used to make classification of survival status of non-small cell lung cancer patients in training set. The model was assessed on the validation data by ROC curve as well as the prediction accuracy.

Methods
Data sets
The study included 186 non-small cell lung cancer (NSCLC) patients from two merged datasets R01 and AMC. The patient characteristics and CT images were obtained from the cancer imaging archive (TCIA) database (https://doi.org/10.7937/K9/TCIA.2017.7hs46erv). Clinical data of all 186 NSCLC patients are provided in Table 1, including the gender, smoking history, histology, treatment, and overall survival data. Additional file 1: Table S1 shows detailed staging information.

Feature extraction
One thousand, two hundred eighteen tumor characteristics were quantified by extracted features from the lesion segmented from patients' CT images. The radiomic features can be categorized into four types such as intensity, shape, texture and wavelet. An open-source package in Python, Pyradiomics was used for various features

Table 1 Demographic characteristics

Characteristic	Number of Patients (%)
Gender	
Male	120 (64.5%)
Female	66 (35.5%)
Smoking Status	
Nonsmoker	39 (20.9%)
Former smoker	117 (62.9%)
Current smoker	30 (16.2%)
Histology	
Adenocarcinoma	154 (82.7%)
Squamous cell carcinoma	29 (15.6%)
NOS	3 (1.7%)
Treatment	
Surgery	33 (17.7%)
Chemotherapy	40 (21.5%)
Radiotherapy	19 (10.2%)
Adjuvant Treatment	40 (21.5%)
Unknown	54 (29.1%)
Overall Survival	
Dead	37 (19.9%)
Alive	149 (80.1%)

NOS not otherwise specified
This table displayed the clinical data of all 186 NSCLC patients, including the gender, smoking history, histology, treatment, and overall survival data

extraction from CT images [17]. A list of 50 quantitative features including first order features, shape features, Gray Level Size Zone Matrix (GLSZM) features, Features Gray Level Run Length Matrix (GLRLM) features and etc. were extracted. The shape descriptors were extracted from the label mask and also not associated with gray value.

Data balance and data splitting
Extracted features were then weighted differently as a result of data balancing. In machine learning, algorithms assume the distributions of groups are similar. In practice, when the disproportion of classes happens, the learning algorithms tend to be biased towards the majority class. But in this study, we are more interested in the minority class with more adverse events take place [18]. Due to sample imbalance (the number of being alive is much less than that of being dead), rather than simply applying over-sampling with replacement for data balance, we conducted a synthetic minority over-sampling (SMOTE) method to increase the size of the minority group. SMOTE can be used when the number of the category is larger than 6 since it generated the new examples by taking samples of the feature space for the target class and its 5 nearest neighbors. SMOTE has an

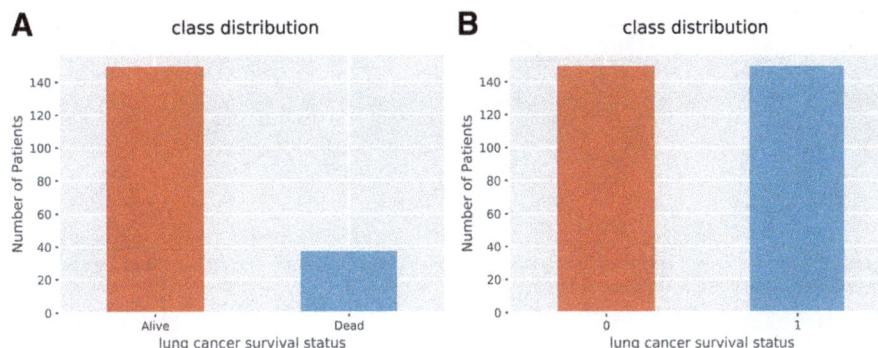

Fig. 1 Survival Status Distribution of Patients. **a** Before oversampling. **b** After oversampling. X axis is the survival status of the patients: the blue bar represents the alive group and the orange bar represents dead group; Y axis is the number of patients in each survival group

advantage of making the decision region of the minority class more general [19, 20]. The final size of the dataset was $n = 298$. Because the minority group was over-sampled thus the dataset was randomized into training set ($n = 223$) and validation set ($n = 75$). The distribution of being alive and dead between training and validation set was also plotted.

Classifier construction

Based on the radiomics features, we aimed to build a radiomics-based survival status prediction model using random forest classifier and hyperparameters tuning in Python [21]. Random forest creates multiple decision trees by randomly choosing subsets of features to make the classification based on the mode (for classification) or the mean (for regression) from all the smaller trees [22, 23]. It has the advantage of being less vulnerable to overfitting problem compared to decision-trees. A generic random forest classifier was constructed first. Parameter estimation using grid search with 10-fold cross-validation was applied to the training data for parameters tunings such as the number of features to consider for the best split (max_feature), the number of trees in the forest (n_estimators), the maximum depth of the tree (max_depth), the minimum number of samples required to split an internal node (min_sample_split). Precision and recall score were used as evaluation standard for parameters tuning respectively. The two best

models with different optimal hyperparameters can be acquired by the top mean precision or recall score respectively. The final preferred model was selected by comparing their performance on the validation data.

Decision threshold adjustment

Instead of directly adopting the absolute predictions, this study also applied for decision value tuning to balance the trade-off between precision and recall. A function of decision values was used to determine the decision threshold of the chosen model to maximize the precision with high recall.

Radiomics model assessment

Model performance was evaluated in terms of the operator characteristic curve (ROC), the area under the curve (AUC) and accuracy, which could quantify the prediction performance of the classifier model.

Results
Class distribution

The class distribution of each class before (Fig. 1a) and after oversampling (Fig. 1b) were presented. It was obvious that after SMOTE method, the number of patient being dead was similar to the number of those being alive. To be note, the sample size after oversampling was 298.

Table 2 Model ranking based on mean precision score

Model	Mean Precision	Mean Recall	Mean Accuracy	Max Depth	Max Features	Min Samples Split	N Estimators
149	0.886	0.892	0.883	15	3	3	1100
252	0.882	0.91	0.888	25	10	3	100
164	0.878	0.901	0.883	15	5	3	500
154	0.878	0.892	0.879	15	3	5	900
233	0.878	0.847	0.861	25	3	10	1100

This table displayed the results of automatic hyper-parameters tuning based on two evaluation standards and ranked the models based on mean precision score. The last four columns represent the values of hyper-parameters of models

Table 3 Model Ranking Based on Mean Recall Score

Model	Mean Precision	Mean Recall	Mean Accuracy	Max Depth	Max Features	Min Samples Split	N Estimators
221	0.886	0.892	0.883	25	3	3	1100
279	0.879	0.892	0.874	25	20	5	700
153	0.884	0.883	0.879	15	3	5	700
225	0.884	0.883	0.879	25	3	5	700
146	0.878	0.883	0.874	15	3	3	500

This table displayed the results of automatic hyper-parameters tuning based on two evaluation standards and ranked the models based on mean recall scores. The last four columns represent the values of hyper-parameters of models

Construction of the survival status prediction model

The construction of the classifier was conducted using a training set consisting of 223 patients with different survive status of NSCLC. Random forest and automatic parameters tuning were applied on the training data to obtain the optimal model. The partial results can be seen in Tables 2 and 3. The confusion matrixes of parameter tuning based on different evaluation standards could be seen in Fig. 2. Comparing the performance of these two models on the validation data, it could draw a conclusion that the model obtained based on recall standard outperformed slightly better than that of precision (The number of correct prediction was slightly larger and false negative was less). The final random forest classifier was constructed using the parameters: 'max_depth': 5, 'max_features': 20, 'min_samples_split': 3 and 'n_estimators': 100. Figure 3 displayed the fifty most important features generated in the random forest by Gini importance. As can be seen from the plot, two large area low gray level emphasis features ranked first and second respectively as the most important features in the prediction model but this did not mean that other features were much less important.

Since when there were multiple correlated features, once a feature was selected the extent to which other features could lead to impurity decreasing dramatically.

Figure 4 listed radiology images from separate body sections of three samples which were chosen randomly and all had certain information and features, such as histology, survival status, first order feature, GLSZM feature and etc. The survival status of (A) was alive, while that of (B) and (C) was dead. In common clinical diagnosis, researchers can make predictions based on the morphology of the lesions. As we can see through picture (A) and (B), size of tumor of (B) was significantly larger than that of (a), and clinicians with few experience could easily make difference of similar cases. However, once there was no distinguishing feature in the radiology images, clinicians hardly could diagnose the illness by naked eye. Through a set of comparison, this study found that a small part of image features had greater ability in prognosis. As a result, features extracted from radiology images were needed for further prognosis. Take (a) and (c) as an example, they are very similar in shape and size, whilst as shown in Table 4, difference in some of their

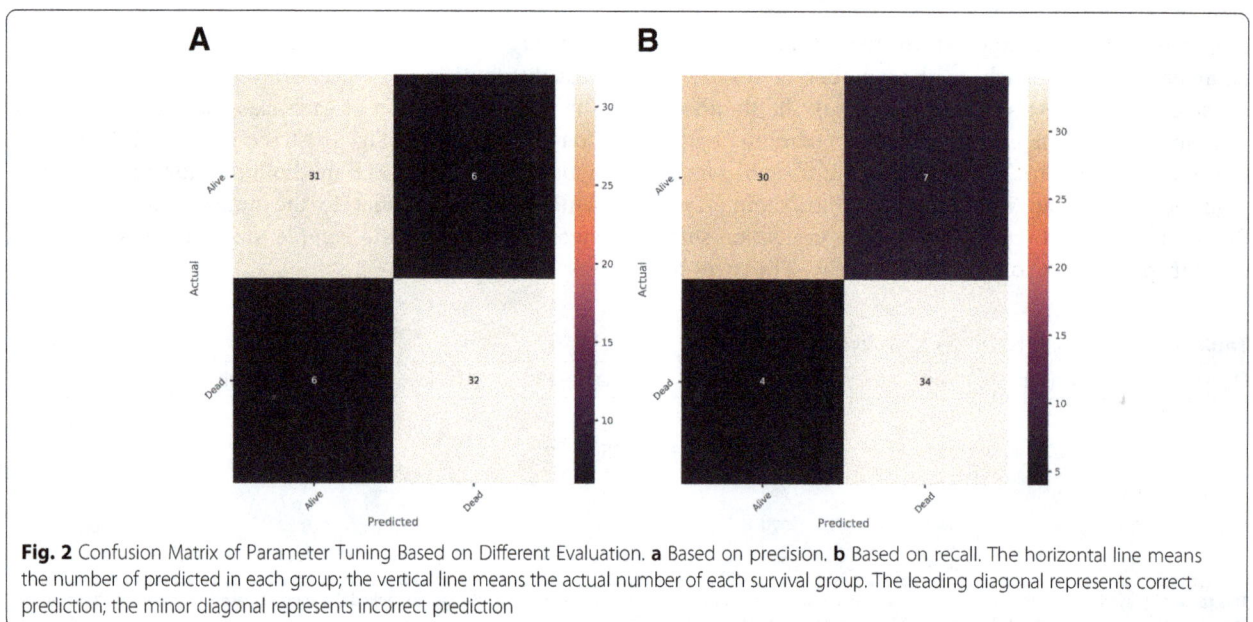

Fig. 2 Confusion Matrix of Parameter Tuning Based on Different Evaluation. **a** Based on precision. **b** Based on recall. The horizontal line means the number of predicted in each group; the vertical line means the actual number of each survival group. The leading diagonal represents correct prediction; the minor diagonal represents incorrect prediction

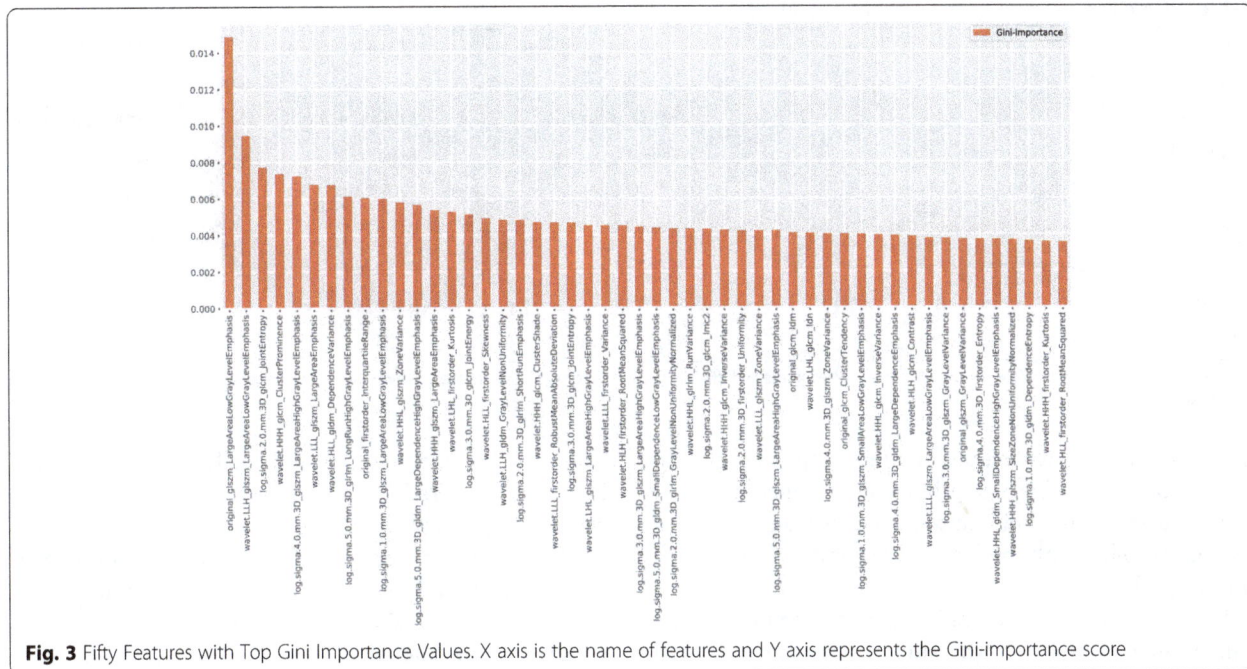

Fig. 3 Fifty Features with Top Gini Importance Values. X axis is the name of features and Y axis represents the Gini-importance score

features, like original_glszm_Large Area Low Gray Level Emphasis, wavelet.LLH_glszm_Large Area Low Gray Level Emphasis, wavelet. HHH_glcm_Cluster Prominence, wavelet.LLL_glszm_Large Area Emphasis and log.sigma. 1.0.mm.3D_glszm_Large AreLowGrayLevelEmphasis is remarkable.

Decision threshold adjustment

After deciding the random forest classifier, we searched for the decision threshold for a trade-off between precision and recall. The default decision threshold in random forest was 0.5. Figure 5 showed precision and recall as a function of decision values, where x represented threshold value and y was the score of precision or recall. The optimal decision threshold was obtained as 0.56 from the intersection point and the precision of the model achieved nearly 90% when recall was around 90%, which was further verified by the precision and recall curve as well as the confusion matrix in Fig. 6.

Performance of Radiomics prediction model

The performance of the classifier constructed was validated according to the receiver operating characteristic (ROC) metrics in the validation set consisting 42 patients. Figure 7 presented the performance results (AUC: area under the ROC curve) obtained in the validation set for the radiomics model. The prediction accuracy was 89.33% (The percentage of correct classification). The AUC score for this model was 0.9296, which meant the model had a great ability of predicting being alive or being dead.

Discussion

Radiomics has gained great attention as a potential method to promote personal medicine. Its image signatures derived from digital images are promising to help diagnostics and prognostics [24]. It has been shown that features such as texture, shape and intensity had prognostic power in independent data of lung and head-and-neck cancer patients since they were able to capture the intratumor heterogeneity [25]. Applying

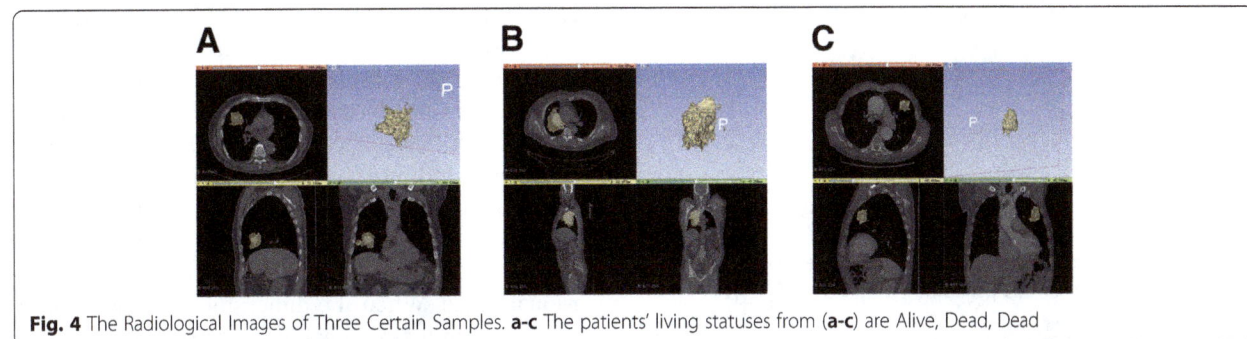

Fig. 4 The Radiological Images of Three Certain Samples. **a-c** The patients' living statuses from (**a-c**) are Alive, Dead, Dead

Table 4 Basic information and the value of certain features of three cases

Features	R01–005	R01–006	R01–129
Case ID			
Histology	Adenocarcinoma	Adenocarcinoma	Adenocarcinoma
Survival Status	Alive	Alive	Dead
original_glszm_LargeAreaLowGrayLevelEmphasis	0.023323	0.330361	100.1903
wavelet.LLH_glszm_LargeAreaLowGrayLevelEmphasis	0.001637	0.008254	2.941066
wavelet.HHH_glcm_ClusterProminence	400.5173	413.4463	8.821475
wavelet.LLL_glszm_LargeAreaEmphasis	2.594846	8.408592	191.8787
wavelet.HLL_gldm_DependenceVariance	0.137999	1.28458	16.99916

It is shown in the table that different survival status corresponds to different level of feature, and it is noteworthy that the difference between them is distinguishing

machine learning techniques on the output data from radiomics has also become a hot topic in oncology, personalized medicine and computer aided diagnosis since its compatibility with the big data generated from digital images [26].

This study intended to predict the non-small cell lung cancer survival status with radiomics features. A total of 1218 features were obtained after feature derivation using Pyradiomics. And those features captured the information about tumor shape, intensity and texture. Data imbalance is always a common problem in classification problem since most interested events like disease, network intrusion and etc. are rare. When sample size is large enough, slight or medium imbalance is not a big problem for training since there is enough information for learning from the minority class. However,

when sample size is small, especially for decision tree the leaves that predict the minority class are likely to be pruned [27]. Thus, in this study, a SMOTE oversampling method was necessary to decrease the training fit error. The model was trained with automatic hyperparameters tuning aiming to make use of the best potential of our model. One common problem with hyperparameter tuning is overfitting, which means that the model performs well on the training data but poorly on the test data. This issue can be amended by using cross-validation where the model performance is evaluated by averaging k models. This study skipped the part of feature selection for two reasons: one was that the sample feature ratio was not low to introduce overfitting and another one was that random forest with parameters tuning was powerful since it optimized the number of tress and selected the best feature at each node. The final result of our study also proved that the model without feature selection had a great generalization on the test data.

Moreover, we studied how the adjustment of decision values impacted the precision and accuracy because a good classification model was not only evaluated on the accuracy. Precision and recall are further standards for model evaluation but there is a trade-off between them. Precision decreases as recall increases [28]. For survival status prediction, it is important to differentiate the death to stratify the patient into high risk group automatically. Thus, it might be more cost expensive to misidentify the high-risk patients. Without further test data validation, the result after decision threshold adjustment could be optimistic. However, this study gave a reference for the decision threshold of a non-small cell patient not being alive based on the radiomic feature. This may indicate that radiomics is promising into automatic computer aided patient risk stratification in a non-invasive way. For hyperparameters tuning, this study used grid search, which performed well in low dimensional space. When the dimension space is large or unknown, random search could be considered [2].

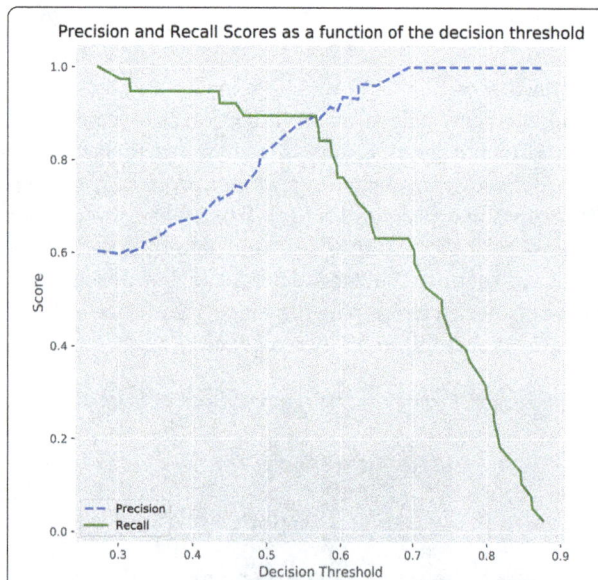

Fig. 5 Precision and Recall Score as a Function of Decision Values. Blue dashed line: precision score; Green line: recall score. Y axis in the score value and X axis is decision threshold value. The intersection of the two curves are the optimal point where the trade-off of precision and recall is achieved

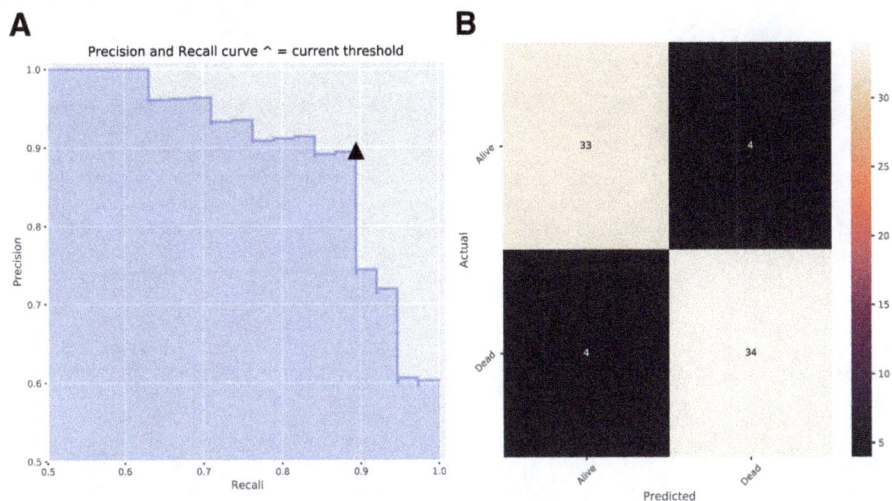

Fig. 6 Precision and Recall with the Determined Decision Threshold. **a** Precision and Recall Curve (This curve shows how recall and precision changes as the decision threshold value changes. The triangle represents the decision threshold we chose). **b** Confusion Matrix. The horizontal line means the number of predicted in each group; the vertical line means the actual number of each survival group. The leading diagonal represents correct prediction; the minor diagonal represents incorrect prediction

Despite of the satisfactory model performance, the study had a few limitations. First, since all training and testing data were acquired from one study, it may not be generalized to all cases [29] with a more heterogeneous dataset, and the accuracy might be lower than the current study. The extents to which the data we used are representative to the real situation also affect how well the trained model could perform in the practical use. Thus, different CT images from different sources are needed to construct a more rigorous and general classification model. The second limitation of the study is disproportion of patients at different disease stages. According to Table 2, the number of people with specific characteristic was far more than the rest, which means patient with a certain stage of the cancer might have more images or more pathologic images. For instance, there were 154 Adenocarcinoma patients, 29 Squamous cell carcinoma patients, and 3 not otherwise specified (NOS) patients.

For future research, more data from diverse patients' background, different databases, and multiple image modalities should be utilized for further testing and validation. Other mathematical model can be developed to improve feature extraction. Our model can be adopted to improve the performance of classifier. The most relevant features can provide useful information for future exploration to develop a better detection method. Also, with larger dataset, different classification criteria can be tuned according to the different types of lung cancer and disease stages.

Conclusion

To conclude, this study intended to construct a survival status classifier with automatic hyperparameters tuning. In order to optimize classification outcomes, the tuning of decision threshold can serve as a reference for future work. Our classification methods has the potential to contribute to a survival prediction model, which is beneficial to better palliative care and treatment decision.

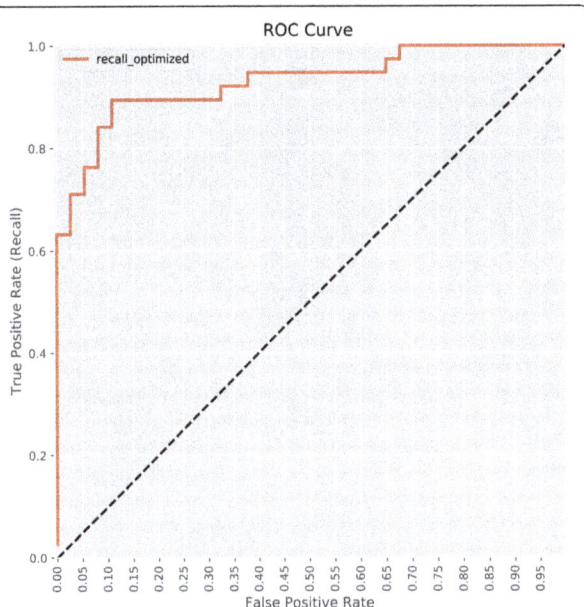

Fig. 7 The ROC curve for Random Forest Model Performance on the Validation Data. X axis represents false positive rate ($\frac{FP}{TN+FP}$) and Y axis is true positive rate ($\frac{TP}{TP+FN}$). The diagonal dashed line means random prediction

Abbreviations

AUC: Area under the curve; GLRLM: Gray Level Run Length Matrix; GLSZM: Gray Level Size Zone Matrix; NSCLC: Non-small cell lung cancer; ROC: Receiver operating characteristic; SMOTE: Synthetic minority over-sampling; TCIA: The cancer imaging archive

Funding

This work was supported by Yunnan Provincial Health Science and Technology Project (2009NS102, 2010NS027, 2011WS0042 & 2012WS0017) and Scientific Research Projects of Research Institutes in Yunnan Medical and Health Units (2017NS037).

Authors' contributions

Substantial contribution to the conception and design of the work: BH + JYP; Analysis and interpretation of the data: DH + ZGZ; Drafting the manuscript: BH + YMJ; Revising the work critically for important intellectual content: WZ; Collection of grants: WZ; Final approval of the work: all authors. All authors read and approved the final manuscript.

Competing interests

The authors declare that they have no competing interests.

Author details

[1]Department of Medical Imaging, the First Affiliated Hospital of Kunming Medical University, No.295 Xichang Road, Kunming 650032, Yunnan, China. [2]Department of Thoracic Surgery, the First Affiliated Hospital of Kunming Medical University, Kunming 650032, Yunnan, China. [3]Department of Pathology, Kunming Medical University, Kunming 650500, Yunnan, China.

References

1. Parmar C, Leijenaar RTH, Grossmann P, Rios Velazquez E, Bussink J, Rietveld D, Rietbergen MM, Haibe-Kains B, Lambin P, Aerts HJWL. Radiomic feature clusters and prognostic signatures specific for lung and head & neck cancer. Sci Rep. 2015;5:11044.
2. Song J, Liu Z, Zhong W, Huang Y, Ma Z, Dong D, Liang C, Tian J. Non-small cell lung cancer: quantitative phenotypic analysis of CT images as a potential marker of prognosis. Sci Rep. 2016;6:38282.
3. Herbst RS, Heymach JV, Lippman SM. Lung cancer. N Engl J Med. 2008;359: 1367-80.
4. Cetin K, Ettinger DS, Hei Y, O'Malley CD. Survival by histologic subtype in stage IV nonsmall cell lung cancer based on data from the surveillance, epidemiology and end results program. Clin Epidemiol. 2011;3:139-48.
5. Miles KA. How to use CT texture analysis for prognostication of non-small cell lung cancer. Cancer Imaging. 2016;16:10.
6. Xu X, Huang Z, Graves D, Pedrycz W. A clustering-based graph Laplacian framework for value function approximation in reinforcement learning. IEEE Trans Cybern. 2014;44:2613-25.
7. Bergstra J, Bengio Y. Random search for hyper-parameter optimization. J Mach Learn Res. 2012;13:281-305.
8. Gillies RJ, Kinahan PE, Hricak H. Radiomics: images are more than pictures, they are data. Radiology. 2016;278:563-77.
9. Leijenaar RT, Carvalho S, Velazquez ER, van Elmpt WJ, Parmar C, Hoekstra OS, Hoekstra CJ, Boellaard R, Dekker AL, Gillies RJ. Stability of FDG-PET Radiomics features: an integrated analysis of test-retest and inter-observer variability. Acta Oncol. 2013;52:1391-7.
10. Kazachkina S, Balakhonova T, Lupanov V, Pogorelova O, Rogoza A, Naumov V. High quality machine-robust image features: identification in nonsmall cell lung cancer computed tomography images. BMC Health Serv Res. 2015;15:1-10.

11. Alic L, Niessen WJ, Veenland JF. Quantification of heterogeneity as a biomarker in tumor imaging: a systematic review. PLoS One. 2014;9:e110300.
12. Segal E, Sirlin CB, Ooi C, Adler AS, Gollub J, Chen X, Chan BK, Matcuk GR, Barry CT, Chang HY. Decoding global gene expression programs in liver cancer by noninvasive imaging. Nat Biotechnol. 2007;25:675.
13. Hui L, Zhu Y, Burnside ES, Drukker K, Hoadley KA, Cheng F, Conzen SD, Whitman GJ, Sutton EJ, Net JM. MR imaging Radiomics signatures for predicting the risk of breast Cancer recurrence as given by research versions of MammaPrint, Oncotype DX, and PAM50 gene assays. Radiology. 2016;281:152110.
14. Huang K, Senthi S, Palma DA, Spoelstra FO, Warner A, Slotman BJ, Senan S. High-risk CT features for detection of local recurrence after stereotactic ablative radiotherapy for lung cancer. Radiother Oncol J Eur Soc Ther Radiol Oncology. 2013;87:S204.
15. Fried DV, Tucker SL, Zhou S, Liao Z, Mawlawi O, Ibbott G, Court LE. Prognostic value and reproducibility of pretreatment CT texture features in stage III non-small cell lung cancer. Int J Radiat Oncol Biol Phys. 2014;90:834-42.
16. Coroller TP, Agrawal V, Narayan V, Hou Y, Grossmann P, Lee SW, Mak RH, Aerts HJ. Radiomic phenotype features predict pathological response in non-small cell lung cancer. Radiother Oncol J Eur Soc Ther Radiol Oncol. 2016;119:480-6.
17. Jjm VG, Fedorov A, Parmar C, Hosny A, Aucoin N, Narayan V, Rgh BT, Fillion-Robin JC, Pieper S, Hjwl A. Computational Radiomics system to decode the radiographic phenotype. Cancer Res. 2017;77:e104.
18. Krawczyk B. Learning from imbalanced data: open challenges and future directions. Prog Artif Int. 2016;5:1-12.
19. Chawla NV, Bowyer KW, Hall LO, Kegelmeyer WP. SMOTE: synthetic minority over-sampling technique. J Artif Intell Res. 2002;16:321-57.
20. Lemaitre G, Nogueira F, Aridas CK. Imbalanced-learn: a python toolbox to tackle the curse of imbalanced datasets in machine learning. J Mach Learn Res. 2017;18(1):559-63.
21. Pedregosa F, Gramfort A, Michel V, Thirion B, Grisel O, Blondel M, Prettenhofer P, Weiss R, Dubourg V, Vanderplas J. Scikit-learn: machine learning in Python. J Mach Learn Res. 2012;12:2825-30.
22. Quadrianto N, Ghahramani Z. A very simple safe-Bayesian random Forest. IEEE Trans Pattern Anal Mach Intell. 2015;37:1297-303.
23. Liu X, Song M, Tao D, Liu Z, Zhang L, Chen C, Bu J. Random forest construction with robust semisupervised node splitting. IEEE Trans Image Process. 2015;24:471-83.
24. Lambin P, Leijenaar RTH, Deist TM, Peerlings J, Jong EECD, Timmeren JV, Sanduleanu S, Larue RTHM, Even AJG, Jochems A. Radiomics: the bridge between medical imaging and personalized medicine. Nat Rev Clin Oncol. 2017;14:749.
25. Aerts HJWL, Velazquez ER, Leijenaar RTH, Parmar C, Grossmann P, Cavalho S, Bussink J, Monshouwer R, Haibekains B, Rietveld D. Decoding tumour phenotype by noninvasive imaging using a quantitative radiomics approach. Nat Commun. 2014;5:4006.
26. Parmar C, Grossmann P, Bussink J, Lambin P, Aerts HJ. Machine learning methods for quantitative Radiomic biomarkers. Sci Rep. 2015;5:13087.
27. SUN Y, AKC WONG, MS KAMEL. Classification of imbalanced data: a review. Int J Pattern Recognit Artif Intell. 2009;23:687-719.
28. Davis J, Goadrich M. The relationship between Precision-Recall and ROC curves. In ICML '06 : Proceedings of the International Conference on Machine Learning. New York: 2006. p. 233-40.
29. Yu KH, Zhang C, Berry GJ, Altman RB, Ré C, Rubin DL, Snyder M. Predicting non-small cell lung cancer prognosis by fully automated microscopic pathology image features. Nat Commun. 2016;7:12474.

7

Childhood asthma is associated with COPD and known asthma variants in COPDGene: a genome-wide association study

Lystra P. Hayden[1,2]* (iD), Michael H. Cho[2,3], Benjamin A. Raby[1,2,3], Terri H. Beaty[4], Edwin K. Silverman[2,3], Craig P. Hersh[2,3] and on behalf of the COPDGene Investigators

Abstract

Background: Childhood asthma is strongly influenced by genetics and is a risk factor for reduced lung function and chronic obstructive pulmonary disease (COPD) in adults. This study investigates self-reported childhood asthma in adult smokers from the COPDGene Study. We hypothesize that childhood asthma is associated with decreased lung function, increased risk for COPD, and that a genome-wide association study (GWAS) will show association with established asthma variants.

Methods: We evaluated current and former smokers ages 45–80 of non-Hispanic white (NHW) or African American (AA) race. Childhood asthma was defined by self-report of asthma, diagnosed by a medical professional, with onset at < 16 years or during childhood. Subjects with a history of childhood asthma were compared to those who never had asthma based on lung function, development of COPD, and genetic variation. GWAS was performed in NHW and AA populations, and combined in meta-analysis. Two sets of established asthma SNPs from published literature were examined for association with childhood asthma.

Results: Among 10,199 adult smokers, 730 (7%) reported childhood asthma and 7493 (73%) reported no history of asthma. Childhood asthmatics had reduced lung function and increased risk for COPD (OR 3.42, 95% CI 2.81–4.18). Genotype data was assessed for 8031 subjects. Among NHWs, 391(7%) had childhood asthma, and GWAS identified one genome-wide significant association in *KIAA1958* (rs59289606, $p = 4.82 \times 10^{-8}$). Among AAs, 339 (12%) had childhood asthma. No SNPs reached genome-wide significance in the AAs or in the meta-analysis combining NHW and AA subjects; however, potential regions of interest were identified. Established asthma SNPs were examined, seven from the NHGRI-EBI database and five with genome-wide significance in the largest pediatric asthma GWAS. Associations were found in the current childhood asthma GWAS with known asthma loci in *IL1RL1*, *IL13*, *LINC01149*, near *GSDMB*, and in the *C11orf30-LRRC32* region (Bonferroni adjusted $p < 0.05$ for all comparisons).

Conclusions: Childhood asthmatics are at increased risk for COPD. Defining asthma by self-report is valid in populations at risk for COPD, identifying subjects with clinical and genetic characteristics known to associate with childhood asthma. This has potential to improve clinical understanding of asthma-COPD overlap (ACO) and enhance future research into ACO-specific treatment regimens.

Trial registration: ClinicalTrials.gov, NCT00608764 (Active since January 28, 2008).

Keywords: Childhood asthma, Genome-wide association study, Chronic obstructive pulmonary disease, Lung function, Genetic epidemiology

* Correspondence: Lystra.Hayden@childrens.harvard.edu
[1]Division of Respiratory Diseases, Boston Children's Hospital, Boston, MA, USA
[2]Channing Division of Network Medicine, Brigham and Women's Hospital,
181 Longwood Avenue, Boston, MA 02115, USA
Full list of author information is available at the end of the article

Background

Asthma is the most common chronic disease of childhood, affecting 8.4% of children in the United States [1]. Childhood asthma is a genetically distinct asthma subtype, with estimated heritability of 68–92% [2–10]. Asthma is a known risk factor for development of reduced lung function and chronic obstructive pulmonary disease (COPD) in adults [11–14]. Asthmatics are often excluded from COPD studies, and thus information on the mechanism of disease and appropriate treatments for asthma-COPD overlap (ACO) remains limited [15].

We have previously examined self-reported history of childhood asthma and ACO in the COPDGene Study, a cohort of more than 10,000 adult smokers with and without COPD. We have shown that a combined history of childhood pneumonia with childhood asthma is a risk factor for developing COPD [16]. We demonstrated that that ACO subjects were younger with a lower lifetime smoking intensity, and that both childhood asthmatics and ACO subjects have increased airways disease on chest computed tomography scan [17–19]. Longitudinal analysis has shown that early-life asthmatics do not have increased rates of lung function decline despite their increased exacerbation frequency [20]. We have not previously examined childhood asthma as an independent risk factor for COPD in this population.

As interest in the long-term outcomes of early-life asthmatics has expanded, a recurring question has risen about the validity of using self-reported asthma history in large adult cohorts recruited for genetic epidemiology studies [21, 22]. This has been particularly important when trying to understand Asthma-COPD Overlap (ACO), as epidemiologic studies of COPD, an adult disease, rely on self-reported history of asthma early in life both for exclusion criteria and for analysis [15, 23]. Our current investigation examines self-reported childhood asthma in adult smokers from the COPDGene Study, to see if they share similar phenotypes and genotypes with those seen in asthmatic subjects from prior studies, including published GWAS [2, 3, 24]. Prior GWAS have implicated genetic susceptibility specific to childhood asthma, including variants in *ORMDL3/GSDMB*, *IL1RL1*, *IL33*, and *RAD50* [4, 7, 24]. We hypothesize that self-reported history of childhood asthma will be associated with decreased lung function and increased risk for COPD in adult smokers, and that a genome-wide association study (GWAS) will show an increased prevalence of known asthma variants among childhood asthmatics, compared to those subjects who never had asthma.

Methods
Subjects
We evaluated 10,199 current and former adult smokers enrolled in the COPDGene Study between 2008 and 2011 (August 31, 2016 dataset). The COPDGene Study is a multicenter, observational study designed to identify genetic and environmental factors associated with COPD. Subjects included were of non-Hispanic (NHW) white or African American (AA) race, between 45 and 80 years of age, and had at least a 10 pack-year history of smoking. We excluded subjects with lung disease other than asthma or COPD, or those who were non-smokers. Subjects were recruited at 21 clinical sites within the U.S. Each site received institutional review board approval and each participant provided informed consent [25]. Details of the study protocol and data forms are available at www.copdgene.org [25, 26].

Data collection
Subject responses to a modified American Thoracic Society Respiratory Epidemiology Questionnaire were used to collect asthma history [26, 27]. A standardized spirometry protocol pre and post-albuterol was completed (ndd EasyOne Spirometer, Zurich, Switzerland). DNA extracted from blood samples was genotyped using HumanOmniExpress arrays (Illumina, San Diego, CA). DNA and single nucleotide polymorphism (SNP) data underwent standard quality control measures [25, 28, 29]. Imputation used 1000 Genomes Phase I v3 reference panels (hg19) to obtain additional genotypes with MaCH and minimac (exomeChip pipelineV1.4) [29–32]. Imputation quality was assessed using Rsq, and SNPs with Rsq > 0.3 were considered to be of acceptable quality. COPD-Gene datasets are publicly available (dbGaP accession number phs000179.v1.p1).

Case identification
Asthma history was assessed by questionnaire response. Subjects were asked if they had ever had asthma, at what age it started, and if it was diagnosed by a doctor or other health professional. Childhood asthma was defined as self-report of asthma diagnosed by a health professional with age of onset at < 16 years or as a child with exact age not known [5, 16, 20, 33]. Subjects were classified as never having asthma if they responded "No" to asthma history on the questionnaire. As in previous COPDGene publications, COPD was defined as Global Initiative for Chronic Obstructive Lung Disease (GOLD) 2007 spirometry grades 2–4, corresponding to post-bronchodilator forced expiratory volume in the first second (FEV_1) to forced vital capacity (FVC) ratio < 0.7 with FEV_1 < 80% predicted [16–18, 20, 34]. Control smokers had normal spirometry, defined as FEV_1/FVC ≥ 0.7 and FEV_1 ≥ 80%.

Statistical analysis
Subjects with childhood asthma were compared to subjects who never had asthma on measures of lung function

Childhood asthma is associated with COPD and known asthma variants...

61

and development of COPD. Subjects with missing or unclassifiable responses were removed from the specific analysis. Statistical analysis used R v3.1.1. Single variable analysis used chi-square tests, Wilcoxon rank sum tests, or t-tests. Multivariable regression analysis was performed, all models were adjusted for number of pack years of smoking history. COPD and FEV_1/FVC models were additionally adjusted for gender, age at enrollment, and race. The FEV_1/FVC model was also adjusted for height; percent predicted FEV_1 and FVC values have these factors accounted for in the baseline variable thus no adjustment was indicated. Logistic regression reported odds ratio (OR) with 95% confidence interval (CI) and linear regression reported absolute difference (β) with standard error (SE).

GWAS were performed comparing those with history of childhood asthma to those who never had asthma using PLINK 1.90 [35]. GWAS were performed in the NHW and AA populations separately using logistic regression adjusted for sex and principal components (PC) for genetic ancestry [28]. SNPs were considered to reach genome-wide significance at the threshold of $p \leq 5 \times 10^{-8}$, and regions of interest were identified at near genome-wide significance with $p \leq 1 \times 10^{-6}$ [36, 37]. The degree of genomic inflation after PC adjustment was assessed [38]. Results from the NHW and AA populations were combined in a fixed effects meta-analysis with inverse variance weighting [35, 39].

Comparison to published asthma GWAS
The childhood asthma GWAS results were examined for association with established asthma SNPs derived from the National Human Genome Research Institute - European Bioinformatics Institute (NHGRI-EBI) Catalog of published genome-wide association studies (Sept 28, 2017 search, https://www.ebi.ac.uk/gwas/search) [2, 3]. A search for the disease/trait "asthma" identified 85 studies, with 600 SNP associations. Eight SNPs were identified in more than one NHGRI-EBI catalog study, and were considered established asthma SNPs: rs10197862 in *IL1RL1*, rs1837253 near *TSLP*, rs2244012 in *RAD50*, rs1295686 in *IL13*, rs7130588 near the *C11orf30-LRRC32* region, rs3894194 in *GSDMA*, rs2305480 and rs11078927 in *GSDMB* [7, 40–50]. Two *GSDMB* SNPs were in high linkage disequilibrium ($r^2 > 0.8$). We selected the SNP that was genotyped in our population, rs2305480, for inclusion, and rs11078927 was excluded, leaving seven established asthma SNPs. These seven established asthma SNPs were examined for association with childhood asthma in the current GWAS, with a Bonferroni correction for seven tests performed, and a significance level of 0.05. Hypergeometric testing was used to calculate the likelihood that the established asthma SNPs were over-represented in this sample.

The childhood asthma GWAS results were additionally examined for association with the five genetic loci found to be associated with pediatric asthma in the largest pediatric asthma GWAS to date (8976 cases, 18,399 controls) from the Trans-National Asthma Genetic Consortium (TAGC): rs4988958 in *IL1RL1*, rs1295685 in *IL13*, rs2596464 in *LINC01149*, rs12551256 in *IL33*, rs8069176 near *GSDMB* [24]. These five TAGC pediatric asthma SNPs were examined for association with childhood asthma in the current GWAS, with a Bonferroni correction for five tests performed, and a significance level of 0.05.

Results
Subject classification
Of 10,199 subjects in the COPDGene study, 730 (7%) had childhood asthma and 7493 (73%) were control subjects without childhood asthma (Table 1). There were 1976 subjects removed from the analysis: 52 with responses to the childhood asthma questions that were not classifiable, 1229 who reported a history of asthma that did not start in childhood, and 695 who reported they did not know if they had asthma (Additional file 1: Figure S1).

Subject characteristics
Compared to subjects without childhood asthma, those with history of childhood asthma were younger and more likely to be AA. Subjects with childhood asthma had increased odds of developing COPD (OR 3.42, 95% CI 2.81–4.18) (Table 2). When compared to those without childhood asthma, adult smokers with asthma during childhood also had reduced lung function measured by FEV_1, FVC and FEV_1/FVC ($p < 0.001$ for all comparisons).

GWAS
Genotype data was assessed in 8031 subjects who met case/control criteria (Additional file 1: Figure S1). Among the 5364 NHWs, there were 385 (7%) childhood asthma

Table 1 Characteristics of childhood asthma subjects compared to subjects without asthma in COPDGene

	Childhood Asthma N = 730	Never Asthma N = 7493	P-value
Male gender (%)[a]	388 (53%)	4255 (57%)	0.06
Mean age, year (SD)[c]	58 (9)	60 (9)	< 0.001
Non-Hispanic white (%)[a]	391 (54%)	5075 (68%)	< 0.001
African American (%)[a]	339 (46%)	2418 (32%)	< 0.001
Pack-years of smoking (SD)[b]	43 (25)	44 (25)	0.09
Current smoking (%)[a]	410 (56%)	4041 (54%)	0.26
History of hay fever (%)[a]	385 (53%)	1727 (23%)	< 0.001

Univariate analysis with [a] Chi-square [b] Wilcoxon rank sum test [c] t-test

Table 2 COPD and lung function in subjects with childhood asthma compared to never asthma subjects

	Childhood Asthma N = 730	Never Asthma N = 7493	Impact of Childhood Asthma		
			OR	95% CI	P-value[a]
COPD (%)[b,d, e]	341 (47%)	2303 (31%)	3.42	(2.81, 4.18)	< 0.001
			β	SE	P-value
FEV$_1$ post-bronchodilator % predicted (SD)[c,d]	69% (25)	80% (26)	−10.44	0.92	< 0.001
FVC post-bronchodilator % predicted (SD)[c,d]	83% (19)	89% (18)	−6.01	0.68	< 0.001
FEV$_1$/FVC post-bronchodilator (SD)[c,d,e,f]	0.64 (0.16)	0.68 (0.16)	−0.06	0.01	< 0.001

Abbreviations: *COPD* chronic obstructive pulmonary disease; *FEV$_1$* forced expiratory volume in the first second; *SD* standard deviation; *FVC* forced vital capacity.
[a]Each row is a separate model: [b]Logistic regression with odds ratio (OR), 95% confidence interval (CI); [c]Linear regression with beta coefficient (β), standard error (SE). Covariates: [d]pack years; [e]gender, age at enrollment, race; [f]height

cases and 4979 (93%) controls without childhood asthma. Among the 2667 AAs, there were 325 (12%) childhood asthma cases and 2342 (88%) controls. NHW and AA GWAS included all SNPs with minor allele frequency (MAF) ≥ 5%, Quantile-Quantile (QQ) and Manhattan plots including can be viewed in Additional file 1: Figure S2 and S3. Lambda values were 1.01 in both NHW and AA populations. Meta-analysis included all SNPs with MAF ≥ 1%, with a lower MAF cutoff used to account for the more modest correlation of variants between ancestries; QQ and Manhattan plots are in Additional file 1: Figure S4 [39, 51].

In the NHW childhood asthma GWAS, one SNP reached the level of genome-wide significance, rs59289606 located in the gene *KIAA1958* ($p = 4.82 \times 10^{-8}$) (Table 3, Fig. 1, Additional file 1: Figure S2). An additional region of interest was identified in *PDZD2* with three SNPs approaching genome-wide significance ($p = 3.9–7.80 \times 10^{-7}$) (Additional file 1: Figure S5). In the AA childhood asthma GWAS, no SNPs reached the level of genome-wide significance, however, regions of interest were identified in *FLJ12825* ($p = 1.75 \times 10^{-7}$) and *PHF14* ($p = 4.94 \times 10^{-7}$) (Additional file 1: Figure S6). Meta-analysis combined the NHW and AA results from this study. No meta-analysis SNPs reached the level of genome-wide significance. However, a region of interest was identified in *SCHIP1* and its read through transcript *IQCJ-SCHIP1* with 14 SNPs approaching genome-wide significance ($p = 2.39–7.84 \times 10^{-7}$) (Fig. 1).

Association testing of established asthma variants
Seven NHGRI-EBI SNPs previously known to be associated with asthma were extracted from the current GWAS results (Table 4). Among the NHW population, the childhood asthma GWAS found association with a known asthma variants in *IL1RL1* (rs10197862, adjusted $p = 0.011$) and approached significance in *GSDMB* (rs2305480, adjusted $p = 0.060$) and near the *C11orf30-LRRC32* region (rs7130588, adjusted $p = 0.054$) (Additional file 1: Figure S7). The meta-analysis of NHW and AA

subjects in our childhood asthma GWAS found association with known asthma variants in *IL1RL1* (rs10197862, adjusted $p = 0.042$), in *IL13* (rs1295686, adjusted $p = 0.043$), and near the *C11orf30-LRRC32* region (rs7130588, adjusted $p = 0.005$) (Additional file 1: Figure S8). There is agreement in direction of effect in these four associated or near associated SNPs in both NHW and AA populations as well as with prior published GWAS [7, 40, 44, 45, 49, 50]. Hypergeometric testing showed that when selecting seven SNPs from the meta-analysis population, the probability of having one or more SNP significant at this level was $p = 0.034$. Among the meta-analysis population, when selecting seven SNPs, the probability of having three or more SNP significant at this level was $p = 1.21 \times 10^{-05}$.

Five SNPs associated with pediatric asthma in the TAGC GWAS were examined within the current GWAS results (Additional file 1: Table S1). Reported *p*-values were Bonferroni corrected for five tests, with a significance level of 0.05. Among the NHW population, the childhood asthma GWAS found association with TAGC pediatric asthma SNPs in *IL1RL1* (rs4988958, adjusted $p = 0.002$), *LINC01149* (rs2596464, adjusted $p = 0.021$), and near the *GSDMB* region (rs8069176, adjusted $p = 0.041$). The meta-analysis of NHW and AA subjects in out childhood asthma GWAS found association with *IL1RL1* (rs4988958, adjusted $p = 0.035$) and *LINC01149* (rs2596464, adjusted $p = 0.017$).

Discussion
This analysis is the first to demonstrate that a self-reported history of childhood asthma is a valid method for defining a population that phenotypically and genetically represent asthmatic subjects among a cohort of adult smokers at risk for COPD. When compared to those who never had asthma, self-reported childhood asthmatics were younger at study enrollment, more likely to be of AA race, and had decreased lung function with greater odds of developing COPD. Three of seven established NHGRI-EBI asthma SNPs and three of five pediatric asthma SNPs from the TAGS GWAS were associated with self-reported childhood

Table 3 Top SNPs from childhood asthma GWAS in COPDGene[e]

	Locus	SNP	Effect Allele	OR	Rsq	Freq (%)	P-value[b,d]	Gene Symbol	Gene Name
NHW[a]	9q32	rs59289606	A	2.06	0.38	20%	4.82E-08	KIAA1958	
(8,900,203 SNPs)	5p13.3	rs439399	C	1.52	0.99	22%	3.90E-07	PDZD2	PDZ domain containing 2
AA[a]	12q13.13	rs7315121	T	2.90	0.45	7%	1.75E-07	FLJ12825	uncharacterized LOC440101
(15,374,350 SNPs)	7p21.3	rs56317450	A	2.11	0.79	8%	4.94E-07	PHF14	PHD finger protein 14

	Locus	SNP	Effect Allele	OR	Rsq NHW, AA	Freq (%) NHW, AA	I^2	P-value[c,d]	Gene Symbol	Gene Name
Meta-analysis (7,658,992 SNPs)	3q25.32-q25.33	rs4679858	G	1.48	0.99, 0.98	14%, 12%	0	2.39E-07	SCHIP1 IQCJ-SCHIP1	schwannomin interacting protein 1 & the readthrough

Abbreviations: *GWAS* genome-wide association study; *NHW* Non-Hispanic Whites; *AA* African American; *SNP* single nucleotide polymorphism; *OR* odds ratio of effect allele; *Rsq* estimation of imputation quality; *Freq* frequency of effect allele; I^2 heterogeneity index; [a] Each population was run as an independent analysis, and then combined in the meta-analysis: [b] Logistic regression based on case control status; [c] Fixed effect meta-analysis weighted by inverse variance. [d] Adjusted for sex, genetic ancestry. [e] Includes the top SNP from each region with GWAS P-value $\leq 1 \times 10-6$

asthma, including SNPs in *IL1RL1*, *IL13*, near the *C11orf30-LRRC32* region, in *LINC01149*, and near *GSDMB*. Additionally, GWAS identified one variant in *KIAA1958* that was associated with childhood asthma among NHWs with genome-wide significance. Regions of interest were identified at near genome-wide significance among NHWs in *PDZD2*, among AAs in *FLJ12825* and *PHF14*, and on meta-analysis in *SCHIP1* and its read-through transcript *IQCJ-SCHIP1*.

There has been a growing interest in the risk of early life asthmatics for developing COPD, and thus ACO, in adulthood [15]. It has been proposed that in some childhood asthmatics, the risk for COPD is the result of the lungs never achieving their expected growth and development in early adulthood [11, 12, 16, 20, 52, 53]. Normal decline in lung function can lead to COPD since expected maximal FEV_1 is never attained. ACO has been recognized as a distinct COPD subtype, with elevated risk for exacerbations, increased health-care burden, and different potential treatment modalities [54]. Research into the mechanisms of disease and genetic susceptibility for ACO subjects has been limited by the traditional exclusion of asthmatic subjects from large COPD studies [15]. Studies of COPD use spirometry as the accepted COPD definition; however, ACO research has been complicated by disagreement on a standard definition for asthma and therefore ACO [15, 34, 54–56]. COPD cohorts often include older adults and in many cases it is not possible to confirm early-life diagnosis of asthma by Global Initiative for Asthma (GINA) spirometry guidelines or by physician records [55, 57]. Once COPD has been diagnosed, it is difficult to use bronchodilator reactivity to define asthma, as this can also be a feature of COPD. Use of self-reported history of asthma has raised concern due to the theoretical risk of misclassification bias [58].

This study confirms that childhood asthmatics who smoke are at increased risk for developing low lung function and COPD as adults, when compared to smokers who never had asthma. This investigation supports self-reported diagnosis of asthma history as a valid method of identifying early-life asthmatics, and a population of ACO subjects, in large population cohorts at risk for COPD. This will be particularly important as researchers further examine the genetic epidemiology of ACO.

There have been a number of prior asthma GWAS conducted in populations of asthmatic subjects, beginning with the GABRIEL Consortium in 2007, which focused on populations of European ancestry, and continuing through the recent TAGC GWAS, a meta-analysis in ethnically diverse populations including 23,948 cases and 118,538 controls; the TAGS GWAS included a pediatric subgroup meta-analysis with 8976 cases and 18,399 controls [4, 24]. These asthma GWAS have used a range of asthma definitions, including physician diagnosis in GABRIEL, electronic medical record information in eMERGE, and physicians' diagnosis and/or standardized questionnaires in the TAGC [4, 24, 47]. A number of prior GWAS have identified distinct genetic susceptibility for pediatric onset asthma, particularly implicating *ORLDM3/GSDMB*, *IL1RL1*, and *IL13*, which were all found to have association with childhood asthma in the current analysis [4, 5, 6, 7, 24, 59]. *C11orf30-LRRC3*, which also has association in this GWAS, has been associated with in pediatric asthma previously, though in prior GWAS the primary link with asthma has been in the setting of allergic disease [33, 60].

This study examined association with seven established asthma SNPs, selected as they were the only SNPs reported by more than one study among 85 studies in the NHGRI-EBI GWAS catalog, and five SNPs from the largest pediatric GWAS to date from the TAGC [2, 3, 24]. Five genes were found to be associated with self-reported childhood asthma in COPDGene: *IL1RL1*, *IL13*, *LINC01149*, near *GSDMB*, and in the *C11orf30-LRRC32* region. *IL1RL1* in the 2q12.1 region is thought to be involved in T-helper cell type 2 (TH2) inflammation including

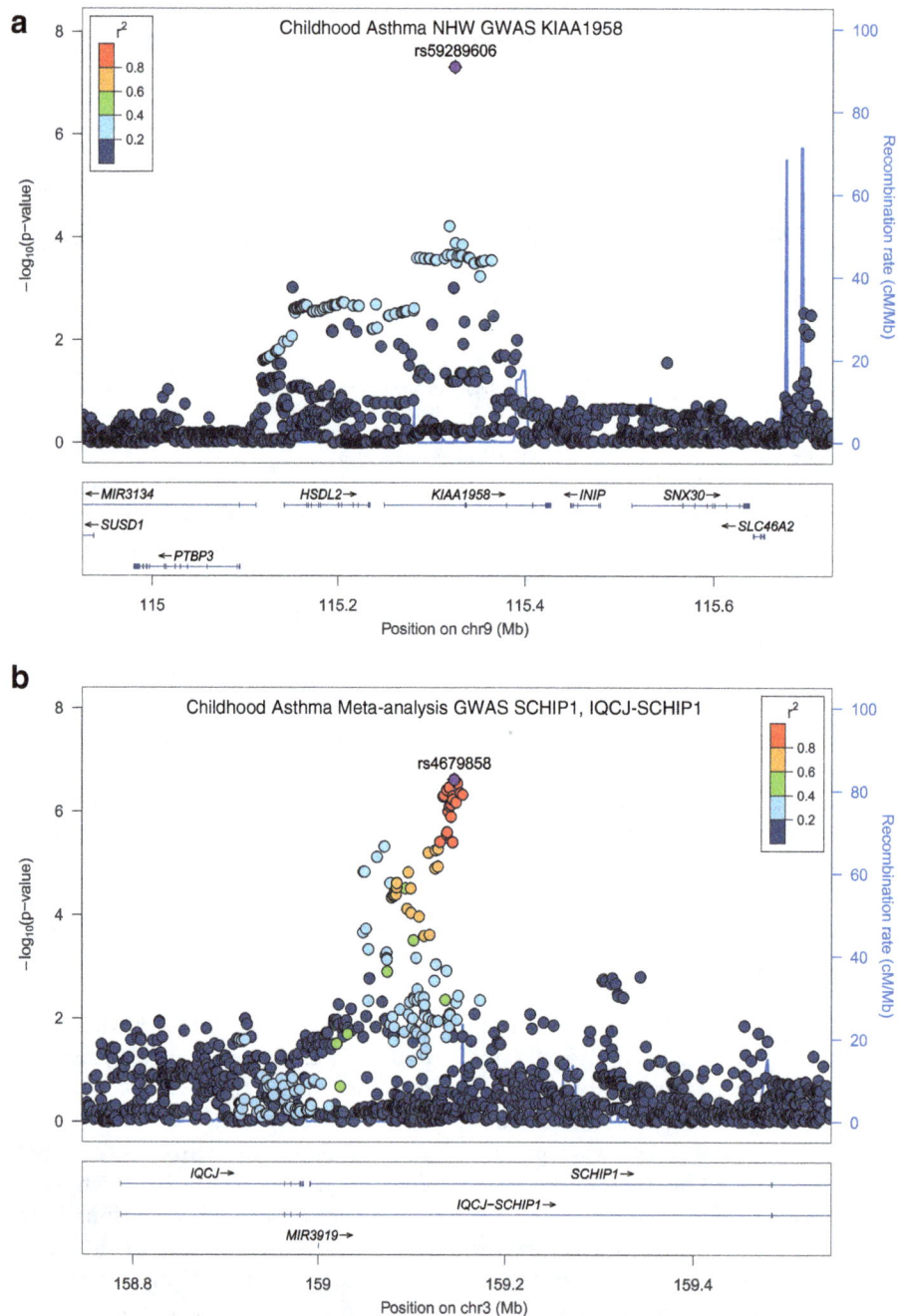

Fig. 1 LocusZoom Plot of childhood asthma GWAS variants **a** from non-Hispanic whites in KIAA1958 and **b** from the meta-analysis in the region near SCHIP1 and its read through transcript IQCJ-SCHIP1

eosinophil activation [42, 44–46, 61–64]. *IL13* is an immunoregulatory cytokine produced by TH2 cells that is critical to the pathogenesis of allergic asthma, operating through mechanisms independent of IgE and eosinophils [65]. *GSDMB* in the established 17q21 childhood asthma risk region is potentially involved in pathogenesis via epithelial cell pyroptosis [4, 7, 41, 44, 47, 49, 50, 66]. In asthmatics, the *C11orf30-LRRC32* region is associated with

total serum IgE levels [67]. We did not see evidence of association from three of the seven established NHGRI-EBI asthma SNPs, those found in *TSLP*, *RAD50*, and *GSDMA*. *TSLP* has a role in TH2 cell responses associated with inflammatory diseases including asthma and COPD [65]. *RAD50* has been implicated in allergic airway inflammation, potentially vial regulation of TH2 cytokine genes, though the exact mechanism remains to be elucidated

Table 4 Associations with NHGRI-EBI asthma SNPs in COPDGene childhood asthma GWAS

NHW[a]	Gene	SNP	Locus	Effect Allele	OR	Rsq	Freq (%)	P-value[b,d]	Adj P-value[e]
(385 cases, 4979 controls)	**IL1RL1**	**rs10197862[f]**	**2q12.1**	**A**	**1.45**	**1.00**	**0.85**	**0.002**	**0.011**
	TSLP	rs1837253[g]	5q22.1	T	1.07	0.75		0.414	1.000
	RAD50	rs2244012[f]	5q31.1	G	1.05	0.78		0.579	1.000
	IL13	rs1295686[f]	5q31.1	T	1.22	0.80		0.026	0.180
	C11orf30-LRRC32	rs7130588[g]	11q13.5	G	1.23	0.64		0.008	0.054
	GSDMB	rs2305480[f]	17q21.1	G	1.22	0.44		0.009	0.060
	GSDMA	rs3894194[f]	17q21.1	A	1.18	0.94	0.47	0.029	0.201
AA[a]	Gene	SNP	Locus	Effect Allele	OR	Rsq	Freq (%)	P-value[b,d]	Adj P-value[e]
(325 cases, 2342 controls)	*IL1RL1*	rs10197862[f]	2q12.1	A	1.10	0.98	0.74	0.344	1.000
	TSLP	rs1837253[g]	5q22.1	C	1.11	0.28	0.283		1.000
	RAD50	rs2244012[f]	5q31.1	G	1.05	0.57		0.603	1.000
	IL13	rs1295686[f]	5q31.1	T	1.16	0.64		0.102	0.717
	C11orf30-LRRC32	rs7130588[g]	11q13.5	G	1.23	0.80		0.035	0.247
	GSDMB	rs2305480[f]	17q21.1	G	1.03	0.13		0.817	1.000
	GSDMA	rs3894194[f]	17q21.1	G	1.02	0.88	0.69	0.846	1.000
Meta-analysis[a]	Gene	SNP	Locus	Effect Allele	OR	I[2]		P-value[c,d]	Adj P-value[e]
(710 cases, 7321 controls)	**IL1RL1**	**rs10197862[f]**	**2q12.1**	**A**	**1.23**	**70**		**0.006**	**0.042**
	TSLP	rs1837253[g]	5q22.1	C	1.01	45		0.910	1.000
	RAD50	rs2244012[f]	5q31.1	G	1.05	0		0.447	1.000
	IL13	**rs1295686[f]**	**5q31.1**	**T**	**1.19**	**0**		**0.006**	**0.043**
	C11orf30-LRRC32	**rs7130588[g]**	**11q13.5**	**G**	**1.23**	**0**		**0.001**	**0.005**
	GSDMB	rs2305480[f]	17q21.1	G	1.17	27		0.018	0.125
	GSDMA	rs3894194[f]	17q21.1	A	1.10	57		0.113	0.794

Abbreviations: *NHGRI-EBI* National Human Genome Research Institute - European Bioinformatics Institute; *SNP* single nucleotide polymorphism; *GWAS* genome-wide association study; *NHW* Non-Hispanic Whites; *AA* African American; *OR* odds ratio of the effect allele; *Rsq* estimation of imputation quality; *Freq* frequency of effect allele; I^2 heterogeneity index; [a] Each population was run as an independent analysis, and then combined in the meta-analysis: [b] Logistic regression based on case control status; [c] Fixed effect meta-analysis weighted by inverse variance. [d] Adjusted for sex, genetic ancestry. [e] Bonferroni correction for seven tests, SNPs with adjusted p < 0.05 in Bold. [f] SNP is in the reported gene, [g] SNP is near the reported gene

[68]. *GSDMA* is along with *GSDMB* and *ORMDL3* part of the complex 17q21.1 locus, more research is needed to understand the specific interactions of variants in this region and their role in asthma pathobiology [69].

There was one novel genome-wide significant SNP associated with childhood asthma in the GWAS, rs59289606, an intron variant in the protein-coding gene *KIAA1958* at locus 9q32; this SNP is imputed with Rsq 0.38, which meets our criteria for imputation quality. *KIAA1958* has not been previously associated with disease pathogenesis [70]. In the AA population, variants of interest were found in *FLJ12825* and *PHF14*. *FLJ12825* is a non-coding RNA, and *PHF14* is a protein coding gene important in regulation of mesenchymal cell proliferation specific to lung fibrosis, that has also been described in newborn respiratory failure and newborn pulmonary hypertension [71, 72]. Meta-analysis identified a region of interest in *SCHIP1* and its read-through transcript *IQCJ-SCHIP1*. *SCHIP1* has been reported along with *IL12A* as a potential systemic

sclerosis gene which functions in immune regulation via T cell activity [73].

Limitations

This childhood asthma GWAS used a cohort of adult smokers at risk for COPD. It is underpowered relative to the large-scale asthma GWAS that have recently been published. However, our objective was not to run a novel asthma GWAS; rather, the goal of this investigation was to examine self-reported asthma in a population of adult smokers at risk for COPD. Ideally, we would have been able to compare this self-reported diagnosis of childhood asthma to a gold-standard diagnosis, such as childhood spirometry or medical records, but this primary data in this cohort of older adults is not available. Notably, when compared to clinical diagnosis, questionnaire reported asthma history has been shown to have relatively good agreement and reliability over time [74–76]. It would have additionally been valuable to use medical records to assess asthma treatment and control; however, we note that many of these subjects had childhood asthma prior to the widespread use of inhaled corticosteroids in the US. Additionally, asthma treatment will not impact the patients' genotype, so the objectivity of that measure is maintained. Since COPDGene includes smokers, we were not able to assess COPD risk among non-smokers; given that this investigation was focused on a population with a high COPD risk, including only smokers is reasonable.

The assessed list of known asthma variants were selected from 600 asthma associations published in the NHGRI-EBI GWAS catalog, where only eight independent SNPs were reported in more than one study. An additional set of five pediatric asthma GWAS SNPs from the TAGC was also examined. We acknowledge that alternative lists of established asthma SNPs could be proposed. It is notable that the established asthma variant list was largely composed of SNPs from European American or NHW populations, and thus the lack of associations in the AA population is not unexpected. This also explains why the combined NHW and AA meta-analysis did not improve power to detect associations for some of the SNPs. It would have been desirable to include other populations with alternative genetic heritage, but COPDGene is limited to NHW and AA subjects.

Conclusions

Self-report of childhood asthma in adult smokers from COPDGene identifies a meaningful population who demonstrate the demographic, clinical, and genetic characteristics known to associate with childhood asthma. Compared to subjects who never had asthma, self-reported childhood asthmatics were younger, more likely to be of AA race, and had increased odds of COPD. We showed associations with known asthma loci in *IL1RL1*, *IL13*, *LINC01149*, near *GSDMB*, and in the *C11orf30-LRRC32* region. This GWAS identified a new variant in *KIAA1958* associated with childhood asthma in NHWs. This study will enhance future genetic epidemiology research in early-life asthmatics at risk for COPD and therefore ACO, by establishing the validity of self-reported asthma in the research setting. This study emphasizes that clinicians need to consider childhood asthma when assessing patients at increased risk for COPD, and that patient self-report is a reliable method of defining ACO.

Additional files

Additional file 1: Figure S1. Subject classification. **Figure S2.** QQ-plot and Manhattan plot of childhood asthma GWAS SNPs in non-Hispanic Whites. **Figure S3.** QQ-plot and Manhattan plot of childhood asthma GWAS SNPs in African Americans. **Figure S4.** QQ-plot and Manhattan plot of childhood asthma GWAS SNPs from meta-analysis of NHW and AA subjects. **Figure S5.** LocusZoom Plots of childhood asthma non-Hispanic white GWAS variants in *PDZD2*. **Figure S6.** LocusZoom Plots of

childhood asthma African American GWAS variants in regions of interest in *FLJ12825* and *PHF14*. **Figure S7.** In non-Hispanic whites the childhood asthma GWAS found association with the known asthma genes *IL1RL1* (rs10197862, adj $p = 0.011$) and *GSDMB* (rs2305480, adj $p = 0.060$). **Figure S8.** Meta-analysis of NHW and AA subjects in this study found association with a known asthma variants in IL13 (rs1295686) and near the *C11orf30-LRRC32* region (rs7130588). **Table S1.** Associations with TAGC Pediatric Asthma GWAS SNPs. (PDF 977 kb)

Abbreviations
AA: African American; ACO: Asthma-COPD overlap; CI: Confidence interval; COPD: Chronic obstructive pulmonary disease; FEV_1: Forced expiratory volume in the first second; FVC: Forced vital capacity; GWAS: Genome-Wide Association Study; LD: Linkage disequilibrium; MAF: Minor allele frequency; NHGRI-EBI: National Human Genome Research Institute - European Bioinformatics Institute; NHW: Non-Hispanic white; OR: Odds ratio; PC: Principal components; QQ: Quantile-Quantile; SE: Standard error; SNP: Single nucleotide polymorphism; TAGC: Trans-National Asthma Genetic Consortium; TH2: T-helper cell type 2

Acknowledgements
COPDGene® Investigators Core Units: Administrative Center: James D. Crapo, MD (PI); Edwin K. Silverman, MD, PhD (PI); Barry J. Make, MD; Elizabeth A. Regan, MD, PhD. Genetic Analysis Center: Terri Beaty, PhD; Ferdouse Begum, PhD; Peter J. Castaldi, MD, MSc; Michael Cho, MD; Dawn L. DeMeo, MD, MPH; Adel R. Boueiz, MD; Marilyn G. Foreman, MD, MS; Eitan Halper-Stromberg; Lystra P. Hayden, MD, MMSc; Craig P. Hersh, MD, MPH; Jacqueline Hetmanski, MS, MPH; Brian D. Hobbs, MD; John E. Hokanson, MPH, PhD; Nan Laird, PhD; Christoph Lange, PhD; Sharon M. Lutz, PhD; Merry-Lynn McDonald, PhD; Margaret M. Parker, PhD; Dandi Qiao, PhD; Elizabeth A. Regan, MD, PhD; Edwin K. Silverman, MD, PhD; Emily S. Wan, MD; Sungho Won, Ph.D.; Phuwanat Sakornsakolpat, M.D.; Dmitry Prokopenko, Ph.D. Imaging Center: Mustafa Al Qaisi, MD; Harvey O. Coxson, PhD; Teresa Gray; MeiLan K. Han, MD, MS; Eric A. Hoffman, PhD; Stephen Humphries, PhD; Francine L. Jacobson, MD, MPH; Philip F. Judy, PhD; Ella A. Kazerooni, MD; Alex Kluiber; David A. Lynch, MB; John D. Newell, Jr., MD; Elizabeth A. Regan, MD, PhD; James C. Ross, PhD; Raul San Jose Estepar, PhD; Joyce Schroeder, MD; Jered Sieren; Douglas Stinson; Berend C. Stoel, PhD; Juerg Tschirren, PhD; Edwin Van Beek, MD, PhD; Bram van Ginneken, PhD; Eva van Rikxoort, PhD; George Washko, MD; Carla G. Wilson, MS. PFT QA Center, Salt Lake City, UT: Robert Jensen, PhD. Data Coordinating Center and Biostatistics, National Jewish Health, Denver, CO: Douglas Everett, PhD; Jim Crooks, PhD; Camille Moore, PhD; Matt Strand, PhD; Carla G. Wilson, MS. *Epidemiology Core, University of Colorado Anschutz Medical Campus, Aurora, CO:* John E. Hokanson, MPH, PhD; John Hughes, PhD; Gregory Kinney, MPH, PhD; Sharon M. Lutz, PhD; Katherine Pratte, MSPH; Kendra A. Young, PhD. *Mortality Adjudication Core:* Surya Bhatt, MD; Jessica Bon, MD; MeiLan K. Han, MD, MS; Barry Make, MD; Carlos Martinez, MD, MS; Susan Murray, ScD; Elizabeth Regan, MD; Xavier Soler, MD; Carla G. Wilson, MS. *Biomarker Core:* Russell P. Bowler, MD, PhD; Katerina Kechris, PhD; Farnoush Banaei-Kashani, Ph.D.
COPDGene® Investigators Clinical Centers: *Ann Arbor VA:* Jeffrey L. Curtis, MD; Carlos H. Martinez, MD, MPH; Perry G. Pernicano, MD. *Baylor College of Medicine, Houston, TX:* Nicola Hanania, MD, MS; Philip Alapat, MD; Mustafa Atik, MD; Venkata Bandi, MD; Aladin Boriek, PhD; Kalpatha Guntupalli, MD; Elizabeth Guy, MD; Arun Nachiappan, MD; Amit Parulekar, MD. *Brigham and Women's Hospital, Boston, MA:* Dawn L. DeMeo, MD, MPH; Craig Hersh, MD, MPH; Francine L. Jacobson, MD, MPH; George Washko, MD. *Columbia University, New York, NY:* R. Graham Barr, MD, DrPH; John Austin, MD; Belinda D'Souza, MD; Gregory D.N. Pearson, MD; Anna Rozenshtein, MD, MPH, FACR; Byron Thomashow, MD. *Duke University Medical Center, Durham, NC:* Neil MacIntyre, Jr., MD; H. Page McAdams, MD; Lacey Washington, MD. *HealthPartners Research Institute, Minneapolis, MN:* Charlene McEvoy, MD, MPH; Joseph Tashjian, MD. *Johns Hopkins University, Baltimore, MD:* Robert Wise, MD; Robert Brown, MD; Nadia N. Hansel, MD, MPH; Karen Horton, MD; Allison Lambert, MD, MHS; Nirupama Putcha, MD, MHS. *Los Angeles Biomedical Research Institute at Harbor UCLA Medical Center, Torrance, CA:* Richard Casaburi, PhD, MD; Alessandra Adami, PhD; Matthew Budoff, MD; Hans Fischer, MD; Janos Porszasz, MD, PhD; Harry Rossiter, PhD; William Stringer, MD. *Michael E. DeBakey VAMC, Houston, TX:* Amir Sharafkhaneh, MD, PhD; Charlie Lan, DO. *Minneapolis VA:* Christine Wendt, MD; Brian Bell, MD.

Morehouse School of Medicine, Atlanta, GA: Marilyn G. Foreman, MD, MS; Eugene Berkowitz, MD, PhD; Gloria Westney, MD, MS. *National Jewish Health, Denver, CO*: Russell Bowler, MD, PhD; David A. Lynch, MB. *Reliant Medical Group, Worcester, MA*: Richard Rosiello, MD; David Pace, MD. *Temple University, Philadelphia, PA*: Gerard Criner, MD; David Ciccolella, MD; Francis Cordova, MD; Chandra Dass, MD; Gilbert D'Alonzo, DO; Parag Desai, MD; Michael Jacobs, PharmD; Steven Kelsen, MD, PhD; Victor Kim, MD; A. James Mamary, MD; Nathaniel Marchetti, DO; Aditi Satti, MD; Kartik Shenoy, MD; Robert M. Steiner, MD; Alex Swift, MD; Irene Swift, MD; Maria Elena Vega-Sanchez, MD. *University of Alabama, Birmingham, AL:* Mark Dransfield, MD; William Bailey, MD; Surya Bhatt, MD; Anand Iyer, MD; Hrudaya Nath, MD; J. Michael Wells, MD. *University of California, San Diego, CA*: Joe Ramsdell, MD; Paul Friedman, MD; Xavier Soler, MD, PhD; Andrew Yen, MD. *University of Iowa, Iowa City, IA*: Alejandro P. Comellas, MD; Karin F. Hoth, PhD; John Newell, Jr., MD; Brad Thompson, MD. *University of Michigan, Ann Arbor, MI:* MeiLan K. Han, MD, MS; Ella Kazerooni, MD; Carlos H. Martinez, MD, MPH. *University of Minnesota, Minneapolis, MN:* Joanne Billings, MD; Abbie Begnaud, MD; Tadashi Allen, MD. *University of Pittsburgh, Pittsburgh, PA*: Frank Sciurba, MD; Jessica Bon, MD; Divay Chandra, MD, MSc; Carl Fuhrman, MD; Joel Weissfeld, MD, MPH. *University of Texas Health Science Center at San Antonio, San Antonio, TX*: Antonio Anzueto, MD; Sandra Adams, MD; Diego Maselli-Caceres, MD; Mario E. Ruiz, MD.

Funding
Supported by National Institutes of Health (NIH) grants K23HL136851 (LPH), K12HL120004 (EKS), R01HL113264 (EKS and MHC), U01HL089856 (EKS), U01HL089897 (JD Crappo), R01HL130512 (CPH), R01HL125583 (CPH), P01HL105339 (EKS). The COPDGene Study (NCT00608764) is also supported by the COPD Foundation through contributions made to an Industry Advisory Board comprised of AstraZeneca, Boehringer Ingelheim, GlaxoSmithKline, Novartis, Pfizer, Siemens and Sunovion. Neither the NIH nor the Industry Advisory Board had a role in the study design, data collection, data analysis, interpretation of the data, writing of the report or the decision to submit the paper for publication. The content is solely the responsibility of the authors and does not necessarily represent the official views of the National Heart, Lung, And Blood Institute or the National Institutes of Health.

Authors' contributions
LPH, MHC, BAR, THB, EKS, CPH contributed to data analysis and interpretation, critical revision of the article, and final approval of the version to be published; they all agree to be accountable for all aspects of the work. LPH, MHC, BAR, THB, EKS, CPH contributed to the study conception and design. EKS, CPH contributed to the acquisition of data. LPH, CPH contributed to drafting of the submitted article. All authors read and approved the final manuscript.

Ethics approval and consent to participate
This study was conducted in accordance with the amended Declaration of Helsinki. This study obtained approval from the Institutional Review Board at Brigham and Women's Hospital and at each of the twenty-one clinical sites. All participants provided written informed consent for their medical data to be used prior to taking part in the study.
Clinical Center and IRB protocol numbers:
Ann Arbor VA, Ann Arbor, MI (PCC 2008–110732).
Baylor College of Medicine, Houston, TX (H-22209).
Brigham and Women's Hospital, Boston, MA (2007-P-000554/2; BWH).
Columbia University, New York, NY (IRB-AAAC9324).
Duke University Medical Center, Durham, NC (Pro00004464).
Health Partners Research Foundation, Minneapolis, MN (07–127).
Johns Hopkins University, Baltimore, MD (NA_00011524).
Los Angeles Biomedical Research Institute at Harbor UCLA Medical Center, Los Angeles, CA (12756–01).
Michael E. DeBakey VAMC, Houston, TX (H-22202).
Minneapolis VA, Minneapolis, MN (4128-A).
Morehouse School of Medicine, Atlanta, GA (07–1029).
National Jewish Health, Denver, CO (HS-1883a).
Reliant Medical Group, Worcester, MA (1143).
Temple University, Philadelphia, PA (11369).
University of Alabama, Birmingham, AL (FO70712014).

University of California, San Diego, CA (70876).
University of Iowa, Iowa City, IA (200710717).
University of Michigan, Ann Arbor, MI (HUM00014973).
University of Minnesota, Minneapolis, MN (0801 M24949).
University of Pittsburgh, Pittsburgh, PA (PRO07120059).
University of Texas Health Science Center at San Antonio, San Antonio, TX (HSC20070644H).

Competing interests
C.P. Hersh reports personal fees from AstraZeneca, grants from Boehringer Ingelheim, personal fees from Mylan, personal fees from Concert Pharmaceuticals, all of which are outside the submitted work. In the past three years, E.K. Silverman received honoraria from Novartis for Continuing Medical Education Seminars and grant and travel support from GlaxoSmithKline unrelated to this manuscript. M.H. Cho has received grant support from GlaxoSmithKline. Authors L.P. Hayden, B.A. Raby, and T.H. Beaty have no conflicts of interest to disclose.

Author details
[1]Division of Respiratory Diseases, Boston Children's Hospital, Boston, MA, USA. [2]Channing Division of Network Medicine, Brigham and Women's Hospital, 181 Longwood Avenue, Boston, MA 02115, USA. [3]Division of Pulmonary and Critical Care Medicine, Brigham and Women's Hospital, Boston, MA, USA. [4]Bloomberg School of Public Health, Johns Hopkins University, Baltimore, MD, USA.

References
1. Asthma Fact Sheet. http://www.who.int/mediacentre/factsheets/fs307/en/. Accessed Jan. 23, 2018.
2. Welter D, MacArthur J, Morales J, Burdett T, Hall P, Junkins H, et al. The NHGRI GWAS catalog, a curated resource of SNP-trait associations. Nucleic Acids Res. 2014;42:D1001–6.
3. The NHGRI-EBI GWAS Catalog of published genome-wide association studies. . https://www.ebi.ac.uk/gwas/. Accessed Sept 28, 2017.
4. Moffatt MF, Kabesch M, Liang L, Dixon AL, Strachan D, Heath S, et al. Genetic variants regulating ORMDL3 expression contribute to the risk of childhood asthma. Nature. 2007;448:470–3.
5. Moffatt MF, Gut IG, Demenais F, Strachan DP, Bouzigon E, Heath S, et al. A large-scale, consortium-based genomewide association study of asthma. N Engl J Med. 2010;363:1211–21.
6. Forno E, Lasky-Su J, Himes B, Howrylak J, Ramsey C, Brehm J, et al. Genome-wide association study of the age of onset of childhood asthma. J Allergy Clin Immunol 2012;130:83–90 e84.
7. Bonnelykke K, Sleiman P, Nielsen K, Kreiner-Moller E, Mercader JM, Belgrave D, et al. A genome-wide association study identifies CDHR3 as a susceptibility locus for early childhood asthma with severe exacerbations. Nat Genet. 2014;46:51–5.
8. Ullemar V, Magnusson PK, Lundholm C, Zettergren A, Melen E, Lichtenstein P, et al. Heritability and confirmation of genetic association studies for childhood asthma in twins. Allergy. 2016;71:230–8.
9. Koeppen-Schomerus G, Stevenson J, Plomin R. Genes and environment in asthma: a study of 4 year old twins. Arch Dis Child. 2001;85:398–400.
10. van Beijsterveldt CE, Boomsma DI. Genetics of parentally reported asthma, eczema and rhinitis in 5-yr-old twins. Eur Respir J. 2007;29:516–21.
11. McGeachie MJ. Childhood asthma is a risk factor for the development of chronic obstructive pulmonary disease. Curr Opin Allergy Clin Immunol. 2017;17:104–9.
12. McGeachie MJ, Yates KP, Zhou X, Guo F, Sternberg AL, Van Natta ML, et al. Patterns of growth and decline in lung function in persistent childhood asthma. N Engl J Med. 2016;374:1842–52.
13. Lange P, Parner J, Vestbo J, Schnohr P, Jensen G. A 15-year follow-up study of ventilatory function in adults with asthma. N Engl J Med. 1998;339:1194–200.
14. Svanes C, Sunyer J, Plana E, Dharmage S, Heinrich J, Jarvis D, et al. Early life origins of chronic obstructive pulmonary disease. Thorax. 2010;65:14–20.

15. Woodruff PG, van den Berge M, Boucher RC, Brightling C, Burchard EG, Christenson SA, et al. American Thoracic Society/National Heart, Lung, and Blood Institute asthma-chronic obstructive pulmonary disease overlap workshop report. Am J Respir Crit Care Med. 2017;196:375–81.

16. Hayden LP, Hobbs BD, Cohen RT, Wise RA, Checkley W, Crapo JD, et al. Childhood pneumonia increases risk for chronic obstructive pulmonary disease: the COPDGene study. Respir Res. 2015;16:115.

17. Hardin M, Silverman EK, Barr RG, Hansel NN, Schroeder JD, Make BJ, et al. The clinical features of the overlap between COPD and asthma. Respir Res. 2011;12:127.

18. Hardin M, Foreman M, Dransfield MT, Hansel N, Han MK, Cho MH, et al. Sex-specific features of emphysema among current and former smokers with COPD. Eur Respir J. 2016;47:104–12.

19. Diaz AA, Hardin ME, Come CE, San Jose Estepar R, Ross JC, Kurugol S, et al. Childhood-onset asthma in smokers. Association between CT measures of airway size, lung function, and chronic airflow obstruction. Ann Am Thorac Soc. 2014;11:1371–8.

20. Hayden LP, Hardin ME, Qiu W, Lynch DA, Strand MJ, van Beek EJ, et al. Asthma is a risk factor for respiratory exacerbations without increased rate of lung function decline: five-year follow-up in adult smokers from the COPDGene study. Chest. 2018;153:368–77.

21. Kesten S, Dzyngel B, Chapman KR, Zamel N, Tarlo S, Malo JL, et al. Defining the asthma phenotype for the purpose of genetic analysis. J Asthma. 1997;34:483–91.

22. Kauppi P, Laitinen LA, Laitinen H, Kere J, Laitinen T. Verification of self-reported asthma and allergy in subjects and their family members volunteering for gene mapping studies. Respir Med. 1998;92:1281–8.

23. Sin DD, Miravitlles M, Mannino DM, Soriano JB, Price D, Celli BR, et al. What is asthma-COPD overlap syndrome? Towards a consensus definition from a round table discussion. Eur Respir J. 2016;48:664–73.

24. Demenais F, Margaritte-Jeannin P, Barnes KC, Cookson WOC, Altmuller J, Ang W, et al. Multiancestry association study identifies new asthma risk loci that colocalize with immune-cell enhancer marks. Nat Genet. 2018;50:42–53.

25. Regan EA, Hokanson JE, Murphy JR, Make B, Lynch DA, Beaty TH, et al. Genetic epidemiology of COPD (COPDGene) study design. COPD. 2010;7:32–43.

26. COPDGene, Phase 1 Study Documents. http://www.copdgene.org/phase-1-study-documents. Accessed Mar. 13, 2015.

27. Ferris BG. Epidemiology standardization project (American Thoracic Society). Am Rev Respir Dis. 1978;118:1–120.

28. Cho MH, Boutaoui N, Klanderman BJ, Sylvia JS, Ziniti JP, Hersh CP, et al. Variants in FAM13A are associated with chronic obstructive pulmonary disease. Nat Genet. 2010;42:200–2.

29. Cho MH, McDonald ML, Zhou X, Mattheisen M, Castaldi PJ, Hersh CP, et al. Risk loci for chronic obstructive pulmonary disease: a genome-wide association study and meta-analysis. Lancet Respir Med. 2014;2:214–25.

30. Genomes Project C, Abecasis GR, Auton A, Brooks LD, DePristo MA, Durbin RM, et al. An integrated map of genetic variation from 1,092 human genomes. Nature. 2012;491:56–65.

31. Howie B, Fuchsberger C, Stephens M, Marchini J, Abecasis GR. Fast and accurate genotype imputation in genome-wide association studies through pre-phasing. Nat Genet. 2012;44:955–9.

32. Li Y, Byrnes AE, Li M. To identify associations with rare variants, just WHaIT: weighted haplotype and imputation-based tests. Am J Hum Genet. 2010;87:728–35.

33. Marenholz I, Esparza-Gordillo J, Ruschendorf F, Bauerfeind A, Strachan DP, Spycher BD, et al. Meta-analysis identifies seven susceptibility loci involved in the atopic march. Nat Commun. 2015;6:8804.

34. Rabe KF, Hurd S, Anzueto A, Barnes PJ, Buist SA, Calverley P, et al. Global strategy for the diagnosis, management, and prevention of chronic obstructive pulmonary disease: GOLD executive summary. Am J Respir Crit Care Med. 2007;176:532–55.

35. Purcell S, Neale B, Todd-Brown K, Thomas L, Ferreira MA, Bender D, et al. PLINK: a tool set for whole-genome association and population-based linkage analyses. Am J Hum Genet. 2007;81:559–75.

36. Hoggart CJ, Clark TG, De Iorio M, Whittaker JC, Balding DJ. Genome-wide significance for dense SNP and resequencing data. Genet Epidemiol. 2008;32:179–85.

37. Risch N, Merikangas K. The future of genetic studies of complex human diseases. Science. 1996;273:1516–7.

38. Yu K, Wang Z, Li Q, Wacholder S, Hunter DJ, Hoover RN, et al. Population substructure and control selection in genome-wide association studies. PLoS One. 2008;3:e2551.

39. Evangelou E, Ioannidis JP. Meta-analysis methods for genome-wide association studies and beyond. Nat Rev Genet. 2013;14:379–89.

40. Ferreira MA, Matheson MC, Duffy DL, Marks GB, Hui J, Le Souef P, et al. Identification of IL6R and chromosome 11q13.5 as risk loci for asthma. Lancet. 2011;378:1006–14.

41. Yan Q, Brehm J, Pino-Yanes M, Forno E, Lin J, Oh SS, et al. A meta-analysis of genome-wide association studies of asthma in Puerto Ricans. Eur Respir J. 2017;49.

42. Barreto-Luis A, Pino-Yanes M, Corrales A, Campo P, Callero A, Acosta-Herrera M, et al. Genome-wide association study in Spanish identifies ADAM metallopeptidase with thrombospondin type 1 motif, 9 (ADAMTS9), as a novel asthma susceptibility gene. J Allergy Clin Immunol. 2016;137:964–6.

43. Hirota T, Takahashi A, Kubo M, Tsunoda T, Tomita K, Doi S, et al. Genome-wide association study identifies three new susceptibility loci for adult asthma in the Japanese population. Nat Genet. 2011;43:893–6.

44. Torgerson DG, Ampleford EJ, Chiu GY, Gauderman WJ, Gignoux CR, Graves PE, et al. Meta-analysis of genome-wide association studies of asthma in ethnically diverse north American populations. Nat Genet. 2011;43:887–92.

45. Ferreira MA, Matheson MC, Tang CS, Granell R, Ang W, Hui J, et al. Genome-wide association analysis identifies 11 risk variants associated with the asthma with hay fever phenotype. J Allergy Clin Immunol. 2014;133:1564–71.

46. Pickrell JK, Berisa T, Liu JZ, Segurel L, Tung JY, Hinds DA. Detection and interpretation of shared genetic influences on 42 human traits. Nat Genet. 2016;48:709–17.

47. Almoguera B, Vazquez L, Mentch F, Connolly J, Pacheco JA, Sundaresan AS, et al. Identification of four novel loci in asthma in European American and African American populations. Am J Respir Crit Care Med. 2017;195:456–63.

48. Li X, Howard TD, Zheng SL, Haselkorn T, Peters SP, Meyers DA, et al. Genome-wide association study of asthma identifies RAD50-IL13 and HLA-DR/DQ regions. J Allergy Clin Immunol. 2010;125:328–335 e311.

49. Weidinger S, Willis-Owen SA, Kamatani Y, Baurecht H, Morar N, Liang L, et al. A genome-wide association study of atopic dermatitis identifies loci with overlapping effects on asthma and psoriasis. Hum Mol Genet. 2013;22:4841–56.

50. Galanter JM, Gignoux CR, Torgerson DG, Roth LA, Eng C, Oh SS, et al. Genome-wide association study and admixture mapping identify different asthma-associated loci in Latinos: the Genes-environments & Admixture in Latino Americans study. J Allergy Clin Immunol. 2014;134:295–305.

51. Morris AP. Transethnic meta-analysis of genomewide association studies. Genet Epidemiol. 2011;35:809–22.

52. Martinez FD. Early-life origins of chronic obstructive pulmonary disease. N Engl J Med. 2016;375:871–8.

53. Hayden LP, Hardin ME, Qiu W, Lynch DA, Strand MJ, van Beek EJ, et al. Asthma is a risk factor for respiratory exacerbations without increased rate of lung function decline: five-year follow-up in adult smokers from the COPDGene study. Chest. 2017.

54. Bujarski S, Parulekar AD, Sharafkhaneh A, Hanania NA. The asthma COPD overlap syndrome (ACOS). Curr Allergy Asthma Rep. 2015;15:509.

55. Global Initiative for Asthma (GINA) Global Initiative for Chronic Obstructive Lung Disease (GOLD). Diagnosis of Diseases of Chronic Airflow Limitation: Asthma COPD and Asthma-COPD Overlap Syndrome (ACOS). 2015.

56. Bonten TN, Kasteleyn MJ, de Mutsert R, Hiemstra PS, Rosendaal FR, Chavannes NH, et al. Defining asthma-COPD overlap syndrome: a population-based study. Eur Respir J. 2017;49.

57. Global Initiative for Asthma (GINA). 2017 GINA Report, Global strategy for asthma management and prevention.

58. Barrecheguren M, Roman-Rodriguez M, Miravitlles M. Is a previous diagnosis of asthma a reliable criterion for asthma-COPD overlap syndrome in a patient with COPD? Int J Chron Obstruct Pulmon Dis. 2015;10:1745–52.

59. Liu Z, Li P, Wang J, Fan Q, Yan P, Zhang X, et al. A meta-analysis of IL-13 polymorphisms and pediatric asthma risk. Med Sci Monit. 2014;20:2617–23.

60. Tamari M, Tanaka S, Hirota T. Genome-wide association studies of allergic diseases. Allergol Int. 2013;62:21–8.

61. Ramasamy A, Kuokkanen M, Vedantam S, Gajdos ZK, Couto Alves A, Lyon HN, et al. Genome-wide association studies of asthma in population-based cohorts confirm known and suggested loci and identify an additional association near HLA. PLoS One. 2012;7:e44008.

62. Gudbjartsson DF, Bjornsdottir US, Halapi E, Helgadottir A, Sulem P, Jonsdottir GM, et al. Sequence variants affecting eosinophil numbers associate with asthma and myocardial infarction. Nat Genet. 2009;41:342–7.

63. Inoue H, Ito I, Niimi A, Matsumoto H, Oguma T, Tajiri T, et al. Association of interleukin 1 receptor-like 1 gene polymorphisms with eosinophilic phenotype in Japanese adults with asthma. Respir Investig. 2017;55:338–47.

64. Gordon ED, Palandra J, Wesolowska-Andersen A, Ringel L, Rios CL, Lachowicz-Scroggins ME, et al. IL1RL1 asthma risk variants regulate airway type 2 inflammation. JCI Insight. 2016;1:e87871.

65. Jenuth JP. The NCBI. Publicly available tools and resources on the web. Methods Mol Biol. 2000;132:301–12.

66. Panganiban RA, Sun M, Dahlin A, Park HR, Kan M, Himes BE, et al. A functional splicing variant associated with decreased asthma risk abolishes the ability of gasdermin B (GSMDB) to induce epithelial cell pyroptosis. J Allergy Clin Immunol. 2018.

67. Li X, Ampleford EJ, Howard TD, Moore WC, Li H, Busse WW, et al. The C11orf30-LRRC32 region is associated with total serum IgE levels in asthmatic patients. J Allergy Clin Immunol. 2012;129:575–8 578 e571–579.

68. Hwang SS, Jang SW, Lee KO, Kim HS, Lee GR. RHS6 coordinately regulates the Th2 cytokine genes by recruiting GATA3, SATB1, and IRF4. Allergy. 2017; 72:772–82.

69. Stein MM, Thompson EE, Schoettler N, Helling BA, Magnaye KM, Stanhope C, et al. A decade of research on the 17q12-21 asthma locus: piecing together the puzzle. J Allergy Clin Immunol. 2018.

70. Kojima KK, Jurka J. Crypton transposons: identification of new diverse families and ancient domestication events. Mob DNA. 2011;2:12.

71. Kitagawa M, Takebe A, Ono Y, Imai T, Nakao K, Nishikawa S, et al. Phf14, a novel regulator of mesenchyme growth via platelet-derived growth factor (PDGF) receptor-alpha. J Biol Chem. 2012;287:27983–96.

72. Huang Q, Zhang L, Wang Y, Zhang C, Zhou S, Yang G, et al. Depletion of PHF14, a novel histone-binding protein gene, causes neonatal lethality in mice due to respiratory failure. Acta Biochim Biophys Sin Shanghai. 2013;45:622–33.

73. Jin J, Chou C, Lima M, Zhou D, Zhou X. Systemic sclerosis is a complex disease associated mainly with immune regulatory and inflammatory genes. Open Rheumatol J. 2014;8:29–42.

74. Toren K, Brisman J, Jarvholm B. Asthma and asthma-like symptoms in adults assessed by questionnaires. A literature review. Chest. 1993;104:600–8.

75. Tisnado DM, Adams JL, Liu H, Damberg CL, Chen WP, Hu FA, et al. What is the concordance between the medical record and patient self-report as data sources for ambulatory care? Med Care. 2006;44:132–40.

76. Mirabelli MC, Beavers SF, Flanders WD, Chatterjee AB. Reliability in reporting asthma history and age at asthma onset. J Asthma. 2014;51:956–63.

8

Proteinase 3; a potential target in chronic obstructive pulmonary disease and other chronic inflammatory diseases

Helena Crisford[1,3]* , Elizabeth Sapey[1] and Robert A. Stockley[2]

Abstract

Chronic Obstructive Pulmonary Disease (COPD) is a common, multifactorial lung disease which results in significant impairment of patients' health and a large impact on society and health care burden. It is believed to be the result of prolonged, destructive neutrophilic inflammation which results in progressive damage to lung structures. During this process, large quantities of neutrophil serine proteinases (NSPs) are released which initiate the damage and contribute towards driving a persistent inflammatory state.

Neutrophil elastase has long been considered the key NSP involved in the pathophysiology of COPD. However, in recent years, a significant role for Proteinase 3 (PR3) in disease development has emerged, both in COPD and other chronic inflammatory conditions. Therefore, there is a need to investigate the importance of PR3 in disease development and hence its potential as a therapeutic target. Research into PR3 has largely been confined to its role as an autoantigen, but PR3 is involved in triggering inflammatory pathways, disrupting cellular signalling, degrading key structural proteins, and pathogen response.

This review summarises what is presently known about PR3, explores its involvement particularly in the development of COPD, and indicates areas requiring further investigation.

Keywords: Proteinase 3/myeloblastin, Serine proteinases, Chronic obstructive pulmonary disease, Lungs, Inflammation

Background

The serine proteinase Proteinase 3 (PR3) is an enzyme released during neutrophilic inflammation and is capable of cleaving many targets including key structural proteins of the lung. Chronic Obstructive Pulmonary Disease (COPD) is an inflammatory condition associated with neutrophilic inflammation. For this reason neutrophil elastase (NE) has long been considered to be a central, proteinase in the pathophysiology as it can replicate many of the structural changes of the disease and hence a potential target for therapeutic manipulation, PR3,another key neutrophil serine proteinase has largely been ignored, even though it may have an important additional role in

the lung as well as other human diseases [1]. This review summarises the current literature to provide an update on the potential role of PR3 in health and disease, with a primary focus on COPD.

Proteinase 3

PR3, alternatively referred to as myeloblastin, azurophil granule protein-7 or p29b, is a highly abundant neutrophil protein which is genetically transcribed in primitive myeloid and monocytic progenitor cells, and expressed in cells of granulocyte and monocyte linage, especially neutrophils but including mast cells and basophils [2–5] and in the neutrophil, it is mainly located within the primary azurophil granules of the mature cell but is also present in specific granules, secretory vesicles, and on the cell surface [6, 7]. It is expressed constitutively on the membrane by naïve neutrophils in peripheral blood of healthy individuals (known as "constitutive" PR3) and is secreted into extracellular medium by activated

* Correspondence: hac795@student.bham.ac.uk
[1]Institute of Inflammation and Ageing, University of Birmingham, Edgbaston, Birmingham B15 2GW, UK
[3]Institute of Inflammation and Ageing, College of Medical and Dental Sciences, Centre for Translational Inflammation Research, University of Birmingham Research Laboratories, Queen Elizabeth Hospital Birmingham, Mindelsohn Way, Birmingham B15 2WB, UK
Full list of author information is available at the end of the article

neutrophils following granule translocation to the cell membrane (known as "induced" PR3) [8–11].

It is encoded by the gene *PRTN3* which is located at human chromosome 19p13.3 and spans 6.57 kb pairs including 5 exons and 4 introns. The gene consists of 222 amino acids that fold to form the 29 kDa glycoprotein PR3 [4].

PR3 is classified within the family of "chymotrypsin"-like neutrophil serine proteinase (NSP) which are identified by their highly conserved catalytic triads (His57, Asp102 and Ser195; using chymotrypsinogen numbering) for proteolytic activity and defined by their active site serine residue [4, 12]. PR3 possesses an enlarged binding site with high specificity and differs from NE by 4 main subsites, S2, S1', S2' and S3' (Fig. 1). which is common to other NSPs, including NE [12]. However, PR3, specificity is further defined by difference in residues which alter subsite specificities (subsites shown in Fig. 1).

These specificities are determined by:

- Amide hydrogens on Gly193 and Ser195 which stabilise charge during catalysis [14].
- 3 charged residues: Lys99, Asp61, Arg143 within the active site region.
- Positioning of the solvent accessible Lys99 (compared to Leu99 in NE), which borders the S2 and S4 sites and makes the S2 subsite deeper and more polar, in addition to reducing its hydrophobicity, which determines preferential binding of negative and polar residues, such as Asp [12, 16, 17].
- Asp61 brings the proteins negatively charged side chain closer to the S1' and S'3 subsites, making the subsites smaller and more polar, which encourages binding of basic residues at P1' and P'3 [12, 16].
- Arg143 (and Pro151) increase the polarity of the S2' subsite which creates a basic S2' subsite that binds acidic residues [12, 16].
- Asp213 (compared to Ala213 in NE) restricts the S1 binding site causing it to preferably bind small

hydrophobic residues at P1, which includes alanine, serine, valine, norvaline, and methionine [12, 14, 16–18].
- Ile217 allows small hydrophobic residues at P4 to bind whilst with Trp218 creating a more hydrophobic S5 subsite [12, 14, 16].

PR3 is initially transcribed as an inactive precursor referred to as a zymogen and then undergoes a two-stage posttranslational modification to become active. Firstly (via signal peptidase), there is N-terminal signal peptide cleavage, followed by cleavage of the N-terminal pro-dipeptide by the cysteine proteinase, cathepsin C which is essential for enzymatic activity. Secondly it undergoes pro-peptide cleavage at the C terminal, which is crucial for granule packaging. This forms the catalytic triad of residues and the final conformation of mature PR3, as shown in Fig. 2, which is stabilised by disulphide bonds and appropriate asparagine-linked glycosylation [4, 12, 20]. PR3 then remains stored within the neutrophil azurophil granules until release.

There is estimated to be 3 pg of PR3 stored in each neutrophil, alongside other key serine proteinases, with a mean PR3 concentration of 13.4 mM in each granule, which is 3–4 fold higher than NE [23]. Once released, either constitutively or via granule translocation, PR3 can act enzymatically in both an intracellular and extracellular manner. Its activity is then controlled through inactivation by inhibitors (both reversibly and irreversibly), including serine proteinase inhibitors (Serpins), chelonianin inhibitors and also alpha-2-macroglobulin [24–26].

PR3 has many functions. Animal transgenic and knockout models have demonstrated that it is able to cleave structural proteins leading to tissue remodelling (as discussed within 'Pathophysiological functions of PR3 in COPD'), through diffusing deeper into tissues than the other NSPs [27–30]. Other functions assist in the defensive immune role of the neutrophil including regulating a variety of cellular processes, cleaving host protein into

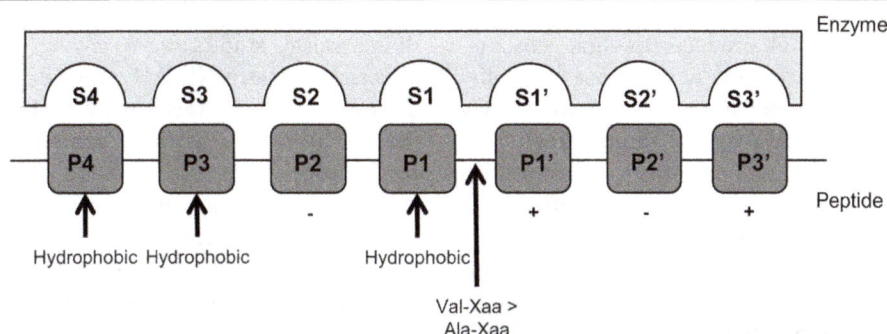

Fig. 1 Diagrammatically demonstrates the substrate binding pockets S4-S3' of PR3 with substrate cleavage positions P4-P3', according to the Schechter and Berger enzyme-ligand binding site numbering convention [19]. The arrows indicate the sites for Val/Ala-containing peptide cleavage and hydrophobic residue binding sites, whilst + indicates positive and − indicates negative residue binding site. Adapted from [13]

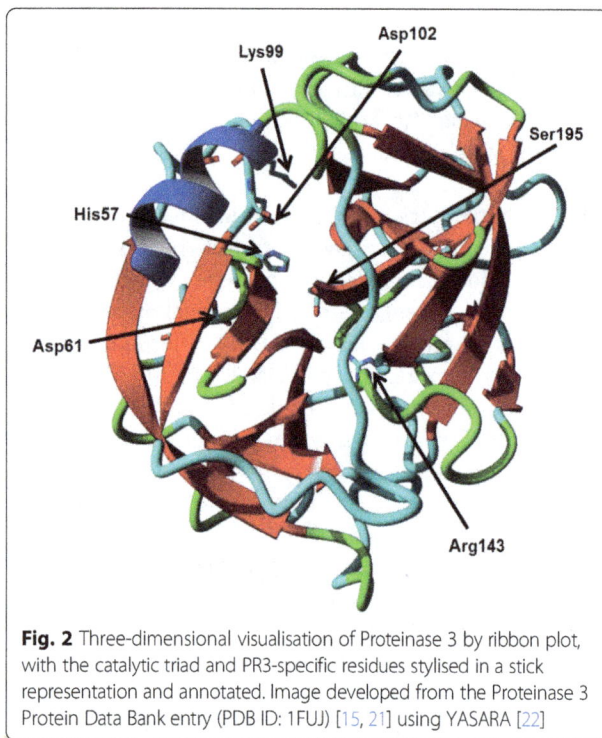

Fig. 2 Three-dimensional visualisation of Proteinase 3 by ribbon plot, with the catalytic triad and PR3-specific residues stylised in a stick representation and annotated. Image developed from the Proteinase 3 Protein Data Bank entry (PDB ID: 1FUJ) [15, 21] using YASARA [22]

antibacterial peptides and activating pro-inflammatory cytokines [31, 32]. Dysfunction of these systems has long been associated with the development or progression of a number of chronic inflammatory diseases including COPD, but often without reference to the potential role of PR3.

Pathophysiological functions of proteinase 3 in COPD

PR3 is likely to have more involvement in the pathophysiology of COPD than previously thought, supported by evidence of increased PR3 activity described in these patients [33–35]. COPD is a progressive, destructive lung disease associated with chronic neutrophilic inflammation and marked by obstruction of airflow, reduced physical activity and breathlessness [36].

The pathophysiology of COPD is considered to reflect an imbalance between proteinases and anti-proteinases in the lung, and Sinden et al. produced the first substantive evidence to support the role of PR3 in a three-dimensional reaction diffusion lung interstitium model [27]. The authors demonstrated that active proteinase diffusion distance following release from a neutrophil varies predominantly depending on concentrations of local physiological inhibitors and that this was greater for PR3 than NE [27]. Generally, activated proteinases have the potential to cause direct lung damage, whereas anti-proteinases provide protection to limit this process. In the lungs, a homeostatic balance is largely maintained, with the exception of a region of quantum proteolysis surrounding migrating and degranulating neutrophils

which is larger in patients with α-1 anti-trypsin deficiency (AATD) explaining the increased susceptibility of these subjects to COPD [37]. This reflects the high concentrations of NSPs released from the granules compared to the immediate concentration of the physiological inhibitors. As the NSPs diffuse away from the neutrophil, the concentration falls exponentially until it equals that of the surrounding inhibitors when activity ceases [37]. It is believed that when levels of NSPs, including PR3, exceed the amount of protective anti-proteinases, such as α-1 anti-trypsin (AAT), excessive damage to lung tissue and other proteinase effects are facilitated [38].

It was previously believed that NE played the key neutrophilic role in tissue damage leading to emphysema, especially in subjects with genetic deficiency of AAT. However, recent data has challenged this concept and supports a potential role for other NSPs including PR3 [33]. Firstly, when a migrating neutrophil degranulates in vitro, it is expected to release more PR3 than NE from the azurophil granules. In vitro some of this becomes membrane bound and more resistant to inhibition, also the free enzyme still has a far greater radius of activity than NE [10, 39, 40]. In addition, although local lung-derived inhibitors are able to inhibit NE the same is not true for PR3, and persistent activity is detectable in lung secretions when NE activity is not [41, 42]. This is important as it implies all the pathological changes in the lung attributed to NE may also be produced by PR3 and potentially to a greater extent.

This theory is supported in vivo by the development of emphysema in hamsters receiving local administration of PR3 and further by recent evidence that SerpinA1-deficient murine models develop spontaneous emphysema [43, 44]. In addition, NSP-knockout murine models are protected against developing emphysema induced by cigarette smoke, whereas mice only deficient in NE are less susceptible, implying that either cathepsin G or PR3 played an important role [30]. Collectively these models suggest that, as well as NE, PR3 is potentially able to contribute to the development of emphysema in humans.

Biochemical studies have shown that PR3 cleaves extracellular matrix (ECM) proteins, including elastin, fibronectin, vitronectin, laminin and collagen, at a GXXPG site within a β-fold conformation resulting in protein degradation [17, 45, 46]. These proteins are important components of tissue structures and, it is the degradation of the extracellular matrix which results in the connective tissue injury in the lung interstitium leading to emphysema, as observed using biomarkers in human COPD and as induced in several animal models [43, 46–48]. Indeed, recent evidence suggests PR3 specific cleavage of elastin is elevated in COPD providing more direct evidence of its role [33].Like other NSPs,

PR3 can also affect mucus clearance by damaging bronchial epithelium and cilia [16]. In addition, PR3 is able to induce mucus production from submucosal gland serous cells and PR3 activity has been implicated in this role in cystic fibrosis (CF) [49]. The net result is excess mucus production in the airways and impaired mucus clearance, which is also a feature of chronic bronchitis, and therefore PR3 is likely to have a similar role in COPD. AATD is a genetic cause of emphysema and chronic bronchitis (in about 30% of patients) and is the result of mutations resulting in little/no production of functional AAT protein. PR3 has a lower association rate with AAT than NE, which means that, in patients with AATD, PR3 is even more poorly regulated, causing a greater proteinase/anti-proteinase imbalance than with NE, and hence potentially mediates more damage to the lungs [4, 27, 50].

As well as causing direct tissue damage, PR3 is also potentially involved in amplifying the inflammation associated with COPD as with other chronic inflammatory diseases.

PR3 is known to modulate a variety of cytokine functions, which impact processes such as metabolism and inflammasome generation [51–53]. The enzyme facilitates an increased production and/or modulation of proinflammatory cytokines and the reduction of anti-inflammatory cytokine production as summarised in Table 1. Many of these cytokines have been implicated in a number of inflammatory diseases, which supports a putative role of PR3 in chronic inflammatory conditions in general as well as COPD with and without AATD.

All these cytokines can act through autocrine, paracrine and endocrine pathways to activate pro-inflammatory cascade responses and upregulate pro-inflammatory genes and transcription factors leading to an inflammatory state [65]. The products of these key inflammatory pathways can further induce feedback loops to enhance chronic inflammation [66–68]. Therefore (similarly to NE) PR3 can potentially play multiple roles in the initiation and amplification as well as the resolution of inflammation, at least as demonstrated in vitro.

More recently, PR3 has been also found to degrade the anti-inflammatory mediator progranulin (PGRN), resulting in generation of granulin (GRN) peptides in vitro [32, 68–70]. PGRN degradation causes increased neutrophil infiltration, activation of reactive oxidative species, pro-inflammatory cytokine production and anti-inflammatory pathway inhibition, sustaining an inflammatory state in other inflammatory disease [71]. GRN molecules are also known to accumulate and release the chemoattractant interleukin (IL)-8 amplifying neutrophil recruitment [70, 72]. In clinically-stable COPD, the concentration of PR3 in airway secretions is a stronger predictor of PGRN levels than NE, because of its greater neutrophil concentration and hence greater secretion activity [69].

PR3 is also able to act in a pro-inflammatory manner by interacting with the complement pathway. It is able to fragment the neutrophil surface complement component 5a (C5a) receptor, resulting in the loss of the N-terminus and an inability to bind C5a [73]. In CF, the lack of C5aR signalling contributes towards inefficient clearance of microbial infections in vitro and also inactivates signalling and stimulates neutrophils to degranulate [73]. This results in a cycle of dysfunctional neutrophils thereby perpetuating the bacterial-stimulated inflammatory signals and further neutrophil recruitment. Although there is no direct evidence, it is likely that C5aR inhibition by PR3 also has a role in COPD with elevated levels of C5a in the sputum of patients and correlations with circulating C5a, physiological gas transfer and the degree of emphysema [74]. Further research is clearly indicated to determine the relevance of this mechanism in COPD.

Despite the potential to impede bacterial clearance, it has also been reported that PR3 itself possesses bactericidal properties through cleavage of the pro-microbicidal protein hCAP-18 (human cathelicidin) into the antibacterial peptide, mucus inducer and neutrophil chemo-attractant LL-37 [51, 75–78]. Furthermore, levels of LL-37 in sputum are related to disease severity in patients with COPD suggesting an indirect role for PR3 which is worthy of further investigation [79].

In addition, PR3 can adhere to neutrophil extracellular traps (NETs) contributing towards the destruction of bacterial virulence factors [80–82]. However, many respiratory-relevant bacteria, such as Streptococcus pneumoniae and Haemophilus influenzae, have evolved NET evasion mechanisms which may overcome this potential clearance mechanism [83, 84]. It has also been noted that patients with Pseudomonas aeruginosa infection are more susceptible to poor outcome when lacking sufficient PR3 inhibition and patients with AATD are at particularly high risk of respiratory infection and lung damage as other natural proteinase inhibitors are unable to compensate for low AAT levels [27, 85]. This is again amplified by the greater neutrophil PR3 content and the fact that the other major lung inhibitor of serine proteinases, secretory leukocyte proteinase inhibitor (SLPI), does not inhibit PR3 [86].

However, PR3 is also able to inactivate SLPI, by cleaving at the Ala-16 site within the N-terminal and preventing SLPI/enzymes complex formation which would indirectly amplify the local activity of other serine proteinases such as NE [86].

Analysis of biopsied lung tissue, from patients with severe emphysema, has shown that cytosolic PR3 interrupts the initiation of anti-inflammatory mechanisms and promotes an apoptotic environment, inducing death of lung epithelial cells which has been implicated in the pathophysiology of emphysema by a further indirect route [87].

An additional mechanism implicated in the pathophysiology of COPD involves the receptor for advanced glycation end-products (RAGE) and soluble RAGE. In prostate cancer cell lines, PR3 has been shown to bind to RAGE both promoting cell activation and preventing its cleavage which escalates inflammation [88, 89]. Furthermore, decreased levels of sRAGE have been implicated in emphysema development [89, 90]. Clearly the relevance of this alternative function also needs to be explored in relation to COPD.

Pathophysiological functions of proteinase 3 in other diseases

The actions discussed above are not just relevant to COPD but are relevant to the pathophysiology of many other diseases. PR3 also has many additional roles which can lead to, or amplify other disease states (see Fig. 3).

As noted in Table 1, PR3 has both a direct and indirect effect on many cytokines and hence can have further downstream influences on diseases beyond or associated with COPD, as outlined in Table 2.

However, although the effects of dysregulation of these cytokines are also implicated in other diseases, PR3 has

not been directly studied in relation to their pathophysiology.

In addition, the interaction between PR3 and PGRN also likely has wider impact than in COPD, through a further role in inflammatory conditions involving PGRN, including lipopolysaccharide-induced acute lung injury, dermatitis and inflammatory arthritis (in murine models), as well as a reported genetic link between loss-of-function mutations in PGRN and the development of neurodegenerative disease [99–104].

It is also suspected that PR3, alongside other NSPs, could have a role in ECM breakdown affecting the pathophysiology of diseases in other organs, such as aneurysms due to vascular remodelling as shown in porcine vasculature; however the relevance has not yet been investigated in detail in humans [105].

PR3 has a role in the efficacy of neutrophil transmigration through interaction with the cell surface receptor NB1 (CD177) which acts with PECAM-1 (CD31) during trans-endothelial migration of neutrophils [106, 107]. In CF, this is supported by a positive relationship between PR3 activity and neutrophil migration effectiveness [20]. The interaction of PR3 with NB1 and PECAM-1 is confirmed in vitro in endothelial cells, where it inhibits activation and upregulation of these adhesion molecules [108].

There is also evidence that PR3 is associated with distortion of cellular signalling pathways and the development of

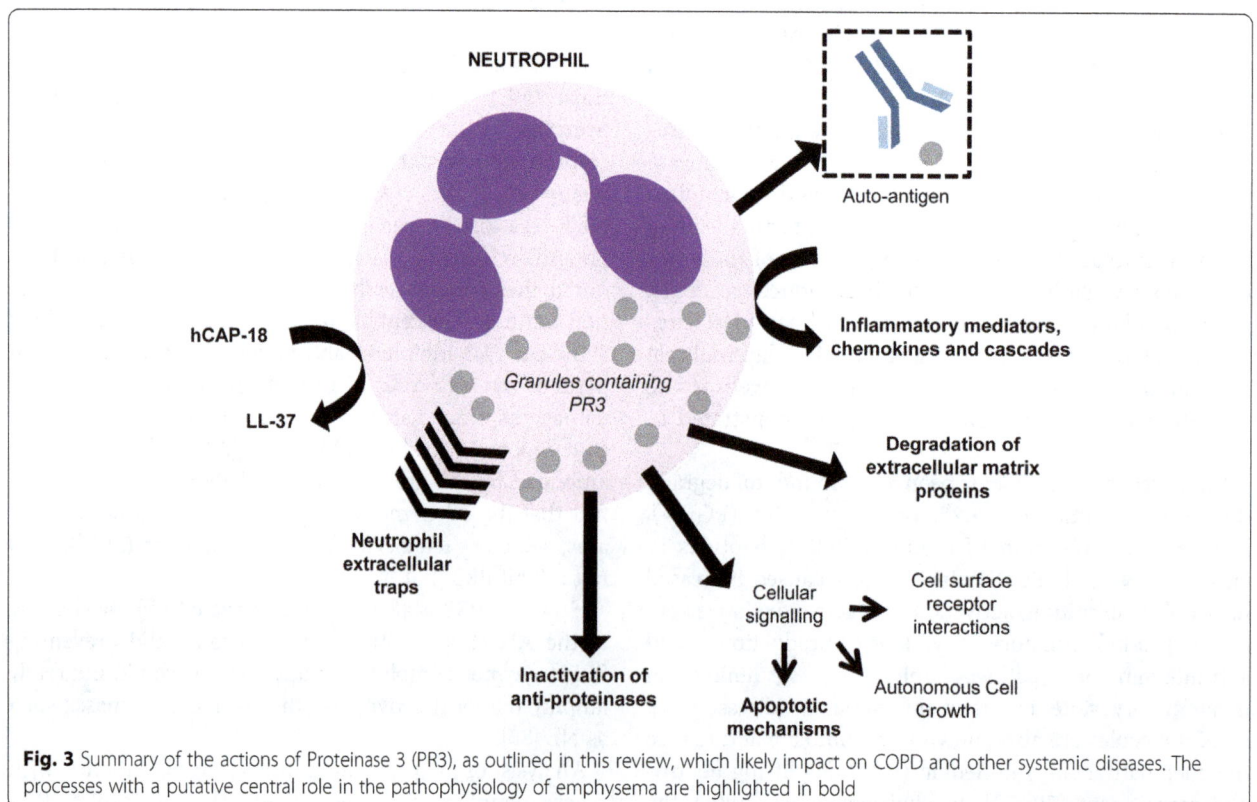

Fig. 3 Summary of the actions of Proteinase 3 (PR3), as outlined in this review, which likely impact on COPD and other systemic diseases. The processes with a putative central role in the pathophysiology of emphysema are highlighted in bold

Table 1 Summary of the cytokines affected by PR3, with the PR3 action on cytokines and the resulting response. The processes relevant to the pathophysiology of COPD are highlighted in bold

Cytokine	Role of PR3	Action of cytokine	References
Interleukin (IL)-1β	Proteolytically activates extracellular pro-forms to be cleaved into active counterparts by Caspase 1 in inflammasomes	• ↑ **neutrophil activation and recruitment** • **canonical NFκB signalling** • ↑ cyclooxygenases [44] and prostaglandin E production • pushes towards T helper cell (Th)17 differentiation	[31, 54–56]
IL-18		• Induces interferon (IFN)-γ and Fas ligand, ↑ differentiation to Th1, Th2 or Th17 responses (dependant on accompanying signals)	[55, 57]
Tumour necrosis factor (TNF)-α	Cleaves precursor to bioactive form (via two hypothesised cleavage sites at Ala15-Leu16 or Val77-Arg78)	• **Activates the caspase and MEK cascades, and PI-3-kinase and canonical NFκB pathway** • **Activates Etk = ↑cellular adhesion, migration and propagation** • ↑ **neutrophil chemotaxis** • **Upregulation of pro-inflammatory genes e.g. IL-8, CCL2, CXCL10, COX-2, and pro-coagulants** • **Recruits apoptosis-inhibiting molecules** • ↓ signalling by cIAP-mediated ubiquitination	[54, 58]
IL-6	Functionally inactivates and degrades the soluble IL-6 receptor (sIL-6R) – exact mechanisms unknown	• Disrupts trans-signalling activity • **Prevents apoptosis** • ↑ **neutrophil recruitment and infiltration**	[59, 60]
IL-8 (CXCL8)	Truncates stored IL-8 (77) into the 10-fold more potent chemo-attractant IL-8 (70) through cleavage of an Ala-Lys bond	• ↑ **respiratory burst** • **Potentiates inflammatory disease cycle** • **Drives neutrophil chemotaxis**	[61]
IL-17 (CTLA8)	Stimulation increases cytokine production	• Directs towards a dominant Th17 environment • T cell hypo-responsiveness	[62]
IL-32	Processes activating cytokines IL-1β, TNF-α and IFN-γ directly or indirectly; cleaves IL-32 at IL-32α to a more bioactive form	• **Activates canonical NFκB and MAPK cascades** • ↑ **production of cytokines incl. TNF-α, IL-8 and CXCL2 production**	[63, 64]

autonomous cell growth. In leukaemia, early expression of PR3 during haematopoiesis is able to induce factor-independent growth and overexpression of PR3 in myeloid leukaemia cells prevents their differentiation into monocytoid cells supporting this mechanism [109–111].

Alternatively to its pro-apoptotic role in COPD, PR3 may paradoxically prevent apoptosis in granulomatosis

Table 2 Cytokines influenced by PR3 (as shown in Table 1) and implicated in disease states other than COPD

Cytokine	Diseases Implicated	References
Interleukin (IL)-1β	• Rheumatoid arthritis • Asthma	[91, 92]
IL-18	• Non-alcoholic fatty liver disease • Type 2 diabetes • Asthma • Rheumatoid arthritis	[92–94]
Tumour necrosis factor (TNF)-α	• Rheumatoid arthritis • Interstitial Lung Disease • Asthma	[95, 96]
IL-6	• Cystic fibrosis	[97]
IL-17 (CTLA8)	• Granulomatosis with polyangiitis	[62]
IL-32	• Psoriasis • Rheumatoid arthritis • Crohn's disease	[98]

with polyangiitis (GPA) by associating with calreticulin, through co-externalisation with phosphatidylserine by phospholipid flip-flop via phospholipid scramblase 1 (PLSCR1), to override the 'eat me' signalling [112].

Finally, PR3 also has a role as an autoantigen in many diseases, including GPA and idiopathic interstitial pneumonias, and is the target of cytoplasmic (c)-anti-neutrophil cytoplasmic antibodies, also referred to as PR3-ANCA in vasculitis [113–115]. Development of disease is dependent on ability of PR3 to associate with the cell membrane [112]. The binding of PR3-ANCA with cell associated PR3 initiates a cascade which amplifies inflammation and results in local cellular and tissue damage [9, 114, 116–118].

It was suspected that PR3-ANCA formation may have a role in COPD development, as more patients with COPD were found to be antinuclear antibody positive than healthy controls [119]. However, despite a reported association with emphysema-dominant disease and lower body mass index, no clear pathophysiological relationship has been established [119]. These wide ranging pro-inflammatory effects of PR3 in other conditions therefore may be also relevant in the pathophysiology of COPD, both directly by tissue damage and indirectly through other multiple pathways of inflammation.

PR3 as a therapeutic target in COPD

There is considerable theoretical evidence and cell-based and animal-model data to support the role of PR3 in the development of COPD. However, as yet, PR3 activity in COPD has been poorly characterised.

To study PR3 in COPD requires the ability to quantify active (uninhibited) PR3 accurately and distinguish it from other NSPs to determine its specific function within biological samples. Reagents for free PR3 activity have only lately become available and until recently, detection required immunofluorescent staining of biopsy specimens, which if positive was followed by a PR3-ANCA specific enzyme-linked immunosorbent assay (ELISA) [120, 121]. Indeed, this was the internationally accepted method for diagnosing PR3-ANCA. Direct PR3 assays have been proposed as a biomarker to determine PR3 presence and production for assisting a diagnosis [122, 123]; however, like immunofluorescence techniques, they do not distinguish the active PR3 from PR3 which has been inactivated by its inhibitors. A similar challenge was seen for the measurement of NE activity and a novel approach to this has been the development of NE specific footprint, which may also be a more relevant approach for PR3 activity in vivo [124].

Whilst there is increasing interest in modifying NSP activity in conditions which predominantly feature neutrophilic inflammation, these have primarily focused on reducing the activity of NE and PR3 has not generally been considered as a relevant target in COPD.

The detection of PR3 activity, directly or indirectly, would improve our understanding of its role in COPD and individual patient's disease activity. It would also potentially allow earlier diagnosis of diseases where PR3 activity was relevant (including COPD) before extensive damage has occurred. Understanding the role of PR3, might therefore allow earlier interventions and therapeutic strategies to be developed with PR3 as a valid target in COPD. Specific inhibitors might serve to reduce disease severity, mortality and the long-term health burdens of COPD. However, clearly the limited data available indicates there is much work to be done to clarify the likely relevance and hence impact of an anti-PR3 strategy.

Conclusions

PR3 has many important functions that are relevant to human physiology and PR3 dysfunction may play a critical role in many processes central to the pathophysiology of COPD and other chronic neutrophilic human diseases. PR3 is the most abundant serine proteinase in the neutrophil, secondarily inhibited to NE, and, in addition to the role in general inflammation, PR3 can also cause direct tissue damage central to structural aspects of diseases such as COPD. This is consistent with the potential for PR3 to produce all the pathological changes of COPD that have traditionally been attributed to NE. Understanding this role and the impact on the inflammatory cascade has major implications for the design of anti-proteinase molecules aimed at restoring proteinase/anti-proteinase balance, ensuring that destructive activity of relevant serine proteinase action and amplification of inflammation is effectively limited, and thereby preventing the development and progression of COPD.

Abbreviations

AAT: α-1 Anti-trypsin; AATD: α-1 Anti-trypsin Deficiency; ANCA: Anti-neutrophil Cytoplasmic Antibodies; C5a: Complement Component 5a; CF: Cystic Fibrosis; COPD: Chronic Obstructive Pulmonary Disease; COX: Cyclooxygenases; D_{LCo}: Diffusing Capacity of the Lungs for Carbon Monoxide; ECM: Extracellular Matrix; ELISA: Enzyme-linked Immunosorbent Assay; GPA: Granulomatosis with Polyangiitis; GRN: Granulin; hCAP-18: Human Cathelicidin; IFN: Interferon; IL: Interleukin; NE: Neutrophil Elastase; NETs: Neutrophil Extracellular Traps; NFkB: Nuclear Factor Kappa-Light-Chain-Enhancer of Activated B Cells; NSP: Neutrophil Serine Proteinase; PGRN: Progranulin; PLSCR1: Phospholipid Scramblase 1; PR3: Proteinase 3; RAGE: Receptor for Advanced Glycation End-products; Serpins: Serine Proteinase Inhibitors; SPLI: Secretory Leukocyte Proteinase Inhibitor; Th: T helper Cells; TNF: Tumour Necrosis Factor

Authors' contributions

All authors met criteria for authorship. HC wrote the initial draft of the manuscript and, ES and RAS revised the manuscript. All authors read and approved the final manuscript.

Competing interests

The authors declare that they have no competing interests.

Author details

[1]Institute of Inflammation and Ageing, University of Birmingham, Edgbaston, Birmingham B15 2GW, UK. [2]University Hospital Birmingham NHS Foundation Trust, Edgbaston, Birmingham B15 2GW, UK. [3]Institute of Inflammation and Ageing, College of Medical and Dental Sciences, Centre for Translational Inflammation Research, University of Birmingham Research Laboratories, Queen Elizabeth Hospital Birmingham, Mindelsohn Way, Birmingham B15 2WB, UK.

References

1. GOLD: Global strategy for the diagnosis, management and prevention of chronic obstructive pulmonary disease. 2017.
2. Baici A, Szedlacsek SE, Fruh H, Michel BA. pH-dependent hysteretic behavior of human Myeloblastin (leucocyte proteinase 3). Biochem J. 1996;317:901–5.
3. Karatepe K, Luo HR. Proteinase 3 is expressed in stem cells and regulates bone marrow hematopoiesis. Blood. 2015;126:1159.
4. Korkmaz B, Moreau T, Gauthier F. Neutrophil elastase, proteinase 3 and Cathepsin G: physiochemical properties, activity and Physiopathologcal functions. Biochemie. 2008;90:227–42.
5. Zimmer M, Medcalf RL, Fink TM, Mattmann C, Lichter P, Jenne DE. Three human elastase-like genes Coordingately expressed in the Myelomonocyte

lineage are organised as a single genetic locus on 19pter. Proc Natl Acad Sci U S A. 1992;89:5.

6. Csernok E, Ernst M, Schmitt W, Bainton DF, Gross WL. Activated neutrophils express proteinase 3 on their plasma membrane In vitro and In vivo. Clin Exp Immunol. 1994;95:244–50.

7. Witko-Sarsat V, Cramer EM, Hieblot C, Guichard J, Nusbaum P, Lopez S, Lesavre P, Halbwachs-Mecarelli L. Presence of proteinase 3 in secretory vesicles: evidence of a novel, highly Mobilizable intracellular Pool distinct from Azurophil granules. Blood. 1999;94:2487–96.

8. Halbwachs-Mecarelli L, Bessou G, Lesavre P, Lopez S, Witko-Sarsat V. Bimodal Distrubution of proteinase 3 (PR3) surface expression reflects a constitutive heterogeneity in the Polymorphonuclear neutrophil Pool. FEBS Lett. 1995;374:29–33.

9. Csernok E, Ludemann J, Gross WL, Bainton DF. Ultrastructural localisation of proteinase 3, the target antigen of anti-cytoplasmic antibodies circulating in Wegener's granulomatosis. Am J Pathol. 1990;137:1113–20.

10. Korkmaz B, Jaillet J, Jourdan M-L, Gauthier A, Gauthier F, Attucci S. Catalytic activity and inhibition of Wegener antigen proteinase 3 on the cell surface of human Polymorphonuclear neutrophils. J Biol Chem. 2009;284:19896–902.

11. Korkmaz B, Lesner A, Letast S, Mahdi YK, Jourdan ML, Dallet-Choisy S, Marchand-Adam S, Kellenberger C, Viaud-Massuard MC, Jenne DE, Gauthier F. Neutrophil proteinase 3 and dipeptidyl peptidase I (cathepsin C) as pharmacological targets in granulomatosis with polyangiitis (Wegener granulomatosis). Semin Immunopathol. 2013;35:411–21.

12. Hajjar E, Broemstrup T, Kantari C, Witko-Sarsat V, Reuter N. Structures of human proteinase 3 and neutrophil elastase - so similar yet so different. FEBS J. 2010;277:2238–54.

13. Hajjar E, Korkmaz B, Gauthier F, Brandsdal BO, Witko-Sarsat V, Reuter N. Inspection of the binding sites of proteinase 3 for the Design of a Highly Specific Substrate. J Med Chem. 2006;49:1248–60.

14. Guarino C, Gruba N, Grzywa R, Dyguda-Kazimierowicz E, Hamon Y, Legowska M, Skorenski M, Dallet-Choisy S, Marchand-Adam S, Kellenberger C, et al. Exploiting the S4-S5 specificity of human neutrophil proteinase 3 to improve the potency of peptidyl Di(chlorophenyl)-phosphonate Ester inhibitors: a kinetic and molecular modeling analysis. J Med Chem. 2018;61:1858–70.

15. Fujinaga M, Chernaia MM, Halenbeck R, Koths K, James MNG. The crystal structure of PR3, a neutrophil serine proteinase antigen of Wegener's granulomatosis antibodies. J Mol Biol. 1996;261:267–77.

16. Korkmaz B, Horwitz MS, Jenne DE, Gauthier F. Neutrophil elastase, proteinase 3, and Cathepsin G as therapeutic targets in human diseases. Pharmacol Rev. 2010;62:726–59.

17. Rao NV, Wehner NG, Marshall BC, Gray WR, Gray BH, Hoidal JR. Characterisation of proteinase 3 (PR-3), a neutrophil serine proteinase: structural and functional properties. J Biol Chem. 1991;266:9540–8.

18. Brubaker MJ, Groutas WC, Hoidal JR, Rao NV. Human neutrophil proteinase 3: mapping of the substrate binding site using peptidyl Thiobenzyl esters. Biochem Biophys Res Commun. 1992;188:1318–24.

19. Schechter I, Berger A. On the size of the active site in proteases. I. Papain. Biochem Biophys Res Commun. 1967;27:157–62.

20. Twigg MS, Brockbank S, Lowry P, FitzGerald SP, Taggart C, Weldon S. The role of serine proteases and Antiproteases in the cystic fibrosis lung. Mediat Inflamm. 2015;2015:10.

21. Berman HM, Westbrook J, Feng Z, Gilliland G, Bhat TN, Weissig H, Shindyalov IN, Bourne PE. The Protein Data Bank. Nucleic Acids Res. 2000;28:235–42.

22. Krieger E, Vriend G. YASARA view - molecular graphics for all devices - from smartphones to workstations. Bioinformatics. 2014;30:2981–2.

23. Campbell EJ, Campbell MA, Owen CA. Bioactive proteinase 3 on the cell surface of human neutrophils: quantification, catalytic activity, and susceptibility to inhibition. J Immunol. 2000;165:3366–74.

24. Loison F, Xu Y, Luo HR. Proteinase 3 and serpin B1: a novel pathway in the regulation of Caspase-3 activation, neutrophil spontaneous apoptosis, and inflammation. Inflamm Cell Signal. 2014;1:1–5.

25. Zani ML, Nobar SM, Lacour SA, Lemoine S, Boudier C, Bieth JG, Moreau T. Kinetics of the inhibition of Neutriophil proteinases by recombinant Elafin and pre-elafin (Trappin-2) expressed in Pichia pastoris. Eur J Biochem. 2004;271:2370–8.

26. Yang L, Mei Y, Fang Q, Wang J, Yan Z, DSong Q, Lin Z, Ye G. Identification and characterization of serine protease inhibitors in a parasitic wasp, Pteromalus puparum. Sci Rep. 2017;7:1-13.

27. Sinden NJ, Baker MJ, Smith DJ, Kreft J-U, Dafforn TR, Stockley RA. Alpha-1-antitrypsin variants and the proteinase/anti-proteinase imbalance in chronic obstructive pulmonary disease. Am J Physiol Lung Cell Mol Physiol. 2015;308:12.

28. Jerke U, Perez Hernandez D, Beaudette P, Korkmaz B, Dittmar G, Kettritz R. Neutrophil Serine Proteases Exert Proteolytic Activity on Endothelial Cells. Kidney Int. 2015;88:764–75.

29. Korkmaz B, Lesner A, Guarino C, Wysocka M, Kellenberger C, Watier H, Specks U, Gauthier F, Jenne DE. Inhibitors and antibody fragments as potential anti-inflammatory therapeutics Targetting neutrophil proteinase 3 in human disease. Pharmacol Rev. 2016;68:603–30.

30. Guyot N, Wartelle J, Malleret L, Todorov AA, Devouassoux G, Pacheco Y, Jenne DE, Belaaouaj A. Unopposed Cathepsin G, neutrophil elastase, and proteinase 3 cause severe lung damage and emphysema. Am J Pathol. 2014;184:2197–210.

31. Joosten LA, Netea MG, Fantuzzi G, Koenders MI, Helsen MM, Sparrer H, Pham CT, van der Meer JW, Dinarello CA, van den Berg WB. Inflammatory Arthritis in Caspase 1 Gene-deficient Mice: Contribution of Proteinase 3 to Caspase 1-independent Production of Bioactive Interleukin-1beta. Arthritis Rheum. 2009;60:3651–62.

32. Kessenbrock K, Frohlich L, Sixt M, Lammermann T, Pfister H, Bateman A, Belaaouaj A, Ring J, Ollert M, Fassler R, Jenne DE. Proteinase 3 and neutrophil elastase enhance inflammation in mice by inactivating anti-inflammatory Progranulin. J Clin Invest. 2008;118:2438–47.

33. Gudmann NS, Manon-Jensen T, Sand JMB, Diefenbach C, Sun S, Danielsen A, Karsdal MA, Leeming DJ. Lung tissue destruction by proteinase 3 and Cathepsin G mediated elastin degradation is elevated in chronic obstructive pulmonary disease. Biochem Biophys Res Commun. 2018;503(3):1284-90.

34. Newby PR, Carter RI, Stockley RA. Aα-Val^{541} a Novel Biomarker of Proteinase 3 Activity. Am J Respir Crit Care Med. 2017;195:A5247.

35. Newby PR, Stockley RA. Neutrophil elastase and proteinase 3 activity in PiSZ Alpha-1 antitrypsin deficiency. Am J Respir Crit Care Med. 2018;197:A4763.

36. Hoenderdos K, Condliffe A. The neutrophil in chronic obstructive pulmonary disease. Too little, too late or too much, too soon? Am J Respir Cell Mol Biol. 2013;48:531–9.

37. Campbell EJ, Campbell MA, Boukedes SS, Owen CA. Quantum proteolysis by neutrophils: implications for pulmonary emphysema in α1-antitrypsin deficiency. CHEST. 2000;117:303S.

38. Stockley RA. Neutrophils and protease/Antiprotease imbalance. Am J Respir Crit Care Med. 1999;160:S49–52.

39. Owen CA, Campbell EJ. The cell biology of leukocyte-mediated proteolysis. J Leukoc Biol. 1999;65:14.

40. Maximova K, Venken T, Reuter N, Trylska J. D-peptides as inhibitors of PR3-membrane interactions. Biomembranes. 1860;2018:458–66.

41. Korkmaz B, Poutrain P, Hazouard E, de Monte M, Attucci S, Gauthier FL. Competition between elastase and related proteases from human neutrophil for binding to α1-protease inhibitor. Am J Respir Cell Mol Biol. 2005;32:553–9.

42. Sinden NJ, Stockley RA. Proteinase 3 activity in sputum from subjects with Alpha-1 anti-trypsin deficiency and COPD. Eur Respir J. 2013;41:1042–50.

43. Kao RC, Wehner NG, Skubitz KM, Gray BH, Hoidal JR. Proteinase 3. A distinct human Polymorphonuclear leukocyte proteinase that produces emphysema in hamsters. J Clin Invest. 1988;82:1963–73.

44. Borel F, Sun H, Zieger M, Cox A, Cardozo B, Li W, Oliveira G, Davis A, Gruntman A, Flotte TR, et al. Editing out five Serpina1 paralogs to create a mouse model of genetic emphysema. Proc Natl Acad Sci U S A. 2018; 115(11):2788-93.

45. Lombard C, Bouchu D, Wallach J, Saulnier J. Proteinase 3 hydrolysis of peptides derived from human elastin exon 24. Amino Acids. 2005;28:403–8.

46. Chelladurai P, Seeger W, Pullamsetti SS. Matrix metalloproteinases and their inhibitors in pulmonary hypertension. Eur Respir J. 2012;40:766–82.

47. Sand JMB, Knox AJ, Lange P, Sun S, Kristensen JH, Leeming DJ, Karsdal MA, Bolton CE, Johnson SR. Accelerated extracellular matrix turnover during exacerbations of COPD. Respir Res. 2015;16:69.

48. Ramaha A, Patston PA. Release and degradation of angiotensin 1 and angiotensin 2 from angiotensinogen by neutrophil serine proteinases. Arch Biochem Biophys. 2002;397:77–83.

49. Witko-Sarsat V, Halbwachs-Mecarelli L, Schuster A, Nusbaum P, Ueki I, Canteloup S, Lenoir G, Descamps-Latscha B, Nadel JA. Proteinase 3, a potent Secretagogue in airways, is present in cystic fibrosis sputum. Am J Respir Cell Mol Biol. 1999;20:729–36.

50. Janciauskiene S, Bals R, Koczulla R, Vogelmeier C, Kohnlein T, Welte T. The discovery of Alpha-1-antitrypsin and its role in health and disease. Respir Med. 2011;105:1129–39.

51. Sorensen OE, Follin P, Johnsen AH, Calafat J, Tjabringa GS, Hiemstra PS, Borregaard N. Human cathelicidin, hCAP-18, is processed to the antimicrobial peptide LL-37 by extracellular cleavage with proteinase 3. Blood J. 2001;97:3951–9.

52. Ren K, Torres R. Role of interleukin-1beta during pain and inflammation. Brain Res Rev. 2009;60:57–64.

53. Popa C, Netea MG, van Riel PLCM, van der Meer JWM, Stalenhoef AFH. The role of TNF-a in chronic inflammatory conditions, intermediary metabolism, and cardiovascular risk. J Lipid Res. 2007;48:751–62.

54. Coeshott C, Ohnemus C, Pilyavskaya A, Ross S, Wieczorek M, Kroona H, Leimer AH, Cheronis J. Converting enzyme-independent release of tumor necrosis factor alpha and IL-1beta from a stimulated human Monocytic cell line in the presence of activated neutrophils or purified proteinase 3. Proc Natl Acad Sci U S A. 1999;96:6261–6.

55. Keyel PA. How is inflammation initiated? Individual influences of IL-1, IL-18 and HMGB1. Cytokine. 2014;69:136-45.

56. Schreiber A, Pham CT, Hu Y, Schneider W, Luft FC, Kettritz R. Neutrophil serine proteases promote IL-1beta generation and injury in necrotizing crescentic glomerulonephritis. J Am Soc Nephrol. 2012;23:470–82.

57. Sugawara A, Uehara A, Nochi T, Yamaguchi T, Ueda H, Sugiyama A, Hanzawa K, Kumagai K, Okamura H, Takada H. Neutrophil proteinase 3-mediated induction of bioactive IL-18 secretion by human Oral epithelial cells. J Immunol. 2001;167:6568–75.

58. Bradley JR. TNF-mediated inflammatory disease. J Pathol. 2008;214:149–60.

59. Hurst SM, Wilkinson TS, McLoughline RM, Jones S, Horiuchi S, Yamamoto N, Rose-john S, Fuller GM, Topley N, Jones SA. IL-6 and its soluble receptor Ochestrate a Temportal switch in the pattern of leukocyte recruitment seen during acute inflammation. Immunity. 2001;14:705–14.

60. McLoughlin RM, Hurst SM, Nowell MA, Harris DA, Horiuchi S, Morgan LW, Wilkinson TS, Yamamoto N, Topley N, Jones SA. Differential regulation of neutrophil-activating chemokines by IL-6 and its soluble receptor isoforms. J Immunol. 2004;172:5676–83.

61. Keatings VM, Collins PD, Scott DM, Barnes PJ. Differences in Interleukin-8 and tumour necrosis factor-alpha in induced sputum from patients with chronic obstructive pulmonary disease or asthma. Am J Respir Crit Care Med. 1996;153:512–21.

62. Rani L, Minz RW, Sharma A, Anand S, Gupta D, Panda NK, Sakhuja VK. Predominance of PR3 specific immune response and skewed Th17 vs. T-regulatory Miliew in active Granfulomatosis with Polyangiitis. Cytokine. 2015;71:7.

63. Kim S-H, Han S-Y, Azam T, Yoon D-Y, Dinarello CA. Interleukin-32: a cytokine and inducer of TNFα. Immunity. 2005;22:131–42.

64. Calabrese F, Baraldo S, Bazzan E, Lunardi F, Rea F, Maestrelli P, Turato G, Lokar-Oliani K, Papi A, Zuin R, Sfriso P. IL-32, a novel Proinflammatory cytokine in chronic obstructive pulmonary disease. Am J Respir Crit Care Med. 2008;178:894–901.

65. Zhang J-M, An J. Cytokines, inflammation and pain. Int Anesthesiol Clin. 2007;45:27–37.

66. Nemeth T, Mocsai A. Feedback amplification of neutrophil function. Cell. 2016;37:412–24.

67. Robache-Gallea S, Morand V, Bruneau JM, Schoot B, Tagat E, Realo E, Chouaib S, Roman-Roman S. In vitro processing of human tumour necrosis factor-alpha. J Biol Chem. 1995;270:23688–92.

68. Kessenbrock K, Dau T, Jenne DE. Tailor-made inflammation: how neutrophil serine proteases modulate the inflammatory response. J Mol Med. 2011;89:23–8.

69. Ungers MJ, Sinden NJ, Stockley RA. Progranulin is a substrate for neutrophil-elastase and Proteinase-3 in the airway and its concentration correlates with mediators of airway inflammation in COPD. Am J Physiol Lung Cell Mol Physiol. 2014;306:L80–7.

70. Couto MA, Harwig SSL, Cullor JS, Hughes JP, Lehrer RI. eNAP-2, a novel cysteine-rich bactericidal peptide from equine leukocytes. Infect Immun. 1992;60:5042–7.

71. Baker M, Mackenzie IR, Pickering-Brown SM, Gass J, Rademakers R, Lindholm C, Snowden J, Adamson J, Sadovnivk AD, Rollinson S, et al. Mutations in Progranulin cause tau-negative frontotemporal dementia linked to chromosome 17. Nature. 2006;442:916–9.

72. Zhu J, Nathan C, Jin W, Sim D, Ashcroft GS, Wahl SM, Lacomis L, Erdujument-Bromage H, Tempst P, Wright CD, Ding A. Conversion of Proepithelin to Epithelins: roles of SLPI and elastase in host defense and wound repair. Cell. 2002;111:867–78.

73. van der Berg CW, Tambourgi DV, Clark HW, Hoong SJ, Spiller OB, McGreal EP. Mechanism of neutrophil dysfunction: neutrophil serine proteases cleave and inactivate the C5a receptor. J Immunol. 2014;192:1787–95.

74. Marc MM, Korosec P, Kosnik M, Kern I, Flezar M, Suskovic S, Sorli J. Complement factors C3a, C4a, and C5a in chronic obstructive pulmonary disease and asthma. Am J Respir Cell Mol Biol. 2004;31:216–9.

75. Zhang Y, Jiang Y, Sun C, Wang Q, Yang Z, Pan X, Zhu M, Xiao W. The human cathelicidin LL-37 enhances airway mucus production in chronic obstructive pulmonary disease. Biochem Biophys Res Commun. 2014;443:103–9.

76. Campanelli D, Detmers PA, Nathan CF, Gabay JE. Azurocidin and a homologous serine protease from neutrophils. Differential antimicrobial and proteolytic properties. J Clin Invest. 1990;85:904–15.

77. Dasaraju PV, Liu C. Infections of the respiratory system. In: Medical Microbiology. 4th ed. Baron S, editor. Texas: University of Texas Medical Branch at Galveston; 1996.

78. Kuroda K, Okumura K, Isogai H, Isogai E. The human cathelicidin antimicrobial peptide LL-37 and mimics are potential anti-Cancer drugs. Front Oncol. 2015;5:10.

79. Jiang Y-Y, Xiao W, Zhu M-X, Yang Z-H, Pan X-J, Zhang Y, Sun C-C, Xing Y. The effect of human antibacterial peptide LL-37 in the pathogenesis of chronic obstructive pulmonary disease. Respir Med. 2012;106:1680–9.

80. Urban CF, Ermert D, Schmid M, Abu-Abed U, Goosmann C, Nacken W, Brinkmann V, Jungblut PR, Sycglinsky A. Neutrophil extracellular traps contain calprotectin, a cytosolic protein complex involved in host defense against Candida albicans. PLoS Pathog. 2009;5:e1000639.

81. Kessenbrock K, Krumbholz M, Schonermarck U, Back W, Gross WL, Werb Z, Grone H-J, Brinkmann V, Jenne DE. Netting Neutrophils in Autoimmune Small-Vessel Vasculitis. Nat Med. 2009;15:623–5.

82. Delgado-Rizo V, Martinez-Guzman MA, Iniguez-Gutierrez L, Garcia-Orozco A, Alvarado-Navarro A, Fafutis-Morris M. Neutrophil extracellular traps and its implications in inflammation: an overview. Front Immunol. 2017;2017:1–20.

83. Beiter K, Wartha F, Albiger B, Normark S, Zychlinsky A, Henriques-Normark B. An endonuclease allows Streptococcus pneumoniae to escape from neutrophil extracellular traps. Curr Biol. 2006;16:401–7.

84. Hong W, Juneau RA, Pang B, Swords WE. Survival of bacterial biofilms within neutrophil extracellular traps promotes Nontypeable Haemophilus influenzae persistence in the Chinchilla model for otitis media. J Innate Immun. 2009;1:215–24.

85. Benarafa C, Priebe GP, Remold-O'Donnell E. The neutrophil serine protease inhibitor SerpinB1 preserves lung Defence functions in Pseudomonas aeruginosa infection. J Exp Med. 2007;204:1901–9.

86. Rao NV, Marshall BC, Gray BH, Hoidal JR. Interaction of secretory leukocyte protease inhibitor with Proteinase-3. Am J Respir Cell Mol Biol. 1993;8:612-6.

87. Kasahara Y, Tuder RM, Cool CD, Lynch DA, Flores SC, Voelkel NF. Endothelial cell death and decreased expression of vascular endothelial growth factor and vascular endothelial growth factor receptor 2 in emphysema. Am J Respir Crit Care Med. 2001;163:737–44.

88. Kolonin AG, Sergeeva A, Staquicini DI, Smith TL, Tarleton CA, Molldrem JJ, Sidman RL, Marchio S, Pasqualini R, Arap W. Interaction between tumour cell surface receptor RAGE and proteinase 3 mediates prostate Cancer Matastasis to bone. Cancer Res. 2017;77:3144–50.

89. Sukkar MB, Ullah MA, Gan WJ, Wark PAB, Chung KF, Hughes JM, Armour CL, Phipps S. RAGE: a new frontier in chronic airways disease. Br J Pharmacol. 2012;167:1161–76.

90. Yonchuk JG, Silverman EK, Bowler RP, Agusti A, Lomas DA, Miller BE, Tal-Singer R, Mayer RJ. Circulating soluble receptor for advanced glycation end products (sRAGE) as a biomarker of emphysema and the RAGE Axis in the lung. Am J Respir Crit Care Med. 2015;192:785–92.

91. Stéhlik C. Multiple IL-1β converting enzymes contribute to inflammatory arthritis. Arthritis Rheum. 2009;60:3524–30.

92. Lee T-H, Song HJ, Park C-S. Role of Inflammasome activation in development and exacerbation of asthma. Asia Pacific Allergy. 2014;4:187–96.

93. Toonen EJ, Mirea AM, Tack CJ, Stienstra R, Ballak DB, van Diepen JA, Hijmans A, Chavakis T, Dokter WH, Pham CT, et al. Activation of proteinase 3 contributes to non-alcoholic fatty liver disease (NAFLD) and insulin resistance. Mol Med. 2016;22:202–14.

94. Gracie JA. Interleukin-18 as a potential target in inflammatory arthritis. Clin Exp Immunol. 2004;136:402–4.

95. Matsumoto T, Kaneko T, Seto M, Wada H, Kobayashi T, Nakatani K, Tonomura H, Tono Y, Ohyabu M, Nobori T, et al. The membrane proteinase 3 expression on neutrophils was downregulated after treatment with infliximab in patients with rheumatoid arthritis. Clin Appl Thromb Hemost. 2008;14:186-92.

96. Armstrong L, Godinho SIH, Uppington KM, Whittington HA, Millar AB. Tumour necrosis factor-α processing in interstitial lung disease: a potential role for exogenous Proteinase-3. Clin Exp Immunol. 2009;156:336–43.

97. McGreal EP, Davies PL, Powell W, Rose-John S, Spiller OB, Doull I, Jones SA, Kotecha S. Inactivation of IL-6 and soluble IL-6 receptor by neutrophil derived serine proteases in cystic fibrosis. Biochim Biophys Acta. 2010;1802:649–58.

98. Dinarello CA, Kim SH. IL-32, a novel cytokine with a possible role in disease. Ann Rheum Dis. 2006;65:4.

99. Zhao Y-P, Tian Q-Y, Liu C-J. Progranulin deficiency exaggerates, whereas Progranulin-derived Atsttrin attenuates, severity of dermatitis in mice. FEBS Lett. 2013;587:6.

100. Tang W, Lu Y, Tian QY, Zhang Y, Guo FJ, Liu GY, Syed NM, Lai Y, Lin EA, Kong L, et al. The growth factor Progranulin binds to TNF receptors and is therapeutic against inflammatory arthritis in mice. Science. 2011;332:7.

101. Guo Z, Li Q, Han Y, Liang Y, Xu Z, Ren T. Prevention of LPS-induced acute lung injury in mice by Progranulin. Mediat Inflamm. 2012;2012:10.

102. Goedert M, Spillantini MG. Frontotemporal lobar degeneration through loss of Progranulin function. Brain Res Rev. 2006;129:2808–10.

103. Bossu P, Salani F, Alberici A, Archetti S, Bellelli G, Galimberti D, Scarpini E, Spalletta G, Caltagirone C, Padovani A, Borroni B. Loss of function mutations in the Progranulin gene are related to pro-inflammatory cytokine dysregulation in frontotemporal lobar degeneration patients. J Neuroinflammation. 2011;8:65–9.

104. Cruts M, van Broeckhoven C. Loss of Progranulin function in frontotemporal lobar degeneration. Trends Genet. 2008;24:186–94.

105. Chow MJ, Choi M, Yun SH, Zhang Y. The effect of static stretch on elastin degradation in arteries. PLoS One. 2013;8:e81951.

106. Kuckleburg CJ, Tilkens SM, Santoso S, Newman PJ. Proteinase 3 contributes to Transendothelial migration of NB1-positive neutrophils. J Immunol. 2012;188:2419–26.

107. Wiedow O, Meyer-Hoffert U. Neutrophil serine proteases: potential key regulators of cell Signalling during inflammation. J Intern Med. 2005;257:319–28.

108. Saragih H, Zilian E, Jaimes Y, Paine A, Figueiredo C, Eiz-Vesper B, Blascysk R, Larmann J, Theilmeier G, Burg-Roderfeld M, et al. PECAM-1-dependent Heme Oxygenase-1 regulation via an Nrf2-mediated pathway in endothelial cells. Thromb Haemost. 2014;111:1077–88.

109. Lutz PG, Houzel-Charavel A, Moog-Lutz C, Cayre YE. Myeloblastin is an Myb target gene: mechanisms of Regulationin myeloid leukemia cells growth-arrested by retinoic acid. Blood Journal. 2001;97:2449–56.

110. Lutz PG, Moog-Lutz C, Coumau-Gatbois E, Kobari L, di Gioia Y, Cayre YE. Myeloblastin is a granulocyte Colony-stimulating factor-responsive gene conferring factor-independent growth to Haematopoietic cells. Proc Natl Acad Sci U S A. 2000;97:1601–6.

111. Bories D, Raynal M-C, Solomon DH, Darzynkiewicz Z, Cayre YE. Down-regulation of a serine protease, Myeloblastin, causes growth arrest and differentiation of Promyelocytic leukemia cells. Cell. 1989;59:959–68.

112. Martin KR, Kantarl-Mimoun C, Yin M, Perderzoll-Ribell M, Angelot-Delettre F, Cerol A, Grauffel C, Benhamou M, Reuter N, Saas P, et al. Proteinase 3 is a phosphatidylserine-binding protein that affects the production and function of microvesicles. J Biol Chem. 2016;291:10476–89.

113. Cerezo LA, Kuklova M, Hulejova H, Vernerova Z, Kasprikova N, Veigl D, Pavelka K, Vencovsky J, Senolt L. Progranulin is associate with disease activity in patients with Rheumatiod arthritis. Mediat Inflamm. 2015;2015:6.

114. Jennette JC, Nachman PH. ANCA glomerulonephritis and Vasculitis. Clin J Am Soc Nephrol. 2017;12:1680–91.

115. Hozumi H, Enomoto N, Oyama Y, Kono M, Fujisawa T, Inui N, Nakamura Y, Suda T. Clinical implication of Proteinase-3-Antineutrophil cytoplasmic antibody in patients with idiopathic interstitial pneumonias. Lung. 2016;194:235–42.

116. Seo P, Stone JH. The Antineutrophilic cytoplasmic antibody-associated Vasulitides. Am J Med. 2004;117:39–50.

117. Falk RJ, Jennette JC. Wegener's granulomatosis systemic Vasculitis, and Antineutrophil cytoplasmic autoantibodies. Annu Rev Med. 1991;42:459–69.

118. Savage COS. Pathogenesis of anti-neutrophil cytoplasmic autoantibody (ANCA)-associated Vasculitis. Clin Exp Immunol. 2011;164:23–6.

119. Bonarius HPJ, Brandsma CA, Kerstjens HAM, Koerts JA, Kerkhof M, Nizankowska-Mogilnicka E, Roozendaal C, Postma DS, Timens W. Antinuclear autoantibodies are more prevalent in COPD in association with low body mass index but not with smoking history. Thorax. 2011;66:101–7.

120. Savige J, Gillis D, Benson E, Davies D, Esnault V, Falk RJ, Hagen EC, Jayne D, Jennette JC, Paspaliaris B, et al. International consensus statement on testing and reporting of Antineutrophil cytoplasmic antibodies (ANCA). Am J Clin Pathol. 1999;111:507–13.

121. Savige J, Dimech W, Fritzler M, Goeken J, Hagen EC, Jennette JC, McEvoy R, Pusey C, Pollock W, Trevisin M, et al. Addendum to the international consensus statement on testing and reporting of Antineutrophil cytoplasmic antibodies. Am J Clin Pathol. 2003;120:312–8.

122. Wong HR, Cvijanovich NZ, Anas N, Allen GL, Thomas NJ, Bigham MT, Weiss SL, Fitzgerald J, Checchia PA, Meyer K, et al. A multibiomarker-based model for estimating the risk of septic acute kidney injury. Crit Care Med. 2015;43:1646–53.

123. Ng LL, Khan SQ, Narayan H, Quinn P, Squire IB, Davies JE. Proteinase 3 and prognosis of patients with acute myocardial infarction. Clin Sci. 2011;120:231–8.

124. Carter RI, Ungers MJ, Mumford RA, Stockley RA. Aa-Val360: a marker of Neurophil elastase and COPD disease activity. Eur Respir J. 2013;41(1):31-8.

9

The prostaglandin D_2 receptor 2 pathway in asthma: a key player in airway inflammation

Christian Domingo[1,2], Oscar Palomares[3], David A. Sandham[4], Veit J. Erpenbeck[5] and Pablo Altman[6*]

Abstract

Asthma is characterised by chronic airway inflammation, airway obstruction and hyper-responsiveness. The inflammatory cascade in asthma comprises a complex interplay of genetic factors, the airway epithelium, and dysregulation of the immune response.

Prostaglandin D_2 (PGD$_2$) is a lipid mediator, predominantly released from mast cells, but also by other immune cells such as T$_H$2 cells and dendritic cells, which plays a significant role in the pathophysiology of asthma. PGD$_2$ mainly exerts its biological functions via two G-protein-coupled receptors, the PGD$_2$ receptor 1 (DP$_1$) and 2 (DP$_2$). The DP$_2$ receptor is mainly expressed by the key cells involved in type 2 immune responses, including T$_H$2 cells, type 2 innate lymphoid cells and eosinophils. The DP$_2$ receptor pathway is a novel and important therapeutic target for asthma, because increased PGD$_2$ production induces significant inflammatory cell chemotaxis and degranulation via its interaction with the DP$_2$ receptor. This interaction has serious consequences in the pulmonary milieu, including the release of pro-inflammatory cytokines and harmful cationic proteases, leading to tissue remodelling, mucus production, structural damage, and compromised lung function. This review will discuss the importance of the DP$_2$ receptor pathway and the current understanding of its role in asthma.

Keywords: Asthma, Airway inflammation, Prostaglandin D_2, Prostaglandin D_2 receptor 2

Background

Asthma affects approximately 358 million people worldwide [1], and is characterised by chronic airway inflammation, reversible airway obstruction and hyper-responsiveness. The heterogeneous nature of this condition may cause difficulty in predicting response to treatment in a particular patient [2, 3].

Despite the availability of clinical practice guidelines and standard-of-care therapy, a large proportion of asthma patients remain symptomatic and experience poor quality-of-life [4, 5]. There is a high unmet need for novel asthma therapies, especially for patients with severe disease. Effective disease control is dependent in part by treatment adherence [6], which can be influenced by route of administration. Adherence to inhaled therapies, particularly maintenance therapies such as

inhaled corticosteroids, is often poor, and is driven by the complexity of the inhaler, as well as errors during device use, such as improper actuation–inhalation coordination [7]. A clinical consequence of poor or non-adherence to inhaled therapies is increase of symptoms and eventually the occurrence of exacerbations [8]. Adherence to oral asthma treatment has been shown to be superior to that of inhaled therapies [9, 10], however oral therapy options for the management of asthma are presently quite limited. Hence, effective new oral therapies may help the management of severe or insufficiently controlled asthma [11, 12], as has been the case with the recent introduction of biological therapies via subcutaneous injection.

A treatment target with a novel mechanism of action that has gained significant interest in recent years and which has promise to be accessible by small molecule-based oral therapies, is the receptor 2 (DP$_2$) of prostaglandin D_2 (PGD$_2$). This receptor is also referred to in the literature as the chemoattractant receptor homologous molecule expressed on T$_H$2 cells (CRT$_H$2) [13], and

* Correspondence: pablo.altman@novartis.com
[6]Novartis Pharmaceuticals Corporation, One Health Plaza East Hanover, East Hanover, NJ 07936-1080, USA
Full list of author information is available at the end of the article

is expressed on the membrane surface of T_H2 cells, type 2 innate lymphoid cells (ILC2), mast cells and eosinophils [14–16]. This review aims to discuss the current understanding of the DP_2 receptor signalling pathway in asthma.

Allergen-dependant and non-allergen-dependent stimulation

The inflammatory cascade in asthma comprises a complex interplay of factors. In a large proportion of patients, asthma is associated with a type 2 immune response (Type 2-high asthma) [17, 18]. Until recently, only the allergen-dependent immune pathway was considered to be an important target for asthma treatment. However, it is now clear that both the non-allergen- and allergen-dependent immune pathways are involved in the pathophysiological and immunological responses in asthma [19]. As PGD_2, a pro-inflammatory lipid mediator, release is stimulated following both non-allergen-dependent (infections, physical stimuli or chemical stimuli) and allergen-dependent immune activation, the DP_2 receptor pathway has relevance in both atopic and non-atopic asthma (Fig. 1) [16, 20].

PGD_2 release from immune cells

PGD_2 is released following activation of the immune system, which can be either non-allergen- or allergen-dependent (Fig. 1); the non-allergen-dependent pathway comprises indirect activation of mast cells via the processing of physical agents, chemical agents or infections by antigen presenting cells, or direct activation via complement, sphingolipids and others. Through the allergen-dependent pathway, inhaled allergens trigger a cascade of events that provoke the release of PGD_2, initiating a signalling cascade through the DP_2 receptor in target cells (T_H2 cells, ILC2 and eosinophils). Inhaled antigens are presented to $CD4^+$ T lymphocytes by allergen presenting cells. In allergic patients, these T lymphocytes differentiate to acquire a T_H2 cell profile, producing significant amounts of IL-4 and IL-13, which promote IgE class-switching in B lymphocytes [21–23]. Mast cells are subsequently activated upon allergen-induced cross-linking of adjacent high-affinity IgE Fc receptor (FcεRI)-bound IgE at the cell surface [24].

PGD_2 is primarily released from mast cells through activation of hematopoietic PGD synthase, resulting in nanomolar local concentrations of the mediator [25]. Mast cells are tissue-resident cells that can be activated

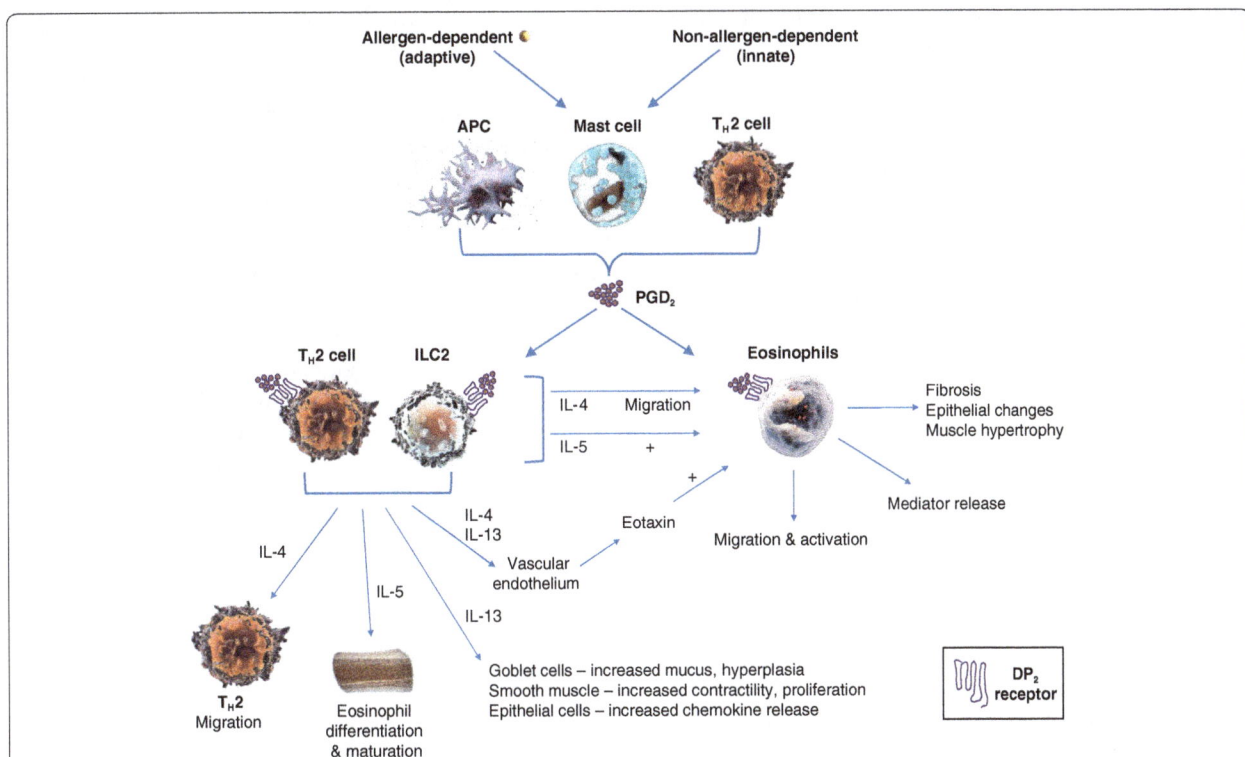

Fig. 1 Overview of the DP_2 receptor-mediated response of immune cells in the inflammatory pathway. Proposed schematic providing an overview of the DP_2 receptor-mediated response of various immune cells, including mast cells, T_H2 cells, ILC2 and eosinophils, and the subsequent effect on inflammation in the asthmatic airways through increased inflammatory cell chemotaxis and cytokine production. Abbreviations, APC: antigen presenting cell; DP_2: prostaglandin D_2 receptor 2; IgE: immunoglobulin E; IL: interleukin; ILC2: type 2 innate lymphoid cell; PGD_2: prostaglandin D_2

and degranulated in minutes [26]. They are widely distributed at mucosal surfaces and in tissues throughout the body, and play a central role in the pathophysiology of asthma, not only by mediating immunoglobulin E (IgE)-dependent allergic responses, but also in non-IgE-mediated mechanisms [27, 28]. Mast cell numbers are similarly increased in both allergic and non-allergic asthma, although response to cyclic adenosine monophosphate (cAMP) is higher in allergic than in non-allergic patients [29].

Aside from mast cells, other cell types can also produce PGD_2 under certain conditions, including biologically meaningful quantities in T_H2 cells [13, 30, 31]. Macrophages [32], and dendritic cells [33, 34] also produce small amounts of PGD_2.

PGD₂ receptors
PGD_2 mainly exerts its biological effect via high affinity interactions with two structurally and pharmacologically distinct receptors (the prostaglandin D_2 receptor 1 [DP_1] and the DP_2 receptor) [13]. At micromolar concentrations, PGD_2 can also stimulate the thromboxane receptor [35].

DP_1, a 359 amino acid, ~40 kDa G-protein-coupled prostaglandin receptor, was the first PGD_2 receptor to be identified [36, 37]. It mediates a range of effects, which are mostly non-inflammatory in nature; vasodilation, inhibition of cell migration, relaxation of smooth muscle, and eosinophil apoptosis [38].

The DP_2 receptor is a 395 amino acid, 43 kDa G-protein-coupled prostaglandin receptor. Binding of PGD_2 to the DP_2 receptor on immune cells induces a myriad of pro-inflammatory downstream effects, which significantly contribute to the recruitment, activation and/or migration of T_H2 cells, ILC2, and eosinophils, thereby fuelling the inflammatory cascade in asthma [14, 38–41]. PGD_2 metabolites (DK-PGD_2, Δ12PGJ2, 15-deoxy- Δ12,14PGD_2, and deoxy- Δ12,14PGJ_2) also activate the DP_2 receptor [42–44].

Cells expressing the DP₂ receptor
The DP_2 receptor plays a key role in the pathophysiology of asthma: it induces and amplifies the inflammatory cascade [16, 25, 45, 46]. This type of receptor can be found in many cell types, however the key cells of the DP_2 receptor pathway include T_H2 cells, ILC2 cells and eosinophils, suggesting a homeostatic role for this receptor (Fig. 1) [14–16, 47]. In addition, type 2 cytotoxic T (Tc2) lymphocytes were recently shown to be activated by PGD_2 acting via the DP_2 receptor, thus contributing to the pathogenesis of eosinophilic asthma [41].

Effects of the DP₂ receptor on T_H2 cells
PGD_2 preferentially upregulates IL-4, IL-5 and IL-13 expression (type 2 cytokines) in T_H2 cells in a dose-dependent manner [48] and induces T_H2 cell migration [46] via its high affinity interaction with the DP_2 receptor (Fig. 1).

DP_2 receptor activation has shown a potent effect on T_H2 cell migration in vitro, highlighting a key function of this receptor in mediating the chemotaxis of T_H2 lymphocytes [49]. As elevated levels of circulating $DP_2{}^+CD_4{}^+$ T cells is a hallmark feature of severe asthma [50], this provides a DP_2 receptor-rich environment upon which already increased levels of PGD_2 levels may act, further perpetuating the inflammatory cascade.

Effects of the DP₂ receptor on ILC2 cells
ILC2 is a cell type that may link the non-allergen- and allergen-dependent responses in asthma. ILC2 cell activation is triggered by inflammatory mediators released from epithelial and immune cells (e.g. IL-33 and PGD_2), and is associated with increased production of type 2 cytokines [51]. Thus, ILC2 cells facilitate a T_H2 immune response that can be independent of the allergen [52].

Secretion of IL-4, IL-5 and IL-13 from ILC2 cells is increased in response to DP_2 receptor stimulation in a dose-dependent manner [16].

In response to IL-33, ILC2 cell activation was initially reported to produce high levels of IL-5 and IL-13 in vitro, but very low levels of IL-4. Interestingly, recent studies have shown that when their DP_2 receptor is stimulated, ILC2 cells produce higher levels of IL-4 [53].

Meanwhile, DP_2 stimulation alone remarkably increases ILC2 cell migration, which is 4.75-fold greater than that of IL-33 [16].

Effects of the DP₂ receptor on eosinophils
Eosinophils are involved in airway hyper-responsiveness, mucus hypersecretion, tissue damage and airway remodelling in asthma. Eosinophil activation is also associated with increased cytokine production, which has various downstream immunomodulatory effects [54]. DP_2 receptor activation at the eosinophil surface facilitates the trans-endothelial migration and influx of eosinophils, increases eosinophil degranulation and induces eosinophil shape change [40, 55, 56]. Eosinophil shape change in response to DP_2 activation [57] is similar to that visualised previously with eotaxin stimulation [58].

Eosinophil influx and activation can cause detrimental effects on the epithelial lining of the lungs of asthma patients. This happens through degranulation and release of harmful mediators such as eosinophil cationic protein, eosinophil peroxidase, eosinophil protein X and cytotoxic major basic protein [19, 59, 60]. Additionally, eosinophils release transforming growth factor (TGF)-ß which induces apoptotic effects upon airway epithelial cells, contributing to airway tissue denudation. Moreover, eosinophils enhance airway smooth muscle cell proliferation, further contributing to structural remodelling of the pulmonary architecture [61]. Charcot-Leyden crystals, a product of activated eosinophils, are detectable in expectorated sputum samples from asthma patients [62]. These crystals are largely comprised of the toxic enzyme lysophospholipase (also known as phospholipase B), and may contribute to eosinophil-driven tissue denudation in the lungs [63].

As mentioned previously, in addition to the direct effects, DP_2 receptor activation also has indirect effects on eosinophils by inducing the release of IL-4, IL-5 and IL-13 from T_H2 cells and ILC2, which affect eosinophil maturation, apoptosis and migration to the lungs.

Effects of DP_2-mediated cytokine release

DP_2 receptor activation increases release of cytokines from ILC2 and T_H2 cells. These cytokines cause some of the characteristic features of asthma, including airway inflammation, IgE production, mucus metaplasia, airway hyper-reactivity, smooth muscle remodelling and eosinophilia [52, 64]. We will review the effects of the key cytokines released:

- IL-4 enhances the migration of eosinophils, which is a key step in the inflammatory cascade. To do this, in synergy with tumour necrosis factor (TNF)-α, IL-4 increases the expression of vascular cell adhesion molecule-1 (VCAM-1) and P selectin on the surface of the vascular endothelium, which facilitates the trans-endothelial passage of eosinophils from the bloodstream into the lung parenchyma [19, 65]. Meanwhile, IL-4 also stimulates the release of eotaxin, a potent and selective eosinophil chemoattractant, from the vascular endothelium (Fig. 1). Eotaxin facilitates eosinophil migration [66, 67]. Differentiation and proliferation of T_H2 cells is also promoted by IL-4 [39].
- IL-5 is directly involved in the differentiation and maturation of eosinophils in the bone marrow, eosinophil chemotaxis to sites of inflammation, and local eosinophilopoiesis [68, 69]. It also inhibits eosinophil apoptosis, leading to the accumulation of these cells at sites of inflammation, which in turn perpetuates and prolongs the inflammatory cycle [70].
- IL-13 is known to induce goblet cell hyperplasia, mucus production, and airway hyper-responsiveness, leading to airway inflammation and tissue remodelling [39, 64]. Furthermore, IL-4 and IL-13 released from T_H2 and ILC2 in response to DP_2 receptor activation promote immunoglobulin class switching from IgM to IgE antibodies in B cells and plasma cells, which leads to further mast cell recruitment, activation and PGD_2 release at sites of inflammation

[16, 20, 71, 72]. It also contributes to the release of eotaxin (together with IL-4), which as mentioned above, facilitates eosinophil migration.
- Levels of other pro-inflammatory cytokines are also increased upon activation of DP_2 receptors, including IL-8, IL-9 and granulocyte–macrophage colony-stimulating factor, which may additionally contribute to excessive immune cell chemotaxis, associated proteases and enhanced airway inflammation in asthma [16].

Results from phase II clinical studies suggest that blocking the activation of the DP_2 receptor pathway with DP_2 receptor antagonists reduces the symptoms associated with asthma, improves pulmonary function and inhibits eosinophil shape change, while showing indirect signs (sputum eosinophil reduction) of the potential to decrease the number of exacerbations experienced by severe asthma patients [73–80].

Further evidence for DP_2 receptor pathway importance in asthma

PGD_2 levels are increased in asthma, with increased levels in patients with severe disease [27, 81], and in response to allergen challenge [82, 83]. The number of DP_2 receptor-positive cells within the submucosal tissue is also significantly higher in patients with severe asthma compared with healthy controls [84]. Interestingly, an association between a single nucleotide polymorphism in the DP_2 receptor (rs533116) and allergic asthma has also been reported [85].

PGD_2 protein and DP_2 receptor expression levels in bronchoalveolar lavage fluid (BALF) from severe asthmatic patients were shown to be significantly higher than from healthy controls or patients with mild or moderate asthma [27, 81]. Interestingly, Murray et al. [82] demonstrated a 150-fold increase in PGD_2 levels in BALF from asthma patients within nine minutes of local antigen (Dermatophagoides pteronyssinus) challenge, demonstrating that allergen-induced PGD_2 release is an early and rapid event. Furthermore, a study by Wenzel and colleagues showed that allergen challenge in atopic asthma patients induced a significant increase in BALF PGD_2 levels compared with atopic patients without asthma [83].

Of significant interest is the sustained activity of PGD_2-derived metabolites despite extensive and rapid PGD_2 metabolism. The PGD_2-derived metabolites PGJ_2 and Δ^{12}-PGJ_2, are themselves known to be potent DP_2 receptor agonists, thereby demonstrating the sustained and prolonged activity of the DP_2 receptor via the metabolites of PGD_2 [45]. Despite the short half-life of PGD_2 in plasma (~30 min), its biological activity towards the DP_2 receptor is maintained through the formation of these metabolites, which are more stable than the parent compound, highlighting their potential role in perpetuating the inflammatory cascade [45].

Blockage of PGD_2 via DP_2 receptor antagonism inhibits inflammatory cell chemotaxis and also reduces type 2 pro-inflammatory cytokine production, which provides further evidence of the vital role played by PGD_2 and its interaction with the DP_2 receptor in asthma [46]. Of note, DP_2 receptor antagonism has also been shown to decrease airway smooth muscle cell mass and chemotaxis of these cells towards PGD_2 [86, 87].

Role of the DP_2 receptor pathway in virus-induced asthma

Viruses, such as rhinovirus (RV), influenza A, and respiratory syncytial virus (RSV), are a major cause of asthma exacerbations and can activate the DP_2 receptor pathway [88]. These respiratory viruses produce double-stranded RNA (dsRNA) during replication, which activates the non-allergen-dependent immune response and results in increased chemokine synthesis from airway epithelial and innate immune cells [88, 89]. A recent study also suggests the involvement of the DP_2 receptor pathway in augmenting virus-mediated airway eosinophilic inflammation [88]. It shows that DP_2 receptor stimulation followed by eosinophil recruitment into the airways is a major pathogenic factor in the dsRNA-induced enhancement of airway inflammation and bronchial hyper-responsiveness [88].

PGD_2 levels have also been found to be increased after viral challenge in asthma patients, which may act synergistically with IL-33 to further drive type 2 cytokine production [90, 91]. The role of PGD_2 in RV16-induced asthma exacerbations was recently investigated in atopic asthma patients [91]. In this study, baseline PGD_2 levels were higher in asthmatic patients versus healthy controls. Furthermore, RV16 infection induced a greater PGD_2 increase in asthmatic patients compared with the healthy participants. The largest RV16-mediated PGD_2 increase was observed in those with severe and poorly-controlled asthma, suggesting a potential role for PGD_2 in driving asthma exacerbations [91].

Polyinosinic:polycytidylic acid (poly I:C) is an immunostimulant; it is structurally similar to double-stranded RNA, which is present in some viruses and is a "natural" stimulant of toll-like receptor 3 (TLR3), which is expressed in the membrane of B-cells, macrophages and dendritic cells. Thus, poly I:C can be considered a synthetic analogue of double-stranded RNA and can simulate viral infections. Early evidence from poly I:C murine asthma models suggests that a selective DP_2 receptor antagonist may dose-dependently block the aforementioned virus-induced T2 response, and may

help to reduce the inflammation caused by virus-mediated asthma exacerbations [92].

Conclusions

The DP_2 receptor pathway is known to play a key role in the pathophysiology of asthma via induction and amplification of the inflammatory cascade by exerting direct effects on immune cells, including T_H2 cella, ILC2 and eosinophils [16, 46, 55]. IL-4, IL-5 and IL-13 release from DP_2 receptor-activated immune cells can have significant effects on immune cell influx, degranulation, tissue remodelling and mucus production in the airways, leading to structural damage, fibrosis and reduced pulmonary function [64]. Additionally, the effect of DP_2 receptor activation on eosinophil activation and migration leads to tissue damage, through release of harmful cationic proteins and enhanced proliferation of airway smooth muscle cells [93].

This review highlights the important pro-inflammatory role of the DP_2 receptor pathway in asthma. Furthermore, multiple DP_2 receptor antagonists are currently under clinical investigation [73–75, 77–80], for asthma therapies. Indeed, in a 12-week study in patients with allergic asthma that was uncontrolled by low-dose ICS, the oral DP_2 receptor antagonist fevipiprant (150 mg once daily or 75 mg twice daily) produced significant improvements in pre-dose FEV_1 compared with placebo [73]. Further, in patients with moderate to severe eosinophilic asthma, fevipiprant significantly reduced mean sputum eosinophil percentage compared with placebo [80]. Initial positive findings have also been reported with timapiprant (OC00459) [78], BI 671800 [77], setipiprant [94] , MK-1029 and ADC-3680 [95] , but not with AZD1981 [75]. Hence, the clinical outcomes of larger, phase III clinical studies involving DP_2 receptor antagonists are eagerly awaited.

Abbreviations
DP_1: Prostaglandin D_2 receptor 1; DP_2: Prostaglandin D_2 receptor 2; IgE: Immunoglobulin E; IL: Interleukin; ILC2: Type 2 innate lymphoid cell; PGD_2: Prostaglandin D_2; Tc2: Type 2 cytotoxic T cell; TGF-β: Transforming growth factor-β; TNF-α: Tumour necrosis factor-α; VCAM-1: Vascular cell adhesion molecule-1

Acknowledgements
The authors thank Gillian Lavelle, PhD, of Novartis Product Lifecycle Services, for providing medical writing support for this article, which was funded by Novartis Pharma AG, Basel, Switzerland in accordance with Good Publication Practice (GPP3) guidelines (http://www.ismpp.org/gpp3).

Funding
This work was funded by Novartis Pharma AG, Basel, Switzerland

Authors' contributions
All authors substantially contributed to the drafting and critical review of all stages of this article. All authors have given final approval of the version to be published and agree to be accountable for all aspects of this work.

Competing interests
Dr. Domingo reports personal fees from Novartis, GSK, AstraZeneca, and Teva, as well as non-financial support from Teva, outside of the submitted work.
Dr. Palomares reports personal fees for giving scientific lectures from Allergy Therapeutics, Amgen, AstraZenenca, Inmunotek S.L, Novartis, and Stallergenes. Dr. Palomares received grants from Inmunotek S.L under collaborative public projects and has participated in advisory boards for Novartis and Sanofi Genzyme. Everything reported is outside the submitted work.
Veit J. Erpenbeck is an employee of Novartis Pharma.
David Sandham is a full-time employee and shareholder of Novartis Institutes for Biomedical Research and Novartis, respectively.
Pablo Altman is a full-time employee of Novartis Pharmaceuticals Corporation.

Author details
[1]Department of Medicine, Universitat Autònoma de Barcelona, Barcelona, Spain. [2]Pulmonary Service, Corporació Sanitària Parc Taulí, Sabadell, Barcelona, Spain. [3]Department of Biochemistry and Molecular Biology, School of Chemistry, Complutense University of Madrid, Madrid, Spain. [4]Novartis Institutes for Biomedical Research, Cambridge, MA, USA. [5]Novartis Pharma AG, Basel, Switzerland. [6]Novartis Pharmaceuticals Corporation, One Health Plaza East Hanover, East Hanover, NJ 07936-1080, USA.

References
1. GBD Chronic Respiratory Disease Collaborators. Global, regional, and national deaths, prevalence, disability-adjusted life years, and years lived with disability for chronic obstructive pulmonary disease and asthma, 1990-2015: a systematic analysis for the Global Burden of Disease Study 2015. Lancet Respir Med. 2017;5:691–706.
2. Boyman O, Kaegi C, Akdis M, Bavbek S, Bossios A, Chatzipetrou A, Eiwegger T, Firinu D, Harr T, Knol E, et al. EAACI IG Biologicals task force paper on the use of biologic agents in allergic disorders. Allergy. 2015;70:727–54.
3. Palomares O, Sanchez-Ramon S, Davila I, Prieto L, Perez de Llano L, Lleonart M, Domingo C, Nieto A. divergEnt: How IgE Axis Contributes to the Continuum of Allergic Asthma and Anti-IgE Therapies. Int J Mol Sci. 2017; 18(16). https://doi.org/10.3390/ijms18061328.
4. Hetherington KJ, Heaney LG. Drug therapies in severe asthma - the era of stratified medicine. Clin Med (Lond). 2015;15:452–6.
5. Price D, Fletcher M, van der Molen T. Asthma control and management in 8,000 European patients: the REcognise Asthma and LInk to Symptoms and Experience (REALISE) survey. NPJ Prim Care Respir Med. 2014;24:14009.
6. Eakin MN, Rand CS. Improving patient adherence with asthma self-management practices: what works? Ann Allergy Asthma Immunol. 2012;109:90–2.
7. Price D, Bosnic-Anticevich S, Briggs A, Chrystyn H, Rand C, Scheuch G, Bousquet J. Inhaler competence in asthma: common errors, barriers to use and recommended solutions. Respir Med. 2013;107:37–46.
8. Williams LK, Peterson EL, Wells K, Ahmedani BK, Kumar R, Burchard EG, Chowdhry VK, Favro D, Lanfear DE, Pladevall M. Quantifying the proportion of severe asthma exacerbations attributable to inhaled corticosteroid nonadherence. J Allergy Clin Immunol. 2011;128:1185–91.
9. Jones C, Santanello NC, Boccuzzi SJ, Wogen J, Strub P, Nelsen LM. Adherence to prescribed treatment for asthma: evidence from pharmacy benefits data. J Asthma. 2003;40:93–101.
10. Rand C, Bilderback A, Schiller K, Edelman JM, Hustad CM, Zeiger RS, Group MSR. Adherence with montelukast or fluticasone in a long-term clinical trial: results from the mild asthma montelukast versus inhaled corticosteroid trial. J Allergy Clin Immunol. 2007;119:916–23.
11. Barnes PJ. New drugs for asthma. Nat Rev Drug Discov. 2004;3:831–44.
12. Barnes PJ. New therapies for asthma: is there any progress? Trends Pharmacol Sci. 2010;31:335–43.
13. Pettipher R. The roles of the prostaglandin D(2) receptors DP(1) and CRTH2 in promoting allergic responses. Br J Pharmacol. 2008;153(Suppl 1):S191–9.
14. Hirai H, Tanaka K, Yoshie O, Ogawa K, Kenmotsu K, Takamori Y, Ichimasa M, Sugamura K, Nakamura M, Takano S, Nagata K. Prostaglandin D2 selectively induces chemotaxis in T helper type 2 cells, eosinophils, and basophils via seven-transmembrane receptor CRTH2. J Exp Med. 2001;193:255–61.
15. Nagata K, Hirai H, Tanaka K, Ogawa K, Aso T, Sugamura K, Nakamura M, Takano S. CRTH2, an orphan receptor of T-helper-2-cells, is expressed on basophils and eosinophils and responds to mast cell-derived factor(s). FEBS Lett. 1999;459:195–9.
16. Xue L, Salimi M, Panse I, Mjosberg JM, McKenzie AN, Spits H, Klenerman P, Ogg G. Prostaglandin D2 activates group 2 innate lymphoid cells through chemoattractant receptor-homologous molecule expressed on TH2 cells. J Allergy Clin Immunol. 2014;133:1184–94.
17. Palomares O, Akdis CA. Chapter 28 - Immunology of the Asthmatic Immune Response. In: Leung D, Szefler S, Bonilla F, Akdis CA, Sampson H, editors. Pediatric Allergy: Principles and Practice, 3rd Edition. London: Elsevier; 2015. p. 250–61.
18. Palomares O, Akdis M, Martin-Fontecha M, Akdis CA. Mechanisms of immune regulation in allergic diseases: the role of regulatory T and B cells. Immunol Rev. 2017;278:219–36.
19. Domingo C. Overlapping Effects of New Monoclonal Antibodies for Severe Asthma. Drugs. 2017;77:1769–87.
20. Townley RG, Agrawal S. CRTH2 antagonists in the treatment of allergic responses involving TH2 cells, basophils, and eosinophils. Ann Allergy Asthma Immunol. 2012;109:365–74.
21. Domingo C, Pacheco A, Hinojosa M, Bosque M. The relevance of IgE in the pathogenesis of allergy: the effect of an anti-IgE drug in asthma and other diseases. Recent Pat Inflamm Allergy Drug Discov. 2007;1:151–64.
22. Domingo C. Omalizumab for severe asthma: efficacy beyond the atopic patient? Drugs. 2014;74:521–33.
23. Peinhaupt M, Sturm EM, Heinemann A. Prostaglandins and Their Receptors in Eosinophil Function and As Therapeutic Targets. Front Med (Lausanne). 2017;4:104.
24. Brightling CE, Bradding P, Pavord ID, Wardlaw AJ. New insights into the role of the mast cell in asthma. Clin Exp Allergy. 2003;33:550–6.
25. Pettipher R, Hansel TT, Armer R. Antagonism of the prostaglandin D2 receptors DP1 and CRTH2 as an approach to treat allergic diseases. Nat Rev Drug Discov. 2007;6:313–25.
26. Matsuda K, Piliponsky AM, Iikura M, Nakae S, Wang EW, Dutta SM, Kawakami T, Tsai M, Galli SJ. Monomeric IgE enhances human mast cell chemokine production: IL-4 augments and dexamethasone suppresses the response. J Allergy Clin Immunol. 2005;116:1357–63.
27. Balzar S, Fajt ML, Comhair SA, Erzurum SC, Bleecker E, Busse WW, Castro M, Gaston B, Israel E, Schwartz LB, et al. Mast cell phenotype, location, and activation in severe asthma. Data from the Severe Asthma Research Program. Am J Respir Crit Care Med. 2011;183:299–309.
28. Amin K. The role of mast cells in allergic inflammation. Respir Med. 2012;106:9–14.
29. Ludviksdottir D, Janson C, Bjornsson E, Stalenheim G, Boman G, Hedenstrom H, Venge P, Gudbjornsson B, Valtysdottir S. Different airway responsiveness profiles in atopic asthma, nonatopic asthma, and Sjogren's syndrome. Allergy. 2000;55:259–65.
30. Vinall SL, Townsend ER, Pettipher R. A paracrine role for chemoattractant receptor-homologous molecule expressed on T helper type 2 cells (CRTH2) in mediating chemotactic activation of CRTH2+ CD4+ T helper type 2 lymphocytes. Immunology. 2007;121:577–84.
31. Tanaka K, Ogawa K, Sugamura K, Nakamura M, Takano S, Nagata K. Cutting edge: differential production of prostaglandin D2 by human helper T cell subsets. J Immunol. 2000;164:2277–80.
32. Tajima T, Murata T, Aritake K, Urade Y, Hirai H, Nakamura M, Ozaki H, Hori M. Lipopolysaccharide induces macrophage migration via prostaglandin D(2) and prostaglandin E(2). J Pharmacol Exp Ther. 2008;326:493–501.
33. Urade Y, Ujihara M, Horiguchi Y, Ikai K, Hayaishi O. The major source of endogenous prostaglandin D2 production is likely antigen-presenting cells. Localization of glutathione-requiring prostaglandin D synthetase in histiocytes, dendritic, and Kupffer cells in various rat tissues. J Immunol. 1989;143:2982–9.
34. Shimura C, Satoh T, Igawa K, Aritake K, Urade Y, Nakamura M, Yokozeki H. Dendritic cells express hematopoietic prostaglandin D synthase and function as a source of prostaglandin D2 in the skin. Am J Pathol. 2010;176:227–37.

35. Coleman RA, Sheldrick RL. Prostanoid-induced contraction of human bronchial smooth muscle is mediated by TP-receptors. Br J Pharmacol. 1989;96:688–92.

36. Hirata M, Kakizuka A, Aizawa M, Ushikubi F, Narumiya S. Molecular characterization of a mouse prostaglandin D receptor and functional expression of the cloned gene. Proc Natl Acad Sci U S A. 1994;91:11192–6.

37. Boie Y, Sawyer N, Slipetz DM, Metters KM, Abramovitz M. Molecular cloning and characterization of the human prostanoid DP receptor. J Biol Chem. 1995;270:18910–6.

38. Kupczyk M, Kuna P. Targeting the PGD2/CRTH2/DP1 Signaling Pathway in Asthma and Allergic Disease: Current Status and Future Perspectives. Drugs. 2017;77:1281–94.

39. Arima M, Fukuda T. Prostaglandin D(2) and T(H)2 inflammation in the pathogenesis of bronchial asthma. Korean J Intern Med. 2011;26:8–18.

40. Sykes DA, Bradley ME, Riddy DM, Willard E, Reilly J, Miah A, Bauer C, Watson SJ, Sandham DA, Dubois G, Charlton SJ. Fevipiprant (QAW039), a Slowly Dissociating CRTh2 Antagonist with the Potential for Improved Clinical Efficacy. Mol Pharmacol. 2016;89:593–605.

41. Xue L, Stöger L, Marchi E, Liu W, Go S, Kurioka A, Leng T, Willberg C, Salimi M, Shrimanker R, et al. Interaction of Type 2 cytotoxic T lymphocytes and mast cell lipid mediators contributes to pathogenesis of eosinophilic asthma. Am J Respir Crit Care Med. 2017;195:A5301.

42. Gazi L, Gyles S, Rose J, Lees S, Allan C, Xue L, Jassal R, Speight G, Gamble V, Pettipher R. Delta12-prostaglandin D2 is a potent and selective CRTH2 receptor agonist and causes activation of human eosinophils and Th2 lymphocytes. Prostaglandins Other Lipid Mediat. 2005;75:153–67.

43. Monneret G, Li H, Vasilescu J, Rokach J, Powell WS. 15-Deoxy-delta 12,14-prostaglandins D2 and J2 are potent activators of human eosinophils. J Immunol. 2002;168:3563–9.

44. Sawyer N, Cauchon E, Chateauneuf A, Cruz RP, Nicholson DW, Metters KM, O'Neill GP, Gervais FG. Molecular pharmacology of the human prostaglandin D2 receptor, CRTH2. Br J Pharmacol. 2002;137:1163–72.

45. Schuligoi R, Schmidt R, Geisslinger G, Kollroser M, Peskar BA, Heinemann A. PGD2 metabolism in plasma: kinetics and relationship with bioactivity on DP1 and CRTH2 receptors. Biochem Pharmacol. 2007;74:107–17.

46. Xue L, Barrow A, Fleming VM, Hunter MG, Ogg G, Klenerman P, Pettipher R. Leukotriene E4 activates human Th2 cells for exaggerated proinflammatory cytokine production in response to prostaglandin D2. J Immunol. 2012;188:694–702.

47. Chang JE, Doherty TA, Baum R, Broide D. Prostaglandin D2 regulates human type 2 innate lymphoid cell chemotaxis. J Allergy Clin Immunol. 2014;133:899–901.

48. Xue L, Gyles SL, Wettey FR, Gazi L, Townsend E, Hunter MG, Pettipher R. Prostaglandin D2 causes preferential induction of proinflammatory Th2 cytokine production through an action on chemoattractant receptor-like molecule expressed on Th2 cells. J Immunol. 2005;175:6531–6.

49. Gyles SL, Xue L, Townsend ER, Wettey F, Pettipher R. A dominant role for chemoattractant receptor-homologous molecule expressed on T helper type 2 (Th2) cells (CRTH2) in mediating chemotaxis of CRTH2+ CD4+ Th2 lymphocytes in response to mast cell supernatants. Immunology. 2006;119:362–8.

50. Palikhe NS, Laratta C, Nahirney D, Vethanayagam D, Bhutani M, Vliagoftis H, Cameron L. Elevated levels of circulating CD4(+) CRTh2(+) T cells characterize severe asthma. Clin Exp Allergy. 2016;46:825–36.

51. Chen R, Smith SG, Salter B, El-Gammal A, Oliveria JP, Obminski C, Watson R, O'Byrne PM, Gauvreau GM, Sehmi R. Allergen-induced Increases in Sputum Levels of Group 2 Innate Lymphoid Cells in Subjects with Asthma. Am J Respir Crit Care Med. 2017;196:700–12.

52. Karta MR, Broide DH, Doherty TA. Insights into Group 2 Innate Lymphoid Cells in Human Airway Disease. Curr Allergy Asthma Rep. 2016;16:8.

53. Lund S, Walford HH, Doherty TA. Type 2 Innate Lymphoid Cells in Allergic Disease. Curr Immunol Rev. 2013;9:214–21.

54. McBrien CN, Menzies-Gow A. The Biology of Eosinophils and Their Role in Asthma. Front Med (Lausanne). 2017;4:93.

55. Gervais FG, Cruz RP, Chateauneuf A, Gale S, Sawyer N, Nantel F, Metters KM, O'Neill GP. Selective modulation of chemokinesis, degranulation, and apoptosis in eosinophils through the PGD2 receptors CRTH2 and DP. J Allergy Clin Immunol. 2001;108:982–8.

56. Sandham DA, Barker L, Brown L, Brown Z, Budd D, Charlton SJ, Chatterjee D, Cox B, Dubois G, Duggan N, et al. Discovery of Fevipiprant (NVP-QAW039), a Potent and Selective DP2 Receptor Antagonist for Treatment of Asthma. ACS Med Chem Lett. 2017;8:582–6.

57. Royer JF, Schratl P, Carrillo JJ, Jupp R, Barker J, Weyman-Jones C, Beri R, Sargent C, Schmidt JA, Lang-Loidolt D, Heinemann A. A novel antagonist of prostaglandin D2 blocks the locomotion of eosinophils and basophils. Eur J Clin Invest. 2008;38:663–71.

58. Willetts L, Ochkur SI, Jacobsen EA, Lee JJ, Lacy P. Eosinophil Shape Change and Secretion. In: Walsh GM, editor. Eosinophils Methods in Molecular Biology (Methods and Protocols) Volume 1178. New York, NY: Humana Press; 2014.

59. Frigas E, Motojima S, Gleich GJ. The eosinophilic injury to the mucosa of the airways in the pathogenesis of bronchial asthma. Eur Respir J Suppl. 1991;13:123s–35s.

60. Carr TF, Berdnikovs S, Simon HU, Bochner BS, Rosenwasser LJ. Eosinophilic bioactivities in severe asthma. World Allergy Organ J. 2016;9:21.

61. Halwani R, Vazquez-Tello A, Sumi Y, Pureza MA, Bahammam A, Al-Jahdali H, Soussi-Gounni A, Mahboub B, Al-Muhsen S, Hamid Q. Eosinophils induce airway smooth muscle cell proliferation. J Clin Immunol. 2013;33:595–604.

62. Dor PJ, Ackerman SJ, Gleich GJ. Charcot-Leyden crystal protein and eosinophil granule major basic protein in sputum of patients with respiratory diseases. Am Rev Respir Dis. 1984;130:1072–7.

63. Weller PF, Goetzl EJ, Austen KF. Identification of human eosinophil lysophospholipase as the constituent of Charcot-Leyden crystals. Proc Natl Acad Sci U S A. 1980;77:7440–3.

64. Farne H, Jackson DJ, Johnston SL. Are emerging PGD2 antagonists a promising therapy class for treating asthma? Expert Opin Emerg Drugs. 2016;21:359–64.

65. Patel KD. Eosinophil tethering to interleukin-4-activated endothelial cells requires both P-selectin and vascular cell adhesion molecule-1. Blood. 1998;92:3904–11.

66. Conroy DM, Williams TJ. Eotaxin and the attraction of eosinophils to the asthmatic lung. Respir Res. 2001;2:150–6.

67. Moore PE, Church TL, Chism DD, Panettieri RA Jr, Shore SA. IL-13 and IL-4 cause eotaxin release in human airway smooth muscle cells: a role for ERK. Am J Physiol Lung Cell Mol Physiol. 2002;282:847–53.

68. Aceves SA, Ackerman SJ. Relationships Between Eosinophilic Inflammation, Tissue Remodeling and Fibrosis in Eosinophilic Esophagitis. Immunology Allergy Clin North Am. 2009;29:197–212.

69. Kouro T, Takatsu K. IL-5- and eosinophil-mediated inflammation: from discovery to therapy. Int Immunol. 2009;21:1303–9.

70. Molfino NA, Gossage D, Kolbeck R, Parker JM, Geba GP. Molecular and clinical rationale for therapeutic targeting of interleukin-5 and its receptor. Clin Exp Allergy. 2012;42:712–37.

71. Punnonen J, Aversa G, Cocks BG, McKenzie AN, Menon S, Zurawski G, de Waal MR, de Vries JE. Interleukin 13 induces interleukin 4-independent IgG4 and IgE synthesis and CD23 expression by human B cells. Proc Natl Acad Sci U S A. 1993;90:3730–4.

72. Vatrella A, Fabozzi I, Calabrese C, Maselli R, Pelaia G. Dupilumab: a novel treatment for asthma. J Asthma Allergy. 2014;7:123–30.

73. Bateman ED, Guerreros AG, Brockhaus F, Holzhauer B, Pethe A, Kay RA, Townley RG. Fevipiprant, an oral prostaglandin DP2 receptor (CRTh2) antagonist, in allergic asthma uncontrolled on low-dose inhaled corticosteroids. Eur Respir J. 2017;50(2). https://doi.org/10.1183/13993003.00670-2017.

74. Santus P, Radovanovic D. Prostaglandin D2 receptor antagonists in early development as potential therapeutic options for asthma. Expert Opin Investig Drugs. 2016;25:1083–92.

75. Kuna P, Bjermer L, Tornling G. Two Phase II randomized trials on the CRTh2 antagonist AZD1981 in adults with asthma. Drug Des Devel Ther. 2016;10:2759–70.

76. Erpenbeck VJ, Popov TA, Miller D, Weinstein SF, Spector S, Magnusson B, Osuntokun W, Goldsmith P, Weiss M, Beier J. The oral CRTh2 antagonist QAW039 (fevipiprant): A phase II study in uncontrolled allergic asthma. Pulm Pharmacol Ther. 2016;39:54–63.

77. Hall IP, Fowler AV, Gupta A, Tetzlaff K, Nivens MC, Sarno M, Finnigan HA, Bateman ED, Rand Sutherland E. Efficacy of BI 671800, an oral CRTh2 antagonist, in poorly controlled asthma as sole controller and in the presence of inhaled corticosteroid treatment. Pulm Pharmacol Ther. 2015;32:37–44.

78. Pettipher R, Hunter MG, Perkins CM, Collins LP, Lewis T, Baillet M, Steiner J, Bell J, Payton MA. Heightened response of eosinophilic asthmatic patients to the CRTH2 antagonist OC000459. Allergy. 2014;69:1223–32.

79. Fowler A, Koenen R, Hilbert J, Blatchford J, Kappeler D, Benediktus E, Wood C, Gupta A. Safety, Tolerability, Pharmacokinetics, and Pharmacodynamics of the Novel CRTH2 Antagonist BI 1021958 at Single Oral Doses in Healthy

Men and Multiple Oral Doses in Men and Women With Well-Controlled Asthma. J Clin Pharmacol. 2017;57:1444–53.

80. Gonem S, Berair R, Singapuri A, Hartley R, Laurencin MF, Bacher G, Holzhauer B, Bourne M, Mistry V, Pavord ID, et al. Fevipiprant, a prostaglandin D2 receptor 2 antagonist, in patients with persistent eosinophilic asthma: a single-centre, randomised, double-blind, parallel-group, placebo-controlled trial. Lancet Respir Med. 2016;4:699–707.

81. Fajt ML, Gelhaus SL, Freeman B, Uvalle CE, Trudeau JB, Holguin F, Wenzel SE. Prostaglandin D(2) pathway upregulation: relation to asthma severity, control, and TH2 inflammation. J Allergy Clin Immunol. 2013;131:1504–12.

82. Murray JJ, Tonnel AB, Brash AR, Roberts LJ 2nd, Gosset P, Workman R, Capron A, Oates JA. Release of prostaglandin D2 into human airways during acute antigen challenge. N Engl J Med. 1986;315:800–4.

83. Wenzel SE, Westcott JY, Larsen GL. Bronchoalveolar lavage fluid mediator levels 5 minutes after allergen challenge in atopic subjects with asthma: relationship to the development of late asthmatic responses. J Allergy Clin Immunol. 1991;87:540–8.

84. Stinson SE, Amrani Y, Brightling CE. D prostanoid receptor 2 (chemoattractant receptor-homologous molecule expressed on TH2 cells) protein expression in asthmatic patients and its effects on bronchial epithelial cells. J Allergy Clin Immunol. 2015;135:395–406.

85. Campos Alberto E, Maclean E, Davidson C, Palikhe NS, Storie J, Tse C, Brenner D, Mayers I, Vliagoftis H, El-Sohemy A, Cameron L. The single nucleotide polymorphism CRTh2 rs533116 is associated with allergic asthma and increased expression of CRTh2. Allergy. 2012;67:1357–64.

86. Saunders RM, Kaul H, Berair R, Singapuri A, Chernyasvsky I, Chachi L, Biddle M, Sutcliffe A, Laurencin M, Bacher G, et al. Fevipiprant (QAW039) reduces airway smooth muscle mass in asthma via antagonism of the prostaglandin D2 receptor 2 (DP2). Am J Respir Crit Care Med. 2017;195:A4677.

87. Parameswaran K, Radford K, Fanat A, Stephen J, Bonnans C, Levy BD, Janssen LJ, Cox PG. Modulation of human airway smooth muscle migration by lipid mediators and Th-2 cytokines. Am J Respir Cell Mol Biol. 2007;37:240–7.

88. Shiraishi Y, Asano K, Niimi K, Fukunaga K, Wakaki M, Kagyo J, Takihara T, Ueda S, Nakajima T, Oguma T, et al. Cyclooxygenase-2/prostaglandin D2/CRTH2 pathway mediates double-stranded RNA-induced enhancement of allergic airway inflammation. J Immunol. 2008;180:541–9.

89. Yu M, Levine SJ. Toll-like receptor, RIG-I-like receptors and the NLRP3 inflammasome: key modulators of innate immune responses to double-stranded RNA viruses. Cytokine Growth Factor Rev. 2011;22:63–72.

90. Barnig C, Cernadas M, Dutile S, Liu X, Perrella MA, Kazani S, Wechsler ME, Israel E, Levy BD. Lipoxin A4 regulates natural killer cell and type 2 innate lymphoid cell activation in asthma. Sci Transl Med. 2013;5(174). 10.1126/scitranslmed.3004812.https://doi.org/10.1126/scitranslmed.3004812.

91. Jackson DJ, Shamji B, Trujillo-Torralbo M-B, Walton RP, Bartlett NW, Edwards MR, Mallia P, Edwards M, Westwick J, Johnston SL. Prostaglandin D2 is induced during rhinovirus-induced asthma exacerbations and related to exacerbation severity in vivo. Am J Respir Crit Care Med. 2014;189:A5351.

92. Sandham D, Asano D, Barker L, Budd D, Erpenbeck V, Knowles I, Mikami T, Profit R, Robb O, Shiraishi Y, et al. Fevipiprant, a potent selective prostaglandin D2 receptor 2 (DP2) antagonist, dose-dependently inhibits pulmonary inflammation in a mouse model of asthma. Am J Respir Crit Care Med. 2018;197:A1418.

93. Russell RJ, Brightling C. Pathogenesis of asthma: implications for precision medicine. Clin Sci (Lond). 2017;131:1723–35.

94. Diamant Z, Sidharta PN, Singh D, O'Connor BJ, Zuiker R, Leaker BR, Silkey M, Dingemanse J. Setipiprant, a selective CRTH2 antagonist, reduces allergen-induced airway responses in allergic asthmatics. Clin Exp Allergy. 2014;44:1044–52.

95. Santini G, Mores N, Malerba M, Mondino C, Macis G, Montuschi P. Investigational prostaglandin D2 receptor antagonists for airway inflammation. Expert Opin Investig Drugs. 2016;25:639–52.

10

A circulating cell population showing both M1 and M2 monocyte/macrophage surface markers characterizes systemic sclerosis patients with lung involvement

Amelia Chiara Trombetta[1†], Stefano Soldano[1†], Paola Contini[2], Veronica Tomatis[1], Barbara Ruaro[1], Sabrina Paolino[1], Renata Brizzolara[1], Paola Montagna[1], Alberto Sulli[1], Carmen Pizzorni[1], Vanessa Smith[3,4] and Maurizio Cutolo[1*] (iD)

Abstract

Background: Systemic sclerosis (SSc) is a disorder characterized by immune system alterations, vasculopathy and fibrosis. SSc-related interstitial lung disease (ILD) represents a common and early complication, being the leading cause of mortality. Monocytes/macrophages seem to have a key role in SSc-related ILD. Interestingly, the classically (M1) and alternatively (M2) activated monocyte/macrophage phenotype categorization is currently under revision.

Our aim was to evaluate if circulating monocyte/macrophage phenotype could be used as biomarker for lung involvement in SSc. To this purpose we developed a wide phenotype characterization of circulating monocyte/macrophage subsets in SSc patients and we evaluated possible relations with lung involvement parameter values.

Methods: A single centre cross-sectional study was performed in fifty-five consecutive SSc patients, during the year 2017. All clinical and instrumental tests requested for SSc follow up and in particular, lung computed tomography (CT) scan, pulmonary function tests (PFTs), Doppler echocardiography with systolic pulmonary artery pressure (sPAP) measurement, blood pro-hormone of brain natriuretic peptide (pro-BNP) evaluation, were performed in each patient in a maximum one-month period. Flow cytometry characterization of circulating cells belonging to the monocyte/macrophage lineage was performed using specific M1 (CD80, CD86, TLR2 and TLR4) and M2 surface markers (CD204, CD163 and CD206). Non-parametric tests were used for statistical analysis.

Results: A higher percentage of circulating CD204$^+$CD163$^+$CD206$^+$TLR4$^+$CD80$^+$CD86$^+$ and CD14$^+$CD206$^+$CD163$^+$CD 204$^+$TLR4$^+$CD80$^+$CD86$^+$ mixed M1/M2 monocyte/macrophage subsets, was identified to characterize patients affected by SSc-related ILD and higher systolic pulmonary artery pressure. Mixed M1/M2 monocyte/macrophage subset showed higher percentages in patients positive for anti-topoisomerase antibody, a known lung involvement predictor.

Conclusions: The present study shows for the first time, through a wide flow cytometry surface marker analysis, that higher circulating mixed M1/M2 monocyte/macrophage cell percentages are associated with ILD, sPAP and anti-topoisomerase antibody positivity in SSc, opening the path for research on their possible role as pathogenic or biomarker elements for SSc lung involvement.

Keywords: Systemic sclerosis, Interstitial lung disease, Pulmonary artery hypertension, Monocyte/macrophage phenotype, M1, M2, Innate immunity, Lung CT scan, Pulmonary function tests, Flow cytometry, Anti-topoisomerase antibody

* Correspondence: mcutolo@unige.it
†Amelia Chiara Trombetta and Stefano Soldano contributed equally to this work.
[1]Research Laboratory and Academic Division of Clinical Rheumatology, Department of Internal Medicine, University of Genova, Polyclinic San Martino Hospital, Genoa, Italy
Full list of author information is available at the end of the article

Background

Systemic sclerosis (SSc) is a rare autoimmune disease, characterized by progressive microvascular damage and fibrosis, involving almost all organs of affected patients and predictable by several biomarkers [1].

Interstitial lung disease (ILD) is a common and early complication in SSc patients, and a certain degree of ILD, in the form of non-specific interstitial pneumonia (NSIP), has been shown in 78% of SSc lung biopsies. Notably, among possible organ involvements in SSc, ILD evolves to the worse prognosis, being the leading cause of mortality in SSc patients [2].

In addition, patients affected by SSc-associated ILD have a high risk to develop cardiopulmonary disease and pulmonary hypertension. After pulmonary hypertension development, severe impairments in both physical and emotional domains of health-related quality of life were demonstrated [3]. The 3-year death rate in SSc patients affected by pulmonary hypertension was calculated to be 44–64% [4, 5].

SSc-associated ILD was demonstrated to be early recognized by lung computed tomography (CT) scan. On the other hand, the wide range of pulmonary function test (PFT) normal values (80–120% of predicted) may determine its reduced sensitivity [6].

Several studies recently highlighted the genetic and epigenetic aberrations involved in the SSc pathogenesis [7, 8]. Importantly, major gene signatures related to phenotype, activation and migration of macrophages demonstrated to be relevant to the progressive pulmonary fibrosis, indicating macrophages as key players [9, 10].

Intriguingly, imbalance in macrophage phenotype features and macrophage activation have been lately considered essential for the development of inflammatory-autoimmune, fibrotic, infective and neoplastic disorders characterized by lung involvement [11–16]. Macrophages have been initially categorized as classically (M1) or alternatively activated (M2), mirroring T cells categories. M1 macrophages express specific phenotype markers, including toll-like receptors (i.e., TLR2 and TLR4) and the co-stimulatory molecules CD80 and CD86, and are involved in triggering intensive inflammation and tissue damage [17]. M2 macrophages primarily express the mannose receptor-1 (CD206) and macrophage scavenger receptors (CD204 and CD163), and they are associated with T helper (Th) 2 response, tissue repair and fibrosis [18, 19].

Recently, classifications based on a wider spectrum of phenotypes of which M1 and M2 subsets would constitute the two extremes have been described [20].

Moreover, it was observed that the majority of alveolar macrophages combine M1 and M2 features in steady state and that the mixed M1/M2 phenotype can be altered by HIV infection [21].

Interestingly, a recent preliminary study demonstrated higher percentages of circulating mixed M1/M2 monocytes/macrophages in SSc patients compared to healthy subjects (HSs) [22]. The aim of the present study was to effectuate a wide phenotype characterization of circulating monocytes/macrophages in consecutive SSc patients stratified according to the severity of lung and right heart involvement, through lung CT scan imaging, PFTs, pro-BNP blood values, and Doppler echocardiography.

Methods

Study design

As part of the regular follow up approved by international guidelines for SSc, all patients underwent clinical examination and instrumental exams over a period of time of up to one month. In particular, lung CT scan, PFT with diffusing capacity of the lungs for carbon monoxide (DLCO), Doppler echocardiography with systolic pulmonary artery pressure (sPAP) measurement, pro-hormone of brain natriuretic peptide (pro-BNP) blood values, were performed for lung-right heart involvement evaluation. The assumption of medications was also considered.

The study was approved by the Ethics Committee of Polyclinic San Martino Hospital, Genoa, Italy (protocol number: 273-reg-2015).

Throughout the manuscript, the investigated cells were defined as circulating "monocytes/macrophages". This is because we wanted to use as much surface markers as possible, including those expressed from mature and polarized macrophages, to better restrict the investigation to monocytes and macrophages, and to study the mixed M1/M2 phenotype, independently from the cell maturation state. In fact, we did not want to exclude also a possible presence of circulating cells in later maturation stages. Therefore, we used different gating strategies, as reported in Additional file 1, including typical markers of immature and mature cells, as previously described [22].

Participants

Fifty-five consecutive SSc patients (50 females and 5 males, mean age 63 ± 13 years), undergoing complete disease staging in a day hospital setting at the Rheumatology Division of Genoa University, were enrolled in the study after written informed consent. Among the enrolled SSc patients, 36 were characterized by a limited cutaneous (lcSSc) disease form and 19 were characterized by a diffused cutaneous (dcSSc) disease form. SSc diagnosis was done according to the American College of Rheumatology (ACR)/European League Against Rheumatism (EULAR) 2013 criteria [23, 24].

Data from blood samples derived from a population of 27 sex and gender matched HSs, analysed in a recent preliminary study, were applied here for comparison with SSc patients, for the most significant results [22].

Lung and right heart involvement parameters

Lung CT scan, PFTs and sPAP, pro-BNP value measurements were performed in each patient in the same period of the other examinations scheduled for SSc follow-up. Results were interpreted by the same operator for each type of diagnostic test.

Afterwards, patients were stratified according to the presence or the absence of any interstitial involvement at lung CT scan (SSc-ILD group versus SSc No-ILD group, respectively). Therefore, patients were stratified also according to the presence or the absence of single CT scan abnormalities, characteristically described in SSc lung involvement: ground glass opacities (defined as an area of increased attenuation in the absence of architectural distortion) of lower lobes, ground glass opacities of upper lobes, peripheral septal thickening, apical fibrotic (architectural distortion with reticular intra-lobular interstitial thickening) changes, diffused fibrotic changes, traction bronchiectasis and bronchiolectasis (dilatation of the airways in the peripheral portion of the lung) and enlarged mediastinal nodes [25].

As regards PFT, forced vital capacity (FVC), DLCO and FVC/DLCO ratio values were reported and analyzed for each SSc patient. In agreement with previous studies, the FVC/DLCO ratio higher than 1.5 was considered suggestive for pulmonary vasculopathy in SSc patients [26].

Flow cytometry

After enrolment, peripheral blood was collected in a lithium-heparin single tube from each SSc patient.

To identify monocyte/macrophage lineage surface markers CD14-APC-Vio770 and CD45-VioGreen antibodies were used. The characterization of M2 phenotype was performed using CD204-PE, CD163-PE-Vio770 and CD206-PeerCP-Vio700, whereas the M1 phenotype was investigated using CD80-APC, CD86-VioBlue, TLR2-PE-Vio615 and TLR4-VioBright-FITC antibodies. CD66b-FITC was used to identify and exclude granulocytes (Miltenyi Biotech, Bergisch Gladbach, Germany).

A total of 0.1 ml of peripheral blood was incubated with 10 μl of antibody for 15 min at room temperature, then erythrocytes were lysed and leucocytes post-fixed. Afterwards, the flow cytometry analysis was performed.

Three initial gating strategies were implemented to investigate circulating monocyte/macrophage phenotype over total leucocyte population and included in the Additional file 1. The first initial gating strategy evaluated the CD14+ cells over total leucocyte population. In this CD14+ cell population, circulating monocytes/macrophages showing an M2 phenotype were characterized based on the expression of CD204, CD163 and CD206. Therefore, a second initial gating strategy evaluated the CD204+ cells in the leucocyte population, excluding lymphocytes, CD66b+ granulocytes, doublets and cellular

debris. In the CD204+ population, circulating cells co-expressing CD163 and CD206 were detected to characterize monocytes/macrophages showing an M2 phenotype. Cells positive for M2 phenotype markers (CD204, CD163, CD206) and M1 phenotype markers (TLR4, CD80 and CD86) were investigated to identify the presence of cells with a mixed M1/M2 phenotype, as recently reported [22]. Although lymphocytes and neutrophils are excluded in the initial gating strategy starting from CD204 + cells, no specific dendritic cell markers were investigated to discriminate these cells and then they might be probably present in a limited percentage in the M1/M2 mixed population.

Finally, a third initial gating strategy was made up to detect monocytes/macrophages showing prominently M1 surface markers CD80, CD86, TLR2 and TLR4 [27].

Flow cytometric analysis was performed using a Navios Flow Cytometer and the Kaluza analysis software (Beckman Coulter, Milan, Italy), evaluating a total of 5×10^6 cells and detecting more than 30 events in the smallest subset investigated, according to consensus guidelines on the minimal residual disease [28].

Statistical analysis

Data were analyzed using IBM SPSS Statistics Version 21.0. (IBM Corp: Armonk, NY). Non-parametric tests were applied for statistical analysis and in particular Mann-Whitney U test was used for comparing data with an ordinal distribution between two independent groups. Kruskal-Wallis test was chosen to assess significantly different distributions of continuous dependent variables by a categorical independent variable with more than two groups. Finally, bivariate Pearson's correlation was calculated to measure linear relationship between two variables with ordinal distribution. A p-value lower than 0.05 was considered as statistically significant. The results were expressed as median ± standard deviation (SD) and graphically represented through box and whisker plots.

Results

Demographics and clinical parameters are summarized in Table 1.

Only 5 males were enrolled among the SSc patient population, consequently the sex variable was not used for the analysis.

Associations between auto-antibody positivity, pro-BNP blood values, disease form, and monocyte/macrophage phenotype

Anti-topoisomerase antibody (Anti-Scl70) positivity was associated with lower FVC% (Scl70 + = 84.5 ± 14% vs. Scl70- = 112.8 ± 22; $p < 0.0001$) and higher pro-BNP values (Scl70+ = 790 ± 883 vs. Scl 70- = 213 ± 243 $p = 0.01$) (Fig. 1a and b).

Table 1 Demographic clinical and imaging data from the whole systemic sclerosis patient population

Demographic, clinical and imaging data in SSc PTs	Mean ± SD OR number-percentage
Age (years, mean ± SD)	63 ± 13
Sex (females/males)	50/5
RP duration (years, mean ± SD)	5.8 ± 10
SSc duration (years, mean ± SD)	8.4 ± 6
SSc form = LcSSc/dcSSc (n = %)	36 = 65.5% / 19 = 34.5%
ANA (n = %)	55 = 100%
ACA (n = %)	20 = 36.4%
Anti-Scl-70 Ab (n = %)	23 = 41.8%
ILD at CT scan (n = %)	37 = 67.3%
Ground glass opacities, lower lobes (n = %)	13 = 23.6%
Ground glass opacities, upper lobes (n = %)	8 = 14.5%
Ground glass opacities, upper and lower lobes (n = %)	8 = 14.5%
Peripheral septal thickening (n = %)	31 = 56.4%
Apical fibrotic changes (n = %)	20 = 36.4%
Diffused fibrotic changes (n = %)	15 = 27.3%
Enlarged mediastinal nodes (n = %)	16 = 29.1%
Traction bronchiectasis and bronchiolectasis (n = %)	16 = 29.1%
FVC% (mean ± SD)	104 ± 24
DLCO/VA% (mean ± SD)	71.5 ± 20
sPAP mmHg (mean ± SD)	34 ± 7
Pro-BNP (pg/ml, mean ± SD)	1423 ± 5119
On immunosuppressive therapy (n = %)	32 = 56.1%
On glucocorticoids (n = %)	9 = 16.4%
On ERAs (n = %)	16 = 28.1%

Data are expressed as means ±standard deviations or numbers = percentages of the total population. *SSc* Systemic sclerosis, *PTs* patients, *RP* Raynaud's phenomenon, *SD* standard deviation, *ILD* interstitial lung disease, *ANA* Anti-nuclear antibody, *ACA*: Anti-centromere antibodies, *Ab anti-Scl70* anti-topoisomerase antibody, *CT* computed tomography, *FVC* forced vital capacity, *DLCO* diffusing capacity of the lungs for carbon monoxide, *sPAP* systolic pulmonary artery pressure, *pro-BNP* prohormone of brain natriuretic peptide, *ERAs* Endothelin 1 receptor antagonists. No other vasomodulating therapies were used by the selected SSc patients

In the circulating CD204$^+$ cell population of Scl70 positive SSc patients, by Mann-Whitney test, several mixed M1/M2 macrophage subsets showed higher percentages compared to Scl70 negative SSc patients: CD204$^+$CD163$^+$CD206$^+$TLR4$^+$CD14$^-$ cells (Scl70+ = 2.4 ± 4.6%, vs. Scl70- = 0.64 ± 7.9%, p = 0.036), CD204$^+$CD163$^+$CD206$^+$TLR4$^+$CD80$^+$ cells (Scl70+ = 8.2 ± 8.2% vs. Scl70- = 0.86 ± 4.4%, p = 0.027, Fig. 1e), CD204$^+$CD163$^+$CD206$^+$TLR4$^+$CD86$^+$ cells (Scl70+ = 2.2 ± 6.9% vs. Scl70- = 0.7 ± 3.6%, p = 0.046), CD204$^+$CD163$^+$CD206$^+$TLR4$^+$CD80$^+$CD86$^+$ cells (Scl70+ = 1.6 ± 6.7% vs. Scl70- = 0.54 ± 3.6%, p = 0.036, Fig. 1c, d, f).

Using HS data, as reported in the Methods section, Kruskal-Wallis test was performed and significantly lower percentages for the same cell populations in HSs were obtained (HSs values for CD204$^+$CD163$^+$CD206$^+$TLR4$^+$CD14$^-$ cells = 0.17 ± 0.41%, p < 0.0001 vs. SSc patients, pairwise comparison: HSs vs Scl70- p = 0.05, HSs vs Scl70+ p < 0.0001; CD204$^+$CD163$^+$CD206$^+$TLR4$^+$CD80$^+$ cells = 0.16 ± 0.48%, p < 0.0001 vs. SSc patients, pairwise comparison: HSs vs Scl70- p = 0.001, HSs vs Scl70+ p < 0.0001; CD204$^+$CD163$^+$CD206$^+$TLR4$^+$CD86$^+$ cells = 0.18 ± 0.36%, p < 0.0001 SSc patients, pairwise comparison: HSs vs Scl70- p = 0.001, HSs vs Scl70+ p < 0.0001; CD204$^+$CD163$^+$CD206$^+$TLR4$^+$CD80$^+$CD86$^+$ cells = 0.08 ± 0.29%, p < 0.0001 SSc patients, pairwise comparison: HSs vs Scl70- p = 0.001, HSs vs Scl70+ p < 0.0001, Additional file 2).

No association was reported between Scl70 Ab positivity and cells expressing exclusively M1 or M2 phenotype markers.

Anti-centromere antibodies (ACA) positivity was associated with older age at the time of the study (ACA+ = 70 ± 7 vs. ACA- = 57 ± 14 years, p = 0.002), longer SSc duration (ACA + = 10 ± 6 vs. ACA- = 7 ± 6 years, p = 0.049), higher FVC percentage (ACA+ = 118 ± 19% vs. ACA- = 94 ± 21%, p < 0.0001), and lower gammaglobulin percentage values (ACA+ = 14.8 ± 3% vs. ACA- = 17.3 ± 3%, p = 0.004).

ACA positive patients showed a higher percentage of CD14$^+$ cells (ACA+ = 7.3 ± 1.9% vs. ACA- 6.3 ± 2.4%, p = 0.022). Several cells more clearly polarized towards an M1 or M2 phenotype segregated with ACA positivity: CD14$^+$TLR2$^+$ (ACA+ = 7.2 ± 2.6% vs. ACA- = 6 ± 3%, p = 0.046), CD14$^+$CD163$^+$ (ACA+ = 7 ± 1.9% vs. ACA- = 5.8 ± 2.6%, p = 0.025), and CD14$^+$CD204$^+$CD163$^+$ (ACA + = 0.18 ± 0.4% vs. ACA- = 0.08 ± 0.3%, p = 0.011).

Only CD204$^+$CD163$^+$CD206$^+$TLR4$^+$CD80$^+$ cells, in the circulating CD204$^+$ cells, showed higher percentages in dcSSc compared to lcSSc patients (dcSSc = 2.96 ± 8% vs. lcSSc = 0.94 ± 5%, p = 0.047). The Kruskal-Wallis test, executed adding HSs data, showed significantly lower CD204$^+$CD163$^+$CD206$^+$TLR4$^+$CD80$^+$ cell percentages in comparison to both lcSSc and dcSSc (0.16 ± 0.48%, p < 0.0001, globally and after pairwise comparison).

Associations between lung disease evaluated at CT scan and monocyte/macrophage phenotype

The only gating strategy that effectively highlighted differences in circulating monocyte/macrophage phenotype between SSc-ILD versus SSc-No ILD group was the one based on initial gating of CD204$^+$ cells (Table 2).

No significant difference was reported for total CD204$^+$ cell percentage, over circulating leukocytes, between SSc-ILD patient and SSc-No ILD patient groups (Table 2).

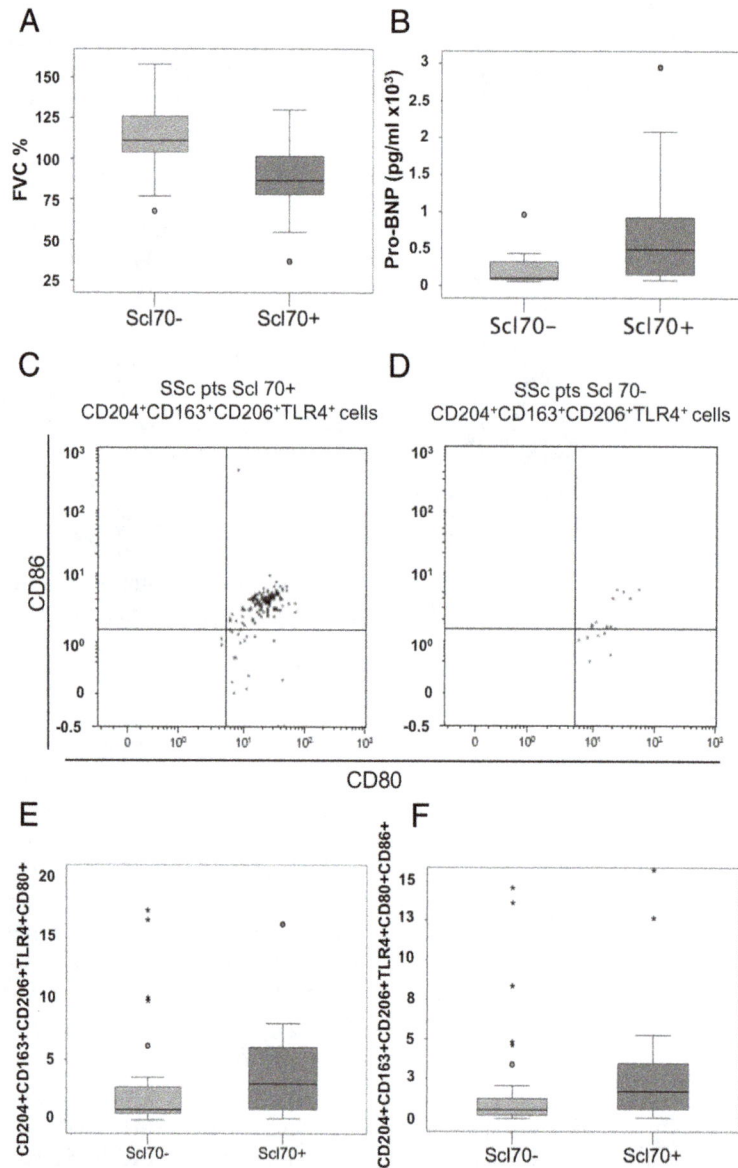

Fig. 1 Ab anti Scl70 positivity: associations with FVC%, Pro-BNP blood values and mixed M1/M2 cells percentages. **a** and **b**, clinical associations of Anti-Scl70 Ab positivity with lower FVC% and higher pro-BNP values are shown. **c** and **d** show the representative dot plots from the flow cytometry analysis of the mixed M1/M2 CD204+CD163+CD206+TLR4+CD80+CD86+ cell subset is shown in patients with positive and negative Ab anti-Scl70. Significant differences ($p = 0.027$) are shown between average percentages of circulating mixed M1/M2 subset CD204+CD163+CD206+TLR4+CD80+ over total CD204+ cells, in Scl70+ vs Scl70- patients (**e**) and between percentage of circulating mixed M1/M2 subset CD204+CD163+CD206+TLR4+CD80+CD86+ over total CD204+ cells, in Scl70+ vs Scl70- patients (**f**). Anti-Scl70 = Anti-topoisomerase; FVC = forced vital capacity; pro-BNP = prohormone of brain natriuretic peptide

Considering the CD204+ cell population, SSc-ILD patients showed a significant increased percentage of circulating CD204+CD163+ cells compared to SSc-No ILD patients (Table 2). Likewise, circulating CD204+CD163+TLR4+ cells, CD204+CD163+CD206+TLR4+ cells, showed significant higher percentages in the SSc-ILD group (Table 2). Among CD204+CD163+TLR4+CD206+ cells, only CD14− and not CD14+ cells showed significantly higher percentages in the SSc-ILD group (Table 2).

Remarkably, in the CD204+CD163+CD206+TLR4+ cell population, mixed M1/M2 phenotype cells expressing CD80 and CD86 markers resulted significantly increased in the SSc-ILD group compared to the SSc-No ILD group (Fig. 2 a, b, c, d and Table 2).

No differences were observed between SSc-ILD and SSc-No ILD patients in the percentage of total circulating CD14+ cells ($6.68 \pm 1.8\%$ and $7.57 \pm 2.5\%$, respectively, $p = 0.18$).

Table 2 The CD204 positive cell population percentages are shown in patients with (SSc-ILD) or without interstitial lung disease (SSc-No ILD) at lung CT scan and healthy subjects (HSs)

Analysis of circulating CD204+ cells	SSc-ILD (37)	SSc-No-ILD (18)	p (MW)	HSs (27)	p (KW)
CD204$^+$ (%)	0.5 ± 0.40	0.8 ± 0.7	$p = 0.13$	0.7 ± 0.3	0.21
CD204$^+$CD163$^+$ (%leukocytes)	0.08 ± 0.22	0.09 ± 0.14	$p = 0.65$	0.03 ± 0.03	**0.001**
CD204$^+$CD163$^+$ (%CD204$^+$)	13.7 ± 15	8.4 ± 13	$p = 0.034$	6.3 ± 3	**< 0.0001**
CD204$^+$CD163$^+$TLR4$^+$ (%leukocytes)	0.03 ± 0.22	0.02 ± 0.15	$p = 0.34$	0.008 ± 0.01	**< 0.0001**
CD204$^+$CD163$^+$TLR4$^+$ (%CD204$^+$)	6.2 ± 16	2.9 ± 15	$p = 0.025$	1.4 ± 1.7	**< 0.0001**
CD204$^+$CD163$^+$CD206$^+$ (%leukocytes)	0.01 ± 0.1	0.01 ± 0.05	$p = 0.65$	0.008 ± 0.01	**0.001**
CD204$^+$CD163$^+$CD206$^+$ (%CD204$^+$)	4 ± 7.4	1.9 ± 5.6	$p = 0.07$	1.1 ± 1.2	**< 0.0001**
CD204$^+$CD163$^+$CD206$^+$TLR4$^+$ (%leukocytes)	0.014 ± 0.1	0.11 ± 0.05	$p = 0.20$	0.003 ± 0.004	**< 0.0001**
CD204$^+$CD163$^+$CD206$^+$TLR4$^+$ (%CD204$^+$)	2.7 ± 7.3	1.1 ± 5.9	$p = 0.013$	0.5 ± 0.6	**< 0.0001**
CD204$^+$CD163$^+$CD206$^+$ TLR4$^+$CD14$^+$(%leukocytes)	0.003 ± 0.014	0.004 ± 0.003	$p = 0.795$	0.001 ± 0.003	**0.008**
CD204$^+$CD163$^+$CD206$^+$ TLR4$^+$CD14$^+$(%CD204$^+$)	0.73 ± 1.4	0.27 ± 0.54	$p = 0.097$	0.20 ± 0.38	**< 0.0001**
CD204$^+$CD163$^+$CD206$^+$ TLR4$^+$CD14$^-$ (%leukocytes)	0.009 ± 0.08	0.006 ± 0.05	$p = 0.092$	0.001 ± 0.002	**< 0.0001**
CD204$^+$CD163$^+$CD206$^+$ TLR4$^+$CD14$^-$ (%CD204+)	1.93 ± 6.56	0.6 ± 5.69	$p = 0.029$	0.17 ± 0.41	**< 0.0001**
CD204$^+$CD163$^+$CD206$^+$ TLR4$^+$CD80$^+$ (%leukocytes)	0.01 ± 0.09	0.004 ± 0.05	$p = 0.041$	0.001 ± 0.003	**< 0.0001**
CD204$^+$CD163$^+$CD206$^+$ TLR4$^+$CD80$^+$ (%CD204$^+$)	2.07 ± 6.83	0.5 ± 5.33	$p = 0.010$	0.16 ± 0.48	**< 0.0001**
CD204$^+$CD163$^+$CD206$^+$ TLR4$^+$CD86$^+$ (%leukocytes)	0.008 ± 0.08	0.005 ± 0.04	$p = 0.082$	0.001 ± 0.002	**< 0.0001**
CD204$^+$CD163$^+$CD206$^+$TLR4$^+$ CD86$^+$ (%CD204$^+$)	1.16 ± 5.8	0.72 ± 4.1	$p = 0.023$	0.19 ± 0.36	**< 0.0001**
CD204$^+$CD163$^+$CD206$^+$TLR4$^+$ CD80$^+$CD86$^+$ (%leukocytes)	0.04 ± 0.08	0.002 ± 0.03	$p = 0.036$	0.0006 ± 0.001	**< 0.0001**
CD204$^+$CD163$^+$CD206$^+$TLR4$^+$ CD80$^+$CD86$^+$ (%CD204$^+$)	1 ± 5.6	0.39 ± 4	$p = 0.021$	0.08 ± 0.2	**< 0.0001**

By Mann-Whitney test, several mixed M1/M2 cell populations were found to show significantly higher percentages (p MW highlighted in bold) in SSc patients affected by ILD, compared to SSc patients with no ILD. On the right, Kruskal-Wallis test was performed adding HSs data, obtaining more significant results (p KW)

No differences were observed between SSc-ILD and SSc-No ILD patients in the percentage of circulating monocytes/macrophages expressing only surface markers considered to be M1 specific.

Monocytes/macrophages phenotype and single CT scan alterations associated with interstitial lung disease, in SSc patients

Interestingly, SSc patients showing fibrotic changes diffused to upper and lower lobes at lung CT scan, seemed to be characterized by a slightly higher percentage of mixed M1/M2 monocytes/macrophages and characterized as CD14$^+$CD206$^+$CD163$^+$CD80$^+$CD86$^+$ compared to patients with less or no lung fibrosis (0.001 ± 0.008 and 0.0006 ± 0.006, $p = 0.044$). Coherently, the same cell population showed higher percentages in patients presenting bronchiectasis or bronchiolectasis (0.002 ± 0.008% and 0.0006 ± 0.006%, $p = 0.021$).

No significant difference was reported in circulating monocyte/macrophage phenotype between patients with reported ground glass opacities localized at lower or upper lung lobes or diffused to both locations at lung CT scan. Similarly, no significant difference was observed in SSc patients for whom peripheral septal thickening, apical fibrotic changes, or enlarged mediastinal nodes were reported at lung CT scan.

Correlations between circulating monocyte/macrophage phenotype, PFTs and sPAP values, in SSc patients

Higher percentages of circulating mixed M1/M2 monocyte/macrophage subset, characterized as CD14$^+$CD206$^+$CD163$^+$CD204$^+$TLR4$^+$CD80$^+$CD86$^+$ cells, showed a weak linear negative correlation with DLCO% ($p = 0.046$, $r = -0.28$, Fig. 3a).

No linear correlations were observed between macrophage subsets phenotype and FVC% values.

A FVC/DLCO ratio higher than 1.5 was associated with several circulating monocyte/macrophage subset percentages, and in particular: CD204$^+$CD163$^+$ cells calculated over total CD204$^+$ cells (FVC/DLCO< 1.5 = 9 ± 15% vs. FVC/DLCO> 1.5 = 13 ± 14%, $p = 0.006$), CD204$^+$CD163$^+$TLR4$^+$ cells calculated over CD204$^+$ cells (FVC/DLCO< 1.5 = 3 ± 15% vs. FVC/DLCO> 1.5 = 6.4 ± 15%, $p = 0.025$), CD204$^+$CD163$^+$TLR4$^+$ cells calculated over total leucocytes (FVC/DLCO< 1.5 = 0.02 ± 0.25%, vs. FVC/DLCO> 1.5 = 0.04 ± 0.02%, $p = 0.039$), CD204$^+$CD163$^+$CD206$^+$TLR4$^+$CD86$^+$ cells calculated over total leucocytes (FVC/DLCO< 1.5 = 0.008 ± 0.03 vs. FVC/DLCO> 1.5 = 0.04 ± 0.09% %, $p = 0.041$, Fig. 3b). As regards cell subsets calculated over total CD14$^+$ cells, significant differences were observed with an FVC/DLCO ratio lower or higher than 1.5: CD14$^+$CD163$^+$ cells (FVC/DLCO< 1.5 = 5.8 ± 2.4% vs. FVC/DLCO> 1.5

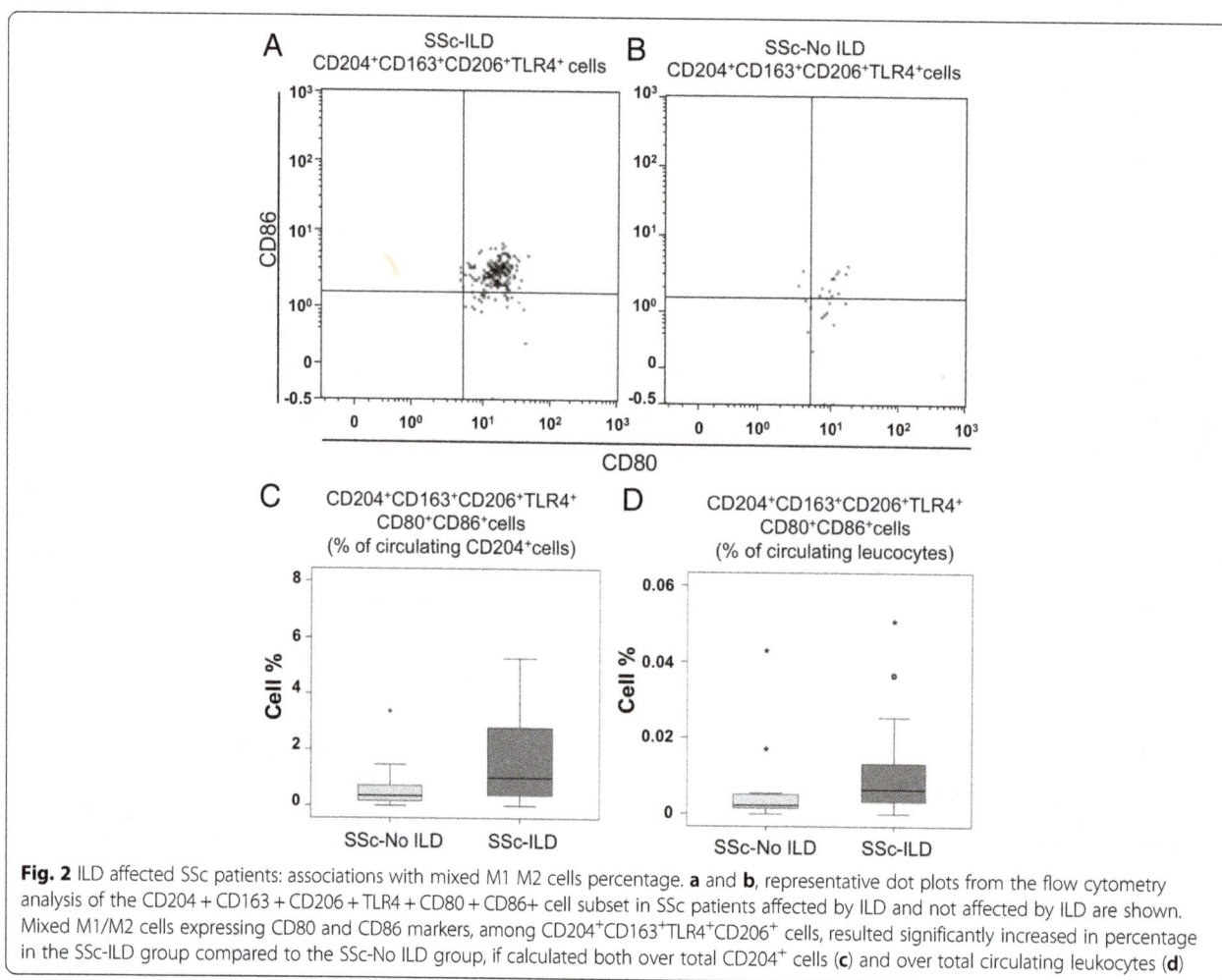

Fig. 2 ILD affected SSc patients: associations with mixed M1 M2 cells percentage. **a** and **b**, representative dot plots from the flow cytometry analysis of the CD204 + CD163 + CD206 + TLR4 + CD80 + CD86+ cell subset in SSc patients affected by ILD and not affected by ILD are shown. Mixed M1/M2 cells expressing CD80 and CD86 markers, among CD204$^+$CD163$^+$TLR4$^+$CD206$^+$ cells, resulted significantly increased in percentage in the SSc-ILD group compared to the SSc-No ILD group, if calculated both over total CD204$^+$ cells (**c**) and over total circulating leukocytes (**d**)

= 6.9 ± 2.3%, p = 0.044), CD14$^+$CD206$^+$ cells (FVC/ DLCO< 1.5 = 6.1 ± 2.8% vs. FVC/DLCO> 1.5 = 7.2 ± 2.8%, p = 0.05), CD14$^+$CD206$^+$CD163$^+$ cells (FVC/DLCO< 1.5 = 5.9 ± 2.7% vs. FVC/DLCO> 1.5 = 6.8 ± 2.7%, p = 0.046), CD14$^+$CD206$^+$CD163$^+$CD86$^+$ cells (FVC/DLCO< 1.5 = 0.01 ± 0.022% vs. FVC/DLCO> 1.5 = 0.03 ± 0.03%, p = 0.034, Fig. 3c), and CD14$^+$CD206$^+$CD163$^+$CD204$^+$ TLR4$^+$CD80$^+$CD86$^+$ cells (FVC/DLCO< 1.5 = 0.0001 ± 0.0005% vs. FVC/DLCO> 1.5 = 0.001 ± 0.005%; p = 0.005, Fig. 3d, Additional file 3). Moreover, the higher percentage of mixed M1/M2 CD14$^+$CD206$^+$CD163$^+$CD204$^+$ TLR4$^+$CD80$^+$CD86$^+$ cell subset correlated positively with the sPAP value (p = 0.028, r = 0.29, Fig. 3e).

Discussion

The results of the present study demonstrated that a population of circulating cells belonging to the monocyte/ macrophage lineage and expressing surface markers of both M1 and M2 phenotypes exists, in significantly high percentages, in SSc patients diagnosed as affected by ILD at CT scan. Additionally, higher percentages of mixed M1/M2 circulating monocytes/macrophages resulted

linearly correlated with lower values of DLCO%, with an FVC/DLCO ratio higher then 1.5, and with higher PAPs values. Finally, mixed M1/M2 cell populations demonstrated to be associated with positivity for Scl-70 antibody, a well-known predictor for lung function decline, and less strictly with diffused disease form [29, 30].

Of note, among the circulating leucocyte population, two initial gating strategies moving from CD204$^+$ cells and CD14$^+$ cells gave significant results in patients affected by SSc-related ILD. On the contrary, no significant results were obtained when investigating CD80$^+$CD86$^+$ cells as initial gating strategy, thus confirming previous studies demonstrating a prevalent presence of markers characteristically linked with the alternately activated macrophage phenotype in SSc patients [31, 32].

The cellular subsets that appear to be correlated with pulmonary involvement seem to be essentially two: the first characterized by the positivity for CD204 and other M2 and M1 surface markers but negative for CD14; the second subset made up of cells positive for CD14 and for other M1 and M2 surface markers, possibly less mature than those positive for CD204. As described by

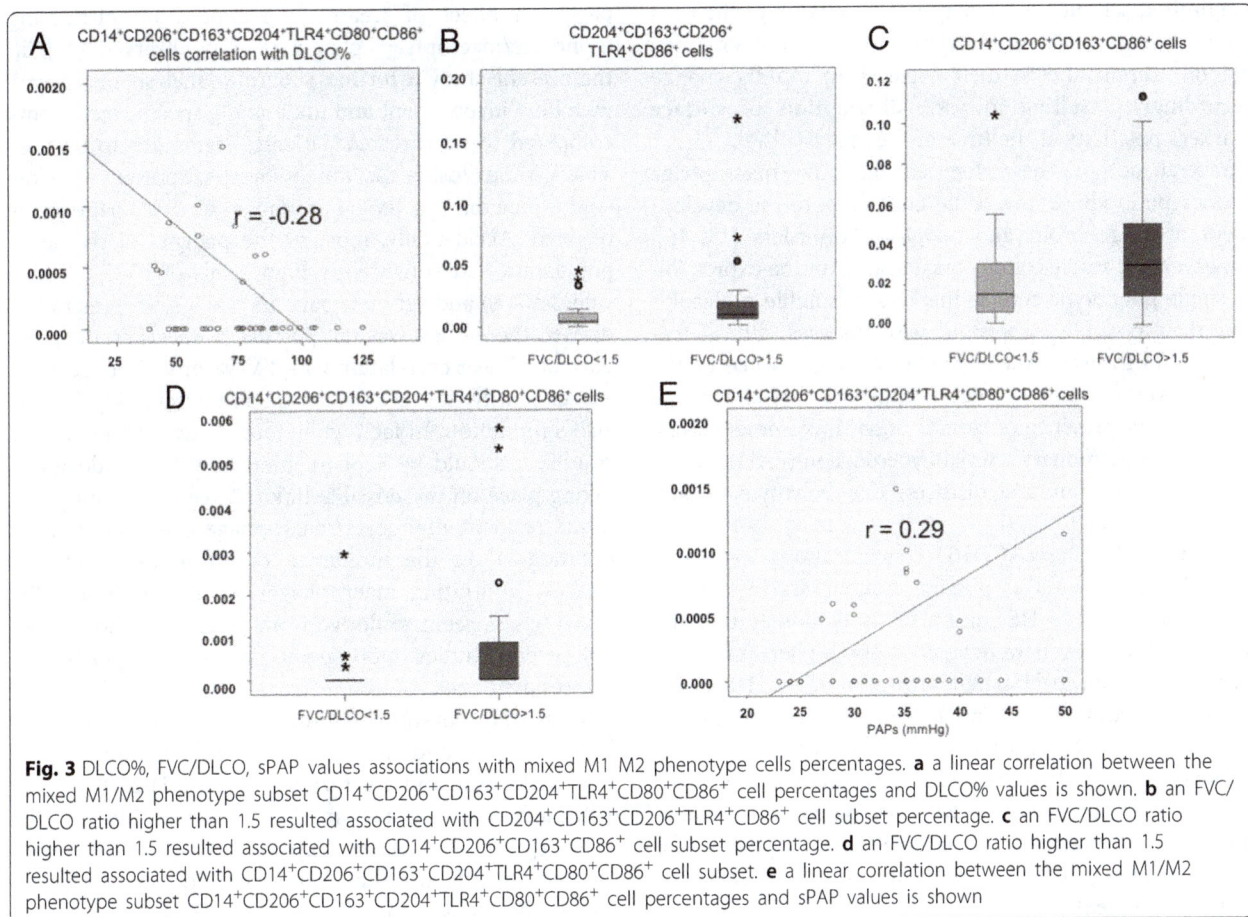

Fig. 3 DLCO%, FVC/DLCO, sPAP values associations with mixed M1 M2 phenotype cells percentages. **a** a linear correlation between the mixed M1/M2 phenotype subset CD14+CD206+CD163+CD204+TLR4+CD80+CD86+ cell percentages and DLCO% values is shown. **b** an FVC/DLCO ratio higher than 1.5 resulted associated with CD204+CD163+CD206+TLR4+CD86+ cell subset percentage. **c** an FVC/DLCO ratio higher than 1.5 resulted associated with CD14+CD206+CD163+CD86+ cell subset percentage. **d** an FVC/DLCO ratio higher than 1.5 resulted associated with CD14+CD206+CD163+CD204+TLR4+CD80+CD86+ cell subset. **e** a linear correlation between the mixed M1/M2 phenotype subset CD14+CD206+CD163+CD204+TLR4+CD80+CD86+ cell percentages and sPAP values is shown

Lambert et al., although the mature circulating monocytes are classically characterized by their expression of CD14, this marker seems not to be considered the hallmark for monocyte identification, in particular in the late phase of maturation, which is accompanied by the expression of CD16 [27]. Moreover, the CD14^{low}CD16^{+} monocyte subset seems to correspond to M2 monocytes/macrophages. Interestingly, in a recent study by Lescoat et al., CD16^{+} monocytes resulted not only associated with pulmonary fibrosis, severity of the restrictive disease and reduction of DLCO but also they were described as precursors of M2 macrophages [33]. Accordingly, even if CD16 was not evaluated in our present study, it may be possible to speculate that the mixed M1/M2 population derived from CD204^{+} monocytes, which is CD14^{-} and associated with ILD, might be positive for CD16.

The presented findings could open to the perspective of a possible role of mixed M1/M2 cells in SSc and SSc-associated ILD pathogenesis, or at least as potential biomarkers for lung involvement in SSc. In a recent study, an integrated genomic approach using a consensus clustering was performed to compare the gene expression profiles of SSc biopsies from different tissues,

including skin, lung and peripheral blood mononuclear cells. The authors described the concept of the immune-fibrotic axis, that is a common pathogenic gene expression signature indicative of the fundamental role of macrophages [34].

In particular, a distinct macrophage signature associated with the alternative activation was observed in SSc-associated pulmonary fibrosis and in the skin of patients with an "inflammatory" SSc gene expression signature, suggesting that there are subtle differences in the macrophage gene expression in lung and skin [34]. Based on these observations, the authors concluded that the plasticity of the monocyte/macrophage lineage is likely to be central to the divergence of fibrotic processes in different SSc-affected tissues and is an important component of an immune-fibrotic axis driving disease pathogenesis [34].

At the same time, the statistics from the present study show the constant presence, in patients affected or not by ILD, of a great variability of cell percentages obtained from the analysis of the various circulating monocyte/macrophages subsets, testified by large standard deviations, and reflecting considerable heterogeneity in cell size. Although this phenomenon could be attributed to the limited sample size, it may also be related to the cells phenotype plasticity in relation with different environmental stimuli and to their capacity to rapidly change accordingly, resulting in wide distribution of surface markers positivity at the time of the analysis [20].

Several authors have focused on how macrophage phenotype modifications could contribute to the development of lung fibrotic and neoplastic disorders [14, 16]. However, the studies often concentrated on the expression of single phenotype surface markers or soluble molecules and their possible association with diseases clinical features. It is the case, for example, of the presence of the M2 markers CD163 or soluble (s)CD163 that showed to be higher in presence of several organ involvements, like in ILD and pulmonary arterial hypertension (PAH), in SSc and other autoimmune diseases, like polymyositis and dermatomyositis [28, 29].

Serum and urinary sCD163 concentrations were very recently investigated as possible biomarkers in SSc patients compared to HSs and a study demonstrated that serum sCD163 levels were significantly higher in SSc patients compared to HSs [35]. However, sCD163 concentrations were not associated with clinical, laboratory, and instrumental characteristics of SSc patients [35].

Other authors described M2 macrophages in SSc patients and their association with several clinical parameters. Higher percentages of circulating cells positive for CD204, CD163, and CD14 were shown to correlate with skin involvement [31].

Circulating alternatively activated CD14$^+$ macrophages, expressing high levels of CD206 were demonstrated to be associated with PAH [32].

A recent study investigated the phenotype of human alveolar macrophages (AMs) in adults living in UK and Malawi, demonstrating that the majority of AMs expressed high levels of M1 and M2 markers simultaneously. As the authors postulate, it is possible that in the healthy lung mucosa, combined M1/M2 features could confer to AMs the ability of maintaining a balance between immune tolerance and protective immunity. On the contrary, a similar circulating phenotype could exert a pathogenic role in SSc patients [21].

Moreover, it was demonstrated that monocyte-derived macrophages co-expressing CD206, CD163 and CD169 were significantly higher in SSc-ILD than in lung cancer or sarcoidosis and that a similar macrophage phenotype was obtained from the analysis of blood-monocytes derived macrophages in SSc patients [36].

However, to our knowledge, no one has so far attempted such a wide phenotype characterization of circulating monocytes/macrophages in connection with the development of SSc-related lung and right heart complications.

This study has several limits. First of all, the relatively small patient population. In fact, even if in a previous

paper an effect of treatment regimens on circulating monocyte/macrophage phenotype was observed [22], in the present study a further subgroup analysis of patients with lung involvement and undergoing specific treatments compared to non-treated patients, seems not to be possible without losing too much statistical power. A follow study including a larger number of SSc patients is planned. Accidentally, most of the patients in the study population had consistently high levels of FVC (average values 104%) and very few patients had a severe restrictive disease, therefore it was not possible to ascertain the presence of a linear correlation with FVC% or with its decline.

Secondarily, the evaluation of only circulating cells is also a limitation. In fact, while interpreting the presented results, it should be kept in mind that a wide debate is taking place on the possible link between circulating and tissue resident monocyte/macrophage cells, questioning the dogma on the monocyte origin of tissue macrophages. Infiltrating macrophages, observed in the diseased tissue, seem to derive from circulating monocytes, but several studies opposed the monocyte origin for tissue resident cells [37, 38].

Moreover, emerging immunological theories attribute to organ and tissues the control of immune system activation and its forms (Th1 or Th2 like) [39]. Although the surface markers investigated in the study (primarily CD204, CD163 and CD206) are considered specific for the characterization of M2 polarized cells, they can also be expressed by dendritic cells [40, 41]. Therefore, based on the gating strategies proposed in our study, a percentage of dendritic cells might be present in the described circulating cell subsets. Monocytes, macrophages and dendritic cells are all members of the mononuclear phagocyte system which is involved in multiple functions during immune responses and, although these cells may be distinguished based on functional and phenotypical characteristics, some cell features are often overlapping and the distinction or classification is challenging [42]. The possible implication of dendritic cells in the development of SSc was recently highlighted in a recent paper by Silvan et al. describing that these cells expressing high levels of PSGL-1 were associated with the presence of interstitial lung disease in SSc patients [43].

Finally, the very low percentage of the newly described circulating cells could make it not easy to use them as a disease biomarker. Evidently, further and larger studies and possibly the sorting of the mixed M1/M2 population will be useful for the evaluation of the importance of this phenotype in both pathogenic, diagnostic or therapeutic perspectives.

Although the identification of these circulating mixed M1/M2 cells was performed through the evaluation of the most investigated and specific markers related to each polarization status and in a previous study they were found significantly increased in SSc patients compared to HSs, the analysis of the marker expression through the detection of the mean fluorescence intensity (MFI), not investigated in this study, might represent a further important aspect that may contribute to understand their possible role in SSc pathogenesis.

In accordance with our results on a possible circulating "scleroderma" macrophage with M1/M2 phenotype, very recently, Moreno-Moral et al. have found in 57 SSc patients, through RNA sequencing and genome-wide genotyping, a mixed macrophage activation signature, characterized by the downregulation of interferon gamma response, attesting for an M2 polarization, but also by the downregulation of the interleukin (IL)-6/JAK/STAT3 signalling pathway, suggesting for a restricted M2 activity [44]. The authors observe that the circulating monocyte/macrophage phenotype could contrast with macrophage signature in tissues such as lung, in which a STAT3-dependent expression of CD163 was associated with pulmonary fibrosis [45].

Interstitial lung disease is a major cause of morbidity and mortality in systemic sclerosis (SSc). Notwithstanding many authors concentrated their attention in this direction, the pathogenic mechanisms of SSc-related ILD remain unknown, and limited therapeutic effects are obtained with the available treatments [46–48].

The knowledge of the mechanisms that initiate the pathogenesis of pulmonary damage or of an easily evaluable biomarker associated with such involvement would be crucial.

Supported by the discovery of interferon (IFN) α, tumor necrosis factor (TNF) α, TLRs, transforming growth factor (TGF) β, platelet derived growth factor (PDGF), genes signatures in SSc, we hypothesized that both Th1 and Th2 activation signals could derive from different damaged tissues, determining the development of circulating mixed M1/M2 cells. At the same time, more polarized responses could possibly develop at tissues level, such as in lungs [39].

Conclusions

In conclusion, it is possible to state that this is the first study showing an association of an M1/M2 monocyte/macrophage phenotype in SSc patients to SSc-related ILD functional and radiological data.

The evaluation of the existence of circulating mixed M1/M2 monocyte/macrophage phenotype and its clinical associations in SSc patients, should be considered as the first step towards a conclusion for a possible role as a pathogenic factor or as an early biomarker for organ involvement in SSc-related ILD. Such a phenotype could be found also in other pulmonary diseases, at the

circulatory or tissue level. The presented acquisitions could therefore be considered as an opening to later studies on a wide phenotype characterization of macrophages at the level of different diseased tissues including lung, kidney, heart, and skin in SSc but also in other fibrotic disorders. Furthermore, isolation and functional study of the described cells are under evaluation for the remarkable values they could have for physiopathology, diagnostic and therapeutic purposes [49].

Additional files

Additional file 1: Gating strategies for the detection of circulating M1, M2 and mixed M1/M2 cells in systemic sclerosis patients and healthy controls. (A) Representative flow cytometry scatter plot and scatter dot plot with median and interquartile range of the initial gating strategy starting from the circulating $CD14^+$cells percentage (%) in the leucocyte population; (B) Representative flow cytometry panels with quadrant regions and scatter dot plot representation of the of circulating $CD14^+CD206^+CD163^+$cells in the $CD14^+$cell population; (C) $CD14^+CD206^+CD163^+CD204^+TLR4^+$cells in the $CD14^+CD206^+CD163^+$cell subset and (D) $CD14^+CD206^+CD163^+CD204^+TLR4^+CD80^+CD86^+$cells in the $CD14^+CD206^+CD163^+TLR4^+$cell subset of healthy subjects (HSs) and systemic sclerosis patients (SSc pts). (E) Representative flow cytometry scatter plot and scatter dot plot with median and interquartile range of the initial gating strategy starting from the circulating $CD204^+$cells percentage (%) in the leucocyte population; (F) Representative flow cytometry panels with quadrant regions and scatter dot plot representation of the of circulating $CD204^+CD163^+CD206^+$cells in the $CD204^+$cell population; (G) $CD204^+CD163^+CD206^+TLR4^+$cells in the $CD204^+CD163^+CD206^+$cell subset; (H) $CD204^+CD163^+CD206^+TLR4^+CD80^+CD86^+$cells and (I) $CD14^+$ and $CD14^-$cells in the $CD204^+ 163^+CD206^+TLR4^+$cell subset of HSs and SSc pts. (J) Representative flow cytometry scatter plot of the initial gating strategy starting from the circulating CD80 + CD86 + cells percentage (%) in the leucocyte population and (L) representative flow cytometry panels with quadrant regions of the of circulating $CD80^+CD86^+TLR2^+TLR4^+$cells in the $CD80^+CD86^+$cell population of HSs and SSc pts. Statistical analysis was performed by Mann-Whitney non-parametric test and p-values lower than 0.05 was considered as statistically significant. (TIF 1646 kb)

Additional file 2: Differences in the percentage of mixed M1/M2 cells in systemic sclerosis patients with or without Ab anti Scl70 positivity and healthy subjects. Cell populations with a mixed M1/M2 phenotype, showing significantly different percentages between Scl70 antibody positive (Scl70 + Pts) and Scl70 antibody negative (Scl70-Pts) patients at Mann-Whitney were then analyzed together with those from age and gender matched healthy subjects (HSs) through Kruskal-Wallis test. HSs showed constantly lower percentages compared to Scl70 + Pts and Scl70-Pts. (TIF 514 kb)

Additional file 3: Differences in the percentage of M2 and mixed M1/M2 cells in systemic sclerosis patients with an FVC/DLCO ratio lower or higher than 1.5. With both gating strategies, one based on CD204 positivity and one based on CD14 positivity, cell populations with an M2 or a mixed M1/M2 phenotype, showed significantly higher percentages in patients with an FVC/DLCO ratio higher then 1.5 compared to patients with an FVC/DLCO ratio lower than 1.5. (DOCX 13 kb)

Abbreviations

Ab anti-Scl70: anti-topoisomerase antibody; ACA: Anti-centromere antibodies; ACR: American College of Rheumatology; ANA: Anti-nuclear antibody; CT: Computed tomography;; dcSSc: Diffused cutaneous systemic sclerosis; DLCO: Diffusing capacity of the lungs for carbon monoxide; EULAR: European League Against Rheumatism; FVC: Forced vital capacity; IL: Interleukin; ILD: Interstitial lung disease; lcSSc: Limited cutaneous systemic sclerosis; MRC1: Gene codifying for c-type mannose receptor 1; NSIP: Non-specific interstitial pneumonia; PFTs: Pulmonary function tests; pro-BNP: Prohormone of brain natriuretic peptide; PTs: Patients; RP: Raynaud's phenomenon; SD: Standard deviation; sPAP: Systolic pulmonary artery pressure; SSc: Systemic sclerosis; Th: T helper; TLR: Toll-like receptors

Acknowledgements
We acknowledge Sara de Gregorio supervising the graphic representation of the data.

Funding
This research did not receive any specific grant from funding agencies in the public, commercial, or not-for-profit sectors.

Authors' contributions
ACT* designed the study, carried out the statistical analysis and wrote the manuscript, SS* designed the study, analysed the data and wrote the manuscript; PC performed the Flow Cytometry analysis; VT and BR enrolled the systemic sclerosis patients and collected the demographic and clinical parameters of the systemic sclerosis patients; RB and PM managed and prepared the samples for the Flow Cytometry analysis; AS, SP and CP supervised the enrolment of the systemic sclerosis patients and healthy subjects and the clinical data collection; VS revised the manuscript; MC supervised the study, wrote and revised the final manuscript. All authors read and approved the final manuscript.

Competing interests
The authors declare that they have no competing interests.

Author details
[1]Research Laboratory and Academic Division of Clinical Rheumatology, Department of Internal Medicine, University of Genova, Polyclinic San Martino Hospital, Genoa, Italy. [2]Clinical Immunology, Department of Internal Medicine, University of Genova, Genoa, Italy. [3]Department of Rheumatology, Ghent University Hospital, Ghent, Belgium. [4]Department of Internal Medicine, Ghent University, Ghent, Belgium.

References
1. Smith V, Riccieri V, Pizzorni C, Decuman S, Deschepper E, Bonroy C, et al. Nailfold capillaroscopy for prediction of novel future severe organ involvement in systemic sclerosis. J Rheumatol. 2013;40:2023–8.
2. Elhai M, Meune C, Boubaya M, Avouac J, Hachulla E, Balbir-Gurman A, et al. Mapping and predicting mortality from systemic sclerosis. Ann Rheum Dis. 2017;76:1897–905.
3. Taichman DB, Shin J, Hud L, Archer-Chicko C, Kaplan S, Sager JS, et al. Health-related quality of life in patients with pulmonary arterial hypertension. Respir Res. 2005;6:92.
4. Hachulla E, Carpentier P, Gressin V, Diot E, Allanore Y, Sibilia J, et al. Risk factors for death and the 3-year survival of patients with systemic sclerosis: the French ItinerAIR-Sclerodermie study. Rheumatology (Oxford). 2009;48:304–8.
5. Zhao J, Wang Q, Liu Y, Tian Z, Guo X, Wang H, et al. Clinical characteristics and survival of pulmonary arterial hypertension associated with three major connective tissue diseases: a cohort study in China. Int J Cardiol. 2017;236:432–7.

6. Goh NS, Desai SR, Veeraraghavan S, Hansell DM, Copley SJ, Maher TM, et al. Interstitial lung disease in systemic sclerosis: a simple staging system. Am J Respir Crit Care Med. 2008;177:1248–54.
7. Luo Y, Wang Y, Wang Q, Xiao R, Lu Q. Systemic sclerosis: genetics and epigenetics. J Autoimmun. 2013;41:161–7.
8. Gourh P, Agarwal SK, Martin E, Divecha D, Rueda B, Bunting H, et al. Association of the C8orf13-BLK region with systemic sclerosis in north-American and European populations. J Autoimmun. 2010;34:155–62.
9. Christmann RB, Sampaio-Barros P, Stifano G, Borges CL, de Carvalho CR, Kairalla R, et al. Association of Interferon- and transforming growth factor beta-regulated genes and macrophage activation with systemic sclerosis-related progressive lung fibrosis. Arthritis Rheumatol. 2014;66:714–25.
10. Hsu E, Shi H, Jordan RM, Lyons-Weiler J, Pilewski JM, Feghali-Bostwick CA. Lung tissues in patients with systemic sclerosis have gene expression patterns unique to pulmonary fibrosis and pulmonary hypertension. Arthritis Rheum. 2011;63:783–94.
11. Enomoto Y, Suzuki Y, Hozumi H, Mori K, Kono M, Karayama M, et al. Clinical significance of soluble CD163 in polymyositis-related or dermatomyositis-related interstitial lung disease. Arthritis Res Ther. 2017;19:9.
12. Jiang Z, Zhu L. Update on the role of alternatively activated macrophages in asthma. J Asthma Allergy. 2016;9:101–7.
13. Bazzan E, Turato G, Tinè M, Radu CM, Balestro E, Rigobello C, et al. Dual polarization of human alveolar macrophages progressively increases with smoking and COPD severity. Respir Res. 2017;18:40.
14. Groves AM, Johnston CJ, Misra RS, Williams JP, Finkelstein JN. Effects of IL-4 on pulmonary fibrosis and the accumulation and phenotype of macrophage subpopulations following thoracic irradiation. Int J Radiat Biol. 2016;92:754–65.
15. Deckman JM, Kurkjian CJ, McGillis JP, Cory TJ, Birket SE, Schutzman LM, et al. Pneumocystis infection alters the activation state of pulmonary macrophages. Immunobiology. 2017;222:188–97.
16. Huang F, Chen Z, Chen H, Lu W, Xie S, Meng QH, et al. Cypermethrin promotes lung Cancer metastasis via modulation of macrophage polarization by targeting MicroRNA-155/Bcl6. Toxicol Sci. 2018. https://doi.org/10.1093/toxsci/kfy039 [Epub ahead of print].
17. Mantovani A, Biswas SK, Galdiero MR, Sica A, Locati M. Macrophage plasticity and polarization in tissue repair and remodelling. J Pathol. 2013;229:176–85.
18. Stifano G, Christmann RB. Macrophage involvement in systemic sclerosis: do we need more evidence? Curr Rheumatol Rep. 2016;18:2.
19. Gundra UM, Girgis NM, Ruckerl D, Jenkins S, Ward LN, Kurtz ZD, et al. Alternatively activated macrophages derived from monocytes and tissue macrophages are phenotypically and functionally distinct. Blood. 2014;123:e110–22.
20. Mosser DM, Edwards JP. Exploring the full spectrum of macrophage activation. Nat Rev Immunol. 2008;8:958–69.
21. Mitsi E, Kamng'ona R, Rylance J, Solórzano C, Jesus Reiné J, Mwandumba HC, et al. Human alveolar macrophages predominately express combined classical M1 and M2 surface markers in steady state. Respir Res. 2018;19:66.
22. Soldano S, Trombetta AC, Contini P, Tomatis V, Ruaro B, Brizzolara R, et al. Increase in circulating cells coexpressing M1 and M2 macrophage surface markers in patients with systemic sclerosis. Ann Rheum Dis Epub ahead of print. Ann Rheum Dis 2018;0:1–3. doi:https://doi.org/10.1136/annrheumdis-2018-213648.
23. van den Hoogen F, Khanna D, Fransen J, Johnson SR, Baron M, Tyndall A, et al. 2013 classification criteria for systemic sclerosis: an American college of rheumatology/European league against rheumatism collaborative initiative. Ann Rheum Dis. 2013;65:2737–47.
24. Hudson M, Fritzler MJ. Diagnostic criteria of systemic sclerosis. J Autoimmun. 2014;48-49:38–41.
25. Kim EA, Johkoh T, Lee KS, Ichikado K, Koh EM, Kim TS, et al. Interstitial pneumonia in progressive systemic sclerosis: serial high-resolution CT findings with functional correlation. J Comput Assist Tomogr. 2001;25:757–63.
26. Sivova N, Launay D, Wémeau-Stervinou L, De Groote P, Remy-Jardin M, Denis G, et al. Relevance of partitioning DLCO to detect pulmonary hypertension in systemic sclerosis. PLoS One. 2013;8:e78001.
27. Lambert C, Preijers FWMB, Yanikkaya Demirel G, Sack U. Monocytes and macrophages in flow: an ESCCA initiative on advanced analysis of monocyte lineage using flow cytometry. Cytometry Part B. 2017;92:180–8.
28. Arroz M, Came N, Lin P, Chen W, Yuan C, Lagoo A, et al. Consensus guidelines on plasma cell myeloma minimal residual disease analysis and reporting. Cytometry Part B. 2016;90:31–9.
29. Briggs DC, Vaughan RW, Welsh KI, Myers A, DuBois RM, Black CM. Immunogenetic prediction of pulmonary fibrosis in systemic sclerosis. Lancet. 1991;338:661–2.

30. Hu PQ, Oppenheim JJ, Medsger TA Jr, Wright TM. T cell lines from systemic sclerosis patients and healthy controls recognize multiple epitopes on DNA topoisomerase. J Autoimmun. 2006;26:258–67.

31. Higashi-Kuwata N, Jinnin M, Makino T, Fukushima S, Inoue Y, Muchemwa FC, et al. Characterization of monocyte/macrophage subsets in the skin and peripheral blood derived from patients with systemic sclerosis. Arthritis Res Ther. 2010;12:R128.

32. Christmann RB, Hayes E, Pendergrass S, Padilla C, Farina G, Affandi AJ, et al. Interferon and alternative activation of monocyte/macrophages in systemic sclerosis–associated pulmonary arterial hypertension. Arthritis Rheum. 2011; 63:1718–28.

33. Lescoat A, Lecureur V, Roussel M, Sunnaram BL, Ballerie A, Coiffier G, et al. CD16-positive circulating monocytes and fibrotic manifestations of systemic sclerosis. Clin Rheumatol. 2017;36:1649–54.

34. Taroni JN, Greene CS, Martyanov V, Wood TA, Christmann RB, Farber HW, et al. A novel multi-network approach reveals tissue-specific cellular modulators of fibrosis in systemic sclerosis. Genome Med. 2017;9:27.

35. Frantz C, Pezet S, Avouac J, Allanore Y. Soluble CD163 as a potential biomarker in systemic sclerosis. Dis Markers. 2018;2018:8509583.

36. Lescoat A, Ballerie A, Augagneur Y, Morzadec C, Vernhet L, Fardel O, et al. Distinct properties of human M-CSF and GM-CSF monocyte-derived macrophages to simulate pathological lung conditions in vitro: application to systemic and inflammatory disorders with pulmonary involvement. Int J Mol Sci 2018;19. pii: E894. doi: https://doi.org/10.3390/ijms19030894.

37. Qian BZ, Li J, Zhang H, Kitamura T, Zhang J, Campion LR, et al. CCL2 recruits inflammatory monocytes to facilitate breast-tumour metastasis. Nature. 2011;475:222–5.

38. Chawla A, Nguyen KD, Goh YP. Macrophage-mediated inflammation in metabolic disease. Nat Rev Immunol. 2011;11:738–49.

39. Matzinger P, Kamala T. Tissue-based class control: the other side of tolerance. Nat Rev Immunol. 2011;11:221–30.

40. Yu X, Wang XY. Antagonizing the innate pattern recognition receptor CD204 to improve dendritic cell-targeted cancer immunotherapy. Oncoimmunology. 2012;1:770–2.

41. Collin M, McGovern N, Haniffa M. Human dendritic cell subsets. Immunology. 2013;140:22–30.

42. Guilliams M, Ginhoux F, Jakubzick C, Naik S, Onai N, Schraml B, et al. Dendritic cells, monocytes and macrophages: a unified nomenclature based on ontogeny. Nat Rev Immunol. 2014;14:571–8.

43. Silván J, González-Tajuelo R, Vicente-Rabaneda E, et al. Deregulated PSGL-1 expression in B cells and dendritic cells may be implicated in human systemic sclerosis development. J Invest Dermatol. 2018;22.

44. Moreno-Moral A, Bagnati M, Koturan S, Ko JH, Fonseca C, Harmston N, et al. Changes in macrophage transcriptome associate with systemic sclerosis and mediate GSDMA contribution to disease risk. Ann Rheum Dis. 2018;77:596–601.

45. Lescoat A, Jégo P, Lecureur V. M-CSF and GM-CSF monocyte-derived macrophages in systemic sclerosis: the two sides of the same coin? Ann Rheum Dis. 2018. https://doi.org/10.1136/annrheumdis-2018-213112 [Epub ahead of print].

46. Johnson ME, Mahoney JM, Taroni J, Sargent JL, Marmarelis E, Wu MR, et al. Experimentally-derived fibroblast gene signatures identify molecular pathways associated with distinct subsets of systemic sclerosis patients in three independent cohorts. PLoS One. 2015;10:e0114017.

47. du Bois RM. Mechanisms of scleroderma-induced lung disease. Proc Am Thorac Soc. 2007;4:434–8.

48. Tan A, Denton CP, Mikhailidis DP, Seifalian AM. Recent advances in the diagnosis and treatment of interstitial lung disease in systemic sclerosis (scleroderma): a review. Clin Exp Rheumatol. 2011;29:S66–74.

49. Burmester GR, Bijlsma JWJ, Cutolo M, McInnes IB. Managing rheumatic and musculoskeletal diseases - past, present and future. Nat Rev Rheumatol. 2017;13:443–8.

11

Significant predictors of medically diagnosed chronic obstructive pulmonary disease in patients with preserved ratio impaired spirometry

Hye Jung Park[1], Min Kwang Byun[1*], Chin Kook Rhee[2], Kyungjoo Kim[2], Hyung Jung Kim[1] and Kwang-Ha Yoo[3]

Abstract

Background: Preserved ratio impaired spirometry (PRISm) is an incompletely understood respiratory condition. We investigated the incidence and significant predictive factors of chronic obstructive pulmonary disease (COPD) in PRISm patients.

Methods: From 11,922 subjects registered in the Korea National Health and Nutrition Examination Survey, never or light smokers, young subjects, and those already medically diagnosed with COPD (defined by ICD-10 code and prescribed medication) were excluded. The 2666 remaining subjects were categorized into PRISm (normal forced expiratory volume in the first second [FEV_1]/force vital capacity [FVC] [≥ 0.7] and low FEV_1 (< 80%); $n = 313$); normal ($n = 1666$); and unrevealed COPD groups (FEV_1/FVC ratio < 0.7; $n = 687$). These groups were compared using matched Health Insurance Review and Assessment Service data over a 3-year follow-up.

Results: COPD incidence in PRISm patients (17/1000 person-year [PY]) was higher than that in normal subjects (4.3/ 1000 PY; $P < 0.001$), but lower than that in unrevealed COPD patients (45/1000 PY; $P < 0.001$). PRISm patients visited hospitals, took COPD medication, and incurred hospitalization costs more frequently than normal subjects, but less frequently than unrevealed COPD patients. In the overall sample, age, FVC, FEV_1, dyspnea, and wheezing were significant predictors of COPD, but in PRISm patients, only age (OR, 1.14; $P = 0.002$) and wheezing (OR, 4.56; $P = 0.04$) were significant predictors.

Conclusion: PRISm patients are likely to develop COPD, and should be monitored carefully, especially older patients and those with wheezing, regardless of lung function.

Keywords: Chronic obstructive pulmonary disorder, Prognosis, Spirometry

Background

Despite the escalating prevalence and economic burden of chronic obstructive pulmonary disease (COPD), many COPD cases remain undiagnosed worldwide [1–3]. A lack of awareness of COPD, lack of educational programs concerning COPD, poor physician adherence to guidelines, and low usage of pulmonary function tests leads to under-diagnosis of COPD [4, 5]. Many studies have reported that

patients with early COPD or even pre-COPD (e.g., smokers or subjects with impaired lung function) have respiratory symptoms and utilize medical support [6, 7]. This has emphasized early-diagnosis and early-treatment of COPD. However, subjects with preserved ratio impaired spirometry (PRISm) are often missed. PRISm patients do not meet COPD criteria [8], with a preserved ratio of force expiratory volume in the first second [FEV_1]/forced vital capacity [FVC] (> 0.7), but have reduced FEV_1 (< 80%, predicted), yet exhibit increased respiratory symptoms, decreased activity, increased comorbidity, and increased mortality [7, 9–14]. Wan et al. described PRISm as a COPD subtype with increased emphysema and gas

---
* Correspondence: littmann@yuhs.ac
[1]Department of Internal Medicine, Gangnam Severance Hospital, Yonsei University College of Medicine, 211 Eonju-ro Gangnam-gu, Seoul 06273, Korea
Full list of author information is available at the end of the article

trapping [15]. Lung density on computed tomography is significantly associated with lung function in PRISm [16]. Thus, some aspects of PRISm are associated with COPD development with worsening of lung function; but the COPD incidence in PRISm patients has rarely been reported.

Tobacco smoking, ageing, air pollution, poor nutritional status, impaired lung function, and underlying asthma are established risk factors for COPD [17, 18]. However, the risk factors associated with COPD in PRISm remain unknown. We sought to elucidate the incidence of COPD in PRISm patients and to identify the significant risk factors for COPD in PRISm, using Korean national cohort data.

Methods
Subjects and study design
We used the cross-sectional the Korea National Health and Nutrition Examination Survey (KNHANES) data of 2007–2009 and KNHANES-matched Health Insurance Review and Assessment (HIRA) cohort data of 2006–2012. A total of 11,922 subjects were available in KNHANES. Among them, never- or light-smokers (< 10 pack-years), young subjects (< 40 years), and patients already medically diagnosed with COPD (based on the ICD-10 code and prescribed medication in HIRA), were excluded ($n = 9256$). We categorized the remaining 2666 subjects into 3 groups based on spirometry (Fig. 1). The normal group ($n = 1666$) had a normal FEV_1/FVC ratio (≥ 0.7) and normal spirometry ($FEV_1 \geq 80\%$ predicted). PRISm subjects ($n = 313$) had a normal FEV_1/FVC ratio (≥ 0.7) and decreased lung

function ($FEV_1 < 80\%$ predicted). Unrevealed COPD subjects had a decreased FEV_1/FVC ratio (< 0.7), regardless of FEV_1 and FVC. KNHANES data did not include post-bronchodilator FEV_1 and FVC, which are recommended in the guidelines [8, 19]; we therefore used pre-bronchodilator FEV_1 and FVC values.

KNHANES and HIRA data
KNHANES data were derived from a national large-scale cross-sectional survey conducted by the Korean government, via the Korea Centers for Disease Control and Prevention. This data were obtained from a well-designed national program with complex, multistage probability sample extraction to reflect the total population of Korea. KNHANES data include age, sex, height, weight, self-reported smoking history, self-reported co-morbidity (answers to the following questions: do you have [the disease, e.g., asthma] diagnosed by a doctor?), results of spirometry tests obtained using Korean classic guidelines [20], and self-reported respiratory symptoms (answers to the following questions: do you have [symptom, e.g., cough for 3 months]?). We enrolled subjects based on age, smoking history (in pack-years, PY), and lung function in the KNHANES data. Other baseline characteristics were also obtained from the KNHANES data.

Subjects enrolled in the KNHANES database have KNHANES-matched HIRA data. HIRA data were obtained from claims from the national health insurance system, which uniquely covers virtually all residents in Korea. It contains the diagnostic code, medical utilization (including

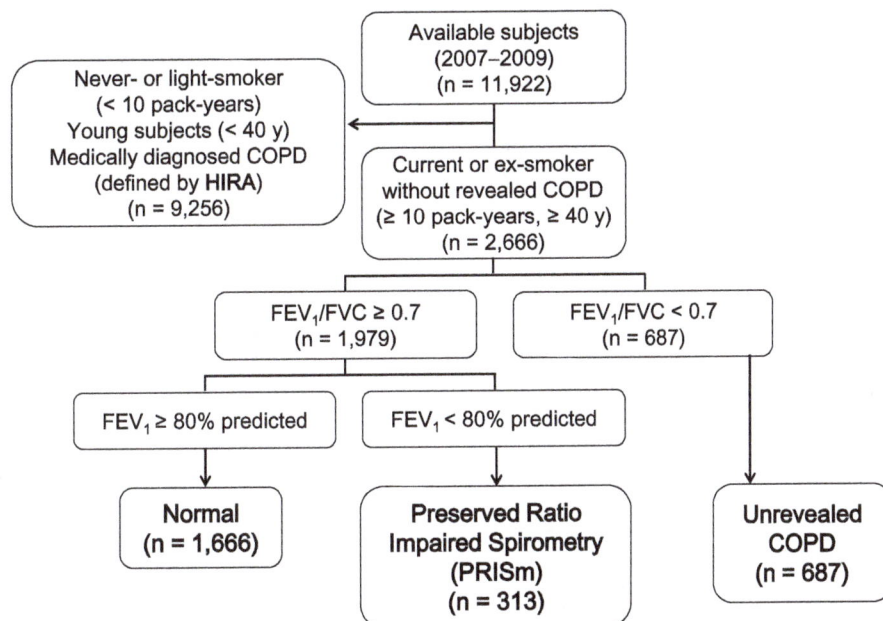

Fig. 1 Subject selection and group assignment based on the KNHANES and HIRA data. KNHANES, Korea National Health and Nutrition Examination Survey; HIRA, Health Insurance Review & Assessment; COPD, chronic obstructive pulmonary disease; FEV₁, forced expiratory volume for 1 s; FVC, forced vital capacity

hospital admission history and prescribed medication), and costs for several years [21].

Parameter definition

Contrary to the established spirometry-based diagnostic criterion for COPD ($FEV_1/FVC < 0.7$), "medically diagnosed COPD" was defined by diagnostic code and prescribed medication [22, 23]. Medically diagnosed COPD patients met all of the following criteria: 1) age ≥ 40 years; 2) ICD-10 codes for COPD or emphysema (J43.0×-J44.x, with the exception of J43.0 as primary or secondary [within fourth position] diagnosis); and 3) the use of more than 1 of the following COPD medications at least twice per year: long-acting muscarinic antagonist, long-acting beta-2 agonist (LABA), fixed-dose inhaled corticosteroid with LABA, short-acting muscarinic antagonist (SAMA), short-acting beta-2 agonist (SABA), SAMA with SABA, phosphodiesterase-4 (PDE-4) inhibitor, systemic beta agonist, or methylxanthine.

Hospitalization cost was defined as any medical utilization costs for inpatient services, confined to admissions with an ICD-10 code for COPD (J43.x–J44.x, except J430) or COPD-related diseases (pneumonia: J12.x–J17.x; pulmonary thromboembolism: I26, I26.0, and I26.9; dyspnea: R06.0; or acute respiratory distress syndrome: J80). Costs were presented in US dollar (USD), using an exchange rate of 1 USD = 1090 Korean Won (exchange rate as on February 9, 2018).

Chronic bronchitis was defined as self-reported chronic cough or sputum persisting for at least 3 months, in at least 2 consecutive years.

Outcomes

We analyzed the 3-year follow-up outcomes from HIRA data (Fig. 2). The incidence of medically diagnosed COPD was the primary outcome. Hospital visits, number and type of prescribed medication, and hospitalization cost were secondary outcomes. Furthermore, we sought to identify significant factors that predicted a COPD diagnosis by group.

Ethics

This study was approved by the Institutional Review Board of Gangnam Severance Hospital (number: 3–2017-0395). The requirement for obtaining informed consent from the patients was waived due to the retrospective nature of this study.

Statistical analyses

We compared the baseline characteristics, COPD incidence, hospital visits, medication use, and hospitalization cost between groups using χ^2 tests (categorized variables) and analysis of variance with Bonferroni post-hoc test (continuous variables). Univariate and multivariate logistic regression analyses were conducted to identify factors that predicted COPD diagnosis. In multivariate analysis, only factors found significant in univariate analysis were included as co-variables. FEV_1/FVC was not used in multivariate analysis, because of increased multicollinearity (variance inflation factor = 23.81). $P < 0.05$ was considered to indicate statistical significance.

Results

Demographics of subjects by group

Unrevealed COPD subjects (64.48 ± 9.54 years) were significantly older than subjects in the normal (54.57 ± 10.52 years; $P < 0.001$) and PRISm (55.97 ± 10.85 years; $P < 0.001$) groups. Most subjects were men, and the sex distribution was similar among groups. Height and weight were less in the unrevealed COPD than in the normal and PRISm subjects. Smoking PY was heavier in the unrevealed COPD group than in the normal and PRISm groups. However, PRISm subjects were more often current-smokers (61.7%) than were normal (51.5%; $P = 0.003$) and unrevealed COPD (53.4%; $P = 0.045$) subjects. Hyperlipidemia was less common in the unrevealed COPD (6.8%) than in the normal group (10.0%; $P = 0.048$). Acute coronary

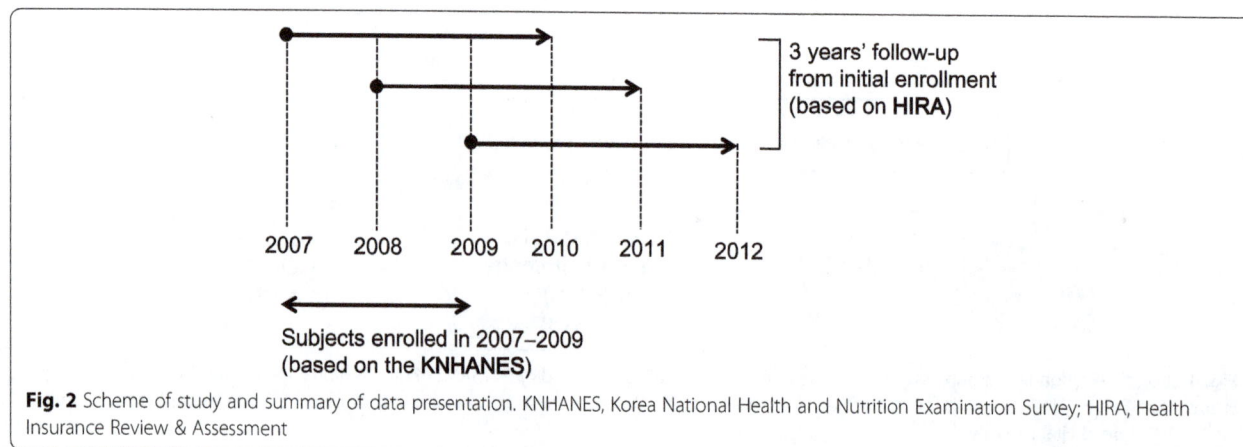

Fig. 2 Scheme of study and summary of data presentation. KNHANES, Korea National Health and Nutrition Examination Survey; HIRA, Health Insurance Review & Assessment

syndrome was more common in the unrevealed COPD (2.3%) than in the normal (1.0%; $P = 0.042$) group. Diabetes mellitus was significantly more prevalent in PRISm (20.1%) than in normal (10.4%; $P < 0.001$) and unrevealed COPD (12.2%; $P = 0.003$) subjects. Pulmonary tuberculosis and asthma was particularly prevalent in the unrevealed COPD group (Table 1).

FVC was significantly lower in the PRISm (72.55 ± 9.45%) than in the normal (92.96 ± 10.02%; $P < 0.001$) and unrevealed COPD (88.51 ± 15.02%; $P < 0.001$) groups. FEV_1 followed a similar pattern. However, the FEV_1/FVC ratio was significantly lower in the unrevealed COPD (0.61 ± 0.09) than in the normal (0.79 ± 0.05, $P < 0.001$) and PRISm (0.77 ± 0.06, $P = 0.035$) groups. Wheezing was more prevalent in PRISm (11.8%) patients than in normal subjects (7.0%; $P = 0.009$), but less prevalent than in the unrevealed COPD group

(22.4%, $P < 0.001$). Other respiratory symptoms followed a similar pattern (Table 1).

COPD incidence, medication and hospital utilization, and cost

The COPD incidence in PRISm subjects (17.0/1000 person year [PY]) was significantly higher than that in normal subjects (4.4/1000 PY; $P < 0.001$); however, that in unrevealed COPD individuals (45.1/1000 PY) was significantly higher than that in PRISm individuals ($P < 0.001$). The PRISm group (13.1%) significantly more often visited the hospital than the normal group (7.3%; $P = 0.002$), but less often than the unrevealed COPD group (24.6%; $P < 0.001$). The type and number of prescribed medications followed a similar pattern. Hospitalization cost in the PRISm group (398.61 ± 1975.51 USD) was almost double that in the normal group (186.17 ± 1411.24 USD; $P = 0.297$); however,

Table 1 Demographics of subjects according to the group

	Normal	PRISm	Unrevealed COPD	P-value	P-value*	P-value+	P-value‡
Age	54.57 ± 10.52	55.97 ± 10.85	64.48 ± 9.54	< 0.001	0.083	< 0.001	< 0.001
Male, n (%)	1560 (93.6)	286 (91.4)	654 (95.2)	0.063	0.426	0.432	0.054
Height (cm)	167.14 ± 6.94	166.79 ± 6.94	165.97 ± 6.56	< 0.001	0.998	<.0.001	0.236
Weight (kg)	68.29 ± 9.91	68.66 ± 11.6	63.7 ± 9.8	< 0.001	0.998	< 0.001	< 0.001
Smoking history							
Current smoking, n (%)	858 (51.5)	193 (61.7)	367 (53.4)	0.004	0.003	0.999	0.045
Pack-years	28.62 ± 17.11	33.20 ± 20.34	36.58 ± 21.14	< 0.001	< 0.001	< 0.001	0.026
Co-morbidity, n (%)							
Hypertension	453 (27.2)	91 (29.1)	209 (30.4)	0.269	0.998	0.336	0.999
Hyperlipidemia	166 (10.0)	34 (10.9)	47 (6.8)	0.035	0.998	0.048	0.092
Stroke	48 (2.9)	14 (4.5)	18 (2.6)	0.252	0.414	0.999	0.368
Acute coronary syndrome	17 (1.0)	8 (2.6)	16 (2.3)	0.019	0.077	0.042	0.999
Diabetes mellitus	174 (10.4)	63 (20.1)	84 (12.2)	< 0.001	< 0.001	0.624	0.003
Pulmonary tuberculosis	124 (7.4)	21 (6.7)	109 (15.9)	< 0.001	0.999	< 0.001	< 0.001
Asthma	20 (1.2)	15 (4.8)	65 (9.5)	< 0.001	< 0.001	< 0.001	0.024
Lung function test							
FVC % predicted	92.96 ± 10.02	72.55 ± 9.45	88.51 ± 15.02	< 0.001	< 0.001	< 0.001	< 0.001
FEV_1% predicted	94.66 ± 9.14	72.8 ± 6.72	74.18 ± 16.57	< 0.001	< 0.001	< 0.001	0.035
FEV_1/FVC	0.79 ± 0.05	0.77 ± 0.06	0.61 ± 0.09	< 0.001	< 0.001	< 0.001	0.006
Respiratory symptoms, n (%)							
Cough for more than 3 months	1 (0.1)	2 (0.6)	19 (2.8)	< 0.001	0.047	< 0.001	0.091
Sputum for more than 3 months	4 (0.2)	2 (0.6)	18 (2.6)	< 0.001	0.999	< 0.001	0.104
Dyspnea	10 (0.6)	3 (1.0)	31 (4.5)	< 0.001	0.999	< 0.001	0.012
Wheezing	116 (7.0)	37 (11.8)	154 (22.4)	< 0.001	0.009	< 0.001	< 0.001
Chronic bronchitis	4 (0.2)	2 (0.6)	21 (3.1)	< 0.001	0.717	< 0.001	0.054
Total	1666	313	687				

Data are presented as mean ± standard deviation or number (percentage)
* P-value for comparison between normal and PRISm group; + P-value for comparison between normal and unrevealed COPD group; ‡ P-value for comparison between PRISm and unrevealed COPD group
PRISm preserved ratio impaired spirometry, COPD chronic obstructive pulmonary disease, FEV_1 forced expiratory volume for 1 s, FVC forced vital capacity

that in the unrevealed COPD group (750.71 ± 3216.02 USD; $P = 0.041$) was larger than that in the PRISm group (Table 2).

Comparison of baseline characteristics, medical utilization, and costs between subjects with and without medically diagnosed COPD

Among the 2666 subjects, 131 patients (4.9%) were medically diagnosed with COPD during the 3 years' follow-up. Subjects with medically diagnosed COPD were older and shorter, weighed less, had a heavier smoking history, and more often had a history of pulmonary tuberculosis and asthma than the remaining patients. Although data are not shown, other co-morbidity was not significantly different between groups. Subjects with medically diagnosed COPD had more markedly impaired lung function and severe symptoms than subjects without medically diagnosed COPD. They also more frequently visited hospitals, more frequently used COPD medication, and had greater hospitalization cost than subjects without medically diagnosed COPD (Table 3).

Significant factors for COPD diagnosis in subjects overall

Multivariate analysis of all subjects showed that the possibility of COPD diagnosis was increased to 10.0% with every year's increase in age (odds ratio [OR], 1.10; 95% confidence interval [CI], 1.07–1.13; $P < 0.001$). A 1% increase in FVC and FEV_1 was significantly associated with a 3% increase

and 5% decrease in COPD diagnosis, respectively (FVC [OR, 1.03; 95% CI, 1.01–1.05; $P = 0.006$] and predicted FEV_1 [OR, 0.95; 95% CI, 0.93–0.96; $P < 0.001$]). Dyspnea (OR, 3.73; 95% CI, 1.23–7.68; $P = 0.017$), and wheezing (OR, 2.90; 95%CI, 1.76–4.78; $P < 0.001$) were significant predictive factors of a COPD diagnosis (Table 4).

Comparison of baseline characteristics, medical utilization, and costs between PRISm patients with and without medically diagnosed COPD

Among the 316 subjects with PRISm, 16 patients were medically diagnosed with COPD during the 3-year follow-up period. Subjects with medically diagnosed COPD were older, shorter, weighed less, more often had asthma and decreased FVC, and more frequently had dyspnea and wheezing. Due to frequent hospital and medical utilization, their hospitalization cost was greater than that of subjects without medically diagnosed COPD (Table 5).

Significant factors for COPD diagnosis in PRISm

In multivariate analysis of subjects with PRISm, the possibility of COPD diagnosis was increased to 14.0% for every year that subjects aged (OR, 1.14; 95% CI, 1.05–1.24; $P = 0.002$). Wheezing (OR, 4.56; 95% CI, 1.08–19.35; $P = 0.040$) was a significant factor for a diagnosis of COPD in PRISm patients (Table 6).

Table 2 COPD incidence, medication and hospital utilization, and cost

	Normal	PRISm	Unrevealed COPD	P-value	P-value*	P-value+	P-value‡
COPD incidence (/1000PY)	4.4	17.0	45.1	< 0.001	< 0.001	< 0.001	< 0.001
OPD visit, n (%)	51 (3.1)	22 (7.0)	131 (19.1)	< 0.001	0.002	< 0.001	< 0.001
No. of OPD visit	0.10 ± 0.91	0.48 ± 2.96	1.86 ± 6.37	< 0.001	0.243	< 0.001	< 0.001
Hospitalization, n (%)	79 (4.7)	29 (9.3)	83 (12.1)	< 0.001	0.004	< 0.001	0.571
ER visit, n (%)	23 (1.4)	12 (3.8)	36 (5.2)	< 0.001	0.008	< 0.001	0.999
ICU admission, n (%)	12 (0.7)	6 (1.9)	19 (2.8)	< 0.001	0.122	< 0.001	0.999
Total hospital visit, n (%)	121 (7.3)	41 (13.1)	169 (24.6)	< 0.001	0.002	< 0.001	< 0.001
ICS, n (%)	4 (0.2)	5 (1.6)	20 (2.9)	< 0.001	0.003	< 0.001	0.651
ICS + LABA, n (%)	2 (0.1)	11 (3.5)	50 (7.3)	< 0.001	< 0.001	< 0.001	0.063
LAMA, n (%)	–	4 (1.3)	44 (6.4)	–	–	–	< 0.001
SAMA, n (%)	12 (0.7)	12 (3.8)	36 (5.2)	< 0.001	< 0.001	< 0.001	0.999
SABA, n (%)	14 (0.8)	11 (3.5)	54 (7.9)	< 0.001	< 0.001	< 0.001	0.029
Systemic bronchodilator, n (%)	28 (1.7)	11 (3.5)	72 (10.5)	< 0.001	0.094	< 0.001	< 0.001
Methylxanthine, n (%)	33 (2.0)	17 (5.4)	101 (14.7)	< 0.001	0.001	< 0.001	< 0.001
Total prescribed medication, n (%)	57 (3.4)	26 (8.3)	127 (18.5)	< 0.001	< 0.001	< 0.001	< 0.001
Hospitalization medical Cost (for 3 years) (USD)	186.17 ± 1411.24	398.61 ± 1975.51	750.71 ± 3216.02	< 0.001	0.297	< 0.001	0.041

Data are presented as mean ± standard deviation or number (percentage)
* P-value for comparison between the normal and PRISm group; + P-value for comparison between normal and unrevealed COPD group; ‡ P-value for comparison between PRISm and unrevealed COPD group
PRISm preserved ratio impaired spirometry, COPD chronic obstructive pulmonary disease, PY person-year, OPD outpatient department, ER emergency room, ICU intensive care unit, ICS inhaled corticosteroid, LABA long-acting beta-2 agonist, LAMA long-acting muscarine antagonist, SAMA short-acting muscarine antagonist, SABA short-acting beta-2 agonist

Table 3 Comparison of baseline characteristics, medical utilization, and costs between subjects with and without medically diagnosed COPD

	Subjects with medically diagnosed COPD	Subjects without medically diagnosed COPD	P-value
Age	68.58 ± 7.77	56.70 ± 11.00	< 0.001
Male, n (%)	123 (93.9)	2377 (93.8)	0.954
Height (cm)	164.04 ± 6.25	166.94 ± 6.86	< 0.001
Weight (kg)	60.35 ± 9.89	67.5 ± 10.2	< 0.001
Smoking history			
Current smoking, n (%)	67 (51.2)	1351 (53.3)	0.631
Pack-years	41.1 ± 23.69	30.7 ± 18.52	< 0.001
Co-morbidity, n (%)			
Pulmonary tuberculosis	28 (21.4)	226 (8.9)	< 0.001
Asthma	3 (26.0)	66 (2.6)	< 0.001
Lung function test			
FVC % predicted	81.14 ± 15.77	89.85 ± 12.85	< 0.001
FEV_1% predicted	66.37 ± 19.36	87.87 ± 14.17	< 0.001
FEV_1/FVC	0.59 ± 0.16	0.75 ± 0.09	< 0.001
Respiratory symptoms, n (%)			
Cough for more than 3 months	14 (10.7)	8 (0.3)	< 0.001
Sputum for more than 3 months	11 (8.4)	13 (0.5)	< 0.001
Dyspnea	23 (17.6)	21 (0.8)	< 0.001
Wheezing	60 (45.8)	247 (9.7)	< 0.001
Chronic bronchitis	14 (10.7)	13 (0.5)	< 0.001
OPD visit, n (%)	116 (88.6)	88 (3.5)	< 0.001
No. of OPD visit	10.88 ± 11.77	0.07 ± 0.59	< 0.001
Hospitalization, n (%)	67 (51.2)	124 (4.9)	< 0.001
ER visit, n (%)	35 (26.7)	36 (1.4)	< 0.001
ICU admission, n (%)	17 (13.0)	20 (0.8)	< 0.001
Total hospital visit, n (%)	131 (100)	200 (7.9)	
ICS, n (%)	25 (19.1)	4 (0.2)	< 0.001
ICS + LABA, n (%)	54 (41.2)	9 (0.4)	< 0.001
LAMA, n (%)	42 (32.1)	6 (0.2)	< 0.001
SAMA, n (%)	44 (33.6)	16 (0.6)	< 0.001
SABA, n (%)	60 (45.8)	19 (0.8)	< 0.001
Systemic bronchodilator, n (%)	75 (57.3)	36 (1.4)	< 0.001
Methylxanthine, n (%)	110 (84.0)	41 (1.6)	< 0.001
Total prescribed medication, n (%)	131 (100.0)	79 (3.1)	–
Hospitalization medical Cost (for 3 years) (USD)	4041.23 ± 6633.39	166.17 ± 1286.46	< 0.001
Total	131	2535	

Data are presented as mean ± standard deviation or number (percentage)
COPD chronic obstructive pulmonary disease, FEV₁ forced expiratory volume for 1 s, FVC forced vital capacity, OPD outpatient department, ER emergency room, ICU intensive care unit, ICS inhaled corticosteroid, LABA long-acting beta-2 agonist, LAMA long-acting muscarine antagonist, SAMA short-acting muscarine antagonist, SABA short-acting beta-2 agonist

Discussion

We investigated the incidence of COPD in PRISm patients and sought to identify significant risk factors of COPD in PRISm patients. We found that PRISm patients were 4 times more likely to receive a COPD diagnosis than a normal group. Sood et al. have also reported a high COPD incidence in PRISm patients (about double that in the normal population) [24]. We also showed that PRISm patients paid more hospital visits, used more prescribed COPD medications, and accounted for an increased

Table 4 Significant factors for COPD diagnosis in all subjects

	Univariate analysis			Multivariate analysis		
	OR	95% CI	P-value	OR	95% CI	P-value
Age (years)	**1.11**	**(1.09,1.13)**	**< 0.001**	**1.10**	**(1.07,1.13)**	**< 0.001**
Male	1.02	(0.49,2.13)	0.954			
Height (cm)	0.95	(0.92,0.97)	< 0.001	1.01	(0.97,1.05)	0.786
Weight (kg)	0.93	(0.91,0.95)	< 0.001	0.98	(0.95,1.01)	0.143
Smoking history						
Current smoking	0.92	(0.65,1.3)	0.631			
Pack-years	1.02	(1.01,1.03)	< 0.001	1.01	(1.00,1.02)	0.059
Co-morbidity						
Pulmonary tuberculosis	2.78	(1.79,4.31)	< 0.001	1.17	(0.66,2.10)	0.587
Asthma	13.11	(8.27,20.79)	< 0.001	1.88	(0.97,3.64)	0.060
Lung function test						
FVC % predicted	**0.95**	**(0.94,0.97)**	**< 0.001**	**1.03**	**(1.01,1.05)**	**0.006**
FEV_1% predicted	**0.93**	**(0.92,0.94)**	**< 0.001**	**0.95**	**(0.93,0.96)**	**< 0.001**
FEV_1/FVC	0.001	(0.001,0.001)	< 0.001			
Self-reported respiratory symptoms						
Cough for more than 3 months	37.80	(15.55,91.87)	< 0.001	2.40	(0.24,24.32)	0.458
Sputum for more than 3 months	17.78	(7.81,40.52)	< 0.001	0.48	(0.02,10.90)	0.647
Dyspnea	**25.49**	**(13.68,47.49)**	**< 0.001**	**3.07**	**(1.23,7.68)**	**0.017**
Wheezing	**7.83**	**(5.42,11.31)**	**< 0.001**	**2.90**	**(1.76,4.78)**	**< 0.001**
Chronic bronchitis	23.21	(10.67,50.5)	< 0.001	2.76	(0.07,109.05)	0.588

Statistically significant data are presented as bold
COPD chronic obstructive pulmonary disease, FEV_1 forced expiratory volume for 1 s, FVC forced vital capacity, OR odds ratio, CI confidence interval

economic burden. Despite not meeting COPD criteria, these patients require careful observation because of their risk for COPD development and concomitant medical utilization. PRISm occurs in about 6.6–17.6% of the general global population [15, 25, 26]; nevertheless, PRISm remains poorly understood. Many clinicians miss this "unclassified" or "non-specific" group, and discharge them without explanation, warning, or follow-up appointment. Detecting and treating these early-stage patients is requisite.

Some subjects with PRISm might have underlying restrictive lung disease. Significantly lower FVC (72.55 ± 9.45%) in PRISm patients than in normal (92.96 ± 10.02; $P < 0.001$) and unrevealed COPD (88.51 ± 15.02; $P < 0.001$) subjects supports this supposition. However, Wan et al. reported that a true restrictive pattern, defined by total lung capacity, was not frequently observed in PRISm [10]. This should be elucidated in further studies.

Subjects in the PRISm group had a heavier smoking history, more severe respiratory symptoms and decreased lung function, and more frequent co-morbidity than the normal population; these differences were less marked when compared to the unrevealed COPD group. However, we found that the prevalence of current smoking in the PRISm group was higher than that in both the

normal and unrevealed COPD groups. It may be that many current-smokers in the PRISm group did not experience respiratory symptoms, did not visit hospitals, and were not warned to stop smoking. Current-smokers in the PRISm group may develop COPD unless they stop smoking, as previously shown [24]. Doctors should check the smoking status in PRISm patients more carefully, and should strongly recommend that they stop smoking.

Although age, lung function, dyspnea, and wheezing are significant predictive factors of COPD in the subjects overall, only age and wheezing were significant predictive factors for a COPD diagnosis in PRISm patients. Both age [27] and wheezing [28] are well-known predictive factors for COPD.

Lung function was not a significant predictive factor of COPD in PRISm. Low FEV_1 was a significant predictive factor of COPD overall, but not in PRISm patients specifically. The preserved ratio which is shown in PRISm means that these patients rarely have an extremely reduced FEV_1. In fact, Table 1 shows a relatively small standard deviation of FEV_1 in PRISm patients, as compared to other groups, although the number of subjects was small. It implies FEV_1 in PRISm has small predictive power for prognosis. Thus, it is necessary to monitor

Table 5 Comparison of baseline characteristics, medical utilization, and costs between PRISm with and without medically diagnosed COPD

	PRISm with medically diagnosed COPD	PRISm without medically diagnosed COPD	P-value
Age	70.06 ± 7.48	55.21 ± 10.49	< 0.001
Male, n (%)	16 (100.0)	270 (90.9)	–
Height (cm)	162.95 ± 6.9	167.0 ± 6.89	0.023
Weight (kg)	61.58 ± 13.13	69.04 ± 11.41	0.012
Smoking history			
Current smoking, n (%)	8 (50.0)	185 (62.3)	0.325
Pack-years	36.63 ± 14.16	33.02 ± 20.62	0.490
Co-morbidity, n (%)			
Pulmonary tuberculosis	1 (6.3)	20 (6.7)	0.940
Asthma	4 (25.0)	11 (3.7)	< 0.001
Lung function test			
FVC % predicted	64.83 ± 10.86	72.96 ± 9.2	< 0.001
FEV_1% predicted	69.77 ± 9.16	72.97 ± 6.55	0.188
FEV_1/FVC	0.76 ± 0.06	0.77 ± 0.06	0.182
Respiratory symptoms, n (%)			
Cough for more than 3 months	0	2 (0.7)	–
Sputum for more than 3 months	0	2 (0.7)	–
Dyspnea	2 (12.5)	1 (0.3)	< 0.001
Wheezing	6 (37.5)	31 (10.4)	0.001
Chronic bronchitis	0	2 (0.7)	–
OPD visit, n (%)	15 (93.8)	7 (2.4)	< 0.001
No. of OPD visit	8.81 ± 10.15	0.03 ± 0.18	< 0.001
Hospitalization, n (%)	9 (56.3)	20 (6.7)	< 0.001
ER visit, n (%)	5 (31.3)	7 (2.4)	< 0.001
ICU admission, n (%)	2 (12.5)	4 (1.4)	0.002
Total hospital visit, n (%)	16 (100.0)	25 (8.4)	–
ICS, n (%)	4 (25.0)	1 (0.3)	< 0.001
ICS + LABA, n (%)	8 (50.0)	3 (1.0)	< 0.001
LAMA, n (%)	4 (25.0)	–	–
SAMA, n (%)	8 (50.0)	4 (1.4)	< 0.001
SABA, n (%)	8 (50.0)	3 (1.0)	< 0.001
Systemic bronchodilator, n (%)	9 (56.3)	2 (0.7)	< 0.001
Methylxanthine, n (%)	11 (68.8)	6 (2.0)	< 0.001
Total prescribed medication, n (%)	16 (100.0)	10 (3.4)	–
Hospitalization medical Cost (for 3 years) (USD)	3647.51 ± 4773.55	223.58 ± 1535.45	0.012
Total	16	297	

Data are presented as mean ± standard deviation or number (percentage)
PRISm preserved ratio impaired spirometry, *COPD* chronic obstructive pulmonary disease, FEV_1 forced expiratory volume for 1 s, *FVC* forced vital capacity, *OPD* outpatient department, *ER* emergency room, *ICU* intensive care unit, *ICS* inhaled corticosteroid, *LABA* long-acting beta-2 agonist, *LAMA* long-acting muscarine antagonist, *SAMA* short-acting muscarine antagonist, *SABA* short-acting beta-2 agonist

PRISm subjects carefully, even in the absence of severe reduced FEV_1.

Additionally, relatively preserved FVC was a significant predictive factor for COPD in the overall cohort using multivariate analysis, but not in PRISm patients. The reasons why preserved FVC is significant risk factor for COPD are as follows. Before adjustment, FVC in subjects with medically diagnosed COPD (81.14 ± 15.77%) was significantly lower than that in subjects without COPD (89.85 ± 12.85%; $P < 0.001$). We can easily assume

Table 6 Significant factors for COPD diagnosis in PRISm

	Univariate analysis			Multivariate analysis		
	OR	95% CI	P-value	OR	95% CI	P-value
Age (years)	**1.14**	**(1.08, 1.21)**	**< 0.001**	**1.14**	**(1.05, 1.24)**	**0.002**
Male						
Height (cm)	0.93	(0.87, 0.99)	0.025	1.03	(0.92, 1.16)	0.564
Weight (kg)	0.94	(0.9, 0.99)	0.013	0.95	(0.89, 1.02)	0.153
Smoking history						
Current smoking	0.61	(0.22, 1.66)	0.329			
Pack-years	1.01	(0.99, 1.03)	0.490			
Co-morbidity						
Pulmonary tuberculosis	0.92	(0.12, 7.35)	0.940			
Asthma	8.67	(2.41, 31.23)	0.001	5.87	(0.94, 36.56)	0.058
Lung function test						
FVC % predicted	0.93	(0.89, 0.97)	0.001	1.01	(0.95, 1.09)	0.694
FEV_1% predicted	0.95	(0.9, 1.01)	0.071			
FEV_1/FVC	0.001	(0.001, 35.7)	0.183			
Self-reported respiratory symptoms						
Cough for more than 3 months						
Sputum for more than 3 months						
Dyspnea	42.29	(3.61, 494.74)	0.003	8.88	(0.65, 121.7)	0.102
Wheezing	**5.15**	**(1.75, 15.14)**	**0.003**	**4.56**	**(1.08, 19.35)**	**0.040**
Chronic bronchitis						

Statistically significant data are presented as bold

COPD chronic obstructive pulmonary disease, PRISm preserved ratio impaired spirometry, FEV_1 forced expiratory volume for 1 s, FVC forced vital capacity, OR odds ratio, CI confidence interval

that preserved FVC will be protective factor for COPD, however results were contrary to that in multivariate analysis with adjustment. This indicates that other associated co-variables affected the findings of FVC in multivariate analysis. We speculated FEV_1 might be contributing factor for this confusing result. The decline in FEV_1 was much larger than that in FVC in Table 3, and FVC is unavoidably influenced by changes in FEV_1. Therefore, we speculated that FEV_1, as a co-variable, might have affected the FVC findings in multivariate analysis with adjustment.

Unrevealed COPD implies a significantly impaired FEV_1/FVC ratio, meeting the standard COPD spirometry criteria for airway obstruction, but without a clinical diagnosis of COPD, no hospital visits, and no use of COPD medication to date. The number of subjects with unrevealed COPD was double that of the PRISm group in this study. Coultas et al. showed a similar proportion of undiagnosed COPD (79.7%) in the USA [3]. Chung et al. have shown that, in Korea, 97% of COPD cases are undiagnosed [2], or misdiagnosed [29]; their diagnosis and treatment should be addressed, because unrevealed COPD also leads to more hospital visits, increased medication use, and an increased economic burden [30].

Woodruff et al. showed that smokers with normal lung function commonly experience respiratory symptoms and exacerbations. They suggested a new entity that includes smoking-related chronic pulmonary disease [6]. Other recent studies also suggest that the pre-COPD stage is clinically and medically important [31, 32]. We assume that PRISm may also be a pre-COPD-stage chronic pulmonary disease. PRISm patients should be advised to have regular check-ups to monitor COPD development, and more so if they have advance aged or wheezing, irrespective of the severity of lung function decrease (FEV_1).

This study had some limitations. First, "medically diagnosed COPD" may be considered artificial. "COPD incidence" is not an accurate term, but in this study reflects the incidence of medically diagnosed COPD as defined by the HIRA data, which includes insurance claims but not pulmonary function test data. However, the previously reported COPD incidence (2.6–9.2/1000 PY) [27, 33–35] is not markedly different from that in this study (4.4/1000 PY in normal; 17.0/1000 PY in PRISm). "Medically diagnosed COPD" with hospital visits and medication use is more relevant than COPD diagnosed based only on impaired lung function ($FEV_1/FVC < 0.7$), without medical utilization. Therefore, this artificial definition may be appropriate for use in this study. Second, this cohort study did not include follow-up pulmonary function tests, because the KNHANES conducted pulmonary function tests in different populations each year.

Conclusions

PRISm is likely to develop into COPD over time, and it leads to frequent hospital visits, increased medication use, and greater hospitalization costs. Subjects with PRISm should be carefully monitored for COPD development, especially when they are older or have wheezing, regardless of lung function.

Abbreviations

CI: confidence interval; COPD: chronic obstructive pulmonary disease; FEV$_1$: forced expiratory volume for 1 s; FVC: forced vital capacity; OR: odds ratio; PRISm: preserved ratio impaired spirometry; PY: pearson-year

Authors' contributions

HJP contributed to the conception and design of this study; analyzed, and interpreted the data; drafted and revised the article, and approved the final version of the article for publication. CKR, HJK, and KHY collected, generated, and analyzed the data; contributed to the draft, revised the article, and approved the final version of the article for publication. KK, as a professional statistician, takes scientific responsibility for the analysis and interpretation of the data. MKB provided constructive criticism on the concept and design of this study, as corresponding author; interpreted the data, and drafted and revised the article, and approved the final version of the article for publication.

Competing interests

All authors declare that they have no competing interests.

Author details

[1]Department of Internal Medicine, Gangnam Severance Hospital, Yonsei University College of Medicine, 211 Eonju-ro Gangnam-gu, Seoul 06273, Korea. [2]Division of Pulmonary, Allergy and Critical Care Medicine, Department of Internal Medicine, Seoul St Mary's Hospital, College of Medicine, The Catholic University of Korea, Seoul, Korea. [3]Department of Internal Medicine, Konkuk University School of Medicine, Seoul, Korea.

References

1. Rhee CK, Kim K, Yoon HK, Kim JA, Kim SH, Lee SH, Park YB, Jung KS, Yoo KH, Hwang YI. Natural course of early COPD. Int J Chron Obstruct Pulmon Dis. 2017;12:663–8.
2. Chung K, Kim K, Jung J, Oh K, Oh Y, Kim S, Kim J, Kim Y. Patterns and determinants of COPD-related healthcare utilization by severity of airway obstruction in Korea. BMC Pulm Med. 2014;14:27.
3. Coultas DB, Mapel D, Gagnon R, Lydick E. The health impact of undiagnosed airflow obstruction in a national sample of United States adults. Am J Respir Crit Care Med. 2001;164:372–7.
4. Cooke CE, Sidel M, Belletti DA, Fuhlbrigge AL. Review: clinical inertia in the management of chronic obstructive pulmonary disease. COPD. 2012;9:73–80.
5. Glaab T, Banik N, Rutschmann OT, Wencker M. National survey of guideline-compliant COPD management among pneumologists and primary care physicians. COPD. 2006;3:141–8.
6. Woodruff PG, Barr RG, Bleecker E, Christenson SA, Couper D, Curtis JL, Gouskova NA, Hansel NN, Hoffman EA, Kanner RE, et al. Clinical significance of symptoms in smokers with preserved pulmonary function. N Engl J Med. 2016;374:1811–21.
7. Vaz Fragoso CA, Gill TM, McAvay G, Yaggi HK, Van Ness PH, Concato J. Respiratory impairment and mortality in older persons: a novel spirometric approach. J Investig Med. 2011;59:1089–95.
8. Vogelmeier CF, Criner GJ, Martinez FJ, Anzueto A, Barnes PJ, Bourbeau J, Celli BR, Chen R, Decramer M, Fabbri LM, et al. Global strategy for the diagnosis, management, and prevention of chronic obstructive lung disease 2017 report: GOLD executive summary. Arch Bronconeumol. 2017;53:128–49.
9. Guerra S, Sherrill DL, Venker C, Ceccato CM, Halonen M, Martinez FD. Morbidity and mortality associated with the restrictive spirometric pattern: a longitudinal study. Thorax. 2010;65:499–504.
10. Wan ES, Hokanson JE, Murphy JR, Regan EA, Make BJ, Lynch DA, Crapo JD, Silverman EK, Investigators CO. Clinical and radiographic predictors of GOLD-unclassified smokers in the COPDGene study. Am J Respir Crit Care Med. 2011;184:57–63.
11. Mannino DM, Ford ES, Redd SC. Obstructive and restrictive lung disease and functional limitation: data from the third National Health and nutrition examination. J Intern Med. 2003;254:540–7.
12. Wan ES, Cho MH, Boutaoui N, Klanderman BJ, Sylvia JS, Ziniti JP, Won S, Lange C, Pillai SG, Anderson WH, et al. Genome-wide association analysis of body mass in chronic obstructive pulmonary disease. Am J Respir Cell Mol Biol. 2011;45:304–10.
13. Soriano JB, Miravitlles M, Garcia-Rio F, Munoz L, Sanchez G, Sobradillo V, Duran E, Guerrero D, Ancochea J. Spirometrically-defined restrictive ventilatory defect: population variability and individual determinants. Prim Care Respir J. 2012;21:187–93.
14. Mannino DM, Holguin F, Pavlin BI, Ferdinands JM. Risk factors for prevalence of and mortality related to restriction on spirometry: findings from the first National Health and nutrition examination survey and follow-up. Int J Tuberc Lung Dis. 2005;9:613–21.
15. Wan ES, Castaldi PJ, Cho MH, Hokanson JE, Regan EA, Make BJ, Beaty TH, Han MK, Curtis JL, Curran-Everett D, et al. Epidemiology, genetics, and subtyping of preserved ratio impaired spirometry (PRISm) in COPDGene. Respir Res. 2014;15:89.
16. Diaz AA, Strand M, Coxson HO, Ross JC, San Jose Estepar R, Lynch D, van Rikxoort EM, Rosas IO, Hunninghake GM, Putman RK, et al. Disease severity dependence of the longitudinal association between CT lung density and lung function in smokers. Chest. 2018;153:638–45.
17. Salvi SS, Barnes PJ. Chronic obstructive pulmonary disease in non-smokers. Lancet. 2009;374:733–43.
18. Zeng G, Sun B, Zhong N. Non-smoking-related chronic obstructive pulmonary disease: a neglected entity? Respirology. 2012;17:908–12.
19. Yoon HK, Park YB, Rhee CK, Lee JH, Oh YM, Committee of the Korean CG. Summary of the chronic obstructive pulmonary disease clinical practice guideline revised in 2014 by the Korean academy of tuberculosis and respiratory disease. Tuberc Respir Dis (Seoul). 2017;80:230–40.
20. Sim YS, Lee JH, Lee WY, Suh DI, Oh YM, Yoon JS, Lee JH, Cho JH, Kwon CS, Chang JH. Spirometry and bronchodilator test. Tuberc Respir Dis (Seoul). 2017;80:105–12.
21. Kim S, Kim J, Kim K, Kim Y, Park Y, Baek S, Park SY, Yoon SY, Kwon HS, Cho YS, et al. Healthcare use and prescription patterns associated with adult asthma in Korea: analysis of the NHI claims database. Allergy. 2013;68:1435–42.
22. Lee J, Lee JH, Kim JA, Rhee CK. Trend of cost and utilization of COPD medication in Korea. Int J Chron Obstruct Pulmon Dis. 2017;12:27–33.
23. Chung SM, Lee SY. Evaluation of appropriate Management of Chronic Obstructive Pulmonary Disease in Korea: based on Health Insurance Review and Assessment Service (HIRA) claims. Tuberc Respir Dis (Seoul). 2017;80:241–6.
24. Sood A, Petersen H, Qualls C, Meek PM, Vazquez-Guillamet R, Celli BR, Tesfaigzi Y. Spirometric variability in smokers: transitions in COPD diagnosis in a five-year longitudinal study. Respir Res. 2016;17:147.
25. Mannino DM, Doherty DE, Sonia Buist A. Global initiative on obstructive lung disease (GOLD) classification of lung disease and mortality: findings from the atherosclerosis risk in communities (ARIC) study. Respir Med. 2006;100:115–22.
26. Quanjer PH, Brazzale DJ, Boros PW, Pretto JJ. Implications of adopting the global lungs initiative 2012 all-age reference equations for spirometry. Eur Respir J. 2013;42:1046–54.
27. Terzikhan N, Verhamme KM, Hofman A, Stricker BH, Brusselle GG, Lahousse L. Prevalence and incidence of COPD in smokers and non-smokers: the Rotterdam study. Eur J Epidemiol. 2016;31:785–92.

28. Smith OO, Helms PJ. Genetic/environmental determinants of adult chronic obstructive pulmonary disease and possible links with childhood wheezing. Paediatr Respir Rev. 2001;2:178–83.

29. Hwang YI, Park YB, Yoo KH. Recent trends in the prevalence of chronic obstructive pulmonary disease in Korea. Tuberc Respir Dis (Seoul). 2017;80:226–9.

30. Labonte LE, Tan WC, Li PZ, Mancino P, Aaron SD, Benedetti A, Chapman KR, Cowie R, FitzGerald JM, Hernandez P, et al. Undiagnosed chronic obstructive pulmonary disease contributes to the burden of health care use. Data from the CanCOLD study. Am J Respir Crit Care Med. 2016;194:285–98.

31. Regan EA, Lynch DA, Curran-Everett D, Curtis JL, Austin JH, Grenier PA, Kauczor HU, Bailey WC, DeMeo DL, Casaburi RH, et al. Clinical and radiologic disease in smokers with Normal spirometry. JAMA Intern Med. 2015;175:1539–49.

32. Tan WC, Bourbeau J, Hernandez P, Chapman KR, Cowie R, FitzGerald JM, Marciniuk DD, Maltais F, Buist AS, O'Donnell DE, et al. Exacerbation-like respiratory symptoms in individuals without chronic obstructive pulmonary disease: results from a population-based study. Thorax. 2014;69:709–17.

33. van Durme Y, Verhamme KMC, Stijnen T, FJA v R, Van Pottelberge GR, Hofman A, Joos GF, Stricker BHC, Brusselle GG. Prevalence, incidence, and lifetime risk for the development of COPD in the elderly: the Rotterdam study. Chest. 2009;135:368–77.

34. Afonso AS, Verhamme KM, Sturkenboom MC, Brusselle GG. COPD in the general population: prevalence, incidence and survival. Respir Med. 2011; 105:1872–84.

35. Garcia Rodriguez LA, Wallander MA, Tolosa LB, Johansson S. Chronic obstructive pulmonary disease in UK primary care: incidence and risk factors. COPD. 2009;6:369–79.

12

Characteristics of lung cancer among patients with idiopathic pulmonary fibrosis and interstitial lung disease – analysis of institutional and population data

Joo Heung Yoon[1]*[iD], Mehdi Nouraie[1], Xiaoping Chen[1], Richard H Zou[1], Jacobo Sellares[1,2], Kristen L Veraldi[1], Jared Chiarchiaro[1], Kathleen Lindell[1], David O Wilson[1], Naftali Kaminski[3], Timothy Burns[4], Humberto Trejo Bittar[5], Samuel Yousem[5], Kevin Gibson[1] and Daniel J Kass[1]

Abstract

Background: Lung Cancer is occasionally observed in patients with Idiopathic Pulmonary Fibrosis (IPF). We sought to describe the epidemiologic and clinical characteristics of lung cancer for patients with IPF and other interstitial lung disease (ILD) using institutional and statewide data registries.

Methods: We conducted a retrospective analysis of IPF and non-IPF ILD patients from the ILD center registry, to compare with lung cancer registries at the University of Pittsburgh as well as with population data of lung cancer obtained from Pennsylvania Department of Health between 2000 and 2015.

Results: Among 1108 IPF patients, 31 patients were identified with IPF and lung cancer. The age-adjusted standard incidence ratio of lung cancer was 3.34 (with IPF) and 2.3 (with non-IPF ILD) (between-group Hazard ratio = 1.4, $p = 0.3$). Lung cancer worsened the mortality of IPF ($p < 0.001$). Lung cancer with IPF had higher mortality compared to lung cancer in non-IPF ILD (Hazard ratio = 6.2, $p = 0.001$). Lung cancer among IPF was characterized by a predilection for lower lobes (63% vs. 26% in non-IPF lung cancer, $p < 0.001$) and by squamous cell histology (41% vs. 29%, $p = 0.07$). Increased incidence of lung cancer was observed among single lung transplant (SLT) recipients for IPF (13 out of 97, 13.4%), with increased mortality compared to SLT for IPF without lung cancer ($p = 0.028$) during observational period.

Conclusions: Lung cancer is approximately 3.34 times more frequently diagnosed in IPF patients compared to general population, and associated with worse prognosis compared with IPF without lung cancer, with squamous cell carcinoma and lower lobe predilection. The causality between non-smoking IPF patients and lung cancer is to be determined.

Keywords: Idiopathic pulmonary fibrosis, Lung cancer

Background

Idiopathic pulmonary fibrosis (IPF) is a fatal pulmonary condition characterized by the accumulation of activated fibroblasts and extracellular matrix within the lung parenchyma that exhibits progressive, but unpredictable disease course [1, 2]. Two medications are currently approved for the treatment of IPF, but their effects on mortality and quality-of-life in IPF are uncertain [3, 4]. IPF is the most common type of the idiopathic interstitial pneumonias [5], and its distinctive radiographic and pathologic characteristics, as well as course of disease differentiate it from other types of interstitial lung disease (ILD) [6, 7]. Although the link between IPF and lung cancer has been known for years [8], estimates of the prevalence of lung cancer among IPF have varied widely [9, 10]. The effect of a lung cancer diagnosis on the prognosis of IPF is also an unsettled question. Some have suggested IPF and lung cancer exhibit no differences

* Correspondence: yoonjh@upmc.edu
[1]Dorothy P. and Richard P. Simmons Center for Interstitial Lung Disease and Division of Pulmonary, Allergy, and Critical Care Medicine, University of Pittsburgh, NW 628 UPMC Montefiore, 3459 Fifth Avenue Pittsburgh, Pittsburgh, PA 15213, USA
Full list of author information is available at the end of the article

in survival rate compared to IPF without lung cancer [11–14], but a more recent study has supported a worse prognosis [15].

In this context, the purpose of our study was to compare primary lung cancers in a large cohort of patients with IPF and non-IPF ILD to lung cancers from population data in order to describe the characteristics of and to estimate the incidence and prevalence of lung cancer in patients with IPF and non-IPF ILD.

Methods
Regulatory approval
The ILD registry at the Dorothy P. and Richard P. Simmons Center for Interstitial Lung Disease and the Lung Cancer registry at the Hillman Cancer Center were approved by the Institutional Review Board at the University of Pittsburgh.

Registries data collection
Data from the Simmons Center for Interstitial Lung Disease were collected from January 2000 to December 2015. The Simmons registry diagnosis was based on established American Thoracic Society and European Respiratory Society clinical criteria [1, 16]. For lung cancer, registry data were obtained from the Hillman Cancer Center during the same observation period. Both registries are linked to providers' clinics, and are actively followed, and vital status is regularly updated from the Social Security Database. Patients from the ILD registry were characterized as having IPF or non-IPF ILD. Non-IPF ILD refers to ILD caused by a disease other than IPF. The combination of the two registries (referred as 'institutional data') according to each disease status of IPF, non-IPF ILD, and lung cancer is shown in Fig. 1. To obtain the radiographic evidence of emphysema among the two institutional registries, natural language process was used to extract keywords including 'emphysema' or 'emphysematous', with its positive and negative terms from the chest computed tomography (CT) radiology reports.

Population data collection
Epidemiologic data of new lung cancer cases were obtained from the Cancer Registry of the Department of Health of the Commonwealth of Pennsylvania, which is a part of the National Program of Cancer Registry. The following queries were used: (1) demographic data: age, gender, ethnicity; (2) Clinical data: age at lung cancer diagnosis, cancer stage according to American Joint Committee on Cancer staging guidelines [17, 18], histology, location, and mortality. The presence of IPF or non-IPF ILD was not identifiable from this data, as they were not collected in this epidemiologic registry. Age-related State Census data was obtained from the Enterprise Data Dissemination Informatics Exchange (EDDIE) for calculating population cancer statistics (http://www.statistics.health.pa.gov/StatisticalResources/EDDIE, last accessed May 15, 2017).

Data management
To extract the data, a standard application programming interface, Microsoft Open Database Connectivity (Microsoft Corporation, Redmond, WA) was used. Lung cancers were classified following the World Health Organization classification [19]. TNM system was used to stage lung cancers at the time of diagnosis. Diagnosis of IPF and other ILDs, as well as lung cancer were based on the codebook of International Classification of Disease, Ninth Edition (ICD-9) at the time of diagnosis. Time of the diagnosis for IPF as well as non-IPF ILD was defined by the first ILD center visit when the ICD-9 code was given. Age-adjusted standard incidence ratio of lung cancer in IPF and non-IPF ILD patients were compared with the DOH data. For the calculation of the survival rate, the time from the time of diagnosis of IPF or non-IPF ILD to death (survival time) were compared. The location of lung

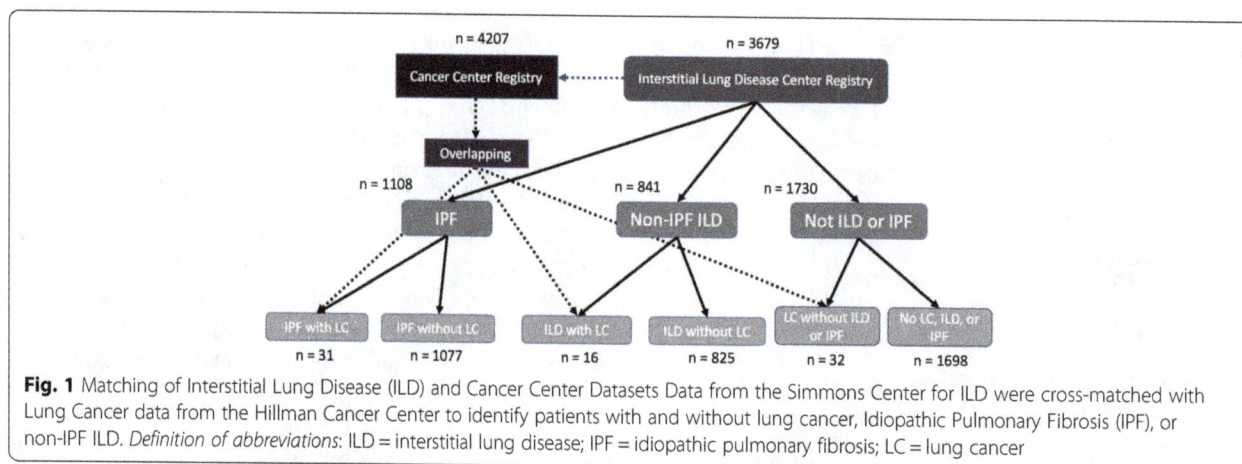

Fig. 1 Matching of Interstitial Lung Disease (ILD) and Cancer Center Datasets Data from the Simmons Center for ILD were cross-matched with Lung Cancer data from the Hillman Cancer Center to identify patients with and without lung cancer, Idiopathic Pulmonary Fibrosis (IPF), or non-IPF ILD. *Definition of abbreviations*: ILD = interstitial lung disease; IPF = idiopathic pulmonary fibrosis; LC = lung cancer

cancers, the histologic phenotypes, and the stage at diagnosis were compared.

Statistical analysis

Continuous and categorical variables were compared between different groups using the Kruskal-Wallis or Fisher's exact test. Log rank test was performed to compare the survival function in lung cancer patients with and without IPF. Standardized incidence ratio was used to compare age-adjusted incidence of lung cancer between IPF patient and lung cancer registry information from Pennsylvania DOH. Age-adjusted standardized incidence ratio was calculated defining each expected and observed cases for group is based on person-years. The person-year was calculated by the sum of the time between the date of diagnosis of IPF or non-IPF ILD and either the date of death, or the end of the observation period (December 31, 2015) for each age bracket. All analyses were performed in STATA 14.2 (StataCorp., College Station, TX).

Results

Patient demographics and characteristics

We identified 1953 patients including 1108 IPF patients and 841 patients with non-IPF ILD diagnosis from the Simmons ILD data (Fig. 1). The baseline demographic profiles of institutional IPF patients were compared to non-IPF ILD patients (Table 1). When compared with non-IPF ILD group, IPF patients were older at diagnosis (median of 69 vs 59 years old), more frequently Caucasian (91% vs 85%), and male (59% vs 38%, all $p < 0.001$). The difference in prevalence of lung cancer between IPF and non-IPF ILD was not statistically significant (2.8 vs 1.9%, $p = 0.12$). More IPF patients than non-IPF ILD patients were smokers (66% vs 57%, $p = 0.001$). All-cause mortality was higher in IPF than non-IPF ILD group (47 vs 12%, $p < 0.001$). From the Hillman Cancer Center Registry, 4207 patients were identified for review for lung cancer of all histologic subtypes including 4176 cases without IPF diagnosis. Following cross-matching of the two registries,

we found 31 patients with both IPF and lung cancer and 16 patients with non-IPF ILD and lung cancer. Primary etiologies included in non-IPF ILD group are summarized in Additional file 1: Table S1.

The demographic characteristics of patients with lung cancer and IPF were compared to lung cancer without IPF from the Hillman Cancer Center Registry, as well as with lung cancer from the population data acquired from Department of Health (DOH) (Table 2). From the DOH data, the total obtained number of lung cancer cases from 2000 to 2015 was 156,032. After excluding duplicated identifiers ($n = 3951$) and non-solid and non-primary (either metastatic disease from other primaries or unknown primary) ($n = 47,127$), 104,954 patients were included in the final analysis.

IPF patients with lung cancer were not significantly different in terms of age (65 vs 67 years, $p = 0.2$), gender (61 vs 48% male, $p = 0.15$), and race (97 vs 88% Caucasian, $p = 0.14$) compared to lung cancer patients without IPF from the Hillman Cancer Center Registry. Fewer IPF patients with lung cancer were former or current smokers compared to lung cancer patients without IPF (77 vs. 90%, $p < 0.001$), with 7 never-smokers (23%) were identified from IPF and lung cancer group. No smoking history data were available from the Pennsylvania Department of Health database. IPF patients with lung cancer were, however, younger compared to the population data for lung cancer (65 vs 69 years, $p = 0.03$). There was no difference in the gender and race between the ILD data and population data. The mortality between lung cancer with IPF and lung cancer without IPF was different when compared within the institution (84 vs 63%, $p = 0.013$). However, this difference was not observed when institutional IPF patients with co-morbid lung cancer were compared to population data (84 vs 75%, $p = 0.2$) over the 15 years of observational period. To better understand the prognosis of IPF with lung cancer, we examined survival time as defined as time interval from the date of lung cancer diagnosis to the date of death. In the institutional cohort,

Table 1 Baseline demographics and clinical characteristics of IPF and non-IPF ILD from institutional registry

Variables	IPF		Non-IPF ILD		p-values
	patients	Results	patients	Results	
Age at diagnosis (years)	1108	69 (62–75)	841	59 (50–68)	< 0.001
Gender (% male)	1108	652 (59%)	841	318 (38%)	< 0.001
Ethnicity (% Caucasian)	1108	1007 (91%)	841	712 (85%)	< 0.001
Smoking – Never	1054	361 (34%)	443	193 (44%)	< 0.001
Former		655 (62%)		224 (51%)	
Current		38 (4%)		26 (6%)	
Prevalence of lung cancer	1108	31 (2.8%)	841	16 (1.9%)	0.20
Mortality over observation period (%)	1108	515 (47%)	841	104 (12%)	< 0.001

Definition of abbreviations: *IPF* idiopathic pulmonary fibrosis, *ILD* interstitial lung disease. Mortality based on patient records as deceased at the time of the review of the registry data

Table 2 Baseline demographics of lung cancer patients with and without idiopathic pulmonary fibrosis (IPF) from institution, and lung cancer in overall population of state of Pennsylvania

Variables	Lung cancer with IPF		Lung cancer without IPF (institutional data)		Lung cancer without IPF (population data)		p-values column 1 vs. 3
	N	Results	N	Results	N	Results	
Age in years, median (IQR)	31	65 (62–71)	4176	67 (60–75)	104,954	69 (61–77)	0.03
Gender (% male)	31	19 (61%)	4176	2023 (48%)	104,954	53,800 (51%)	0.16
Ethnicity (% Caucasian)	31	30 (97%)	4176	3679 (88%)	104,954	89,643 (85%)	0.07
Smoking – never	31	7 (23%)	4176	395 (10%)	NA		< 0.001 (column 1 vs 2)
former		24 (77%)		2362 (57%)			
current		0		1361 (33%)			
Mortality over observation period (%)	31	26 (84%)	4176	2644 (63%)	104,954	78,254 (75%)	0.2
Survival time in months, median (IQR)	26	5 (1–10)	4176	13 (6–26)	NA	NA	0.002 (column 1 vs 2)

Definition of abbreviations: IQR Interquartile range. Column 1 = Lung cancer with IPF; column 2 = Lung cancer with non-IPF ILD; column 3 = Lung cancer in general population in Pennsylvania. *NA* not available. Survival time was calculated by the time from lung cancer diagnosis to the date of expiration, or the time of registry data review

patients with lung cancer without IPF had a significantly longer survival time, compared to lung cancer patients with IPF (median survival time 5 vs 13 months, $p = 0.002$).

Cumulative incidence of lung cancer in IPF and non-IPF ILD

We next examined the cumulative incidence of lung cancer in IPF and non-IPF ILD patients. The median time to the discovery of lung cancer after the diagnosis of IPF was 53 months (interquartile range (IQR) 25–77 months), and 55 months (IQR 44–62 months) in non-IPF ILD. Although there was no observed difference in the median time to the discovery of lung cancer between these groups, there did appear to be increased incidence of lung cancer in the first 2 years after diagnosis in the IPF group which persisted until year four (Fig. 2).

Age-adjusted incidence of lung cancer among IPF compared to general population in Pennsylvania

Observed incidence of lung cancer (Table 3) in general population was calculated within different age brackets, and showed that the rate among IPF patients was 3.34 times higher (95% confidence interval 2.3–4.7) and in non-IPF ILD patients 2.3 times higher (95%CI 1.3–3.6) compared to general population. To drill down the cancer risk in non-IPF ILD cases, the non-IPF ILD group was subdivided further into ILD associated with autoimmunity, hypersensitivity pneumonitis (HP), pneumoconiosis, and smoking-related ILDs (eosinophilic granuloma, respiratory bronchiolitis-associated interstitial lung disease, and desquamative interstitial pneumonia). No lung cancers were observed in the HP or pneumoconiosis groups. Among non-IPF ILD patients, 508 patients with ILD related to autoimmunity (including systemic sclerosis, rheumatoid arthritis, polymyositis/dermatomyositis, Sjogren's disease, and mixed connective tissue disease) were identified, among them 12 lung cancer cases diagnosed within the

observation period. When the autoimmunity group is considered alone, the age-adjusted incidence of lung cancer was 4.95 times higher than general population (95% CI 2.7–8.4). The rate of non-smokers among autoimmune-related ILD patients were 47% (123 out of 261 known history of smoking). Among patients with HP ($n = 109$), no lung cancer was identified, in which 48% (28 out of 58 known history of smoking) were smokers. From a small group of patients ($n = 47$) with smoking-related ILDs, two cases of lung cancer were found.

Survival estimates of lung cancer in IPF

The survival probabilities for IPF without lung cancer ($n = 1077$) and IPF with lung cancer ($n = 31$) were compared over time. Figure 3 illustrates Kaplan-Meier curves for institutional data - IPF without lung cancer and IPF with lung cancer groups, where statistically significant ($p < 0.001$) lower survival rate over time was observed for IPF and lung cancer patients compared to IPF patients without lung cancer. The trend in cumulative incidences between the two groups showed no major differences across 15 years of accumulated follow-up period of variable lengths of observed individual cases.

Clinical characteristic of lung cancer patients with IPF compared to non-IPF ILD and the Department of Health data

The clinical characteristics of lung cancer with a diagnosis of IPF and non-IPF ILD are described in Table 4. The primary site of the lung cancer for IPF patients showed more frequent lower lobe predilection compared to population lung cancer data (63% vs. 36%, $p < 0.001$). On the other hand, lung cancer diagnosed from institutional non-IPF ILD patients demonstrated no statistically significant differences in location compared to population lung cancer data ($p = 0.2$). The most common type of lung cancer

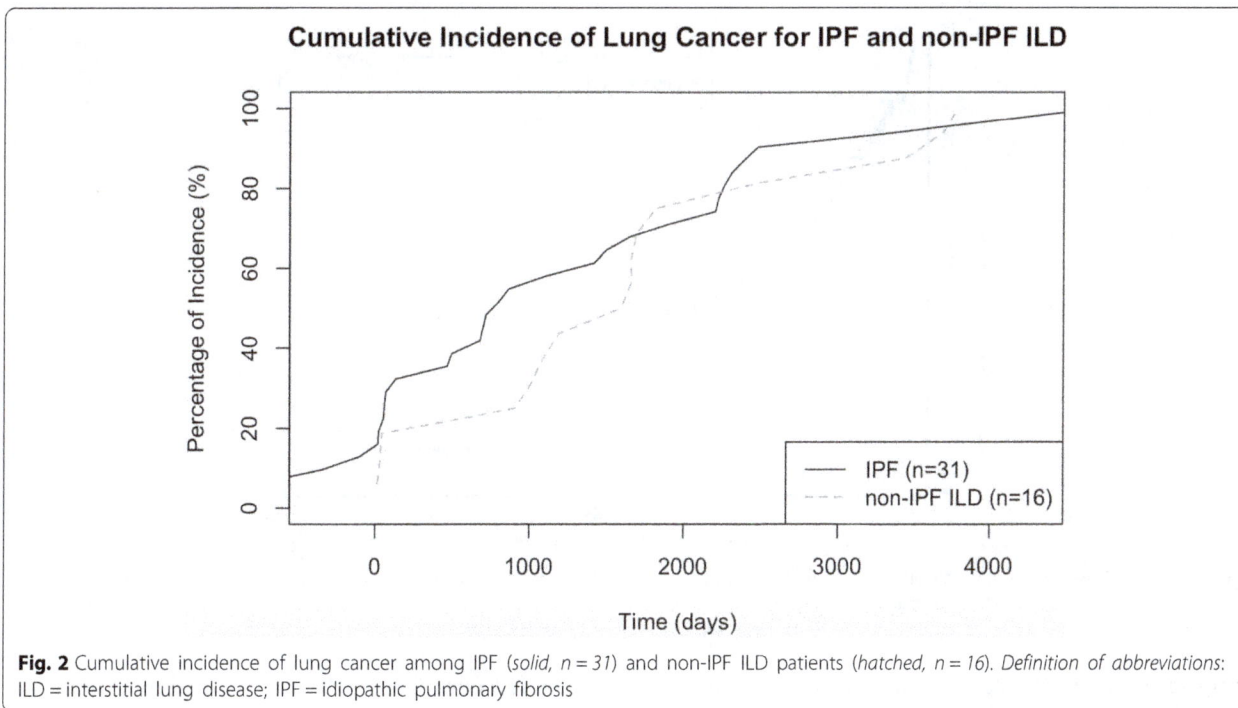

Fig. 2 Cumulative incidence of lung cancer among IPF (*solid, n = 31*) and non-IPF ILD patients (*hatched, n = 16*). *Definition of abbreviations*: ILD = interstitial lung disease; IPF = idiopathic pulmonary fibrosis

in IPF patient to be squamous cell cancer, higher in IPF patients (41%) compared to non-IPF ILD patients (19%) with lung cancer within the institution. Squamous cancer in IPF was also more common compared with squamous cell cancer ratio in population data (29%) but not reaching statistical significance (p = 0.07). The histology of lung cancer was not significantly different between non-IPF ILD patients and general population (p = 0.4). No significant differences in distribution of lung cancer stage in IPF compared to patients with lung cancer without IPF were identified in the DOH data (p = 0.6). The similarity in the cancer stage distribution also exists when compared with the institutional non-IPF ILD patients with lung cancer data (p = 0.8), nor with the population data (p = 0.6). Lung cancer patients with non-IPF ILD also demonstrated no differences compared to population data. Individual level descriptive analysis for all 31 patients diagnosed with IPF and lung cancer are available (Additional file 1: Table S2).

Among our 1108 IPF patients, 233 (21%) cases were found to have emphysema as a comorbid condition during the clinic encounters. From 841 non-IPF ILD patients, 156 (19%) had a diagnosis of emphysema. For the patients diagnosed with lung cancer along with IPF, 17 patients had a diagnosis of emphysema. We observed that radiologic emphysema was overrepresented in IPF patients with lung cancer (OR 5.2) compared to non-IPF patients from Hillman Cancer Center data.

Transplantation and immunosuppression have been associated with an increased rate of cancer development. This is especially true as single lung transplant has been known for higher rate of lung cancer in native lung, ranging from 6.9–9.8% [20, 21]. To estimate the effect of single lung transplant on development of lung cancer for IPF patients, a subgroup analysis was performed (Additional file 1: Table S3) within the institutional registry data. With the data collected until 2014, a total of 97 IPF with single lung transplanted patients were enrolled in our registry. Among them, 13 cases of lung cancer

Table 3 Age-adjusted standardized incidence rate of Idiopathic pulmonary fibrosis (IPF), and non-IPF interstitial lung disease (ILD) and lung cancer from combined registries, compared to Department of Health lung cancer registry and Pennsylvania census data, based on 1000 person-year for each expected and observed age group. Observed incidence of lung cancer in general population was calculated within different age brackets, as well as lung cancer occurrence in IPF and ILD population

Case number	Registry IPF and LC over population	Registry non-IPF ILD and LC over population
	Observed / Expected cases	Observed / Expected cases
	31 / 9.28	16 / 7.05
SIR (95% CI)	3.34 (2.31–4.68)	2.27 (1.34–3.61)

Definition of abbreviations: *SIR* standardized incidence ratio, *CI* confidence interval, *IPF* idiopathic pulmonary fibrosis, *LC* lung cancer

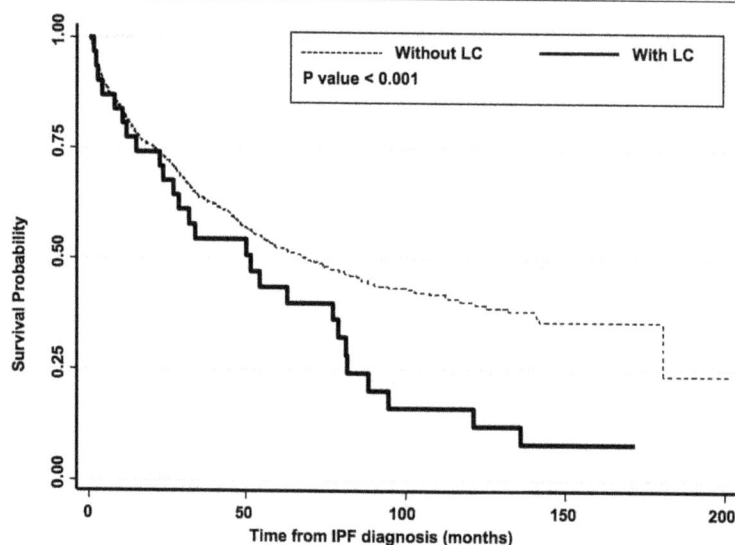

Fig. 3 Comparison of survival probabilities of IPF patients with and without co-morbid lung cancer (between the two institutional datasets). *Definition of abbreviations*: IPF = idiopathic pulmonary fibrosis; LC = lung cancer

were identified in the native lung (13.4%) following single lung transplant (SLT). There was no difference in age, gender, ethnicity, or smoking history, but the mortality of single lung transplant recipients who developed lung cancer (12 out of 13 patients, 92%) were significantly higher than single lung transplant without lung cancer (49 out of 84, 59%, *p* = 0.028) during follow-up period.

Discussion

The association between IPF and lung cancer has been observed for years, although estimates of the risk have

Table 4 Characteristics of lung cancer in patients with IPF or non-IPF ILD compared to Pennsylvania state data

Variables	Lung cancer with IPF		Lung cancer with non-IPF ILD		Lung cancer in general population in Pennsylvania		*p*-value (column 1 vs. 3)
	N	Results	N	Results	N	Results	
Laterality	31		16		100,949		0.4
Left		14 (45%)		7 (44%)		41,745 (41%)	
Right		16 (52%)		7 (44%)		57,566 (57%)	
Bilateral		1 (3%)		2 (12%)		1638 (2%)	
Primary site	27		13		85,087		< 0.001
Upper lobe		8 (27%)		6 (46%)		53,288 (63%)	
Lower lobe		17 (63%)		6 (46%)		30,422 (36%)	
Others		2 (7%)		1 (8%)		1377 (2%)	
Histology	27		16		104,954		0.07
SCC		11 (41%)		3 (19%)		30,596 (29%)	
Adenocarcinoma		7 (26%)		10 (63%)		49,217 (47%)	
Other		9 (33%)		3 (19%)		25,141 (24%)	
Stage	29		16		83,994		0.6
I		9 (31%)		4 (25%)		19,000 (23%)	
II		2 (7%)		1 (6%)		4312 (5%)	
III		7 (24%)		6 (38%)		21,730 (26%)	
IV		11 (38%)		5 (31%)		38,952 (46%)	

Definition of abbreviations: *SCC* squamous cell cancer, *NA* not available. Column 1 = Lung cancer with IPF; column 2 = Lung cancer with non-IPF ILD; column 3 = Lung cancer in general population in Pennsylvania

varied widely. Co-morbid lung cancer represents a very challenging problem for the clinician. In this study, we sought to identify the clinical characteristics of lung cancer among patients with IPF and non-IPF ILD from our institutional data and to compare these data from population data. In our study, which represents the largest review in the United States, we have found that patients with IPF exhibited a 3.34-fold higher incidence of lung cancer compared to the general population who developed lung cancer. IPF patients showed a statistically significant worse mortality rate over observation period compared to lung cancer patients without IPF. Consistent with several previous studies, lung cancer in IPF was observed more frequently in the lower lobes, with a borderline association between IPF and the squamous cell carcinoma histology, as observed previously [22–25]. Overall, our data suggest that lung cancer in IPF is phenotypically distinctive from "sporadic" lung cancer, and exhibits worse prognosis compared to IPF without lung cancer, or lung cancer without IPF.

We found that single lung transplant patients from IPF exhibited a higher prevalence of lung cancer, and the development of lung cancer in this group was associated with higher mortality during follow-up period. When the native IPF lung is exposed to immunosuppressive medications to prevent rejection from lung transplant, the risk of cancer may be accentuated by loss of immune-mediated "tumor surveillance" [20]. This raises the question if single lung transplant represents an additional risk factor for the development of lung cancer in IPF. While our numbers are small, the suggestion is that indeed, transplant enhances the risk of lung cancer. Furthermore, it begs the highly speculative question if IPF patients should undergo double lung transplant as a potential "cure" to the lung cancer risk. Additional study of single lung transplant for all indications might help elucidate the specific risk of lung cancer in IPF associated with immunosuppression.

The subject of IPF and lung cancer has been studied in diverse ethnic groups and health care systems. One of the largest studies of health care databases identified a relative risk 7.3 for lung cancer in IPF patients in the United Kingdom (UK) [12], which was validated by analysis of an overlapping UK database where 1064 IPF patients were studied identifying a nearly fivefold increased rate of lung cancer [9]. Our estimate for incidence of lung cancer among IPF was lower at 3.3, showing little change after controlling for smoking in the British study [12]. While smoking rates were similar in the UK studies between IPF and control patients, smoking was less common in IPF patients with lung cancer compared to patients with lung cancer alone in our institutional data. These data corroborate the idea that IPF is a risk factor for lung cancer independent of smoking. It is possible that smoking may

account for the observed prevalence of lung cancer in IPF of 13% in an Italian cohort [15], which is significantly higher than our observed prevalence of 2.8%. The number of never smokers in our cohort is at least three-fold higher than the Italian cohort. Another UK study cohort [26] showed that most IPF patients with lung cancer diagnosed had smoking histories (never smoker $n = 2$, 4.5%), along with other IPF and lung cancer studies [13, 27, 28]. In our analysis, the IPF patients without a history of smoking did not exhibit an increased risk of lung cancer, which suggests that cigarette smoking could be an important contributor of lung cancer development. The role of genetics in IPF could play a pivotal role in the development of lung cancer [29], but the mechanistic pathway has not been fully elucidated. Another factor that could drive the prevalence of lung cancer in pulmonary fibrosis cohort would be combined pulmonary fibrosis with emphysema (CPFE) [30]. Despite the higher lung cancer rate for IPF patients with radiologic emphysema (OR 5.2), the distribution of radiologic diagnosis of emphysema varied from 12 years before to 3 months after the diagnosis of lung cancer, and definitive quantification of impact of emphysema was hard to estimate from our results. In addition, concern of surveillance bias exists in our data because of the frequency of chest CTs in this population. Further study is needed to determine a dose-response effect for lung cancer risk in IPF possibly based on volumetric CT analysis.

Cancer risk in the non-IPF ILD population is well known. Some phenotypes of non-IPF ILD including polymyositis/dermatomyositis [31], rheumatoid arthritis [32], and systemic sclerosis [33] are known to be associated with increased risk for lung cancer. We found a prevalence of lung cancer in 1.9% among non-IPF ILD patients. This appears to be lower than some previously published estimates [34, 35], as well as a recent comprehensive study [36]. Thus, the molecular underpinnings of lung cancer risk in non-IPF ILD may be different than in IPF. Among non-IPF ILD patients, our analysis showed 4.95-fold increased age-adjusted incident rate of lung cancer among autoimmune disease-related ILD within the observation period. However, it is difficult to determine if the increased risk of lung cancer is associated with an autoimmune process versus immunosuppressive therapy which is needed to treat autoimmune disease. Further study is needed to quantify these risks at both the population level and at the molecular level.

Previous studies have suggested that mortality of patients with lung cancer and IPF was no greater than for IPF patients without lung cancer [23, 37]. More recent studies, however, have argued there that the mortality of lung cancer in IPF patients is higher than for lung cancer alone [15, 25] and that the presence of IPF is associated with a prognosis worse than lung cancer. We found that lung cancer worsened the prognosis of IPF. Based on the Simmons data and DOH data, however, having IPF did not increase the overall mortality of lung cancer in the general population in a statistically significant way. What explains this discrepancy? This observation may be influenced by other important prognostic information in the general population that are not available to us for study such as smoking status. The clinically relevant question here would be whether a screening process for lung cancer among IPF patients would yield survival benefit. However, there are no current recommendations to guide clinicians how to diagnose and manage lung cancer in IPF. It is unclear how treatment decisions should be made at an individual level. Does impaired pulmonary function affect treatment decisions? Stage at diagnosis did not differ between IPF and non IPF patients. These data highlight many of the unanswered questions surrounding lung cancer and IPF.

Recently, the anti-cancer effect of IPF therapy has been suggested in recent studies [38–40]. This could raise an interesting question, whether the risk of lung cancer could be affected for our registry population with the use of pirfenidone. However, because IPF therapy was officially approved by the United States Food and Drug Administration in November 2014, and most of our patients' data were collected beforehand, we cannot determine if therapy changes lung cancer risk in IPF. Thus, the direct effect of pirfenidone in our registry data on the development cannot be assessed in this study.

Limitations

We recognize that there are several limitations to this study. This single-center study with retrospective database review may underrepresent the IPF and lung cancer population. Conversely, referral bias may inflate the prevalence as sicker and more complicated patients seek care at the tertiary specialty center. Surveillance bias for lung cancer could exist, with IPF or non-IPF ILD patients tend to visit clinic more often for diagnostic work-up or symptoms, while early-stage lung cancers may be asymptomatic. Evolving diagnostic criteria for IPF and ILD over the last 15 years may be associated with misclassification, with no clear unifying interpretation present for the changing criteria [41]. These factors may have potentially affected our analysis on the prevalence and survival trajectories because the possibility of misclassification over time. Third, some of our referrals were from out-of-state and might not be represented by the PA population data. The population data for lung cancer obtained from the Pennsylvania Department of Health lack smoking history and the exact time of lung cancer diagnosis (data only has year of diagnosis). For these reasons, assessment of risk factors for lung cancer and head-to-head survival analysis between institutional and the DOH data were not possible in this study.

Conclusions

The incidence of lung cancer was higher among IPF patients compared to general population or ILD patients. Lung cancers in IPF was observed more commonly in never smokers and demonstrated predilection for the lower lobe, and the squamous cell histology may predominate. In addition, lung cancer negatively impacts the prognosis of IPF. Further study is needed to elucidate how the IPF phenotype alters the lung cancer phenotype and if screening for lung cancer in this population will ultimately impact the course of the disease.

Acknowledgements

The authors wish to acknowledge the efforts of Karla Stewart, BS, CTR, Thoracic Research Registrar with the UPMC Network Cancer Registry. Population data were supplied by the Bureau of Health Statistics & Registries, Pennsylvania Department of Health, Harrisburg, Pennsylvania. The Pennsylvania Department of Health specifically disclaims responsibility for any analyses, interpretations or conclusions.

Funding

This study was supported in part by the National Institute of Health (NIH) funding R01-HL126990 (DJK). Registry Information Services from Hillman Cancer Center is managed with funding from NIH P30CA047904.

Authors' contributions

JHY, MN, KG, NK, and DJK participated in the concept and design of the study. JHY, XC, RZ, KV, KL, TB, KG, and DJK participated in the acquisition of the data. JHY, MN, XC performed the data analysis. JHY, MN, DJK drafted the initial manuscript. All authors critically revised the manuscript and approved the final version for submission.

Competing interests

JHY, MN, XC, JC, KV, KL, DOW and SY have nothing to disclose. JS reports grants from Boehringer, grants and personal fees from Roche, personal fees from Rovi, outside the submitted work. TB reports personal fees from AbbVIE and Regeneron, outside the submitted work. NK reports grant and personal fees from Biogen Idec, personal fees from MMI, non-financial support from Actelion, non-financial support from Miragen, non-financial support from Astra Zeneca, non-financial support from GSK, personal fees from Pilant, and is a consultant to Samumed, Numedii, which are outside the submitted work. NK is also a member of the Scientific Advisory Committee, the Research Advisory Forum, and the Board of the Pulmonary Fibrosis Foundation, as well as serving as Deputy Editor of Thorax and BMJ. KG reports personal fees from Bayer, outside the submitted work. DJK reports research grant funding from Regeneron, outside the submitted work.

Author details

[1]Dorothy P. and Richard P. Simmons Center for Interstitial Lung Disease and Division of Pulmonary, Allergy, and Critical Care Medicine, University of Pittsburgh, NW 628 UPMC Montefiore, 3459 Fifth Avenue Pittsburgh, Pittsburgh, PA 15213, USA. [2]Interstitial Lung Diseases Program, Servei de Pneumologia, Institut Clinic Respiratori, Barcelona, Spain. [3]Section of Pulmonary, Critical Care and Sleep Medicine, Yale University, New Haven, CT, USA. [4]Division of Hematology and Oncology, University of Pittsburgh, Pittsburgh, PA, USA. [5]Department of Pathology, University of Pittsburgh, Pittsburgh, PA, USA.

References

1. Raghu G, Collard HR, Egan JJ, Martinez FJ, Behr J, Brown KK, Colby TV, Cordier JF, Flaherty KR, Lasky JA, Lynch DA, Ryu JH, Swigris JJ, Wells AU, Ancochea J, Bouros D, Carvalho C, Costabel U, Ebina M, Hansell DM, Johkoh T, Kim DS, King TE Jr, Kondoh Y, Myers J, Muller NL, Nicholson AG, Richeldi L, Selman M, Dudden RF, Griss BS, Protzko SL, Schunemann HJ, Fibrosis AEJACIP. An official ATS/ERS/JRS/ALAT statement: idiopathic pulmonary fibrosis: evidence-based guidelines for diagnosis and management. Am J Respir Crit Care Med. 2011;183:788–824.
2. Ley B, Collard HR. Epidemiology of idiopathic pulmonary fibrosis. Clin Epidemiol. 2013;5:483–92.
3. King TE Jr, Bradford WZ, Castro-Bernardini S, Fagan EA, Glaspole I, Glassberg MK, Gorina E, Hopkins PM, Kardatzke D, Lancaster L, Lederer DJ, Nathan SD, Pereira CA, Sahn SA, Sussman R, Swigris JJ, Noble PW, Group AS. A phase 3 trial of pirfenidone in patients with idiopathic pulmonary fibrosis. N Engl J Med. 2014;370:2083–92.
4. Richeldi L, du Bois RM, Raghu G, Azuma A, Brown KK, Costabel U, Cottin V, Flaherty KR, Hansell DM, Inoue Y, Kim DS, Kolb M, Nicholson AG, Noble PW, Selman M, Taniguchi H, Brun M, Le Maulf F, Girard M, Stowasser S, Schlenker-Herceg R, Disse B, Collard HR, Investigators IT. Efficacy and safety of nintedanib in idiopathic pulmonary fibrosis. N Engl J Med. 2014;370:2071–82.
5. Wuyts WA, Cavazza A, Rossi G, Bonella F, Sverzellati N, Spagnolo P. Differential diagnosis of usual interstitial pneumonia: when is it truly idiopathic? Eur Respir Rev. 2014;23:308–19.
6. Flaherty KR, Toews GB, Travis WD, Colby TV, Kazerooni EA, Gross BH, Jain A, Strawderman RL 3rd, Paine R, Flint A, Lynch JP 3rd, Martinez FJ. Clinical significance of histological classification of idiopathic interstitial pneumonia. Eur Respir J. 2002;19:275–83.
7. Nicholson AG, Colby TV, du Bois RM, Hansell DM, Wells AU. The prognostic significance of the histologic pattern of interstitial pneumonia in patients presenting with the clinical entity of cryptogenic fibrosing alveolitis. Am J Respir Crit Care Med. 2000;162:2213–7.
8. Meyer EC, Liebow AA. Relationship of interstitial pneumonia honeycombing and atypical epithelial proliferation to cancer of the lung. Cancer. 1965;18:322–51.
9. Le Jeune I, Gribbin J, West J, Smith C, Cullinan P, Hubbard R. The incidence of cancer in patients with idiopathic pulmonary fibrosis and sarcoidosis in the UK. Respir Med. 2007;101:2534–40.
10. Matsushita H, Tanaka S, Saiki Y, Hara M, Nakata K, Tanimura S, Banba J. Lung cancer associated with usual interstitial pneumonia. Pathol Int. 1995;45:925–32.
11. Araki T, Katsura H, Sawabe M, Kida KA. Clinical study of idiopathic pulmonary fibrosis based on autopsy studies in elderly patients. Intern Med (Tokyo, Japan). 2003;42:483–9.
12. Hubbard R, Venn A, Lewis S, Britton J. Lung cancer and cryptogenic fibrosing alveolitis. A population-based cohort study. Am J Respir Crit Care Med. 2000;161:5–8.
13. Ozawa Y, Suda T, Naito T, Enomoto N, Hashimoto D, Fujisawa T, Nakamura Y, Inui N, Nakamura H, Chida K. Cumulative incidence of and predictive factors for lung cancer in IPF. Respirol (Carlton, Vic). 2009;14:723–8.
14. Stack BH, Choo-Kang YF, Heard BE. The prognosis of cryptogenic fibrosing alveolitis. Thorax. 1972;27:535–42.
15. Tomassetti S, Gurioli C, Ryu JH, Decker PA, Ravaglia C, Tantalocco P, Buccioli M, Piciucchi S, Sverzellati N, Dubini A, Gavelli G, Chilosi M, Poletti V. The impact of lung cancer on survival of idiopathic pulmonary fibrosis. Chest. 2015;147:157–64.
16. American Thoracic Society. Idiopathic pulmonary fibrosis: diagnosis and treatment. International consensus statement. American Thoracic Society (ATS), and the European Respiratory Society (ERS). Am J Respir Crit Care Med. 2000;161:646–64.
17. AJCC Cancer Staging Manual / American Joint Committee on Cancer. 5th. Philiadelphia, : Lippincott-Raven; 1997.
18. AJCC Cancer Staging Manual / American Joint Committee on Cancer. 6th. New York: Springer; 2002.
19. Travis WD, Brambilla E, Nicholson AG, Yatabe Y, Austin JH, Beasley MB, Chirieac LR, Dacic S, Duhig E, Flieder DB, Geisinger K, Hirsch FR, Ishikawa Y, Kerr KM, Noguchi M, Pelosi G, Powell CA, Tsao MS, Wistuba I. The 2015 World Health Organization classification of lung tumors: impact of genetic, clinical and radiologic advances since the 2004 classification. J Thorac Oncol. 2015;10:1243–60.
20. Dickson RP, Davis RD, Rea JB, Palmer SM. High frequency of bronchogenic carcinoma after single-lung transplantation. J Heart Lung Transplant. 2006; 25:1297–301.
21. Yserbyt J, Verleden GM, Dupont LJ, Van Raemdonck DE, Dooms C. Bronchial carcinoma after lung transplantation: a single-center experience. J Heart Lung Transplant. 2012;31:585–90.
22. Nagai A, Chiyotani A, Nakadate T, Konno K. Lung cancer in patients with idiopathic pulmonary fibrosis. Tohoku J Exp Med. 1992;167:231–7.
23. Aubry MC, Myers JL, Douglas WW, Tazelaar HD, Washington Stephens TL, Hartman TE, Deschamps C, Pankratz VS. Primary pulmonary carcinoma in patients with idiopathic pulmonary fibrosis. Mayo Clin Proc. 2002;77:763–70.
24. Lee T, Park JY, Lee HY, Cho YJ, Yoon HI, Lee JH, Jheon S, Lee CT, Park JS. Lung cancer in patients with idiopathic pulmonary fibrosis: clinical characteristics and impact on survival. Respir Med. 2014;108:1549–55.
25. Kanaji N, Tadokoro A, Kita N, Murota M, Ishii T, Takagi T, Watanabe N, Tojo Y, Harada S, Hasui Y, Kadowaki N, Bandoh S. Impact of idiopathic pulmonary fibrosis on advanced non-small cell lung cancer survival. J Cancer Res Clin Oncol. 2016;142:1855–65.
26. Harris JM, Johnston ID, Rudd R, Taylor AJ, Cullinan P. Cryptogenic fibrosing alveolitis and lung cancer: the BTS study. Thorax. 2010;65:70–6.
27. Khan KA, Kennedy MP, Moore E, Crush L, Prendeville S, Maher MM, Burke L, Henry MT. Radiological characteristics, histological features and clinical outcomes of lung cancer patients with coexistent idiopathic pulmonary fibrosis. Lung. 2015;193:71–7.
28. Park J, Kim DS, Shim TS, Lim CM, Koh Y, Lee SD, Kim WS, Kim WD, Lee JS, Song KS. Lung cancer in patients with idiopathic pulmonary fibrosis. Eur Respir J. 2001;17:1216–9.
29. Guyard A, Danel C, Theou-Anton N, Debray MP, Gibault L, Mordant P, Castier Y, Crestani B, Zalcman G, Blons H, Cazes A. Morphologic and molecular study of lung cancers associated with idiopathic pulmonary fibrosis and other pulmonary fibroses. Respir Res. 2017;18:120.
30. Koo HJ, Do KH, Lee JB, Alblushi S, Lee SM. Lung Cancer in combined pulmonary fibrosis and emphysema: a systematic review and meta-analysis. PLoS One. 2016;11:e0161437.
31. Huang YL, Chen YJ, Lin MW, Wu CY, Liu PC, Chen TJ, Chen YC, Jih JS, Chen CC, Lee DD, Chang YT, Wang WJ, Liu HN. Malignancies associated with dermatomyositis and polymyositis in Taiwan: a nationwide population-based study. Br J Dermatol. 2009;161:854–60.
32. Simon TA, Thompson A, Gandhi KK, Hochberg MC, Suissa S. Incidence of malignancy in adult patients with rheumatoid arthritis: a meta-analysis. Arthritis Res Ther. 2015;17:212.
33. Enomoto Y, Inui N, Yoshimura K, Nishimoto K, Mori K, Kono M, Fujisawa T, Enomoto N, Nakamura Y, Iwashita T, Suda T. Lung cancer development in patients with connective tissue disease-related interstitial lung disease: a retrospective observational study. Medicine. 2016;95:e5716.
34. Bouros D, Hatzakis K, Labrakis H, Zeibecoglou K. Association of malignancy with diseases causing interstitial pulmonary changes. Chest. 2002;121:1278–89.
35. Saijo A, Hanibuchi M, Goto H, Toyoda Y, Tezuka T, Nishioka Y. An analysis of the clinical features of lung cancer in patients with connective tissue diseases. Respir Investig. 2017;55:153–60.
36. Watanabe S, Saeki K, Waseda Y, Murata A, Takato H, Ichikawa Y, Yasui H, Kimura H, Hamaguchi Y, Matsushita T, Yamada K, Kawano M, Furuichi K, Wada T, Kasahara K. Lung cancer in connective tissue disease-associated interstitial lung disease: clinical features and impact on outcomes. J Thorac Dis. 2018;10:799–807.
37. Song DH, Choi IH, Ha SY, Han KM, Lee JJ, Hong ME, Jeon K, Chung MP, Kim J, Han J. Usual interstitial pneumonia with lung cancer: clinicopathological analysis of 43 cases. Korean J Pathol. 2014;48:10–6.
38. Kozono S, Ohuchida K, Eguchi D, Ikenaga N, Fujiwara K, Cui L, Mizumoto K, Tanaka M. Pirfenidone inhibits pancreatic cancer desmoplasia by regulating stellate cells. Cancer Res. 2013;73:2345–56.
39. Polydorou C, Mpekris F, Papageorgis P, Voutouri C, Stylianopoulos T. Pirfenidone normalizes the tumor microenvironment to improve chemotherapy. Oncotarget. 2017;8:24506–17.
40. Iwata T, Yoshino I, Yoshida S, Ikeda N, Tsuboi M, Asato Y, Katakami N, Sakamoto K, Yamashita Y, Okami J, Mitsudomi T, Yamashita M, Yokouchi H, Okubo K, Okada M, Takenoyama M, Chida M, Tomii K, Matsuura M, Azuma A, Iwasawa T, Kuwano K, Sakai S, Hiroshima K, Fukuoka J, Yoshimura K, Tada H, Nakagawa K, Nakanishi Y. A phase II trial evaluating the efficacy and safety of perioperative pirfenidone for prevention of acute exacerbation of idiopathic pulmonary fibrosis in lung cancer patients undergoing pulmonary resection: West Japan oncology group 6711 L (PEOPLE study). Respir Res. 2016;17:90.

13

Upregulation of microRNA-17-5p contributes to hypoxia-induced proliferation in human pulmonary artery smooth muscle cells through modulation of p21 and PTEN

Guangjie Liu[1][*][†], Peng Hao[2,3,4][†], Jie Xu[1], Liming Wang[2,3,4], Yuchuan Wang[2,3,4], Ruifang Han[2,3,4], Ming Ying[2,3,4], Shuangshuang Sui[3], Jinghua Liu[3] and Xuan Li[2,3,4][*] (iD)

Abstract

Background: Pulmonary arterial smooth muscle cell (PASMC) proliferation in response to hypoxia plays an important role in the vascular remodelling that occurs in hypoxic pulmonary hypertension. MicroRNAs (miRs) are emerging as important regulators in the progression of pulmonary hypertension. In this study, we investigated whether the expression of miR-17-5p is modulated by hypoxia and is involved in the hypoxia-induced proliferation of PASMCs.

Methods: Human PASMCs were cultured under hypoxic conditions. miR-17-5p expression was determined by real-time RT-PCR. A BrdU incorporation assay and time-lapse recording were utilized to determine cell proliferation and migration.

Results: PASMC proliferation was increased by moderate hypoxia (3% oxygen) but was reduced by severe hypoxia (0.1% oxygen) after 48 h. Moderate hypoxia induced miR-17-5p expression. Overexpression of miR-17-5p by transfection with miR-17-5p enhanced cell proliferation and migration in normoxia, whereas knockdown of miR-17-5p with anti-miR-17-5p inhibitors significantly reduced cell proliferation and migration. The expression of miR-17-5p target genes, specifically phosphatase and tensin homologue (PTEN) and cyclin-dependent kinase inhibitor 1 (p21WAF1/Cip1, p21), was reduced under moderate hypoxia in PASMCs. Under normoxia, overexpression of miR-17-5p in PASMCs reduced the expression of PTEN and p21.

Conclusion: Our data indicate that miR-17-5p might play a significant role in hypoxia-induced pulmonary vascular smooth muscle cell proliferation by regulating multiple gene targets, including PTEN and p21, and that miR-17-5p could be a novel therapeutic target for the management of hypoxia-induced PH.

Keywords: Hypoxia, Pulmonary hypertension, miR-17-5p, PTEN, p21

Background

Pulmonary hypertension (PH) is a life-threatening disease characterized by increased pulmonary vascular resistance and pulmonary arterial pressure leading to right heart failure. Chronic obstructive pulmonary disease (COPD) is one of the most common causes of secondary PH. Pulmonary vascular remodelling in COPD is the main cause of the increase in pulmonary artery pressure and is thought to result from the combined effects of hypoxia, inflammation and a loss of capillaries in severe emphysema. The aetiology and pathogenesis of PH are complex, and factors that contribute to vascular smooth muscle cell proliferation play a central role in disease pathogenesis [1]. It is known that hypoxia is a potent stimulus associated with enhanced proliferation of pulmonary artery smooth muscle

* Correspondence: lguj2016@126.com; xuanli08@yahoo.com
†Guangjie Liu and Peng Hao contributed equally to this work.
[1]Department of Respiratory Medicine, Beijing Tongren Hospital, Capital Medical University, Beijing 100730, China
[2]Tianjin Eye Hospital, Tianjin Eye Institute, Tianjin Key Lab of Ophthalmology and Visual Science, Tianjin 300020, China
Full list of author information is available at the end of the article

cells (PASMCs), which is a major contributor to the development of hypoxic PH. Hypoxic PH is characterized by a decreased apoptosis/proliferation ratio in PASMCs and a thickened, disordered adventitia [1, 2].

MicroRNAs (miRNAs) are small noncoding transcripts of 19 to 25 nucleotides that post-transcriptionally regulate gene expression by targeting messenger RNAs (mRNAs). Their expression can be regulated in a transcriptional or post-transcriptional fashion. Following transcription and processing in the nucleus, mature miRNAs downregulate the expression of specific target mRNAs by interacting with the 3′ untranslated region (3′-UTR) of mRNA. MiRNAs regulate gene expression post-transcriptionally by either degrading target mRNAs or inhibiting their translation. It has been estimated that approximately 1,400 distinct miRNAs are encoded by the human genome and that approximately 1/3 of human genes can be regulated by miRNAs [2]. MiRNAs play important roles in the regulation of diverse cellular processes, including proliferation, differentiation, and apoptosis. Aberrant expression of miRNAs is closely associated with pathophysiologic processes, including diabetes, cancer, and cardiovascular disease [3]. Emerging data indicate that hypoxia exerts important modulatory effects on miRNAs at multiple levels of biogenesis [4]. A handful of dysregulated miRNAs have been reported in PH lung specimens from humans and animal models [5].

The miR-17-92 cluster (miR-17, miR-18a, miR-19a, miR-19b, miR-20a, and miR-92a) has been confirmed to be involved in biological development, and miR-17-5p, a member of the miR-17-19 cluster, regulates cell proliferation and migration in various cancers [6–8]. Mir-17-5p has been reported to be upregulated in various cancers and functions as an oncogenic miRNA [9]. It is strongly expressed in embryonic stem cells and has essential roles in vital processes such as cell cycle regulation, proliferation and apoptosis [10, 11]. It has been reported that miR-17-92 is downregulated in PASMCs isolated from patients with PH [12]. In addition, miR-17 and miR-20 have been reported to target bone morphogenetic protein receptor type II (BMPR2) via the STAT3-miR-17/92-BMPR2 pathway [13]. These findings suggest that miR-17 plays an important role in the regulation of PH pathogenesis. However, the mechanism of miR-17-5p modulation in PASMC proliferation in hypoxia is still unclear. In this study, we investigated the role of miR-17-5p in hypoxia-induced cellular responses in human PASMCs. We provide evidence that hypoxia upregulates the transcription of miR-17-5p and that miR-17-5p may modulate PASMC proliferation and migration via targeting phosphatase and tensin homologue (PTEN) and p21. Inhibition of miR-17-5p attenuates hypoxia-induced PASMC proliferation and migration. These data further our understanding of the regulatory

function of miR-17-5p on cell proliferation and suggest that miR-17-5p could be developed as a potential therapeutic target for PH.

Methods

Cell culture

Human pulmonary arterial smooth muscle cells (PASMCs) were purchased from Lonza. PASMCs were cultured as previously described [14]. Briefly, PASMCs from passages 3–6 were subjected to serum starvation for 24 h before being used for the experiments. The cells were grown to 70% confluence and then incubated in normoxia (21% O_2) or hypoxia (3% O_2 or 0.1% O_2) with 5% CO_2 for 24–72 h, as described in previously published studies [15, 16].

BrdU incorporation assay

A BrdU assay was conducted according to the standard protocol of the manufacturer. Cellular proliferation was evaluated by cell count directly before the assay was performed with a kit from Roche that monitors the incorporation of BrdU into newly synthesized DNA. BrdU was detected using an anti-BrdU peroxidase conjugate in accordance with the manufacturer's instructions. The amount of BrdU incorporated was determined by measuring the absorbance at 450 nm.

Cell viability evaluation

A cell count was performed using a haemocytometer after trypan blue staining. Cell viability and proliferation were evaluated using thiazolyl blue tetrazolium bromide (MTT, Sigma-Aldrich, Inc., USA) according to the manufacturer's instructions. MTT reagent was added to each sample and incubated for 3 h to allow the formation of MTT formazan. The resulting formazan was dissolved with dimethyl sulfoxide (DMSO, Sigma-Aldrich, Inc., USA), and the absorbance of each solution was measured at a wavelength of 595 nm with a microplate reader in triplicate (BioTek ELX-800 Absorbance Reader, USA).

Cell migration assay

Cell migration was monitored with a Cytation 5 Cell Imaging Multi-Mode Reader (BioTek Instruments, Inc., Winooski, VT, USA). Cytation 5 offers image capturing and time-lapse recording. Cells culture inserts (Ibidi GmbH, Martinsried, Germany) were used as barriers to create linear/rectangular gaps (500 μm × 50 μm) in sheets of PASMCs without physical wounding. The insert was then removed using a pair of sterilized forceps with one swift pull. The area devoid of cells was imaged at 2-h intervals until the cells from both sides of the bare area merged. All wound closure assays were performed in quadruplicate.

Western blot analysis

Cell lysates were prepared with RIPA buffer containing a complete protease mix (Roche). Total protein was assayed for the expression of p21, PCNA, and PTEN by western blot analysis as previously described [14]. Briefly, 50 µg of protein was subjected to SDS-PAGE and electrotransferred to a PVDF membrane. Membranes were processed as described by the manufacturer of the antibodies. The immunoreactive bands were detected by chemiluminescence (Millipore) and quantified by densitometry.

Real-time reverse transcription PCR

Total RNA was extracted using TRIzol (Invitrogen, Carlsbad, CA, USA). The amount of RNA was quantitatively determined using a Nanodrop spectrophotometer (Thermo Scientific, NJ, USA), and the total RNA was then converted to cDNA with a MultiScribe Reverse Transcriptase Kit (Applied Biosystems, Foster City, CA). The cDNA was quantified using SYBR Green Real-time PCR Master Mix (QPK-201, Toyobo, Tokyo, Japan) in an ABI 7900 PCR system (Applied Biosystems, Foster City, CA). Relative mRNA expression was normalized to GAPDH mRNA expression using the $\Delta\Delta$Ct method.

Quantification of mature miR-17-5p

Total RNA was extracted from cell samples with a mirVana Isolation Kit (Applied Biosystems, Foster City, CA). Quantitative RT-PCR was performed with a TaqMan microRNA Assay Kit using the manufacturer's protocol. Relative expression of miRNA was normalized to RNU48 expression using the $\Delta\Delta$Ct method. The primer sequences were as follows: HmiR-17-5p-forward, GCCGCCAAAGTGCT TACA, HmiR-17-5p-reverse, AGAGCAGGGTCCGAGGT; U6-forward, CTCGCTTCGGCAGCACA, U6-reverse, AA CGCTTCACGAATTTGCGT.

PASMC transfection

The miR-17-5p antagomir, the miR-17-5p agomir and their respective negative controls (NC) were obtained from GenePharma (Shanghai, China). Transfection of primary PASMCs was performed using Lipofectamine RNAiMAX Reagent (Invitrogen, Carlsbad, CA) according to the manufacturer's instructions. The microRNA agomir and antagomir were used in this experiment. The agomir of miR-17-5p used for overexpression was double stranded with the following sequence: sense ACCUGCACUGUAAGCACUUUGTT and antisense CAAAGUGCUUACAGUGAGGUAG. The miR-17-5p antagomir was single stranded with the following sequence: 5'-CUACCUGCACUGUAAGCACUUUG-3'. PASMCs were cultured in six-well plates at 70% confluence at the time of transfection.

Statistics

The data were tested for normality with Shapiro Wilk's test or the Kolmogorov-Smirnov test. All quantitative data are reported as the means ± SD. Student's t-test was used to assess differences between two means. If multiple means had to be assessed, one-way or two-way ANOVA followed by Bonferroni's post hoc test was performed. If the n number was not sufficient for normality testing, nonparametric tests (the Mann-Whitney U-test or one-way ANOVA followed by Dunn's test) were used. All statistical analyses were performed using GraphPad Prism (version 7). Statistical significance was defined as $P < 0.05$.

Results

Moderate hypoxia increases PASMC proliferation and upregulates miR-17-5p

Hypoxia plays an important role in regulating vascular smooth muscle cell proliferation. We examined the effects of oxygen tension on the proliferation of PASMCs, and our data showed that moderate hypoxia (3% oxygen) significantly increased cell proliferation as assessed by both the MTT assay and the BrdU assay (Fig. 1a and b). Figure 1b shows that moderate hypoxia induced a 26% increase in cell proliferation after 24 h and a 30% increase after 48 h compared with normoxia. However, severe hypoxia (0.1% O_2) significantly decreased cell viability at 48 h (Fig. 1a). Therefore, we investigated the effect of moderate hypoxia (3% O_2) in the following study.

To explore the role of miR-17-5p on PASMC proliferation in response to hypoxia, we performed qRT-PCR to detect the levels of miR-17-5p in PASMCs under hypoxic conditions. Compared with the expression under normoxia, the expression of miR-17-5p was significantly increased under moderate hypoxia in PASMCs (Fig. 1c). In addition, severe hypoxia (0.1% oxygen) significantly reduced miR-17-5p expression in PASMCs.

miR-17-5p plays a role in PASMC proliferation and migration

Since vascular SMC proliferation and migration are known to contribute to vascular remodelling in PH, we investigated whether miR-17-5p plays a relevant role in the regulation of PASMC proliferation and migration. We transfected PASMCs with miR-17-5p or its negative control (NC) and studied the effects of overexpressing miR-17-5p on PASMC proliferation and migration. As shown in Fig. 2a, transfection of miR-17-5p substantially increased miR-17-5p expression. Overexpression of miR-17-5p resulted in increased cell proliferation compared with that of controls, as measured by the BrdU incorporation assay (Fig. 2b). Moreover, overexpression of miR-17-5p induced proliferating cell nuclear antigen (PCNA) expression (Fig. 2c). Densitometric measurements of western blots showed that

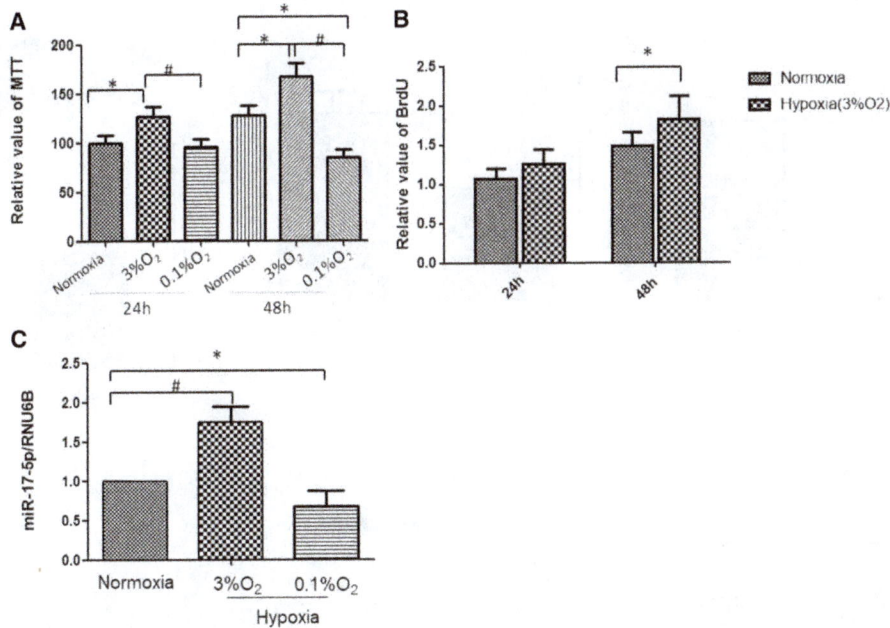

Fig. 1 Moderate hypoxia increases PASMC proliferation and upregulates miR-17-5p. **a** Cell viability was assayed by MTT assay after PASMCs were incubated under hypoxic conditions for 24 h and 48 h. **b** Cell proliferation was examined by BrdU assay. Moderate hypoxia (3% O2) stimulated PASMC proliferation. The results are the means ± SD of three independent experiments, and in each experiment, three parallel samples were analysed per group. **c** miR-17-5p levels were quantified by real-time PCR and normalized to RNU48 expression after hypoxia stimulation for 48 h. The results are the means ± SD, and the experiments were performed in triplicate and were repeated a minimum of three times. *$P < 0.05$, #$P < 0.01$

miR-17-5p overexpression significantly increased PCNA protein levels by ∼ 50%. To further confirm the effect of miR-17-5p on PASMC proliferation, we transfected cells with an miR-17-5p antagomir to inhibit miR-17-5p. Treatment with the miR-17-5p inhibitor reduced PASMC proliferation (Fig. 2d). Additionally, the expression of PCNA was decreased after transfection of PASMCs with the miR-17-5p antagomir (Fig. 2e).

To investigate the role of miR-17-5p in PASMC migration, we used a non-traumatic migration assay under a time-lapse microscope. As shown in Fig. 3, the upregulation of miR-17-5p promoted PASMC migration compared to the migration of control cells. MiR-17-5p overexpression induced an ∼ 16% increase in the cell-covered area after 12 h, whereas the downregulation of miR-17-5p expression inhibited migration by ∼ 10% after 12 h (Fig. 3a, b, c and d). These results indicated that miR-17-5p plays a role in PASMC proliferation and migration.

miR-17-5p regulates the expression of proteins involved in cell cycle progression, cell proliferation and apoptosis in PASMCs in vitro

PTEN, p21, BIM (Bcl-2-like protein 11, Bcl2l11), and BMPR2 have been reported as miR-17-92 cluster targets [13, 17–19]. We found that the inhibition of miR-17-5p by transfection with an miR-17-5p inhibitor caused the upregulation of PTEN, p21, BIM, and BMPR2 in

PASMCs at the mRNA level. Western blot analysis also showed that the protein levels of PTEN and p21 were increased by transfection with the miR-17-5p inhibitor (Fig. 4a and b). In contrast, overexpression of miR-17-5p in PASMCs resulted in the downregulation of PTEN and p21 at the protein level under normoxic or hypoxic conditions (Fig. 4c and d). Importantly, further studies showed that transfection of an miR-17-5p agomir into PASMCs induced the expression of proliferation-related genes, including Cyclin D1, Cyclin-dependent kinase (CDK) 4, CDK6, Ki67, and PCNA (Fig. 4f). These results indicated that miR-17-5p could mediate PASMC proliferation by regulating its targets, PTEN, BMPR2, and p21, which negatively control cell growth. In addition, inhibition of miR-17-5p reduced the expression of collagen type I and collagen type III in PASMCs, suggesting the potential of miR-17-5p to act as a target for the prevention of pulmonary vascular remodelling.

Effect of hypoxia on miR-17-5p predicted targets

Moderate hypoxia increases PASMC proliferation by regulating some genes involved in cell proliferation and apoptosis. Gene expression profiling was used to identify hypoxia-modulated genes. As shown in Fig. 5a, we found that moderate hypoxia induced the upregulation of pro-proliferative genes, including ki67 and MAPK2; several anti-proliferative genes, including p21, BMP2, and

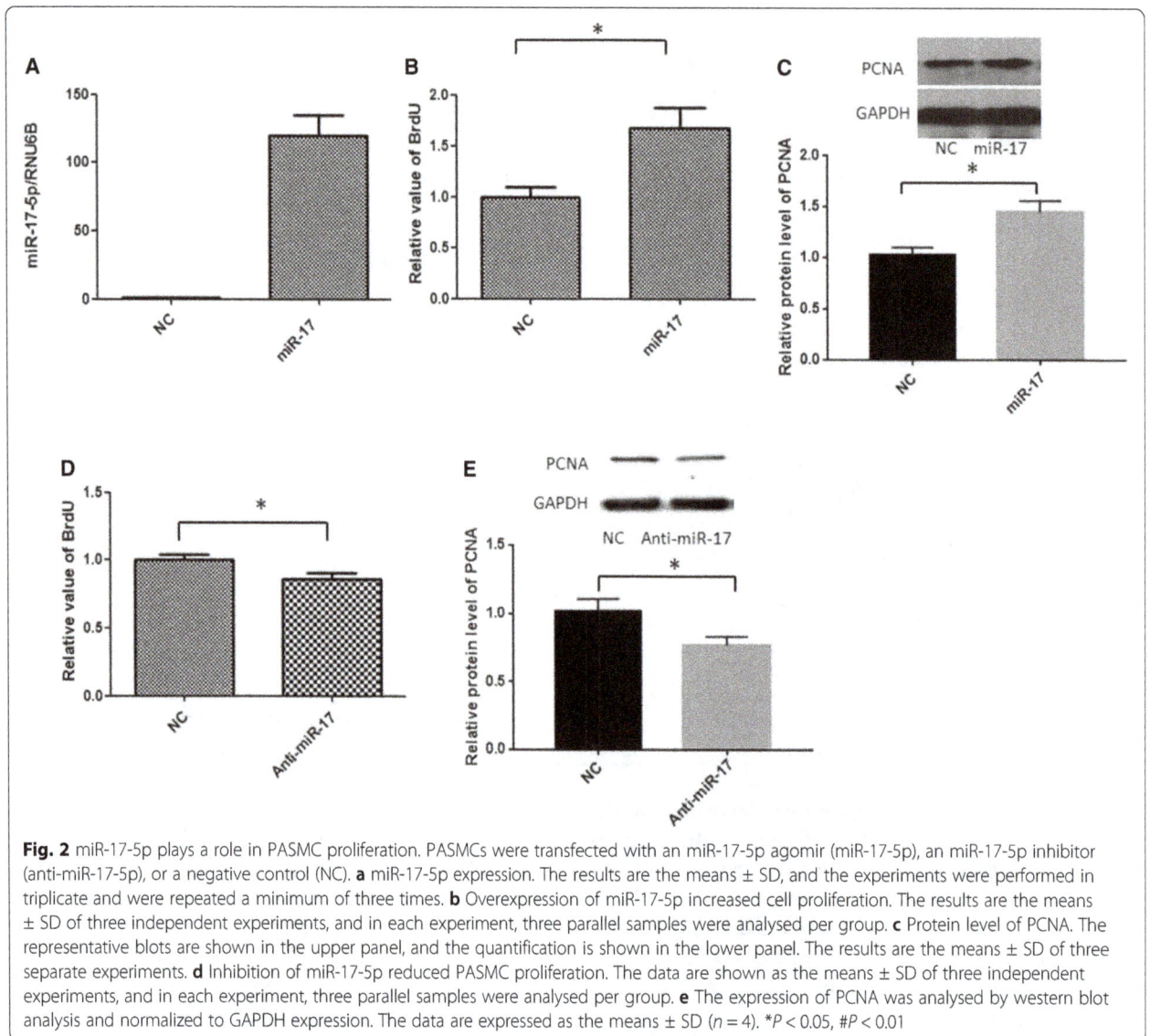

Fig. 2 miR-17-5p plays a role in PASMC proliferation. PASMCs were transfected with an miR-17-5p agomir (miR-17-5p), an miR-17-5p inhibitor (anti-miR-17-5p), or a negative control (NC). **a** miR-17-5p expression. The results are the means ± SD, and the experiments were performed in triplicate and were repeated a minimum of three times. **b** Overexpression of miR-17-5p increased cell proliferation. The results are the means ± SD of three independent experiments, and in each experiment, three parallel samples were analysed per group. **c** Protein level of PCNA. The representative blots are shown in the upper panel, and the quantification is shown in the lower panel. The results are the means ± SD of three separate experiments. **d** Inhibition of miR-17-5p reduced PASMC proliferation. The data are shown as the means ± SD of three independent experiments, and in each experiment, three parallel samples were analysed per group. **e** The expression of PCNA was analysed by western blot analysis and normalized to GAPDH expression. The data are expressed as the means ± SD ($n = 4$). *$P < 0.05$, #$P < 0.01$

PTEN, were downregulated. Exposure to moderate hypoxia caused PASMC proliferation accompanied by the upregulation of miR-17-5p and the downregulation of p21, PTEN, and BMP2. The results showed that the expression of miR-17-5p was negatively correlated with the levels of anti-proliferation genes, including p21, PTEN, and BMP2, in PASMCs under hypoxia stimulation. Among these genes, both PTEN and p21 have been identified as miR-17-5p target genes. We therefore measured the protein levels of these two miR-17 targets in cell lysates obtained from PASMCs exposed to normoxia or hypoxia. As shown in Fig. 5b, hypoxia significantly reduced the protein levels of p21 and PTEN. In addition, inhibition of miR-17-5p reduced cell proliferation in both normoxia and hypoxia (Fig. 5c). In accordance with the results of the BrdU assay, PCNA protein expression, as determined by western blot analysis, was increased in

PASMCs under hypoxia stimulation (3% O2). Furthermore, the expression of PCNA was increased in PASMCs when miR-17-5p was overexpressed using the miR-17-5p agomir. On the other hand, inhibition of miR-17-5p by the miR-17-5p antagomir transfection decreased PCNA expression in PASMCs (Fig. 5d). These results suggested that miR-17-5p might play an important role in mediating hypoxia-induced PASMC proliferation and migration via targeting p21 and PTEN.

Discussion

The miR-17-92 cluster is located in the locus of the non-protein-coding gene MIR17HG (the miR-17/92 cluster host gene, also known as C13orf25) [20]. The miR-17-92 cluster has been well studied in various cancer cells. It is known that C-MYC is involved in activating MIR17HG transcription. The miR-17-92 cluster is

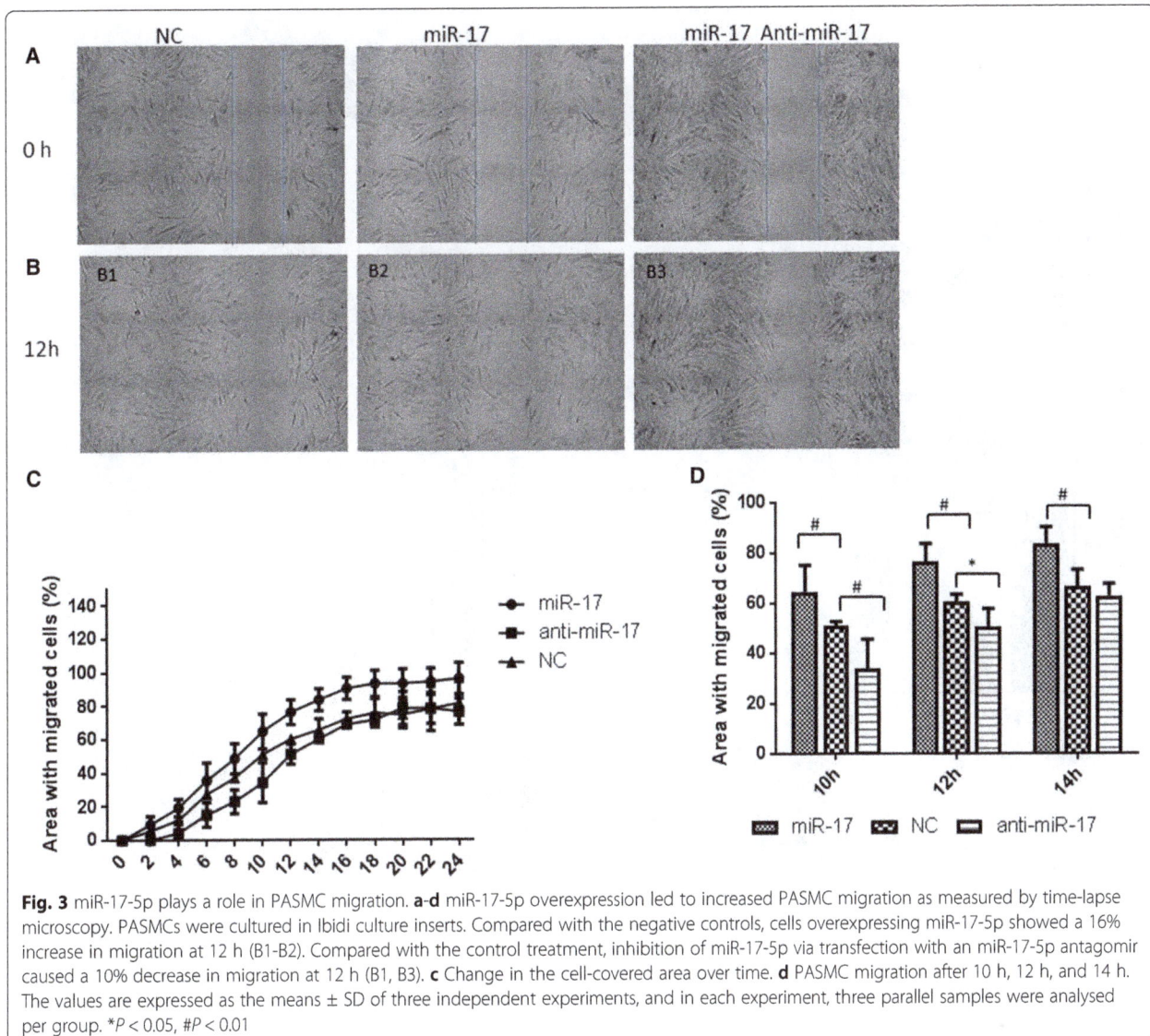

Fig. 3 miR-17-5p plays a role in PASMC migration. **a-d** miR-17-5p overexpression led to increased PASMC migration as measured by time-lapse microscopy. PASMCs were cultured in Ibidi culture inserts. Compared with the negative controls, cells overexpressing miR-17-5p showed a 16% increase in migration at 12 h (B1-B2). Compared with the control treatment, inhibition of miR-17-5p via transfection with an miR-17-5p antagomir caused a 10% decrease in migration at 12 h (B1, B3). **c** Change in the cell-covered area over time. **d** PASMC migration after 10 h, 12 h, and 14 h. The values are expressed as the means ± SD of three independent experiments, and in each experiment, three parallel samples were analysed per group. *$P < 0.05$, #$P < 0.01$

important in cell cycle progression, proliferation, apoptosis and other pivotal processes [9, 21]. The miR-17-92 cluster has been linked to vascular pathogenesis, including that of coronary artery disease and PH [5, 12]. However, the function of this locus in PASMCs is still unclear. In the present study, we demonstrated that miR-17-5p, a single miRNA from this locus, induces PASMC proliferation and migration. Previous studies have indicated that miR-17-5p is often upregulated in various cancers and is correlated with cell cycle progression, apoptosis and proliferation [11, 22]. Here, we found that miR-17-5p was upregulated in PASMCs by hypoxia stimulation. Hypoxia is a well-known stimulus for the development of PH. Hypoxia promotes pulmonary arterial wall remodelling via the induction of cell proliferation in all three layers, particularly in smooth muscle cells. Our data provide evidence that hypoxia induces the

upregulation of miR-17-5p in PASMCs. miR-17-5p promotes PASMC proliferation and migration, while inhibiting miR-17-5p attenuates PASMC proliferation and collagen synthesis. These findings are consistent with those of a previous study reporting that the miR-17-92 cluster can induce both PASMC proliferation and differentiation and that SMC-specific knockout of miR-17-92 attenuates hypoxia-induced PH in mice [12]. However, the roles of miR-17-5p in PASMCs may be more complex than previously assumed, and further in vivo functional studies are needed to establish its specific role in PH pathogenesis.

The expression patterns of miRNAs are regulated by many factors, among which hypoxia is well known to alter the expression of a number of miRNAs [4, 23]. Caruso et al. reported that chronic hypoxia reduced the expression of Dicer. Dicer is involved in miRNA

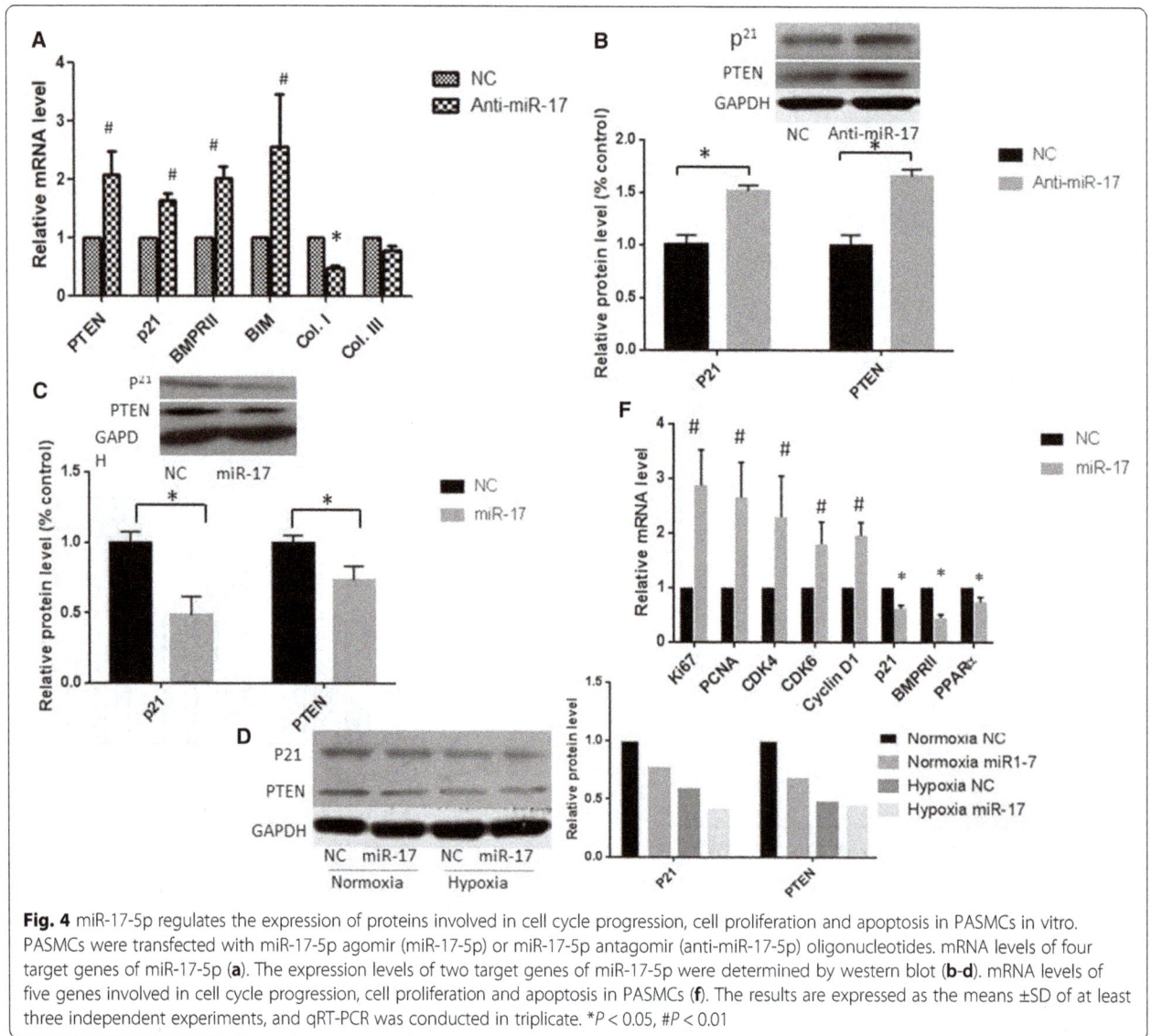

Fig. 4 miR-17-5p regulates the expression of proteins involved in cell cycle progression, cell proliferation and apoptosis in PASMCs in vitro. PASMCs were transfected with miR-17-5p agomir (miR-17-5p) or miR-17-5p antagomir (anti-miR-17-5p) oligonucleotides. mRNA levels of four target genes of miR-17-5p (**a**). The expression levels of two target genes of miR-17-5p were determined by western blot (**b-d**). mRNA levels of five genes involved in cell cycle progression, cell proliferation and apoptosis in PASMCs (**f**). The results are expressed as the means ±SD of at least three independent experiments, and qRT-PCR was conducted in triplicate. *$P < 0.05$, #$P < 0.01$

processing and may cause the downregulation of a number of miRNAs in rat PH induced by hypoxia and monocrotaline (MCT) [24]. Abnormal miR-17-92 expression in PH has been reported in previous studies [12, 13, 25]. Chen T and coworkers reported that miR-17-92 is downregulated in PASMCs isolated from patients with PH, and the reduced expression of miR-17-97 is associated with decreased levels of the dedifferentiated smooth muscle cell phenotype [12]. Pullamsetti and colleagues reported that miR-17 is transiently upregulated in the hypoxia-induced PH mouse model [25]. Consistent with this report, miR-17-5p was found to be upregulated under hypoxia at 48 h in PASMCs in vitro in this study. These results implied that the regulation of miRNAs by hypoxia might be different according to the details of the experimental conditions, cell types, and both the duration and the degree of reduced oxygen tension. Our

results demonstrate that miR-17-5p expression increases after acute hypoxia in PASMCs in vitro and that overexpression of miR-17-5p promotes PASMC proliferation. Therefore, it appears that the miR-17 cluster is upregulated in the initial stage and serves as a promoter for vascular smooth muscle cell proliferation during the remodelling phase. Further studies should investigate the time course of miR-17-5p expression in PH models in vivo.

Hypoxia is thought to be a cause of pulmonary vascular remodelling and PASMC proliferation. Cell cycle progression is dependent on the expression and activation of specific CDK enzymes, which form complexes with their regulatory subunits, the cyclins. The cyclin-CDK complexes formed in cell cycle progression are regulated by CDK inhibitors, such as p21/Cip1 and p27/Kip1. p21 is a cell cycle inhibitor that inhibits the

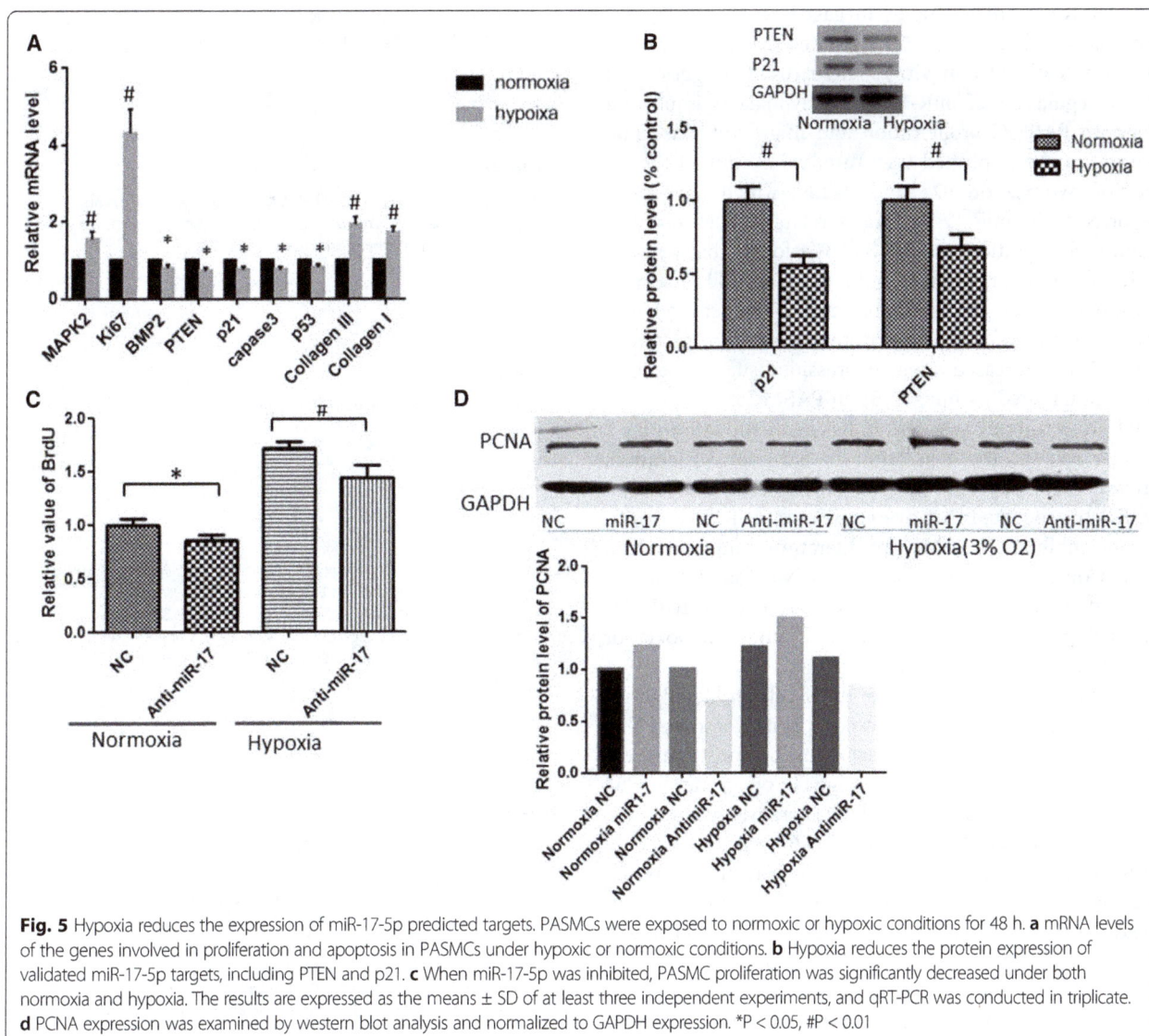

Fig. 5 Hypoxia reduces the expression of miR-17-5p predicted targets. PASMCs were exposed to normoxic or hypoxic conditions for 48 h. **a** mRNA levels of the genes involved in proliferation and apoptosis in PASMCs under hypoxic or normoxic conditions. **b** Hypoxia reduces the protein expression of validated miR-17-5p targets, including PTEN and p21. **c** When miR-17-5p was inhibited, PASMC proliferation was significantly decreased under both normoxia and hypoxia. The results are expressed as the means ± SD of at least three independent experiments, and qRT-PCR was conducted in triplicate. **d** PCNA expression was examined by western blot analysis and normalized to GAPDH expression. *P < 0.05, #P < 0.01

activity of cyclin-CDK2, CDK1, and CDK4/6. Current research implies that p21 may represent a major target for new therapies targeting PASMC proliferation during the progression of PH [26]. Moderate hypoxia has been found to enhance the proliferation of PASMCs via the p21 pathway, whereas severe hypoxia (0.1% oxygen) leads to cell cycle arrest via the p53-p21 pathway [27]. Consistent with previous reports, our present study demonstrated that 3% oxygen induced PASMC proliferation and migration accompanied by decreased expression of p21. In addition, we found that 3% oxygen induced the expression of miR-17-5p. The miR-17-92 cluster has been reported to be a target for p53-mediated transcriptional repression under severe hypoxia [16]. In line with this finding, we found that 0.1% oxygen reduced miR-17-5p expression. These results suggest that miR-17-5p is involved in mediating hypoxia-induced cell proliferation and apoptosis. The

miR-17-5p target p21 may regulate moderate hypoxia-induced cell proliferation.

We demonstrated that moderate hypoxia caused PASMC proliferation accompanied by the upregulation of miR-17 and downregulation of p21, PTEN, and BMP2. It has been reported that PTEN, p21, and BMPRII are the targets of the miR-17-92 cluster [17, 18, 28]. There is evidence indicating that miR-17 represses BMP signalling by targeting BMPRII [28]. PTEN and p21 have been identified as anti-proliferation genes. Furthermore, it has been reported that BMP2 inhibits cell proliferation via p21 in human aortic smooth muscle cells. Additionally, BMP2 has been reported to induce PTEN expression in PASMCs under hypoxia [29–31]. Our results are consistent with the findings of these studies.

The migration of proliferating vascular smooth muscle cells is a crucial factor in PH. In this study, we found that miR-17-5p plays an important role in the migration of PASMCs. Similar studies in gastric cancer cells [32] have shown that miR-17-5p regulates the gastric cancer cell line SGC-7901 in vitro. These results suggest that the upregulation of miR-17-5p in hypoxia is important for both PASMC proliferation and migration. Based on reports in the published literature, we examined the effect of hypoxia on p21 and PTEN, which have been reported to be miR-17-5p targets related to cell proliferation and migration [17, 18, 33]. We found that hypoxia reduced the expression of both p21 and PTEN. Under normoxia, overexpression of miR-17-5p caused decreased expression of these proteins, and knockdown of miR-17-5p increased their expression, suggesting that they are targeted by miR-17-5p in PASMCs.

PTEN, a tumour suppressor, has been shown to play a crucial role in the regulation of adhesion, migration, growth and apoptosis. Jianhua Huang and Christopher D. Kontos reported that overexpression of PTEN significantly inhibited PASMC proliferation and migration [34]. Consistent with these results, we found that decreased expression of PTEN was correlated with increased proliferation and migration under hypoxia or after transfection with miR-17-5p.

We examined the mRNA levels of cell proliferation-related genes in PASMCs transfected with an miR-17-5p antagomir or agomir. Consistent with the constitutive expression of miR-17-5p being potentially oncogenic [9, 35], the mRNA expression of pro-proliferative genes (ki67, PCNA, cyclin D1, CDK4, and CDK6) was increased in miR-17-5p-overexpressing PASMCs, representing a proliferative signal. Inhibition of miR-17-5p significantly upregulated the mRNA levels of genes including p21, PTEN, and BMPR2, which are confirmed as targets of miR-17-5p. The suppression of these target genes is consistent with the pro-proliferative phenotype observed in PASMCs overexpressing miR-17-5p.

Conclusion

In summary, miR-17-5p, a single miRNA, could drive a proliferative phenotype in PASMCs. Moderate hypoxia increases the expression of miR-17-5p, which is involved in cell proliferation and migration via the targeting the PTEN and p21 genes in PASMCs. Inhibition of miR-17-5p attenuates hypoxia-induced PASMC proliferation and migration. These data further our understanding of the regulatory function of miR-17-5p on cell proliferation and suggest that miR-17-5p could be developed as a potential therapeutic target for PH.

Acknowledgements
We are grateful to Xi Chen for technical assistance during the experiments.

Funding
This study was supported by grants from the Beijing Natural Science Foundation (7153164), the National Natural Science Foundation of China (81170828), the Tianjin Science & Technology Foundation (15JCZDJC35300), and the Tianjin Health and Family Planning Communication Foundation (14KG133).

Authors' contributions
Acquisition of data: GL, PH, LW, RH, YW, MY, SS, and JL. Analysis and interpretation of data: GL and JX. Drafting of manuscript: XL and GL. All authors read and approved the final manuscript.

Competing interests
The authors declare that they have no competing interests.

Author details
[1]Department of Respiratory Medicine, Beijing Tongren Hospital, Capital Medical University, Beijing 100730, China. [2]Tianjin Eye Hospital, Tianjin Eye Institute, Tianjin Key Lab of Ophthalmology and Visual Science, Tianjin 300020, China. [3]Clinical College of Ophthalmology, Tianjin Medical University, Tianjin 300020, China. [4]Nankai University Affiliated Eye Hospital, Tianjin 300020, China.

References
1. Hanze J, Weissmann N, Grimminger F, Seeger W, Rose F. Cellular and molecular mechanisms of hypoxia-inducible factor driven vascular remodeling. Thromb Haemost. 2007;97:774–87.
2. Esteller M. Non-coding RNAs in human disease. Nat Rev Genet. 2011;12: 861–74. https://doi.org/10.1038/nrg3074.
3. Cordes KR, Srivastava D. MicroRNA regulation of cardiovascular development. Circ Res. 2009;104:724–32. https://doi.org/10.1161/CIRCRESAHA.108.192872.
4. Nallamshetty S, Chan SY, Loscalzo J. Hypoxia: a master regulator of microRNA biogenesis and activity. Free Radic Biol Med. 2013;64:20–30. https://doi.org/10.1016/j.freeradbiomed.2013.05.022.
5. Bienertova-Vasku J, Novak J, Vasku A. MicroRNAs in pulmonary arterial hypertension: pathogenesis, diagnosis and treatment. J Am Soc Hypertens. 2015;9:221–34. https://doi.org/10.1016/j.jash.2014.12.011.
6. Concepcion CP, Bonetti C, Ventura A. The microRNA-17-92 family of microRNA clusters in development and disease. Cancer J. 2012;18:262–7. https://doi.org/10.1097/PPO.0b013e318258b60a.
7. Gu R, et al. MicroRNA-17 family as novel biomarkers for cancer diagnosis: a meta-analysis based on 19 articles. Tumour Biol. 2016;37:6403–11. https://doi.org/10.1007/s13277-015-4484-x.
8. Zhou G, Chen T, Raj JU. MicroRNAs in pulmonary arterial hypertension. Am J Respir Cell Mol Biol. 2015;52:139–51. https://doi.org/10.1165/rcmb.2014-0166TR.
9. Jin HY, et al. MicroRNA-17~92 plays a causative role in lymphomagenesis by coordinating multiple oncogenic pathways. EMBO J. 2013;32:2377–91. https://doi.org/10.1038/emboj.2013.178.
10. Lu Y, Okubo T, Rawlins E, Hogan BL. Epithelial progenitor cells of the embryonic lung and the role of microRNAs in their proliferation. Proc Am Thorac Soc. 2008;5:300–4. https://doi.org/10.1513/pats.200710-162DR.
11. Dellago H, Bobbili MR, Grillari J. MicroRNA-17-5p: at the crossroads of Cancer and aging - a mini-review. Gerontology. 2017;63:20–8. https://doi.org/10.1159/000447773.
12. Chen T, et al. Loss of microRNA-17 approximately 92 in smooth muscle cells attenuates experimental pulmonary hypertension via induction of PDZ and LIM domain 5. Am J Respir Crit Care Med. 2015;191:678–92. https://doi.org/10.1164/rccm.201405-0941OC.

Upregulation of microRNA-17-5p contributes to hypoxia-induced proliferation in human pulmonary...

129

13. Brock M, et al. Interleukin-6 modulates the expression of the bone morphogenic protein receptor type II through a novel STAT3-microRNA cluster 17/92 pathway. Circ Res. 2009;104:1184–91. https://doi.org/10.1161/CIRCRESAHA.109.197491.

14. Liu G, et al. PPARdelta agonist GW501516 inhibits PDGF-stimulated pulmonary arterial smooth muscle cell function related to pathological vascular remodeling. Biomed Res Int. 2013;2013:903947. https://doi.org/10.1155/2013/903947.

15. Mizuno S, Toga H, Ishizaki T. Current Basic and Pathological Approaches to the Function of Muscle Cells and Tissues – From Molecules to Humans Chapter 17 Hypoxic Pulmonary Vascular Smooth Muscle Cell Proliferation. 2012. p. 379-90.

16. Yan HL, et al. Repression of the miR-17-92 cluster by p53 has an important function in hypoxia-induced apoptosis. EMBO J. 2009;28:2719–32. https://doi.org/10.1038/emboj.2009.214.

17. Wu SY, et al. MicroRNA-17-5p post-transcriptionally regulates p21 expression in irradiated betel quid chewing-related oral squamous cell carcinoma cells. Strahlentherapie und Onkologie : Organ der Deutschen Rontgengesellschaft. 2013;189:675–83. https://doi.org/10.1007/s00066-013-0347-9.

18. Fang L, et al. MicroRNA-17-5p promotes chemotherapeutic drug resistance and tumour metastasis of colorectal cancer by repressing PTEN expression. Oncotarget. 2014;5:2974–87. https://doi.org/10.18632/oncotarget.1614.

19. Meng XW, Kaufmann SH. Bim regulation miRrors microRNA 17 approximately 92 cluster expression in endothelial cells in vivo. Cell Death Differ. 2014;21:1665–6. https://doi.org/10.1038/cdd.2014.127.

20. Mogilyansky E, Rigoutsos I. The miR-17/92 cluster: a comprehensive update on its genomics, genetics, functions and increasingly important and numerous roles in health and disease. Cell Death Differ. 2013;20:1603–14. https://doi.org/10.1038/cdd.2013.125.

21. Marrone AK, et al. MicroRNA-17~92 is required for nephrogenesis and renal function. J Am Soc Nephrol. 2014;25:1440–52. https://doi.org/10.1681/ASN.2013040390.

22. Hao J, et al. Induction of microRNA-17-5p by p53 protects against renal ischemia-reperfusion injury by targeting death receptor 6. Kidney Int. 2017; 91:106–18. https://doi.org/10.1016/j.kint.2016.07.017.

23. Bandara V, Michael MZ, Gleadle JM. Hypoxia represses microRNA biogenesis proteins in breast cancer cells. BMC Cancer. 2014;14:533. https://doi.org/10.1186/1471-2407-14-533.

24. Caruso P, et al. Dynamic changes in lung microRNA profiles during the development of pulmonary hypertension due to chronic hypoxia and monocrotaline. Arterioscler Thromb Vasc Biol. 2010;30:716–23. https://doi.org/10.1161/atvbaha.109.202028.

25. Pullamsetti SS, et al. Inhibition of microRNA-17 improves lung and heart function in experimental pulmonary hypertension. Am J Respir Crit Care Med. 2012;185:409–19. https://doi.org/10.1164/rccm.201106-1093OC.

26. Abid S, et al. P21-dependent protective effects of a carbon monoxide-releasing molecule-3 in pulmonary hypertension. Arterioscler Thromb Vasc Biol. 2014;34:304–12. https://doi.org/10.1161/atvbaha.113.302302.

27. Mizuno S, et al. Hypoxia regulates human lung fibroblast proliferation via p53-dependent and -independent pathways. Respir Res. 2009;10:17. https://doi.org/10.1186/1465-9921-10-17.

28. Mao S, et al. miR-17 regulates the proliferation and differentiation of the neural precursor cells during mouse corticogenesis. FEBS J. 2014;281:1144–58. https://doi.org/10.1111/febs.12680.

29. Pi W, Guo X, Su L, Xu W. BMP-2 up-regulates PTEN expression and induces apoptosis of pulmonary artery smooth muscle cells under hypoxia. PLoS One. 2012;7:e35283. https://doi.org/10.1371/journal.pone.0035283.

30. Waite KA, Eng C. BMP2 exposure results in decreased PTEN protein degradation and increased PTEN levels. Hum Mol Genet. 2003;12:679–84.

31. Wong GA, Tang V, El-Sabeawy F, Weiss RH. BMP-2 inhibits proliferation of human aortic smooth muscle cells via p21Cip1/Waf1. Am J Physiol Endocrinol Metab. 2003;284:E972–9. https://doi.org/10.1152/ajpendo.00385.2002.

32. Chen P, et al. MicroRNA-17-5p promotes gastric cancer proliferation, migration and invasion by directly targeting early growth response 2. Am J Cancer Res. 2016;6:2010–20.

33. Li JF, et al. Hypoxia-induced miR-17-5p ameliorates the viability reduction of astrocytes via targeting p21. Eur Rev Med Pharmacol Sci. 2016;20:3051–9.

34. Huang J, Niu XL, Pippen AM, Annex BH, Kontos CD. Adenovirus-mediated intraarterial delivery of PTEN inhibits neointimal hyperplasia. Arterioscler Thromb Vasc Biol. 2005;25:354–8. https://doi.org/10.1161/01.ATV.0000151619.54108.a5.

35. Kim K, et al. Identification of oncogenic microRNA-17-92/ZBTB4/specificity protein axis in breast cancer. Oncogene. 2012;31:1034–44. https://doi.org/10.1038/onc.2011.296.

14

Efficacy and safety of antagonists for chemoattractant receptor-homologous molecule expressed on Th2 cells in adult patients with asthma

Jing Yang[1,2†], Jian Luo[1†], Ling Yang[1], Dan Yang[1], Dan Wang[1], Bicui Liu[1], Tingxuan Huang[1], Xiaohu Wang[1], Binmiao Liang[1*] and Chuntao Liu[1] (iD)

Abstract

Background: Chemoattractant receptor-homologous molecule expressed on Th2 cells (CRTH2) antagonists are novel agents for asthma but with controversial efficacies in clinical trials. Therefore, we conducted a meta-analysis to determine the roles of CRTH2 antagonists in asthma.

Methods: We searched in major databases for RCTs comparing CRTH2 antagonists with placebo in asthma. Fixed- or random-effects model was performed to calculate mean differences (MD), risk ratio (RR) or risk difference (RD) and 95% confidence interval (CI).

Results: A total of 14 trails with 4671 participants were included in our final analysis. Instead of add-on treatment of CRTH2 antagonists to corticosteroids, CRTH2 antagonist monotherapy significantly improved pre-bronchodilator FEV_1 (MD = 0.09, 95% CI 0.04 to 0.15, $P = 0.0005$), FEV_1% predicted (MD = 3.65, 95% CI 1.15 to 6.14, $P = 0.004$), and AQLQ (MD = 0.25, 95% CI 0.09 to 0.41, $P = 0.002$), and reduced asthma exacerbations (RR = 0.45, 95% CI 0.23 to 0.85, $P = 0.01$). Rescue use of SABA was significantly decreased in both CRTH2 antagonist monotherapy (MD = − 0.04, 95% CI -0.05 to − 0.03, $P < 0.00001$) and as add-on to corticosteroids (MD = − 0.78, 95% CI -1.47 to − 0.09, $P = 0.03$). Adverse events were similar between the intervention and placebo groups.

Conclusions: CRTH2 antagonist monotherapy can safely improve lung function and quality of life, and reduce asthma exacerbations and SABA use in asthmatics.

Keywords: Asthma, CRTH2 antagonist, Lung function, Adverse events, Meta-analysis, Systematic review

Introduction

Asthma is a common respiratory disease characterized by chronic airway inflammation, airway hyperresponsiveness, and reversible airflow limitation, which affects more than 300 million people worldwide and imposes a considerable social and economic burdens [1]. Most of patients can be effectively controlled by inhaled corticosteroids, the first-line therapy as recommended by the Global Initiative for Asthma (GINA) guideline [2], however, at least 40% of asthmatics remain inadequately controlled in spite of treatment with high dose of inhaled corticosteroids [3]. Moreover, a clear association between risk of adverse effects and long-term use of corticosteroid has also been observed [4], therefore, novel therapeutics is warranted to improve symptoms control and avoid overuse of steroids.

The chemoattractant receptor-homologous molecule expressed on Th2 cells (CRTH2) is a G-protein coupled

* Correspondence: liangbm0202@yahoo.com; ChuntaoLiu2018@163.com
†Jing Yang and Jian Luo contributed equally to this work.
[1]Department of Respiratory and Critical Care Medicine, West China School of Medicine and West China Hospital, Sichuan University, No.37, Guoxue Alley, Chengdu 610041, China
Full list of author information is available at the end of the article

receptor, and it is reported to be crucial in asthma development due to the chemotaxis of type 2 helper T cells and eosinophils, delay in cell apoptosis, as well as production of proinflammatory cytokines including interleukin-4, 5, and 13 by the activation of prostaglandin D_2 (PGD_2) [5–7]. Accumulating evidence has shown that the blockade of CRTH2 receptor significantly reduces allergic airway inflammation in animal models [8–10], but inconsistent efficacy and safety profiles of CRTH2 antagonists are noticed in clinical trials. Barnes and his colleagues [11] for the first time reported that OC000459, a CRTH2 antagonist, significantly improved quality of life but had no effect on lung function and airway inflammation in patients with asthma, while a significant improvement of forced volume in one second (FEV_1) [12] and inhibition of post-allergen increase in sputum eosinophils [13] but no relief of asthma symptoms in symptomatic controller-naïve asthmatics [14] were reported by subsequent studies.

Based on the current controversial and ambiguous findings in the treatment of patients with asthma by CRTH2 antagonists, we conducted a meta-analysis and systematic review of all available randomized controlled trials (RCTs) to further determine the roles of CRTH2 antagonists in asthmatics.

Methods

Search strategies

A comprehensive computer search was conducted in Cochrane Central Register of Controlled Trials (CENTRAL), Pubmed, Medline, Embase, ISI Web of Science and American College of Physician (ACP) between 1946 and September 2018 by using the keywords of "CRTH2" or "chemoattractant receptor-homologous molecule expressed on TH2 cells" or "chemoattractant receptor expressed on TH2 cells" or "DP2" or "prostaglandin D2 receptor" and "antagonist" or "inhibitor" and "asthma". Publication type and species were limited to RCTs and humans, respectively, but we did not limit the publication language. References listed in each identified article were checked and the related articles were searched manually to identify all eligible studies and minimize the potential publication bias.

Inclusion and exclusion criteria

Eligible clinical trials were identified based on the following criteria: 1) asthma was diagnosed by physicians according to the GINA guideline [2] with the evidence of airway hyperresponsiveness (the provocation concentration of methacholine causing a 20% fall in FEV_1 (methacholine PC_{20}) < 16 mg/mL) and/or bronchodilator responsiveness (an increase of FEV_1% predicted > 12% and FEV_1 > 200 mL following inhalation of 200 µg salbutamol); 2) age was not less than 18 and smoking history was no more than 10 pack-years; 3) study designs were randomized placebo-controlled trials; 4) intervention

treatment was oral CRTH2 antagonists regardless of dose, frequency, and durations; 5) outcomes included but not limited to lung function, asthma control and quality of life scores, sputum and blood eosinophil count, fractional exhaled nitric oxide (FeNO), asthma exacerbations, rescue use of short-acting β_2 agonists (SABA), and adverse events. Retrospective, observational, cohort or case control studies were excluded.

Study selection

Two investigators independently performed the study selection in two phases. First, they screened the titles and abstracts of all identified studies to discard duplicated and nonrandomized controlled studies. Then, eligible studies were extracted by reviewing full texts according to the previously defined study inclusion and exclusion criteria. Disagreements were resolved by consensus or consulting a third investigator.

Data extraction and quality assessment

Two investigators independently and separately conducted the data extraction and quality assessment. Data from eligible studies were extracted in a standard form recommended by Cochrane [15] including authors, publication year, study design, participant characteristics, population, interventions, concomitant treatment, outcome measures and study results. Cochrane risk of bias tool was used to assess the risk of bias in estimating the study outcomes. Each study was assessed for: 1) random sequence generation; 2) allocation concealment; 3) blinding of participants and personnel; 4) blinding of related outcomes assessment; 5) incomplete outcome data; 6) selective reporting; and 7) other biases. For any missing data or information, we contacted corresponding authors by e-mail to request the full original data. Any divergence was resolved by mutual consensus in the presence of a third investigator.

Statistical analysis

Statistical analysis was accomplished by an independent statistician using Cochrane systematic review software Review Manager (RevMan; Version 5.3.5, the Cochrane Collaboration) and Stata (version 14.0, Stata Corporation, USA). P value < 0.05 was defined as statistical significance and the results were showed in forest plots. We conducted a systematic review when data could not be pooled in meta-analysis.

Continuous variables were expressed as mean and standard deviation (SD), while dichotomous variables were shown as frequency and proportion. Mean differences (MD) and 95% confidence interval (CI) were calculated for continuous data, and risk ratio (RR) or risk difference (RD) combined with 95% CI for dichotomous data. If a study presents more than two interventions, they were combined into a single intervention group according to the Cochrane handbook [15]. Heterogeneity was quantified by I^2 statistic and chi-squared test with $P < 0.1$ and $I^2 > 50\%$ indicating significant heterogeneity. Random-effects model was applied in the statistical heterogeneity; otherwise fixed-effects model was used. Publication bias was tested by Funnel plot with Egger's and Begg's tests. All analyses were conducted based on the intention-to-treat principle. The potential influence of pre-specified factors, such as types of CRTH2 antagonists, presence of concomitant treatment, treatment duration, asthma severity, on the effect estimates was further explored via random-effects model meta-regression when an outcome of interest was reported by at least three RCTs in each subgroup.

Results

A total of 659 potentially relevant articles were identified, and 490 articles were screened for eligibility after removal of 169 duplicate records. After reviewing the titles and abstracts, we identified and retrieved 34 studies for later full-text assessment due to the discard of non-RCTs $(n = 253)$, animal experiments $(n = 90)$, non-CRTH2 antagonists $(n = 87)$, non-asthmatic patients $(n = 18)$, and others going against our inclusion criteria $(n = 8)$. Finally, 14 studies were included for our systematic review and meta-analysis because 20 studies were excluded owing to abstract form of included studies $(n = 12)$ and insufficient data for analysis $(n = 8)$. (Fig. 1).

Study characteristics

The characteristics of included RCTs and baseline characteristics of the patients enrolled were summarized in Table 1 and Table 2, respectively. There were eleven [11, 12, 14, 16–23]parallel and three [13, 24, 25] crossover RCTs, and twelve RCTs were designed as multicenter trials [11–14, 16–18, 21–25]. Overall, 4671 participants were included, among which 2581 patients were assigned to receive CRTH2 antagonists, while 2090 patients were administered placebo. Different trials reported inconsistent types of CRTH2 antagonists: 3 for OC000459 [11–13], 3 for Fivipiprant (QAW039) [16, 18, 20], 2 for BI 671800 [14, 25] and AZD1981 [21, 23], and 1 for Setipiprant [24], AMG 853 [17], ARRY-502 [22], and BI 1021958 [19]. Corticosteroids were used as concomitant treatments by all participants in seven trials [14, 16, 17, 20, 21, 23, 25] and SABA was allowed if necessary in all trails. Treatment duration ranged from 5 days to 12 weeks and follow-up varied from 15 days to about 24 weeks.

The mean age of the participants ranged from 33.1 to 50 years old, and the mean $FEV_1\%$ predicted values at baseline was between 64.2 and 85.2%. Body mass index (BMI) was reported to be from 24.2 to 32.0 kg/m^2 in 11 studies [14, 16–25], and FeNO varied from 30.0 to

51.6 ppb in 5 studies [13, 17, 18, 20, 24]. All participants were non-smokers or ex-smokers with a smoking history ≤10 pack-years. One study [24] only included male participants, and eight studies [11, 13, 16, 18, 21–24] enrolled allergic asthmatics. Four studies [17, 20, 21, 23] involved patients with moderate-to-severe asthma, eight studies [11–14, 18, 19, 22, 25] included patients with mild to moderate asthma, and the remaining three studies [16, 21, 24] did not specify asthma severity.

Quality assessment

Based on the six domains, all the included studies showed low risk of bias (Fig. 2). The method used in randomization sequence generation and allocation concealment was clearly described in all the studies except seven studies [13, 17–19, 22–24]. All the 13 studies were double-blinded and reported complete outcome data.

Outcomes
FEV_1

Ten studies [11–14, 17, 20–23, 25] examined the effect of CRTH2 antagonists compared with placebo on FEV_1, of which eight studies [11–13, 17, 20–23] reported FEV_1 in liters (L) and four [13, 14, 17, 25] in $FEV_1\%$ predicted. In terms of pre- and post-bronchodilator FEV_1, eight studies [11–13, 17, 20–23] and four studies [13, 14, 17, 24] showed pre-bronchodilator FEV_1 (L) and $FEV_1\%$ predicted, while three studies [17, 20, 21] and one study [17] evaluated post-bronchodilator FEV_1 (L) and $FEV_1\%$ predicted, respectively. The mean difference in pre-bronchodilator FEV_1 (L) from baseline was computed for five studies [11–13, 21, 22] of no corticosteroids use and four studies [17, 20, 21, 23] of corticosteroids use.

No statistical heterogeneity ($I^2 = 0\%$, $P = 0.70$) (Fig. 3) or publication bias (Begg's test = 0.754, Egger's test = 0.307) (Additional file 1: Figure S1) were detected in the assessment of pre-bronchodilator FEV_1 (L). Compared with placebo, CRTH2 antagonists significantly improved pre-bronchodilator FEV_1 (L) (MD = 0.06, 95% CI 0.03 to 0.09, $P = 0.0004$). Meta-regression indicated that the pooled effect of pre-bronchodilator FEV_1 (L) was associated with neither treatment duration ($P = 0.994$) (Additional file 1: Figure S2), asthma severity ($P = 0.150$) (Additional file 1: Figure S3), nor concomitant treatment ($P = 0.146$) (Additional file 1: Figure S4). The limited number of studies precluded further assessment of the impacts of different CRTH2 types on pre-bronchodilator FEV_1 (L), but we could separately extract patients treated with CRTH2 antagonists alone or CRTH2 antagonist combined with corticosteroids. In such a subgroup analysis, we found CRTH2 antagonists monotherapy, instead of CRTH2 antagonists as an add-on treatment to corticosteroids,

Efficacy and safety of antagonists for chemoattractant receptor-homologous molecule...

133

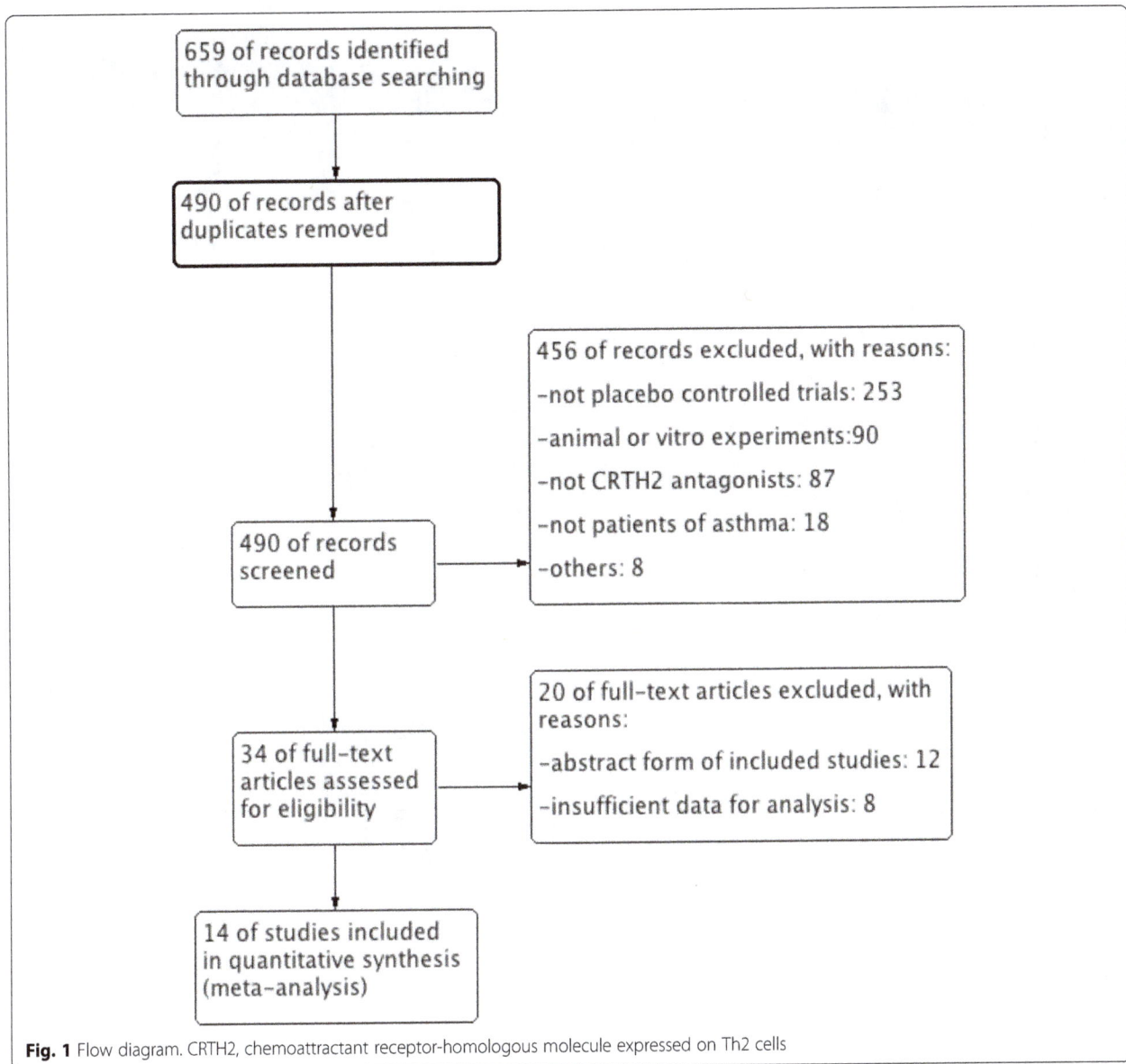

Fig. 1 Flow diagram. CRTH2, chemoattractant receptor-homologous molecule expressed on Th2 cells

significantly improved pre-bronchodilator FEV$_1$ (L) (MD = 0.09, 95% CI, 0.04 to 0.15, P = 0.0005) (Fig. 3).

Similarly, pre-bronchodilator FEV$_1$% predicted could be significantly improved in asthmatics with CRTH2 antagonists monotherapy (MD = 3.65, 95% CI 1.15 to 6.14, P = 0.004) rather than CRTH2 antagonists as add-on treatment to corticosteroids therapy (MD = 1.03, 95% CI -0.83 to 2.90, P = 0.28), however, moderate statistical heterogeneity (I^2 = 63%, P = 0.07) was found in combination therapy of CRTH2 antagonists and corticosteroids but not in CRTH2 antagonists alone (I^2 = 0%, P = 0.82). In the pooled analysis, we found no superior effect of CRTH2 antagonists compared to the placebo on pre-bronchodilator FEV$_1$% predicted (MD = 1.75, 95% CI -0.04 to 3.53, P = 0.06), but it also showed moderate statistical heterogeneity (I^2 = 63%, P = 0.03) (Additional file 1: Figure S5).

As for the post-bronchodilator FEV$_1$ (L) and FEV$_1$% predicted, no effect of CRTH2 antagonists was observed neither in the pooled (FEV$_1$ (L): MD = 0.05, 95% CI -0.07 to 0.17, P = 0.44) nor subgroup analysis of CRTH2 antagonists as add-on treatment to corticosteroids therapy (FEV$_1$ (L): MD = 0.06, 95% CI -0.09 to 0.22, P = 0.42; FEV$_1$% predicted: MD = – 0.09, 95% CI -1.65 to 1.47, P = 0.91), but moderate-to-high statistical heterogeneity of FEV$_1$ (L) was found in asthmatics with CRTH2 antagonists as add-on treatment to corticosteroids (I^2 = 75%, P = 0.04) and pooled asthmatics (I^2 = 52%, P = 0.13) (Additional file 1: Figure S6).

Forced vital capacity (FVC)
Two studies with three trials [11, 21] reported the effect of CRTH2 antagonists compared to placebo on FVC, of

Table 1 Characteristics of randomized controlled trials included

Source	Study Design	Participants characteristics	Population	Intervention (Drug, Dose, Frequency)	Control	Concomitant treatments	Duration	Follow-up	Outcomes*
Barnes 2012 [11]	Multi-center, parallel-group, RCT	Steroid-free, moderate persistent asthma	132	OC000459, 200 mg, Twice daily	Placebo	SABA	4 weeks	10 weeks	(1)(5)(6)(7)(9)(11)(12)(16)(19)
Pettipher 2014 [12]	Multi-center, parallel-group, RCT	Mild-to-moderate persistent steroid-free asthma	482	OC000459, 25 mg, Once daily; OC000459, 200 mg, Once daily; OC000459, 100 mg, Twice daily	Placebo	SABA	12 weeks	20–22 weeks	(1)(5)(16)(17)(18)
Singh 2013 [13]	Multi-center, two-period, cross-over, RCT	Steroid-naïve mild allergic asthma	21	OC000459, 200 mg, Twice daily	Placebo	SABA	16 days	35–41 days	(1)(13)(14)(15)(16)
Hall (trial 1) 2015 [14]	Multi-center, parallel-group, RCT	Symptomatic, mild-to-moderate, steroid-naïve asthma	317	BI 671800, 50 mg, Twice daily; BI 671800, 200 mg, Twice daily; BI 671800, 400 mg, Twice daily	Placebo	SABA	6 weeks	10 weeks	(3)(6)(12)(18)(19)
Hall (trial 2) 2015 [14]	Multi-center, parallel-group	Symptomatic, mild-to-moderate asthmatic patients on ICS	176	BI 671800, 400 mg, Twice daily	Placebo	SABA, ICS		10–12 weeks	(3)(6)(17)(18)(19)
Bateman 2017 [16]	Multi-center, parallel-group, RCT	Allergic asthma inadequately controlled with low-dose ICS	901	Fevipiprant, 1 mg/3 mg/10 mg or 2 mg, Once daily or twice daily; Fevipiprant, 30 mg/50 mg/75 mg or 25 mg, Once daily or twice daily; Fevipiprant, 150 mg/300 mg or 75 mg/150 mg, Once daily or twice daily; Fevipiprant, 450 mg, Once daily	placebo	SABA or ICS	12 weeks	22–24 weeks and 2 days	(11)(14)(16)(18)(19)
Busse 2013 [17]	Multi-center, parallel-group, RCT	Inadequately controlled, moderate-to-severe asthma	396	AMG 853, 5 mg, Twice daily; AMG 853, 25 mg, Twice daily; AMG 853, 100 mg, Twice daily; AMG 853, 200 mg, Twice daily	Placebo	SABA, ICS	12 weeks	18 weeks	(1)(2)(3)(4)(5)(6)(8)(9)(10)(11)(12)(14)(16)(17)(18)(19)

Table 1 Characteristics of randomized controlled trials included (*Continued*)

Source	Study Design	Participants characteristics	Population	Intervention (Drug, Dose, Frequency)	Control	Concomitant treatments	Duration	Follow-up	Outcomes*
Erpenbeck 2016 [18]	Multi-center, parallel-group, RCT	mild-to-moderate persistent allergic asthma	170	Fevipiprant, 500 mg, Twice daily	Placebo	SABA	4 weeks	8 weeks	⑧⑩⑯⑰
Fowler 2017 [19]	Single-center, parallel-group, RCT	Well controlled mild asthma	84	BI 1021958, 5/20/60/200 mg or 40/150/400 mg, Twice daily or once daily	Placebo	SABA	15 days	15 days	⑯⑰⑱⑲
Gonem 2016 [20]	Single-center, parallel-group, RCT	Persistent, moderate-to-severe eosinophilic asthma	61	Fevipiprant, 225 mg, Twice daily	Placebo	SABA, ICS, LABA, or oral prednisone	12 weeks	20 weeks	①②⑧⑨⑫⑬⑭⑯⑰
Kuna (trial 1) 2016 [21]	Multi-center, parallel-group, RCT	Stable asthma withdrawn from ICS	113	AZD1981, 1000 mg, Twice daily	Placebo	SABA	4 weeks	8 weeks	①②⑤⑥⑩⑫⑬⑭⑯⑰⑱⑲
Kuna (trial 2) 2016 [21]	Multi-center, parallel-group, RCT	Uncontrolled moderate-to-severe asthma despite moderate-to-high dose of ICS	368	AZD1981, 50 mg, Twice daily; AZD1981, 400 mg, Twice daily; AZD1981, 1000 mg, Twice daily	Placebo	SABA, ICS	4 weeks	8 weeks	①⑦⑩⑯⑰⑱⑲
Wenzel 2014 [22]	Multi-center, parallel-group, RCT	Steroid-free, mild atopic asthma	184	ARRY-502, 200 mg, Twice daily	Placebo	SABA	4 weeks	6 weeks	①⑧⑨⑪⑯⑲
Bateman 2018 [23]	Multi-center, parallel-group, RCT	Persistent allergic asthma	1144	AZD1981, 80/200 mg, once daily, or 10/40/100 mg, twice daily	Placebo	ICS, LABA, SABA	12 weeks	15 weeks	①⑧⑪⑯⑰⑱
Diamant 2014 [24]	Multi-center, two-period, cross-over, RCT	Stable, allergic asthma	14	Setipiprant, 1000 mg, Twice daily	Placebo	SABA	5 days	37 days	③④⑮
Miller 2017 [25]	Multi-center, three-period, cross-over, RCT	Mild-to-moderate symptomatic asthma	108	BI 671800, 400 mg, Once daily (a.m)	Placebo	SABA, ICS	12 weeks	16–18 weeks	③⑧⑯⑰⑱⑲

*Outcomes include: ① change of pre-bronchodilator FEV_1, ② change of post-bronchodilator FEV_1, ③ change of pre-bronchodilator FEV_1, % predicted, ④ change of post-bronchodilator FEV_1, % predicted, ⑤ change of morning PEF, ⑥ change of evening PEF, ⑦ change of FVC, ⑧ change of ACQ scores, ⑨ change of AQLQ scores, ⑩ change of SABA use, ⑪ incidence of asthma exacerbation, ⑫ change of sputum eosinophils, ⑬ change of blood eosinophils, ⑭ change of FeNO, ⑮ change of methacholine PC_{20}, ⑯ incidence of adverse events, ⑰ incidence of severe adverse events, ⑱ incidence of treatment related adverse events, ⑲ incidence of adverse events leading to treatment withdrawal

ACQ asthma control questionnaire, AQLQ asthma quality of life questionnaire, FeNO fractional exhaled nitric oxide, FEV_1 forced expiratory volume in one second, FVC forced vital capacity, Methacholine PC_{20} the provocation concentration of methacholine causing a 20% fall in FEV_1, NM not mentioned, PEF peak expiratory flow, RCT randomized controlled trial, SABA short-acting beta-agonists

Table 2 Baseline characteristics of patients in each enrolled trial

Source	No.	Age (years)*	Female (%)	BMI (kg/m²)*	Smoking (Pack-year)	Pre-bronchodilator FEV₁% predicted*	FeNO (ppb)*	Positive atopic status (%)	Diagnosis or duration of asthma (years)*
Barnes 2012 [11]	65	43.4 (18–55)**	41.53	NM	≤10	NM	NM	100	6.5 (6.29)
Pettipher 2014 [12]	125	40.4 (11.4)	70	NM	<10	71.5 (6.1)	NM	NM	NM
	123	39.7 (10.2)	81	NM	<10	71.0 (6.2)	NM	NM	NM
	117	38.9 (11.4)	76	NM	<10	71.5 (6.9)	NM	NM	NM
Singh 2013 [13]	21	31.1 (7.1)	14.3	NM	<10	87.4 (12.0)	32.7 (21.8)	100	NM
Hall (trial 1) 2015 [14]	77	39.1 (11.5)	53.2	27.0 (4.6)	<10	71.4 (7.3)	NM	75.3	NM
	83	35.1 (11.1)	50.6	25.9 (4.3)	<10	73.3 (7.3)	NM	78.3	NM
	79	37.5 (12.2)	54.4	26.5 (4.7)	<10	73.6 (6.9)	NM	84.8	NM
Hall (trial 2) 2015 [14]	81	41.8 (12.7)	61.7	27.6 (4.1)	<10	72.6 (7.6)	NM	82.7	NM
Bateman 2017 [16]	201	45.2 (12.1)	59.2	28.1 (5.7)	0	64.4 (9.6)	NM	100	20.5 (14.9)
	219	45.6 (12.1)	54.34	26.9 (5.0)	0	64.1 (10.1)	NM	100	20.5 (14.9)
	212	43.5 (12.3)	60.85	27.4 (5.5)	0	64.5 (9.7)	NM	100	18.4 (14.0)
	133	45.8 (12.5)	54.89	27.8 (5.0)	0	63.7 (10.5)	NM	100	21.2 (15.0)
Busse 2013 [17]	79	44.7 (11.5)	65.8	29.6 (6.2)	<10	68.2 (7.9)	31.9 (21.4)	93.7	28.0 (14.1)
	79	45.0 (11.3)	58.2	32.0 (6.5)	<10	67.1 (7.9)	30.9 (30.5)	91.1	24.8 (13.2)
	79	44.6 (11.4)	69.8	31.9 (8.0)	<10	66.7 (8.5)	28.3 (23.2)	91.1	28.9 (14.5)
	80	43.7 (11.4)	40.0	31.4 (7.2)	<10	66.1 (8.9)	33.5 (31.6)	95.0	27.3 (12.8)
Erpenbeck 2016 [18]	82	41 (12.9)	24	28.5 (5.81)	<10	71.5 (7.11)	32 (NM)	100	NM
Fowler 2017 [19]	63	33.1 (10.9)	NM	24.2 (2.9)	<10	85.2 (15.0)	NM	NM	NM
Gonem 2016 [20]	30	50 (17)	40	31.0 (5.9)	NM	72.5 (23.8)	30 (24)	87	32 (16)
Kuna (trial 1) 2016 [21]	57	38.4 (NM)	16	26.3 (NM)	<10	82.6 (NM)	NM	100	13 (NM)
Kuna (trial 2)2016 [21]	95	43.3 (NM)	28	26.9 (NM)	<10	66.2 (NM)	NM	72	11.1 (NM)
	90	43.0 (NM)	21	27.0 (NM)	<10	68.5 (NM)	NM	77	12.1 (NM)
	92	43.5 (NM)	37	27.2 (NM)	<10	69.0 (NM)	NM	64	10 (NM)
Wenzel 2014 [22]	93	35 (18–68)**	49	26.0 (19.3–34.6)**	<10	73.4 (60–84)***	47.5 (26–244)**	100	NM
Bateman 2018 [23]	976	41.0 (NM)	49.5	27.5 (NM)	≤10	NM	NM	100	18.2 (NM)
Diamant 2014 [24]	18	30.6 (21–46)**	0	25.58 (NM)	<10	NM	51.6 (38.5)	100	NM
Miller 2017 [25]	108	41.1 (12.4)	53.7	28.8 (4.8)	<10	72.8 (7.6)	NM	63.9	28.2 (12.9)

Data was expressed as * mean (SD), ** mean (range), *** median (range)
BMI body mass index, FeNO fractional exhaled nitric oxide, FEV, forced expiratory volume in one second, NM not mentioned

which two trials [11, 21] administered CRTH2 antagonists alone. FVC could not be significantly improved by either overall CRTH2 antagonists (MD = 0.03, 95% CI -0.12 to 0.19, $P = 0.67$) or CRTH2 antagonist monotherapy (MD = 0.05, 95% CI -0.14 to 0.24, $P = 0.61$) even though no statistical heterogeneities were detected ($I^2 = 0\%$, $P = 0.79$) (Additional file 1: Figure S7). One trial [21] used CRTH2 antagonist as add-on treatment to corticosteroids, but the result showed no improvement in FVC.

Peak expiratory flow (PEF)
PEF was reported as morning and evening PEF in four [12, 13, 17, 21] and three [11, 17, 21] studies, respectively. Three studies [11, 12, 21] assessed the effect of CRTH2 antagonists monotherapy, while one study [17] also showed CRTH2 antagonists as add-on treatment. No statistical heterogeneities were found except for that in morning PEF in the pooled analysis ($I^2 = 55\%$, $P = 0.08$) (Fig. 4). No significant improvements of morning and evening PEF were shown in asthmatics with CRTH2 antagonists monotherapy (morning PEF: MD = 0.01, 95% CI -0.00 to 0.02, $P = 0.17$; evening PEF: MD = 10.01, 95% CI -7.74 to 27.75, $P = 0.27$) or in pooled analysis (morning PEF: MD = - 2.75, 95% CI -11.04 to 5.54, $P = 0.52$; evening PEF: MD = - 3.84, 95% CI -12.65 to 4.97, $P = 0.85$). However, subgroup analysis indicated that CRTH2 antagonists as add-on treatment to corticosteroid could reduce morning PEF (MD = - 12.35, 95% CI -22.04 to - 2.66, $P = 0.01$) instead of evening PEF (MD = - 8.38, 95% CI -18.53 to 1.78, $P = 0.11$).

Asthma control questionnaire (ACQ)
The effect of CRTH2 antagonists on ACQ scores was reported in six studies [17, 18, 20, 22, 23, 25], of which four [17, 20, 23, 25] in asthmatics with CRTH2 antagonists as add-on treatment and two [18, 22] with CRTH2 antagonists monotherapy. Moderate statistical heterogeneity was noticed in CRTH2 antagonists monotherapy ($I^2 = 72\%$, $P = 0.06$) , and the results showed that CRTH2 antagonists in general could significantly reduce ACQ score in asthmatics (MD = - 0.12, 95% CI -0.21 to - 0.03, $P = 0.009$), but little effect was observed in asthmatics with CRTH2 antagonists used as neither monotherapy (MD = - 0.23, 95% CI -0.48 to 0.02, $P = 0.08$) nor add-on treatment to corticosteroids (MD = - 0.07, 95% CI -0.14 to 0.001, $P = 0.045$) (Fig. 5).

Asthma quality of life questionnaire (AQLQ)
Four studies [11, 17, 20, 22] reported AQLQ score in asthmatic patients with treatment of CRTH2 antagonists, and we did not find statistical heterogeneities except for CRTH2 antagonists used as add-on treatment to corticosteroids ($I^2 = 76\%$, $P = 0.04$). CRTH2 antagonists were shown to significantly improve AQLQ score

compared to placebo (MD = 0.23, 95% CI 0.07 to 0.39, $P = 0.005$), however, in the subgroup analysis, it resulted in significant improvement of AQLQ score in patients with CRTH2 antagonists monotherapy (MD = 0.25, 95% CI 0.09 to 0.41, $P = 0.002$) rather than CRTH2 antagonists as add-on treatment (MD = 0.29, 95% CI -0.23 to 0.82, $P = 0.27$) (Fig. 6).

Rescue use of SABA
Three studies [17, 18, 21] reported the effect of CRTH2 antagonists on the rescue use of SABA, and we found that CRTH2 antagonists significantly reduced SABA usage (MD = - 0.04, 95% CI -0.05 to - 0.03, $P < 0.00001$), regardless of monotherapy (MD = - 0.04, 95% CI -0.05 to - 0.03, $P < 0.00001$) or serving as an add-on therapy to corticosteroids (MD = - 0.78, 95% CI -1.47 to - 0.09, $P = 0.03$) (Fig. 7).

Asthma exacerbations
Six studies [11, 12, 16, 17, 22, 23] presented data on asthma exacerbations, and they all included patients with exacerbations based on a decline of more than 30% from the baseline in morning PEF on two or more consecutive mornings, or a worsening of asthma symptoms requiring treatment with systemic corticosteroids or increased doses of rescue medication, and/or the need for asthma-related hospitalization/emergency room visit. The pooled analysis showed no significant difference in the incidence of asthma exacerbations (RR = 0.76, 95% CI 0.52 to 1.13, $P = 0.18$) between asthmatics treated with CRTH2 antagonists and placebo, however, in the subgroup analysis, we found asthma exacerbations were significantly reduced in CRTH2 monotherapy (RR = 0.45, 95% CI 0.23 to 0.85; $P = 0.01$) rather than CRTH2 antagonists as add-on treatment (RR = 1.05, 95% CI 0.63 to 1.75, $P = 0.86$) (Fig. 8). No statistical heterogeneities were detected in pooled ($I^2 = 0$, $P = 0.52$) and subgroup (monotherapy: $I^2 = 0$, $P = 0.85$; add-on treatment: $I^2 = 0$, $P = 0.99$) analysis.

Adverse events
Adverse events were reported in thirteen studies [11-14, 16-23, 25], of which ten [12, 14, 16-21, 23, 25], eight [12, 14, 16, 17, 19, 21, 23, 25] and eight [11, 14, 16, 17, 19, 21, 22, 25] studies further examined severe adverse events, treatment related adverse events, and adverse events leading to treatment withdrawal, respectively. The most commonly reported adverse events were nasopharyngitis, headache, asthma, infections and gastrointestinal disorders. Each type of adverse events was pooled into our meta-analysis, and no significant statistical heterogeneities were found either in overall or subgroup analysis (Fig. 9 and Additional file 1: Figures S8–S10). In terms of adverse events, severe adverse events and treatment related

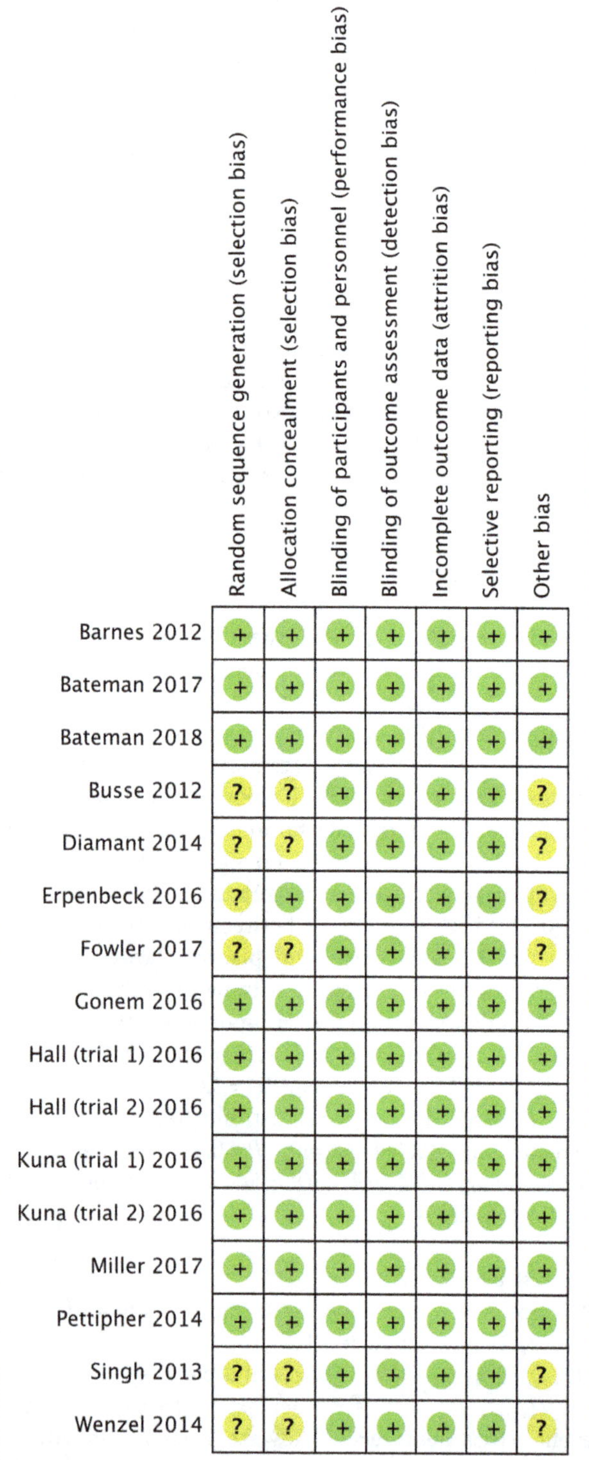

Fig. 2 Risk of bias summary

CI 0.75 to 1.34, $P = 0.97$) as well as CRTH2 antagonists monotherapy (adverse events: RR = 0.98, 95% CI 0.87 to 1.11, $P = 0.76$; severe adverse events: RD = − 0.01, 95% CI -0.02 to 0.01, $P = 0.23$; treatment related adverse events: RR = 0.89, 95% CI 0.63 to 1.25, $P = 0.49$) and add-on treatment to corticosteroids (adverse events: RR = 1.00, 95% CI 0.90 to 1.11, $P = 0.99$; severe adverse events: RD = − 0.00, 95% CI -0.01 to 0.01, $P = 0.93$; treatment related adverse events: RR = 1.16, 95% CI 0.77 to 1.74, $P = 0.48$) (Fig. 9 and Additional file 1: Figure S8 and S9). However, significantly lower incidence of adverse events leading to treatment withdrawal was found in CRTH2 antagonists treatment compared to placebo (RD = − 0.02, 95% CI -0.04 to − 0.00; $P = 0.03$), and subgroup analysis showed significantly lesser adverse events leading to treatment withdrawal in CRTH2 antagonists monotherapy (RD = − 0.04, 95% CI -0.08 to − 0.01; $P = 0.02$) rather than CRTH2 antagonists as add-on treatment (RD = − 0.01, 95% CI -0.04 to 0.01; $P = 0.29$) (Additional file 1: Figure S10). Further analysis also demonstrated no evidence of publication bias (Egger's test = 0.758, Begg's test = 0.767) (Additional file 1: Figure S11) and no association either between treatment duration and the incidence of adverse events ($P = 0.139$) (Additional file 1: Figure S12) or between concomitant therapy ($P = 0.827$) (Additional file 1: Figure S13) or asthma severity ($P = 0.415$) (Additional file 1: Figure S14) and the incidence of adverse events.

Sputum and blood eosinophils

Five studies [11, 13, 17, 20, 21] presented data on sputum eosinophils in patients with CRTH2 antagonists treatment, and three studies [20, 21, 24] reported blood eosinophils. However, we could not conduct individual synthesized analysis of each outcome due to the inconsistently reported data, in which eosinophils levels were presented either as amount per gram or percent of the whole white cells, and we were unable to extract mean change of eosinophils after treatment from only mean (range) or geometric mean (95% CI).

Table 3 summarized available studies with sputum or blood eosinophils. Ambiguous results were noticed in sputum eosinophils as some studies [13, 20] showed significant reduction of sputum eosinophils in patients with CRTH2 antagonists treatment compared to placebo while some studies [11, 17, 21] did not find any significant differences. As for blood eosinophils, all three available studies showed that CRTH2 antagonists treatment could not significantly reduce blood eosinophils compared to placebo regardless of being as monotherapy or an add-on treatment to corticosteroids.

FeNO and methacholine PC$_{20}$

Similar to sputum and blood eosinophils, data of FeNO and methacholine PC$_{20}$ from available studies could not

adverse events, we found similar incidence between CRTH2 antagonists and placebo in pooled analysis (adverse events: RR = 0.99, 95% CI 0.92 to 1.07, $P = 0.86$; severe adverse events: RD = − 0.00, 95% CI -0.01 to 0.00, $P = 0.43$; treatment related adverse events: RR = 1.01, 95%

Fig. 3 — The effect of CRTH2 antagonists vs placebo on FEV₁

Study or Subgroup	Experimental Mean	SD	Total	Control Mean	SD	Total	Weight	Mean Difference IV, Fixed, 95% CI
1.1.1 asthmatics with CRTH2 antagonists monotherapy								
Barnes 2012	0.17	0.49	64	0.09	0.46	67	4.1%	0.08 [-0.08, 0.24]
Kuna (trial 1) 2016	0.07	0.948	57	0.02	0.9123	56	0.9%	0.05 [-0.29, 0.39]
Pettipher 2014	0.149	0.408	361	0.057	0.359	116	18.2%	0.09 [0.01, 0.17]
Singh 2013	0	0.6745	16	-0.16	0.7451	16	0.5%	0.16 [-0.33, 0.65]
Wenzel 2014	0.1199	0.2971	93	0.0171	0.2971	91	14.9%	0.10 [0.02, 0.19]
Subtotal (95% CI)			591			346	38.6%	0.09 [0.04, 0.15]

Heterogeneity: Chi² = 0.20, df = 4 (P = 1.00); I² = 0%
Test for overall effect: Z = 3.48 (P = 0.0005)

Study or Subgroup	Experimental Mean	SD	Total	Control Mean	SD	Total	Weight	Mean Difference IV, Fixed, 95% CI
1.1.2 asthmatics with CRTH2 antagonists as add-on to corticosteroids therapy								
Bateman 2018	0.1728	0.3515	976	0.1393	0.3515	161	32.0%	0.03 [-0.03, 0.09]
Busse 2012	0.0283	0.3578	317	0.019	0.2844	79	20.0%	0.01 [-0.06, 0.08]
Gonem 2016	0.08	0.3539	27	0.004	0.5222	30	2.1%	0.08 [-0.15, 0.31]
Kuna (trial 2) 2016	0.21	0.5191	277	0.0845	0.5193	91	7.3%	0.13 [0.00, 0.25]
Subtotal (95% CI)			1597			361	61.4%	0.04 [-0.00, 0.08]

Heterogeneity: Chi² = 2.65, df = 3 (P = 0.45); I² = 0%
Test for overall effect: Z = 1.76 (P = 0.08)

Total (95% CI) 2188   707   100.0%   0.06 [0.03, 0.09]
Heterogeneity: Chi² = 5.52, df = 8 (P = 0.70); I² = 0%
Test for overall effect: Z = 3.54 (P = 0.0004)
Test for subgroup differences: Chi² = 2.67, df = 1 (P = 0.10), I² = 62.5%

(Forest plot axis: -0.5, -0.25, 0, 0.25, 0.5; Favours [control] / Favours [experimental])

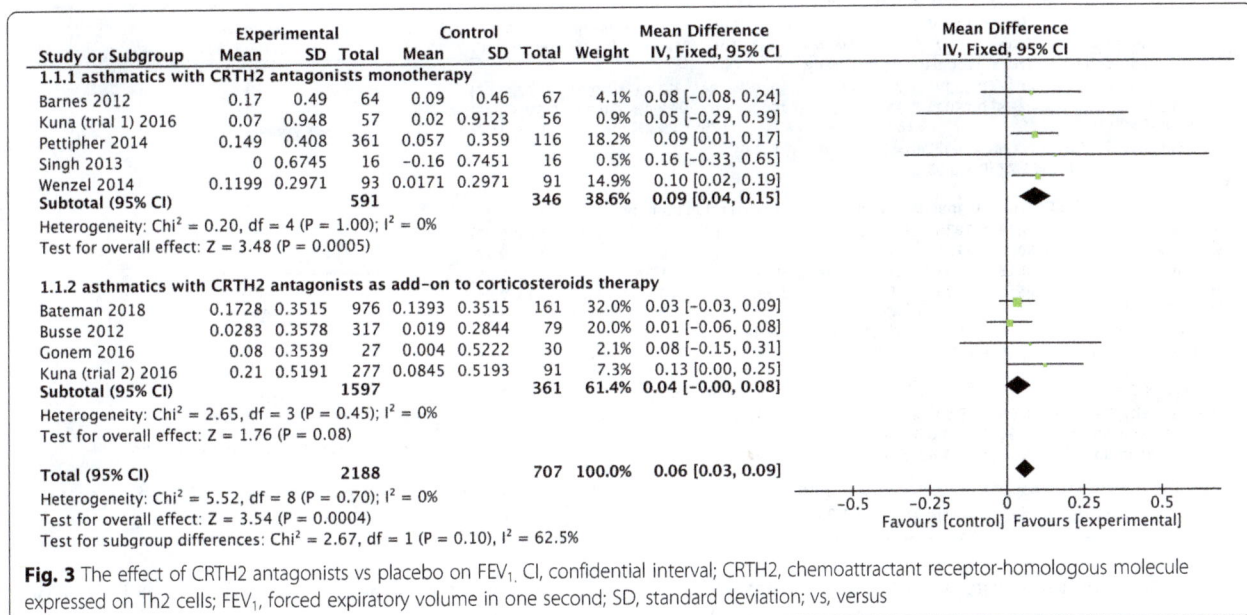

Fig. 3 The effect of CRTH2 antagonists vs placebo on FEV₁. CI, confidential interval; CRTH2, chemoattractant receptor-homologous molecule expressed on Th2 cells; FEV₁, forced expiratory volume in one second; SD, standard deviation; vs, versus

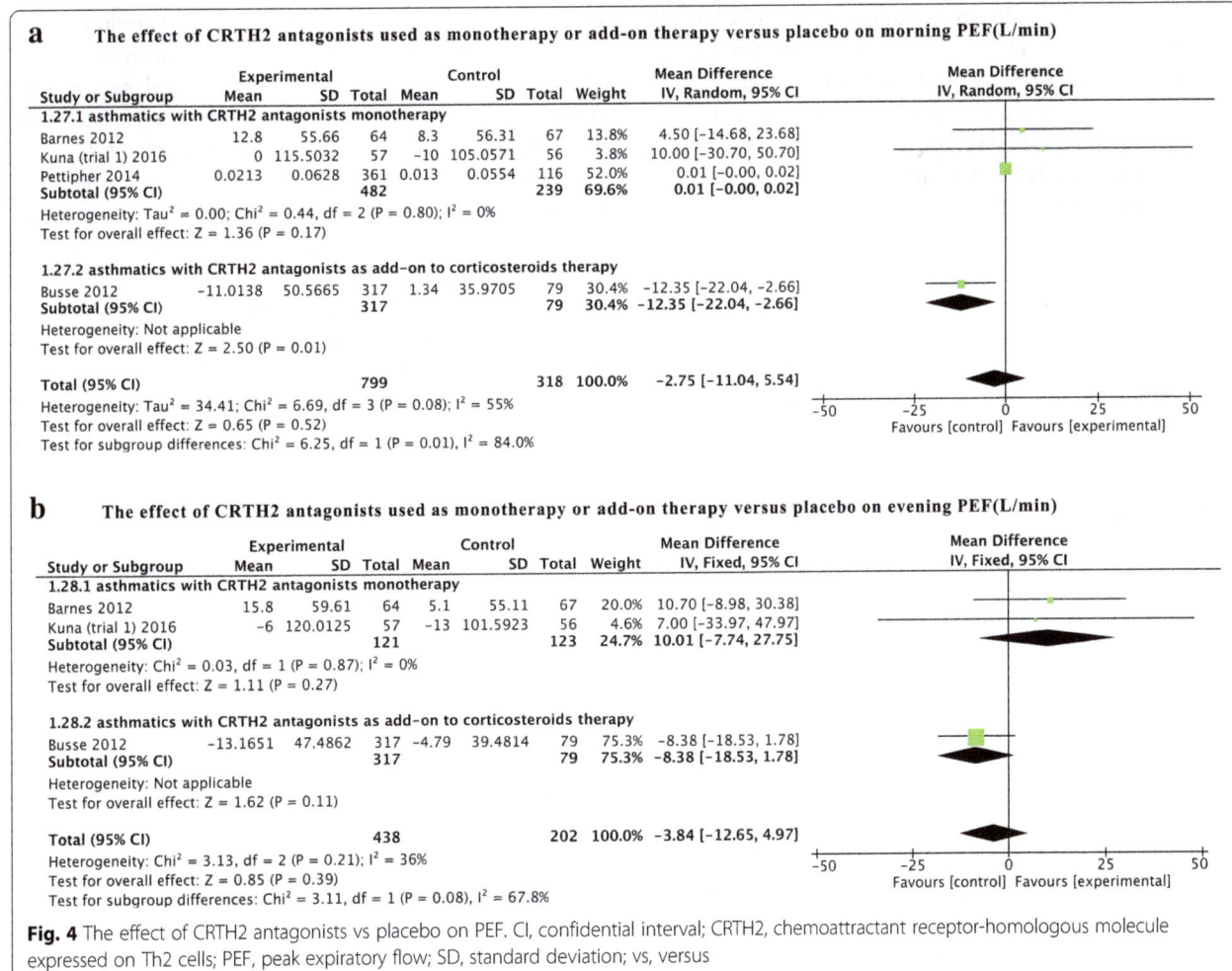

a   The effect of CRTH2 antagonists used as monotherapy or add-on therapy versus placebo on morning PEF(L/min)

Study or Subgroup	Experimental Mean	SD	Total	Control Mean	SD	Total	Weight	Mean Difference IV, Random, 95% CI
1.27.1 asthmatics with CRTH2 antagonists monotherapy								
Barnes 2012	12.8	55.66	64	8.3	56.31	67	13.8%	4.50 [-14.68, 23.68]
Kuna (trial 1) 2016	0	115.5032	57	-10	105.0571	56	3.8%	10.00 [-30.70, 50.70]
Pettipher 2014	0.0213	0.0628	361	0.013	0.0554	116	52.0%	0.01 [-0.00, 0.02]
Subtotal (95% CI)			482			239	69.6%	0.01 [-0.00, 0.02]

Heterogeneity: Tau² = 0.00; Chi² = 0.44, df = 2 (P = 0.80); I² = 0%
Test for overall effect: Z = 1.36 (P = 0.17)

Study or Subgroup	Experimental Mean	SD	Total	Control Mean	SD	Total	Weight	Mean Difference IV, Random, 95% CI
1.27.2 asthmatics with CRTH2 antagonists as add-on to corticosteroids therapy								
Busse 2012	-11.0138	50.5665	317	1.34	35.9705	79	30.4%	-12.35 [-22.04, -2.66]
Subtotal (95% CI)			317			79	30.4%	-12.35 [-22.04, -2.66]

Heterogeneity: Not applicable
Test for overall effect: Z = 2.50 (P = 0.01)

Total (95% CI) 799   318   100.0%   -2.75 [-11.04, 5.54]
Heterogeneity: Tau² = 34.41; Chi² = 6.69, df = 3 (P = 0.08); I² = 55%
Test for overall effect: Z = 0.65 (P = 0.52)
Test for subgroup differences: Chi² = 6.25, df = 1 (P = 0.01), I² = 84.0%

(Forest plot axis: -50, -25, 0, 25, 50; Favours [control] / Favours [experimental])

b   The effect of CRTH2 antagonists used as monotherapy or add-on therapy versus placebo on evening PEF(L/min)

Study or Subgroup	Experimental Mean	SD	Total	Control Mean	SD	Total	Weight	Mean Difference IV, Fixed, 95% CI
1.28.1 asthmatics with CRTH2 antagonists monotherapy								
Barnes 2012	15.8	59.61	64	5.1	55.11	67	20.0%	10.70 [-8.98, 30.38]
Kuna (trial 1) 2016	-6	120.0125	57	-13	101.5923	56	4.6%	7.00 [-33.97, 47.97]
Subtotal (95% CI)			121			123	24.7%	10.01 [-7.74, 27.75]

Heterogeneity: Chi² = 0.03, df = 1 (P = 0.87); I² = 0%
Test for overall effect: Z = 1.11 (P = 0.27)

Study or Subgroup	Experimental Mean	SD	Total	Control Mean	SD	Total	Weight	Mean Difference IV, Fixed, 95% CI
1.28.2 asthmatics with CRTH2 antagonists as add-on to corticosteroids therapy								
Busse 2012	-13.1651	47.4862	317	-4.79	39.4814	79	75.3%	-8.38 [-18.53, 1.78]
Subtotal (95% CI)			317			79	75.3%	-8.38 [-18.53, 1.78]

Heterogeneity: Not applicable
Test for overall effect: Z = 1.62 (P = 0.11)

Total (95% CI) 438   202   100.0%   -3.84 [-12.65, 4.97]
Heterogeneity: Chi² = 3.13, df = 2 (P = 0.21); I² = 36%
Test for overall effect: Z = 0.85 (P = 0.39)
Test for subgroup differences: Chi² = 3.11, df = 1 (P = 0.08), I² = 67.8%

(Forest plot axis: -50, -25, 0, 25, 50; Favours [control] / Favours [experimental])

Fig. 4 The effect of CRTH2 antagonists vs placebo on PEF. CI, confidential interval; CRTH2, chemoattractant receptor-homologous molecule expressed on Th2 cells; PEF, peak expiratory flow; SD, standard deviation; vs, versus

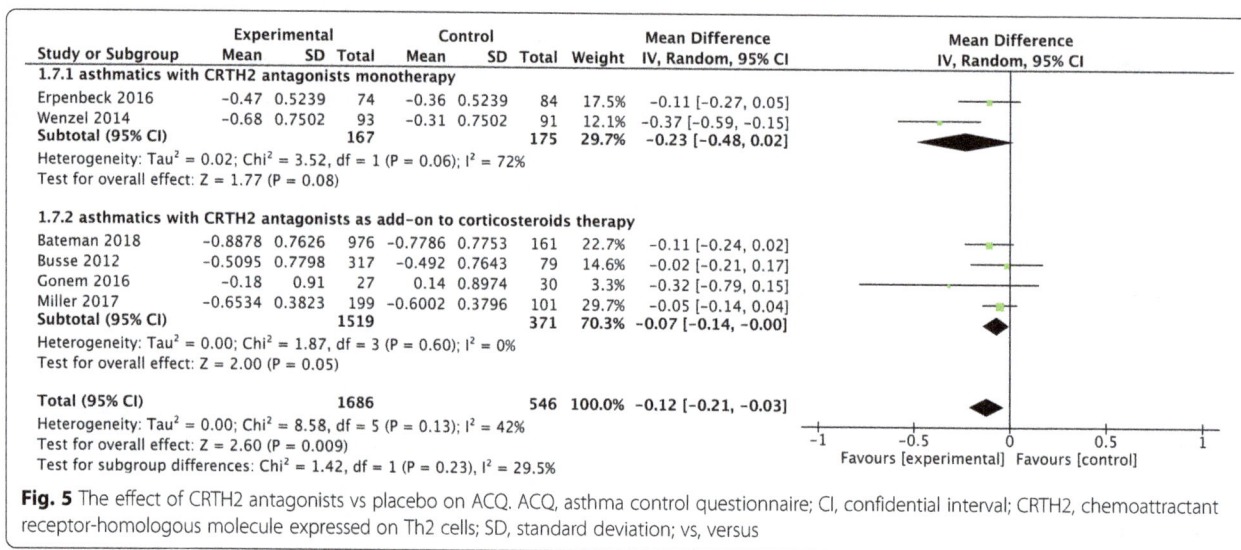

Fig. 5 The effect of CRTH2 antagonists vs placebo on ACQ. ACQ, asthma control questionnaire; CI, confidential interval; CRTH2, chemoattractant receptor-homologous molecule expressed on Th2 cells; SD, standard deviation; vs, versus

be pooled in meta-analysis. In total, six studies [13, 16, 17, 20, 21, 24] and two studies [13, 24] depicted change of FeNO and methacholine PC_{20}, respectively. No significant difference in FeNO was found between CRTH2 antagonists and placebo even in CRTH2 antagonists monotherapy or as add-on treatment to corticosteroids. However, Diamant et al. [24] showed that Setipiprant monotherapy significantly stablized methacholine PC_{20} in stable allergic steroid-free asthma compared to placebo, which was not observed in the study by Singh et al. [13] in stable allergic steroid-naïve asthmatics treated with OC000459 monotherapy.

Discussion

In our study, we found that CRTH2 antagonists, compared to placebo, significantly improved pre-bronchodilator FEV_1 (L) and AQLQ scores, reduced ACQ scores and SABA use in adults with asthma, which was also true in the treatment of CRTH2 antagonists monotherapy except for no effect on

ACQ scores but improved pre-bronchodilator $FEV_1\%$ predicted and reduced asthma exacerbations. However, CRTH2 antagonists as add-on treatment to corticosteroids did not show any obvious superior advantages over placebo. CRTH2 antagonists monotherapy was associated with lesser adverse events leading to treatment withdrawal, but CRTH2 antagonists, regardless of monotherapy or as add-on treatment to corticosteroids, showed similar incidence of adverse events, severe adverse events, and treatment related adverse events compared with placebo.

Reversible airflow limitation and airway hyperresponsiveness are the key traits in asthma pathophysiology, and FEV_1, PEF as well as Methacholine PC_{20} are the most widely used parameters to assess asthma severity and control, and predict future risk of asthma exacerbations [26, 27]. Our study found that CRTH2 antagonists monotherapy could significantly improve pre-bronchodilator FEV_1 and $FEV_1\%$ predicted, which might be attributed to the potential anti-inflammation effects of CRTH2 antagonists [5–7]. As

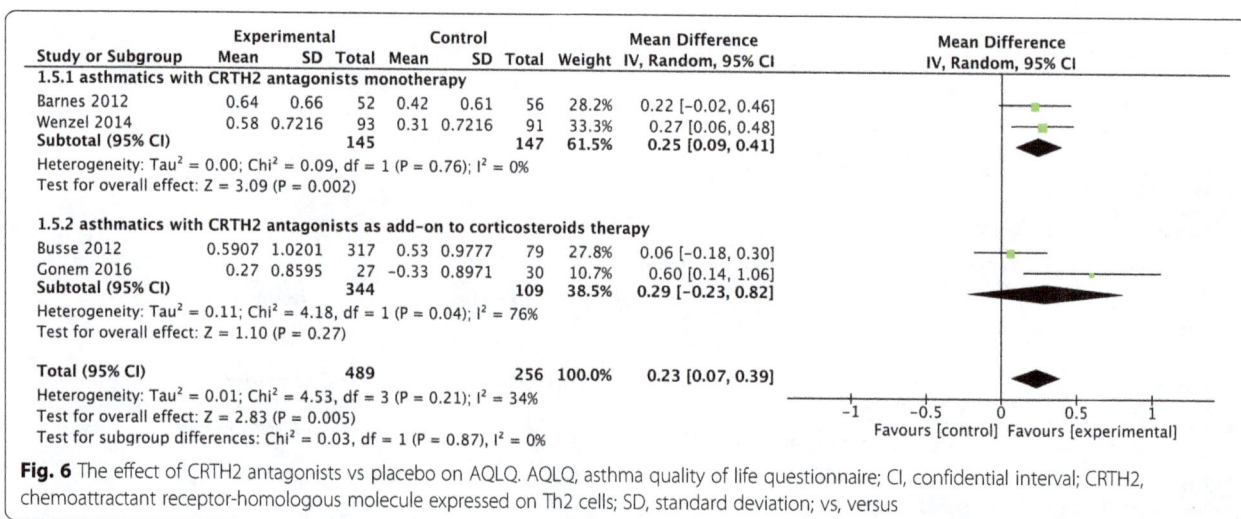

Fig. 6 The effect of CRTH2 antagonists vs placebo on AQLQ. AQLQ, asthma quality of life questionnaire; CI, confidential interval; CRTH2, chemoattractant receptor-homologous molecule expressed on Th2 cells; SD, standard deviation; vs, versus

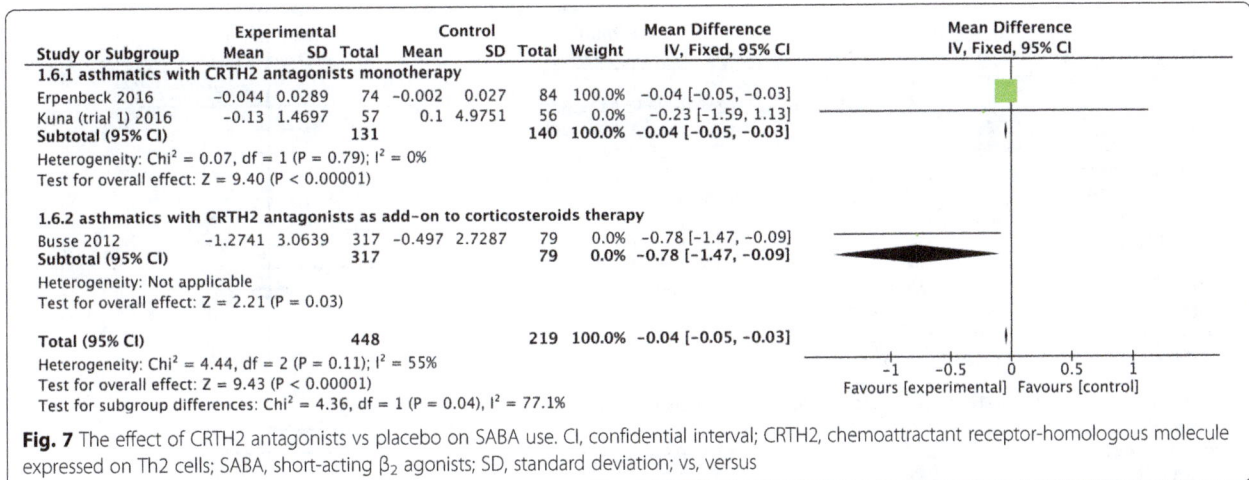

Fig. 7 The effect of CRTH2 antagonists vs placebo on SABA use. CI, confidential interval; CRTH2, chemoattractant receptor-homologous molecule expressed on Th2 cells; SABA, short-acting β_2 agonists; SD, standard deviation; vs, versus

mentioned above, the binding of PGD2 to CRTH2 induces respiratory burst and degranulation of eosinophils as well as increases release of type 2 cytokines, leukotrienes and cationic proteins, which may damage airway epithelia, thus resulting in airway narrowing and development of airway hyperresponsiveness [7, 28–30]. Furthermore, it has been demonstrated that production of type 2 cytokines is associated with greater decline in lung functions [31]. However, in our study, no additional synergistic effects were observed when CRTH2 antagonists were used as add-on treatment to corticosteroids. With consideration of the meta-regression analysis, which indicated no association between pre-bronchodilator FEV_1 and either asthma severity, concomitant treatment, or treatment duration, the non-superiority of add-on treatment of CRTH2 antagonists to corticosteroids might result from: 1) the difference

in CRTH2 antagonists types and doses with various bio-availability, pharmacokinetics and pharmacodynamics; 2) the true benefit of CRTH2 antagonists being covered by the potent effects of concurrent corticosteroids use. For example, Hall et al. [14] also found that in steroids-naïve rather than steroids-on-use asthmatics 400 mg of BI 671800 could improve lung function [25].

In terms of PEF, our pooled and subgroup analysis revealed no improvement of morning and evening PEF in asthmatics with CRTH2 antagonists treatment. Moreover, one study [17] even reported that CRTH2 antagonists together with corticosteroids could reduce morning PEF. The poor relationship between FEV_1 and PEF might relate to the disassociation of the effect of CRTH2 antagonists on these two parameters [32, 33]. However, the effect of CRTH2 antagonists on PEF should be

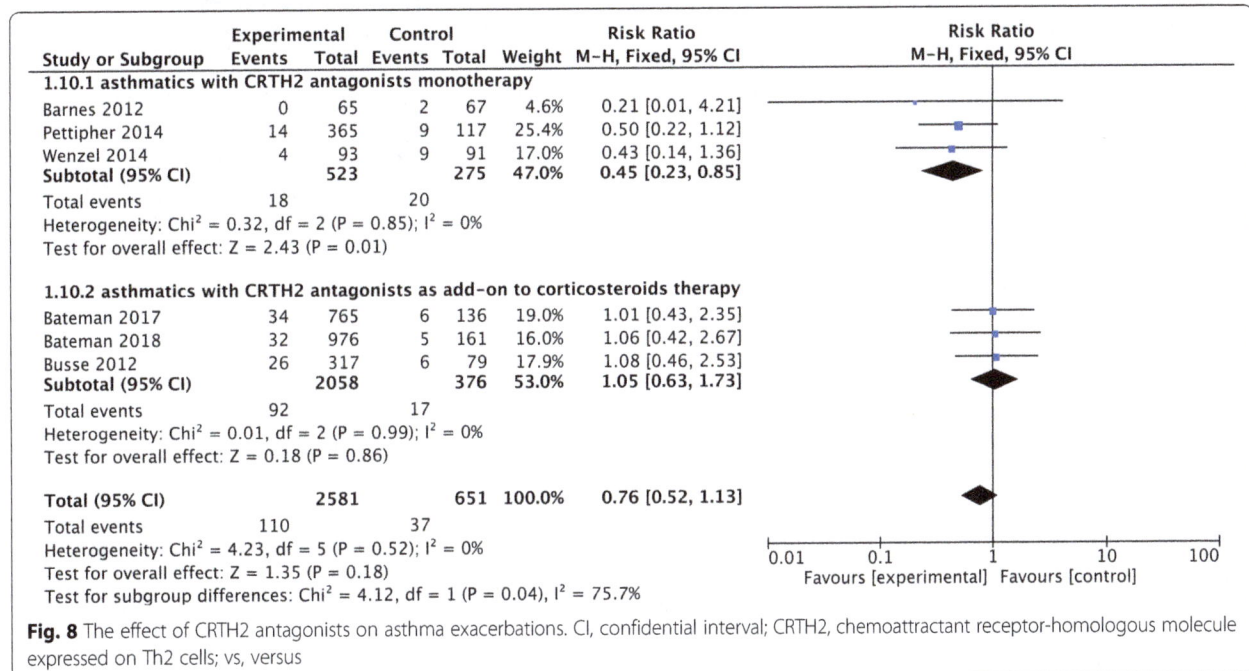

Fig. 8 The effect of CRTH2 antagonists on asthma exacerbations. CI, confidential interval; CRTH2, chemoattractant receptor-homologous molecule expressed on Th2 cells; vs, versus

Study or Subgroup	Experimental Events	Total	Control Events	Total	Weight	Risk Ratio IV, Fixed, 95% CI
1.11.1 asthmatics with CRTH2 antagonists monotherapy						
Barnes 2012	14	65	15	67	1.5%	0.96 [0.51, 1.83]
Erpenbeck 2016	29	82	25	88	3.2%	1.24 [0.80, 1.94]
Fowler 2017	53	63	15	21	7.4%	1.18 [0.88, 1.58]
Hall (trial 1) 2015	109	239	32	78	6.9%	1.11 [0.82, 1.50]
Kuna (trial 1) 2016	29	57	26	56	4.3%	1.10 [0.75, 1.60]
Pettipher 2014	106	296	53	123	9.7%	0.83 [0.64, 1.07]
Singh 2013	13	20	14	19	3.6%	0.88 [0.58, 1.34]
Wenzel 2014	35	93	45	91	5.6%	0.76 [0.54, 1.06]
Subtotal (95% CI)		915		543	42.2%	0.98 [0.87, 1.11]
Total events	388		225			

Heterogeneity: Chi^2 = 7.73, df = 7 (P = 0.36); I^2 = 9%
Test for overall effect: Z = 0.30 (P = 0.76)

1.11.2 asthmatics with CRTH2 antagonists as add–on to corticosteroids therapy						
Bateman 2017	367	765	68	136	18.6%	0.96 [0.80, 1.15]
Bateman 2018	283	977	49	163	9.7%	0.96 [0.75, 1.24]
Busse 2012	178	317	36	79	9.3%	1.23 [0.95, 1.60]
Gonem 2016	21	29	25	32	7.4%	0.93 [0.69, 1.24]
Hall (trial 2) 2015	28	81	43	95	4.5%	0.76 [0.53, 1.11]
Kuna (trial 2) 2016	83	277	24	91	4.2%	1.14 [0.77, 1.67]
Miller 2017	60	205	27	104	4.2%	1.13 [0.76, 1.66]
Subtotal (95% CI)		2651		700	57.8%	1.00 [0.90, 1.11]
Total events	1020		272			

Heterogeneity: Chi^2 = 5.82, df = 6 (P = 0.44); I^2 = 0%
Test for overall effect: Z = 0.02 (P = 0.99)

Total (95% CI)		3566		1243	100.0%	0.99 [0.92, 1.07]
Total events	1408		497			

Heterogeneity: Chi^2 = 13.60, df = 14 (P = 0.48); I^2 = 0%
Test for overall effect: Z = 0.18 (P = 0.86)
Test for subgroup differences: Chi^2 = 0.06, df = 1 (P = 0.81), I^2 = 0%

Favours [experimental] Favours [control]

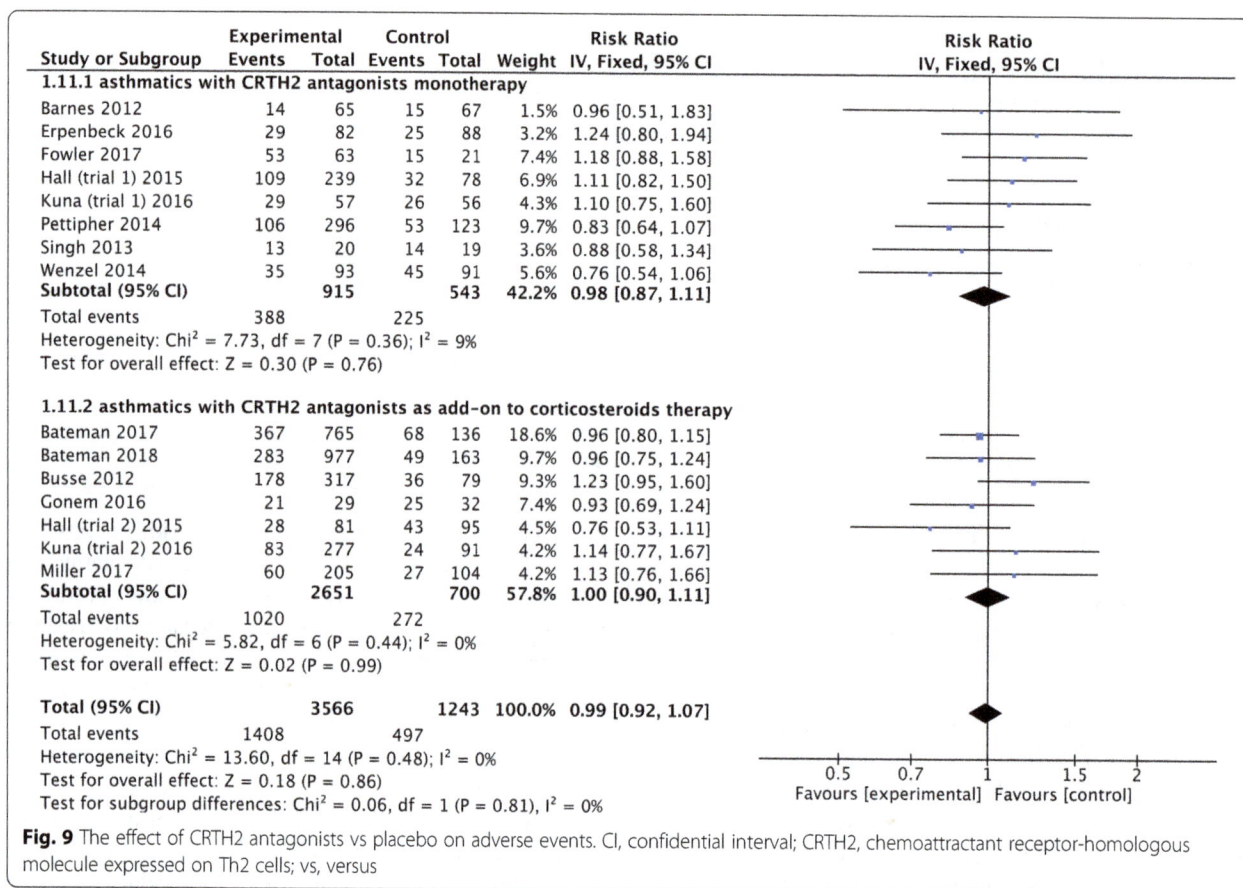

Fig. 9 The effect of CRTH2 antagonists vs placebo on adverse events. CI, confidential interval; CRTH2, chemoattractant receptor-homologous molecule expressed on Th2 cells; vs, versus

interpreted cautiously because of the moderate heterogeneity and limited studies included, which is also true for Methacholine PC$_{20}$. Thus, further studies are needed to clarify the effect of CRTH2 antagonists on PEF and Methacholine PC$_{20}$.

It is recommended by GINA that asthma assessment should focus on asthma symptom control and future exacerbations risk reduction [2]. ACQ and AQLQ are both commonly used self-evaluation questionnaires for asthma symptoms and quality of life [34, 35], and our meta-analysis showed that CRTH2 antagonists therapy could reduce ACQ scores and increase AQLQ scores. SABA is one of the most important quick relievers for asthma onset, and the number of its rescue use has already been elucidated to be associated with asthma exacerbations [2]. Our meta-analysis also found that CRTH2 antagonists, either used as monotherapy or add-on therapy to corticosteroids, could reduce SABA use. Asthma exacerbations are associated with the poor asthma control [2] and is the major cause of morbidity and mortality in asthmatics [36]. In our meta-analysis, significant reduction in asthma exacerbations was found in the asthmatics with CRTH2 antagonist monotherapy rather than add-on therapy to corticosteroids. Therefore, based on the above positive findings, CRTH2 antagonists

may serve as an efficacious surrogate for corticosteroids and reduce the use or adverse events of corticosteroids. However, future studies are still warranted due to the inconsistent of CRTH2 antagonists types, doses, and durations, as well as the potential heterogeneities and limited studies.

It is reported that sputum or blood eosinophil level is associated with high incidence of asthma attacks, and they are also one of the important markers for asthma phenotyping [37, 38]. Meanwhile, blockade of CRTH2 has been recognized to down-regulate Th2 cytokines production [8], decrease eosinophils release from bone marrow [7, 39], chemotaxis and respiratory burst [28]. Therefore, eosinophil might be a potential indicator for treatment effectiveness and asthma phenotyping may also help to identify the better responsive subgroup. However, inconsistent data from the included studies disabled us to pool in meta-analysis, and our systematic review also showed inconclusive results. FeNO is believed to be an indirect marker for eosinophilic airway inflammation [40], and our systematic review found that CRTH2 antagonists could not decrease FeNO. However, more studies are necessitated before we can draw a clear conclusion because the role of FeNO itself in asthma airway inflammation is still not clarified and controversial

Table 3 Results of sputum and blood eosinophils, FeNO and Methacholine PC_{20}

Source	Groups	Baseline	Treatment endpoint	Change after treatment	P value (Intervention vs Placebo)	Significant Difference
Sputum eosinophils (10^6/g)						
Singh 2013 [13]	Intervention	NM	0.4##	NM	0.002	Yes
	Control	NM	0.75##	NM		No
Kuna (trial 1) 2016 [21]	Intervention	0.024 (0.00 to 0.53)§	0.004 (0.00 to 0.53)§	NM	NM	No
	Control	0.033 (0.00 to 1.21)§	0.014 (0.00 to 0.73)§	NM		
Sputum eosinophils (%)						
Barnes 2012 [11]	Intervention	2.1 (NM)‡	0.7 (NM)‡	3.1 (1.1, 8.8)§§	0.37	No
	Control	1.8(NM)‡	1.2 (NM)‡	1.5 (0.4, 5.3)§§		
Singh 2013 [13]	Intervention	6.0 (1.5, 23.9)‡	18.1 (10.0, 33.2)‡	NM	0.002	Yes
	Control	6.0 (1.5, 23.9)‡	5.6 (2.7, 11.6)‡	NM		
Busse 2013 [17]	Intervention	2.0 (0 to 93)§	NM	−3.5 (−93 to 5)§	NM	No
		1.0 (0 to 69)§	NM	−0.5 (−68 to 36)§	NM	
		1.0 (0 to 91)§	NM	0.0 (−72 to 6)§	NM	
		1.0 (0 to 80)§	NM	0.0 (−24 to 4)§	NM	
	Control	0.0 (0 to 53)§	NM	2.0 (−2.3 to 84)§	–	
Gonem 2016 [20]	Intervention	5.4 (3.1, 9.6)‡	1.1 (0.7, 1.9)‡	0.22 (0.13, 0.39)§§	0.0014	Yes
	Control	4.6 (2.5–8.7)‡	3.9 (2.3–6.7)‡	0.78 (0.45, 1.33)§§		
Blood eosinophils (10^9/L)						
Gonem 2016 [20]	Intervention	0.29 (95.03)#	0.29 (0.23–0.36)‡	1.01 (0.79, 1.28)§§	0.44	No
	Control	0.28 (80.63)#	0.32 (0.25, 0.41)‡	1.13 (0.89, 1.43)§§		
Kuna (trial 1) 2016 [21]	Intervention	NM	NM	NM	NM	No
	Control	NM	NM	NM		
Diamant 2014 [24]	Intervention	NM	NM	NM	NM	No
	Control	NM	NM	NM		
FeNO (ppb)						
Singh 2013 [13]	Intervention	33.9 (22.4)*	26.3 (23.7)*	NM	NM	No
	Control	39.3 (23.9)*	23.3 (22.8)*	NM		
Bateman 2017 [16]	Intervention	NM	NM	NM	> 0.05	No
		NM	NM	NM	> 0.05	
		NM	NM	NM	> 0.05	
	Control	NM	NM	NM	–	

Table 3 Results of sputum and blood eosinophils, FeNO and Methacholine PC_{20} (Continued)

Source	Groups	Baseline	Treatment endpoint	Change after treatment	P value (Intervention vs Placebo)	Significant Difference
Busse 2013 [17]	Intervention	31.9 (21.4)*	NM	0.221	> 0.05	No
		30.9 (30.5)*	NM	2.368	> 0.05	
		28.3 (23.2)*	NM	−0.080	> 0.05	
		33.5 (31.6)*	NM	1.333	> 0.05	
	Control	28.1 (22.0)*	NM	−7.000	–	
Gonem 2016 [20]	Intervention	37.72 (4.75)†	34.88 (3.97)†	−5.82 (−13.79, 2.16)**	0.49	No
	Control	43.67 (6.97)†	38.48 (4.32)†	−2.21 (−10.90, 6.48)**		
Kuna (trial 1) 2016 [21]	Intervention	NM	NM	NM	NM	No
	Control	NM	NM	NM		
Diamant 2014 [24]	Intervention	51.6 (38.5)*	NM	NM	NM	No
	Control	71.0 (36.5)*	NM	NM		
Methacholine PC_{20} (mg/mL)						
Singh 2013 [13]	Intervention	1.48 (3.2)*	0.31*	NM	NM	No
	Control	1.48 (3.2)*	0.39*			
Diamant 2014 [24]	Intervention	0.91 (2.21)††	0.97 (1.98)††	NM	0.038	Yes
	Control	1.00 (2.19)††	0.49 (2.19)††			

Methacholine PC_{20}, the provocation concentration of methacholine causing a 20% fall in FEV_1; NM, not mentioned

findings showed that the specific inhibition of inducible nitric oxide synthase did not affect airway hyperresponsiveness and airway inflammation [41].

In our meta-analysis, we found similar adverse events between CRTH2 antagonists treatment and placebo, and no treatment related severe adverse events and deaths were reported, which indicated a general safety profile of CRTH2 antagonists in the treatment of asthma patients. Although CRTH2 antagonists were reported to cause some adverse events, but most of them were mild and moderate such as nasopharyngitis, headache, asthma, infections and gastrointestinal disorders. However, use with cautions, especially for some elderly patients with concomitant diseases, should always be addressed.

Several potential limitations require consideration in interpreting our study results. First of all, although some parameters, such as pre-bronchodilator FEV_1, ACQ and AQLQ scores, have been improved in patients with CRTH2 antagonists, the clinical importance of these improvements need to be questioned because they are less than minimal clinical importance difference [35, 42, 43]. Secondly, asthma exacerbations in the trials included were not defined consistently and even not defined explicitly in one trial [22]. Thirdly, a small scale of some studies and limited number of RCTs included in several outcomes analysis may affect the power to explore the real outcome. Finally, the heterogeneities among the studies might cause inaccurate results in some outcomes. Although we have classified the studies into subgroups based on the intervention therapies and we found no statistical heterogeneities in most of the outcomes, but the baseline asthma severity and phenotypes varied among studies, which makes it necessary for further studies to clarify which subgroups of asthmatics can benefit this treatment. Moreover, given the variety of CRTH2 antagonists in selectivity, specificity and affinity, such as the dual affinity of AMG 853 to both DP2 and DP1, the interpretation of our results should also be cautious and it is hard to decide the optimal types of CRTH2 antagonists, dose, and treatment duration. Therefore, future studies involving and dealing with these issues are urgently needed.

Conclusions

In patients with asthma, CRTH2 antagonists especially being administered as monotherapy were well tolerated and efficacious in improving lung function and quality of life , as well as reducing rescue use of SABA and asthma exacerbations. CRHT2 antagonists might be suitable surrogates for corticosteroids in patients who are contraindicated to steroids treatment or who require steroids limitation to avoid related adverse events. However, further trials are necessitated, particularly in different asthma phenotypes as well as in comparison between CRTH2 antagonists and corticosteroids monotherapy, to identify the potential asthma subgroups with best treatment responses and determine the optimal administration strategy of CRTH2 antagonists.

Additional file

Additional file 1: Figure S1. Begg's test for publication bias on pre-bronchodilator FEV1 (L). Figure S2. Meta-regression plot of mean difference for pre-bronchodilator FEV_1 (L) predicted by treatment duration. Figure S3. Meta-regression plot of mean difference for pre-bronchodilator FEV_1 (L) predicted by asthma severity. Figure S4. Meta-regression plot of mean difference for pre-bronchodilator FEV_1 (L) predicted by concomitant treatment. Figure S5. The effect of CRTH2 antagonists used as monotherapy or add-on therapy versus placebo on pre-bronchodilator FEV_1% predicted. Figure S6. The effect of CRTH2 antagonists used as monotherapy or add-on therapy versus placebo on post-bronchodilator FEV_1 (L). Figure S7. The effect of CRTH2 antagonists used as monotherapy or add-on therapy versus placebo on FVC. Figure S8. The effect of CRTH2 antagonists used as monotherapy or add-on therapy versus placebo on severe adverse events. Figure S9. The effect of CRTH2 antagonists used as monotherapy or add-on therapy versus placebo on treatment related adverse events. Figure S10. The effect of CRTH2 antagonists used as monotherapy or add-on therapy versus placebo on adverse events leading to treatment withdrawal. Figure S11. Begg's test for publication bias on adverse event. Figure S12. Meta-regression plot of risk ratio for adverse events predicted by treatment duration. Figure S13. Meta-regression plot of risk ratio for adverse events predicted by concomitant treatment. Figure S14. Meta-regression plot of risk ratio for adverse events predicted by asthma severity. (DOCX 10650 kb)

Abbreviations

ACQ: Asthma control questionnaire; AQLQ: Asthma quality of life questionnaire; CI: Confidence interval; CRTH2: Chemoattractant receptor-homologous molecule expressed on Th2 cells; FeNO: Fractional exhaled nitric oxide; FEV_1: Forced volume in one second; FVC: Forced vital capacity; GINA: Global Initiative for Asthma; MD: Mean differences; Methacholine PC_{20}: The provocation concentration of methacholine causing a 20% fall in FEV_1; PEF: Peak expiratory flow; RCT: Randomized controlled trial; RD: Risk difference; RR: Risk ratio; SABA: Short-acting β_2 agonists; SD: Standard deviation

Acknowledgements
not applicable.

Funding
This study was supported by the National Science Foundation of China (81770035).

Authors' contributions

JY serve as a guarantor and take responsibility for the content of the manuscript, including data and analysis. JY and JL contributed to the design of the study, data analysis and interpretation and drafted the manuscript; LY and T–XH conducted the literature search and data extraction; DY and B–CL conducted quality assessment; DW, X–HW revised the manuscript critically for important intellectual content; C-TL made the decision to submit the report for publication. All authors read and approved the final manuscript.

Competing interests

the authors declare that they have no competing interests.

Author details

[1]Department of Respiratory and Critical Care Medicine, West China School of Medicine and West China Hospital, Sichuan University, No.37, Guoxue Alley, Chengdu 610041, China. [2]Department of Respiratory Medicine, Mianyang Central Hospital, Mianyang 621099, China.

References

1. Masoli M, Fabian D, Holt S, Beasley R. The global burden of asthma: executive summary of the GINA Dissemination Committee report. Allergy. 2004;59(5):469–78.
2. Global Strategy for Asthma Management and Prevention, 2017. Available from: http://www.ginasthma/.org.
3. Price D, Fletcher M, van der Molen T. Asthma control and management in 8,000 European patients: the REcognise asthma and LInk to symptoms and experience (REALISE) survey. Npj Primary Care Respiratory Medicine. 2014;24.
4. Stead RJ, Cooke NJ. Adverse effects of inhaled corticosteroids. Bmj. 1989; 298:403–4.
5. Hirai H, Tanaka K, Yoshie O, Ogawa K, Kenmotsu K, Takamori Y, Ichimasa M, Sugamura K, Nakamura M, Takano S, Nagata K. Prostaglandin D2 selectively induces chemotaxis in T helper type 2 cells, eosinophils, and basophils via seven-transmembrane receptor CRTH2. J Exp Med. 2001;193:255–61.
6. Xue L, Barrow A, Pettipher R. Novel function of CRTH2 in preventing apoptosis of human Th2 cells through activation of the phosphatidylinositol 3-kinase pathway. J Immunol. 2009;182:7580–6.
7. Xue L, Gyles SL, Wettey FR, Gazi L, Townsend E, Hunter MG, Pettipher R. Prostaglandin D2 causes preferential induction of proinflammatory Th2 cytokine production through an action on chemoattractant receptor-like molecule expressed on Th2 cells. J Immunol. 2005;175:6531–6.
8. Lukacs NW, Berlin AA, Franz-Bacon K, Sasik R, Sprague LJ, Ly TW, Hardiman G, Boehme SA, Bacon KB. CRTH2 antagonism significantly ameliorates airway hyperreactivity and downregulates inflammation-induced genes in a mouse model of airway inflammation. Am J Phys Lung Cell Mol Phys. 2008; 295:L767–79.
9. Stebbins KJ, Broadhead AR, Correa LD, Scott JM, Truong YP, Stearns BA, Hutchinson JH, Prasit P, Evans JF, Lorrain DS. Therapeutic efficacy of AM156, a novel prostanoid DP2 receptor antagonist, in murine models of allergic rhinitis and house dust mite-induced pulmonary inflammation. Eur J Pharmacol. 2010;638:142–9.
10. Uller L, Mathiesen JM, Alenmyr L, Korsgren M, Ulven T, Hogberg T, Andersson G, Persson CGA, Kostenis E. Antagonism of the prostaglandin D-2 receptor CRTH2 attenuates asthma pathology in mouse eosinophilic airway inflammation. Respir Res. 2007;8.
11. Barnes N, Pavord I, Chuchalin A, Bell J, Hunter M, Lewis T, Parker D, Payton M, Collins LP, Pettipher R, et al. A randomized, double-blind, placebo-controlled study of the CRTH2 antagonist OC000459 in moderate persistent asthma. Clin Exp Allergy. 2012;42:38–48.
12. Pettipher R, Hunter MG, Perkins CM, Collins LP, Lewis T, Baillet M, Steiner J, Bell J, Payton MA. Heightened response of eosinophilic asthmatic patients to the CRTH2 antagonist OC000459. Allergy. 2014;69:1223–32.
13. Singh D, Cadden P, Hunter M, Pearce Collins L, Perkins M, Pettipher R, Townsend E, Vinall S, O'Connor B. Inhibition of the asthmatic allergen challenge response by the CRTH2 antagonist OC000459. Eur Respir J. 2013; 41:46–52.
14. Hall IP, Fowler AV, Gupta A, Tetzlaff K, Nivens MC, Sarno M, Finnigan HA, Bateman ED, Sutherland ER. Efficacy of BI 671800, an oral CRTH2 antagonist, in poorly controlled asthma as sole controller and in the presence of inhaled corticosteroid treatment. Pulm Pharmacol Ther. 2015;32:37–44.
15. Higgins J, Green S (2013) Cochrane handbook for systematic reviews of interventions version 5.1. 0, the Cochrane collaboration, 2011.
16. Bateman ED, Guerreros AG, Brockhaus F, Holzhauer B, Pethe A, Kay RA, Townley RG. Fevipiprant, an oral prostaglandin DP2 receptor (CRTH2) antagonist, in allergic asthma uncontrolled on low-dose inhaled corticosteroids. Eur Respir J. 2017;50.
17. Busse WW, Wenzel SE, Meltzer EO, Kerwin EM, Liu MC, Zhang N, Chon Y, Budelsky AL, Lin J, Lin SL. Safety and efficacy of the prostaglandin D2 receptor antagonist AMG 853 in asthmatic patients. J Allergy Clin Immunol. 2013;131:339–45.
18. Erpenbeck VJ, Popov TA, Miller D, Weinstein SF, Spector S, Magnusson B, Osuntokun W, Goldsmith P, Weiss M, Beier J. The oral CRTH2 antagonist QAW039 (fevipiprant): a phase II study in uncontrolled allergic asthma. Pulmonary Pharmacology and Therapeutics. 2016;39:54–63.
19. Fowler A, Koenen R, Hilbert J, Blatchford J, Kappeler D, Benediktus E, Wood C, Gupta A. Safety, tolerability, pharmacokinetics, and pharmacodynamics of the novel CRTH2 antagonist BI 1021958 at single Oral doses in healthy men and multiple Oral doses in men and women with well-controlled asthma. J Clin Pharmacol. 2017;57:1444–53.
20. Gonem S, Berair R, Singapuri A, Hartley R, Laurencin MFM, Bacher G, Holzhauer B, Bourne M, Mistry V, Pavord ID, et al. Fevipiprant, a prostaglandin D-2 receptor 2 antagonist, in patients with persistent eosinophilic asthma: a single-Centre, randomised, double-blind, parallel-group, placebo-controlled trial. Lancet Respiratory Medicine. 2016;4:699–707.
21. Kuna P, Bjermer L, Tornling G. Two phase II randomized trials on the CRTh2 antagonist AZD1981 in adults with asthma. Drug Design Development and Therapy. 2016;10:2759–70.
22. Wenzel SE, Hopkins R, Saunders M, Chantry D, Anderson L, Aitchison R, Eberhardt C, Bell S, Cole J, Wolfe J, et al: Safety and efficacy of ARRY-502, a potent, selective, Oral CRTh2 antagonist, in patients with mild to moderate Th2-driven asthma. J Allergy Clin Immunol 2014, 133:AB4-AB4.
23. Bateman ED, O'Brien C, Rugman P, Luke S, Ivanov S, Uddin M. Efficacy and safety of the CRTh2 antagonist AZD1981 as add-on therapy to inhaled corticosteroids and long-acting beta$_2$-agonists in patients with atopic asthma. Drug Design, Development and Therapy. 2018;12:1093–106.
24. Diamant Z, Sidharta PN, Singh D, O'Connor BJ, Zuiker R, Leaker BR, Silkey M, Dingemanse J. Setipiprant, a selective CRTH2 antagonist, reduces allergen-induced airway responses in allergic asthmatics. Clin Exp Allergy. 2014;44: 1044–52.
25. Miller D, Wood C, Bateman E, LaForce C, Blatchford J, Hilbert J, Gupta A, Fowler A. A randomized study of BI 671800, a CRTH2 antagonist, as add-on therapy in poorly controlled asthma. Allergy and Asthma Proceedings. 2017; 38:157–64.
26. Frey U, Brodbeck T, Majumdar A, Taylor DR, Town GI, Silverman M, Suki B. Risk of severe asthma episodes predicted from fluctuation analysis of airway function. Nature. 2005;438:667–70.
27. O'Byrne PM, Inman MD. Airway hyperresponsiveness. Chest. 2003;123: 411s–6s.
28. Royer JF, Schratl P, Lorenz S, Kostenis E, Ulven T, Schuligoi R, Peskar BA, Heinemann A. A novel antagonist of CRTH2 blocks eosinophil release from bone marrow, chemotaxis and respiratory burst. Allergy. 2007;62:1401–9.
29. Gleich GJ. Mechanisms of eosinophil-associated inflammation. J Allergy Clin Immunol. 2000;105:651–63.
30. Larche M, Robinson DS, Kay AB. The role of T lymphocytes in the pathogenesis of asthma. J Allergy Clin Immunol. 2003;111:450–63.
31. Atamas SP, Yurovsky VV, Wise R, Wigley FM, Goter Robinson CJ, Henry P, Alms WJ, White B. Production of type 2 cytokines by CD8+ lung cells is associated with greater decline in pulmonary function in patients with systemic sclerosis. Arthritis Rheum. 1999;42:1168–78.
32. Llewellin P, Sawyer G, Lewis S, Cheng S, Weatherall M, Fitzharris P, Beasley R. The relationship between FEV$_1$ and PEF in the assessment of the severity of airways obstruction. Respirology. 2002;7:333–7.
33. Aggarwal AN, Gupta D, Jindal SK. The relationship between FEV$_1$ and peak expiratory flow in patients with airways obstruction is poor. Chest. 2006;130: 1454–61.
34. Juniper EF, Guyatt GH, Epstein RS, Ferrie PJ, Jaeschke R, Hiller TK. Evaluation of impairment of health related quality of life in asthma: development of a questionnaire for use in clinical trials. Thorax. 1992;47:76–83.
35. Juniper EF, Svensson K, Mork AC, Stahl E. Measurement properties and interpretation of three shortened versions of the asthma control questionnaire. Respir Med. 2005;99:553–8.
36. Masoli M, Fabian D, Holt S, Beasley R. The global burden of asthma: executive summary of the GINA dissemination committee report. Allergy. 2004;59:469–78.
37. Tran TN, Khatry DB, Ke X, Ward CK, Gossage D. High blood eosinophil count is associated with more frequent asthma attacks in asthma patients. Ann Allergy Asthma Immunol. 2014;113:19–24.
38. Simpson JL, Scott R, Boyle MJ, Gibson PG. Inflammatory subtypes in asthma: assessment and identification using induced sputum. Respirology. 2006;11:54–61.
39. Xue L, Salimi M, Panse I, Mjosberg JM, McKenzie AN, Spits H, Klenerman P, Ogg G. Prostaglandin D2 activates group 2 innate lymphoid cells through chemoattractant receptor-homologous molecule expressed on TH2 cells. J Allergy Clin Immunol. 2014;133:1184–94.

15

High-flow nasal cannula in adults with acute respiratory failure and after extubation

Zhiheng Xu[1,2†], Yimin Li[1,2†], Jianmeng Zhou[1], Xi Li[1,2], Yongbo Huang[1,2], Xiaoqing Liu[1], Karen E. A. Burns[3,4,5*], Nanshan Zhong[1] and Haibo Zhang[1,2,3,4,5*]

Abstract

Background: High-flow nasal cannula (HFNC) can be used as an initial support strategy for patients with acute respiratory failure (ARF) and after extubation. However, no clear evidence exists to support or oppose HFNC use in clinical practice. We summarized the effects of HFNC, compared to conventional oxygen therapy (COT) and noninvasive ventilation (NIV), on important outcomes including treatment failure and intubation/reintubation rates in adult patients with ARF and after extubation.

Methods: We searched 4 electronic databases (Pubmed, EMBASE, Scopus, and Web of Science) to identify randomized controlled trials (RCTs) comparing the effects of HFNC with either COT or NIV on rates of 1) treatment failure and 2) intubation/reintubation in adult critically ill patients.

Results: We identified 18 RCTs ($n = 4251$ patients) in pooled analyses. As a primary mode of support, HFNC treatment reduced the risk of treatment failure [Odds Ratio (OR) 0.65; 95% confidence interval (CI) 0.43–0.98; $p = 0.04$; $I^2 = 32\%$] but had no effect on preventing intubation (OR, 0.74; 95%CI 0.45–1.21; $p = 0.23$; $I^2 = 0\%$) compared to COT. When used after extubation, HFNC (vs. COT) treatment significantly decreased reintubation rate (OR 0.46; 95%CI 0.33–0.63; $p < 0.00001$; $I^2 = 30\%$) and extubation failure (OR 0.43; 95%CI 0.25–0.73; $p = 0.002$; $I^2 = 66\%$). Compared to NIV, HFNC significantly reduced intubation rate (OR 0.57; 95%CI 0.36–0.92; $p = 0.02$; $I^2 = 0\%$) when used as initial support, but did no favorably impact clinical outcomes post extubation in few trials.

Conclusions: HFNC was superior to COT in reducing treatment failure when used as a primary support strategy and in reducing rates of extubation failure and reintubation when used after extubation. In few trials, HFNC reduced intubation rate compared to NIV when used as initial support but demonstrated no beneficial effects after extubation.

Keywords: Conventional oxygen therapy, Noninvasive ventilation, Extubation

Background

Acute respiratory failure (ARF) is one of the most common causes of intensive care unit (ICU) mortality [1–3]. Oxygen therapy is a main stay of treatment for patients with hypoxemic respiratory failure. Several devices can be used to administer conventional oxygen treatments

* Correspondence: BurnsK@smh.ca; zhangh@smh.ca
†Zhiheng Xu and Yimin Li contributed equally to this work.
[3]Interdepartmental Division of Critical Care Medicine, University of Toronto, Toronto, ON, Canada
[1]State Key Laboratory of Respiratory Diseases, National Clinical Research Center for Respiratory Disease, Guangzhou Institute for Respiratory Health, Guangzhou, China
Full list of author information is available at the end of the article

(COT), including nasal cannula, simple face masks, Venturi masks, and high-concentration reservoir masks [4]. The maximal flow rate that can be achieved with COT is 15 L/min which is lower than the inspiratory flow of most patients with ARF. Room air is often added to increase flow but at the expense of reducing the final concentration of oxygen delivered to patients at the alveolar level [5, 6]. Additionally, insufficient moisture and a lack of warm air during COT can induce discomfort for patients who require supplemental oxygen [7, 8].

High-flow nasal cannula (HFNC) delivers heated and humidified oxygen gas through the nasal or tracheal route with flow rates as high as 60 L/min in adults [6]. Several clinical trials have reported that HFNC improves oxygenation prior to intubation and reduces episodes of severe hypoxemia during intubation [9], post-cardiothoracic surgery [10], during bronchoscopy [11] and after extubation from invasive mechanical ventilation (IMV) in patients with ARF [12, 13]. Despite encouraging results from preliminary randomized controlled trials (RCTs), clarity is lacking regarding specific patient populations who may benefit from HFNC use [14–17]. To address this deficiency in the literature, we performed the current meta-analysis to compare the effect of HFNC, COT and noninvasive ventilation (NIV) on clinical outcomes of patients receiving either initial ARF treatment or respiratory support after extubation.

Methods

Inclusion and exclusion criteria

We included prospective RCTs involving adult patients comparing HFNC with either COT or NIV as an initial support strategy in patients with ARF or after extubation. We limited publications to adult patients (using author's definitions) and the English language. We excluded crossover trials, before-after studies, abstract publications, conference presentations, case reports, editorials, and trials that included fewer than 20 patients in either treatment arm.

Search strategy

To increase the sensitivity of our search strategy, we combined the terms "high flow oxygen" with "noninvasive ventilation" or "oxygen inhalation therapy" as key words or Medical Subject Headings (MeSH) terms. We searched 4 databases (Pubmed, EMBASE, Scopus, and Web of Science) from electronic databases inception to September, 1st, 2018. We systematically screened abstracts and full text publications for studies that met our eligibility criteria.

Definitions

ARF was defined as the requirement for oxygen therapy to maintain peripheral capillary oxygen saturation (SpO_2) > 92% or PaO_2/FiO_2 (P/F ratio) > 300, symptoms of respiratory distress (including tachypnea > 22 breaths/min, labored breathing, use of intercostal muscles, and/or dyspnea at rest) or using 'authors' definitions. HFNC was defined as respiratory support that delivered a high flow (> 15 L/min) of heated and humidified oxygen (37 °C) administered through nasal cannula. COT was referred to relatively low flow oxygen (≤ 15 L/min) through nasal cannula, a simple face mask, a Venturi mask, or a high-concentration reservoir mask. NIV included bilevel positive airway pressure and continuous positive airway pressure (CPAP). Treatment failure was defined as switching to a higher level respiratory support, (e.g., from HFNC or COT to NIV or IMV, or from HFNC or NIV to IMV).

Extubation failure was defined as the need for NIV or reintubation within 72 h after HFNC use.

Outcomes

The primary outcomes of this review were treatment failure and intubation (alternatively, reintubation rate in trials comparing alternative treatments after extubation) reflecting the efficacy of HFNC therapy (i.e., HFNC vs. COT, HFNC vs. NIV). Secondary outcomes included ICU and hospital mortality, ICU and hospital length of stay (LOS), patient comfort, respiratory rate (RR), and P/F ratio.

The four main comparisons in our review include (a) HFNC versus COT as initial support for patients with ARF; (b) HFNC versus COT to prevent extubation failure; (c) HFNC versus NIV in patients with ARF and (d) HFNC versus NIV after extubation. In a pre-specified subgroup analysis, we sought to compare the effect on intubation rate of HFNC vs. NIV in studies involving patients with severe hypoxemia (P/F ratio < 200 mmHg).

Data abstraction

Three investigators (ZX, XL and JZ), working in pairs, independently reviewed and abstracted data from each retrieved article and supplement, where indicated. Discrepancies were resolved by discussion and consensus.

Quality assessment

We assessed the quality of all included trials based on review of published trial protocols identified on trial registration sites ID (ClinicalTrials.gov; Australia New Zealand Clinical Trials Registry, Thai Clinical Trials Registry, International Standard Randomized Controlled Trial Number Registry) and the details in the method section and supplements of included trials. We appraised trial quality using the Cochrane collaboration tool for assessing risk of bias (RoB) [18] including assessment of random sequence generation, allocation concealment, blinding (of interventions and outcome measurement or assessment), incomplete outcome data, selective reporting bias and other potential sources of bias (e.g., industry funding). For each criterion, we appraised the RoB to be either of low, high, or unclear risk (e.g., insufficient details). Three authors (ZX, JZ, XL), working in pairs, independently assessed study quality and disagreements were resolved by consensus.

Assessment of heterogeneity

We used the I^2 statistic to evaluate the impact of heterogeneity on pooled results. An I^2 value of greater than 50% indicated substantial heterogeneity [18]. We used fixed-effects models to pool data when heterogeneity was insignificant and the random effects models to pool data when significant heterogeneity was identified.

Statistical analysis

Categorical data and continuous data were pooled using the odds ratios (ORs) and mean difference (MD), with the 95% confidence intervals (CIs). The Grading of Recommendation, Assessment, Development and Evaluation (GRADE) criteria were used to assess the quality of the evidence for HFNC on rates of intubation/reintubation since GRADE assigns high, moderate, low and very low classification based on assessment of study limitations, inconsistency, indirectness, imprecision, and publication bias [19]. Statistical analyses were conducted with Review Manager (RevMan) Version 5.3 (Copenhagen: The Nordic Cochrane Centre, The Cochrane Collaboration, 2014), and two-sided p values < 0.05 were considered statistically significant.

Results

Description of studies

We identified 551 potentially eligible studies. After exclusion of duplicate and irrelevant articles, 28 trials were retrieved to be reviewed in greater detail. Of these, we excluded 10 studies that did not meet our eligibility criteria and thus included 18 trials in our review (Fig. 1, Additional files 1 and 2: Table S1). Of the 18 RCTs (n = 4251 including 2129 HFNC treated patients), 6 trials (n = 871) compared HFNC to COT [20–25] and 2 trials (n = 420) compared HFNC to NIV [24, 26] as an initial support strategy. For post-extubation use, 9 trials (n = 1731) compared HFNC to COT [12, 13, 27–33] and 2 trials (n = 1434) compared HFNC to NIV [10, 34]. Of these, 1 trial [24] compared HFNC, COT, and NIV treatment and data from this post-extubation trial were included in comparisons of HFNC vs. COT and HFNC vs. NIV. Two trials [25, 33] reported neither treatment failure nor intubation rate but included other secondary outcomes of interest.

Risk of bias of included studies

The RCTs included were all assessed to be at low risk of bias with respect to randomization and allocation concealment except for 3 trials [25, 31, 32] for which selection bias was deemed unclear. The same 3 trials also were assessed to be at unclear risk of bias with regard to blinded outcome assessment, completeness of outcomes data, selective outcomes reporting, and other potential sources of bias [25, 31, 32]. All trials were deemed to be at high risk of performance bias as blinding of patients, physicians, and research personnel to treatment allocation was not feasible (Fig. 2).

Primary outcomes

Trials comparing HFNC versus COT

HFNC versus COT as an initial support strategy Five of 6 trials (n = 831) comparing HFNC and COT as an

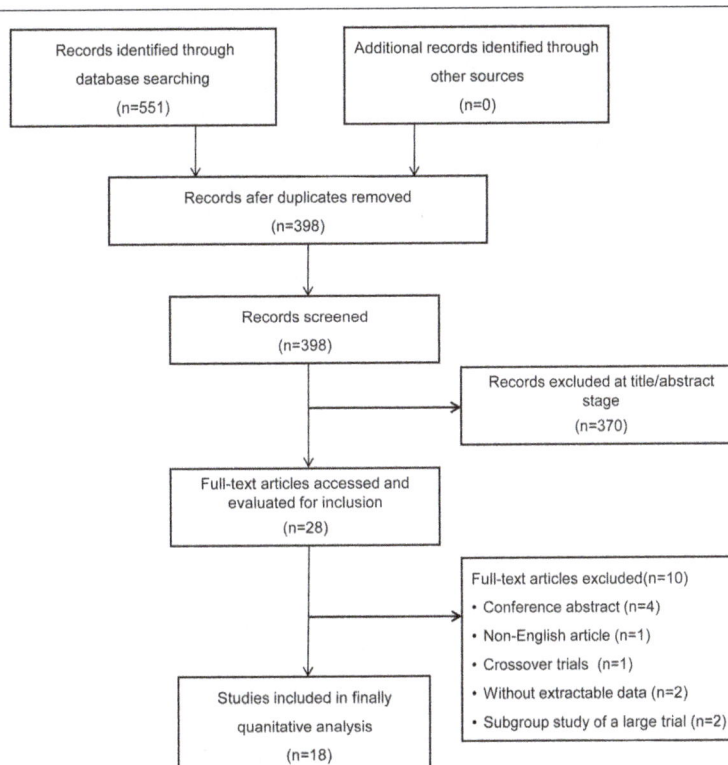

Fig. 1 Search strategy of meta-analysis on selecting patients for inclusion

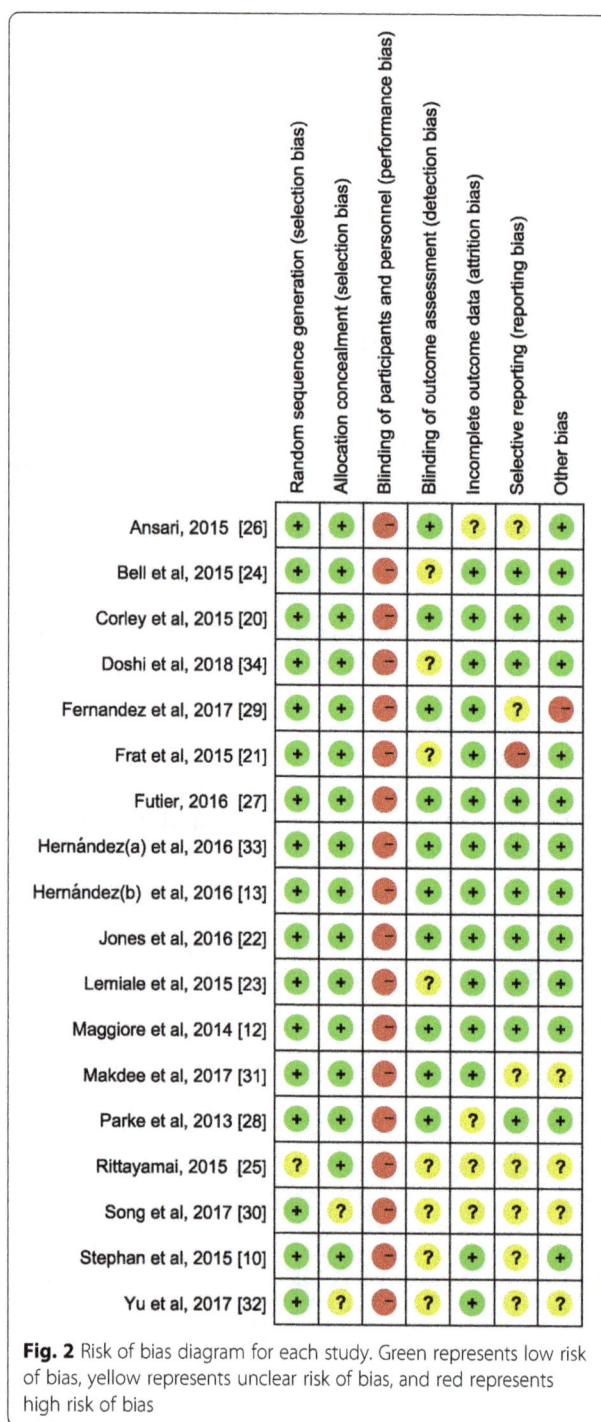

Fig. 2 Risk of bias diagram for each study. Green represents low risk of bias, yellow represents unclear risk of bias, and red represents high risk of bias

effects of the alternative support strategies on rates of extubation failure and reintubation [12, 27–33]. Compared to COT, HFNC significantly reduced the risk of extubation failure (OR 0.43; 95%CI 0.25–0.73; $p = 0.002$; $I^2 = 66\%$) (Fig. 4) and reintubation (OR 0.46; 95%CI 0.33–0.63; $p < 0.00001$; $I^2 = 30\%$) (Fig. 5).

Trials comparing HFNC versus NIV

HFNC versus NIV as an initial support strategy We pooled 2 trials ($n = 420$) that compared HFNC to NIV as an initial support strategy [24, 26]. Although HFNC had no effect on the rate treatment failure (OR 1.00; 95%CI 0.36–2.76; $p = 1.00$; $I^2 = 82\%$), it significantly reduced intubation rate in patients with ARF (OR 0.57; 95%CI 0.36–0.92; $p = 0.02$; $I^2 = 0\%$) (Additional file 2: Figure S1A).

HFNC versus NIV after Extubation In 2 trials ($n = 1434$) comparing the effects of HFNC and NIV after extubation [10, 34], there was no significant difference in rates of treatment failure (OR 0.96; 95%CI 0.75–1.24; $p = 0.77$; $I^2 = 0\%$) and reintubation (OR 1.00; 95%CI 0.76–1.32; $p = 0.98$; $I^2 = 0\%$) (Additional file 2: Figure S1B).

Secondary outcomes
Mortality and length of stay
We did not find differences in ICU and hospital mortality or lengths of stay when HFNC was compared to COT/NIV (Table 1).

Patient comfort
Due to variability in reporting of scales used to assess comfort, we were unable to pool this data quantitatively. Qualitatively, 5 trials [12, 22–24, 31] found that HFNC was more comfortable than COT. Conversely, 3 trials [20, 25, 30] reported that COT was more comfortable than HFNC and 2 trials [21, 29] noted similar comfort ratings between HFNC and COT treated patients. In trials comparing HFNC and NIV, only 2 trials reported comfort scores with 1 study reporting greater comfort with HFNC [21] for patients with ARF and 1 trial [10] reporting similar comfort scores in patients after extubation (Additional file 2: Table S2).

Physiologic outcomes
We were unable to pool related to respiratory rate and P/F ratio due to variability in measuring and reporting these outcomes (Additional file 1). The results from trials were summarized in Additional file 2: Figures S3 and S4 and Tables S4 and S5.

Subgroup analysis
In 2 trials including 640 patients with severe hypoxemia (P/F < 200 mmHg) [10, 24], HFNC had similar effects on

initial support strategy reported intubation and treatment failure rates [20–24]. Although HFNC had no effect on intubation (OR 0.74; 95%CI 0.45–1.21; $p = 0.23$; $I^2 = 0\%$), HFNC significantly reduced treatment failure (OR 0.65; 95%CI 0.43–0.98; $p = 0.04$; $I^2 = 32\%$) (Fig. 3).

HFNC versus COT after Extubation Eight of 9 trials ($n = 1672$) comparing HFNC with COT reported the

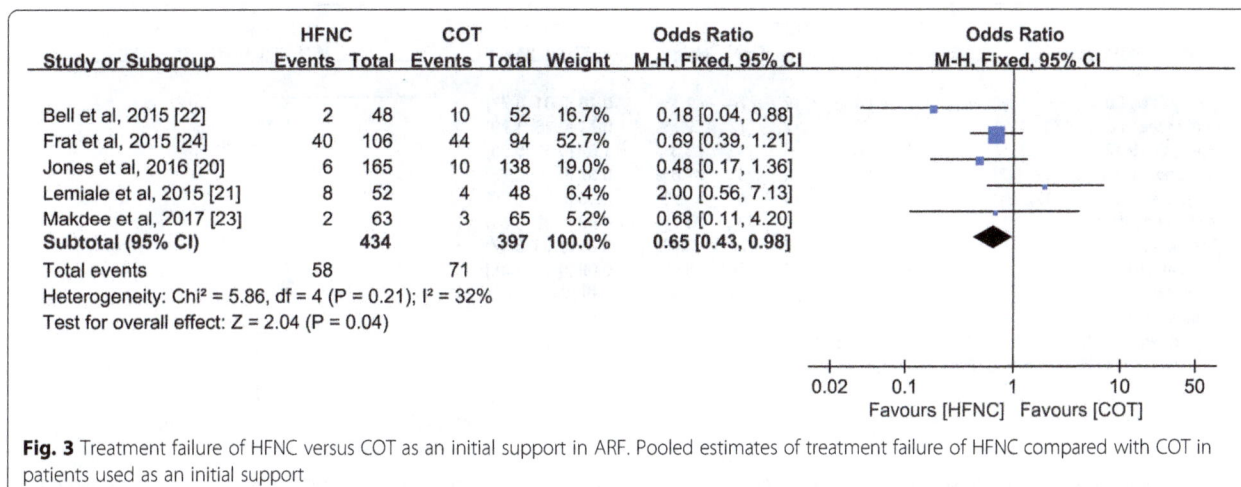

Fig. 3 Treatment failure of HFNC versus COT as an initial support in ARF. Pooled estimates of treatment failure of HFNC compared with COT in patients used as an initial support

intubation compared to NIV (OR 0.69; 95%CI 0.24–1.99; $p = 0.49$; $I^2 = 87\%$) (Additional file 2: Figure S2).

Quality assessment

The strength of the evidence comparing HFNC to COT in ARF patients on treatment failure and intubation rate was of low quality, whereas for the comparison of HFNC with COT in extubation patients, the evidence on treatment failure and reintubation rate was of moderate quality. When comparing HFNC to NIV, both the intubation rate in ARF and reintubation rate in extubation patients were of low quality (Table 2).

Discussion

We found that HFNC was superior to COT in reducing treatment failure when used as an initial support strategy and reduced rates of extubation failure, and reintubation when used after extubation. In few trials, HFNC reduced intubation rate compared to NIV when used as initial

support strategy but did not impact rates of treatment failure and reintubation when used after extubation.

To date meta-analyses have shown different effects of HFNC on intubation in patients with ARF [35–41]. The meta-analysis by Maitra et al. included 7 trials ($n = 1699$) found no benefit of HFNC compared to COT or NIV [35]. Subsequently, Monro-Somerville et al. combined data from 9 trials ($n = 2507$) comparing HFNC to other forms of respiratory support, including COT and NIV (as usual care), found no significant differences between treatment strategies in intubation and mortality rates [36]. Similarly, the review of Nedel and colleagues included 9 trials ($n = 1552$) of critically ill patients with or at risk of ARF found that HFNC therapy was not superior to COT or NIV [37]. In 2 trials ($n = 495$), a meta-analysis comparing HFNC in cardiac surgery patients, found that HFNC reduced escalation of respiratory support compared to COT [38]. Conversely, a recent meta-analysis by Ni et al. pooled 8 studies ($n = 1084$) including RCTs and retrospective studies and identified that

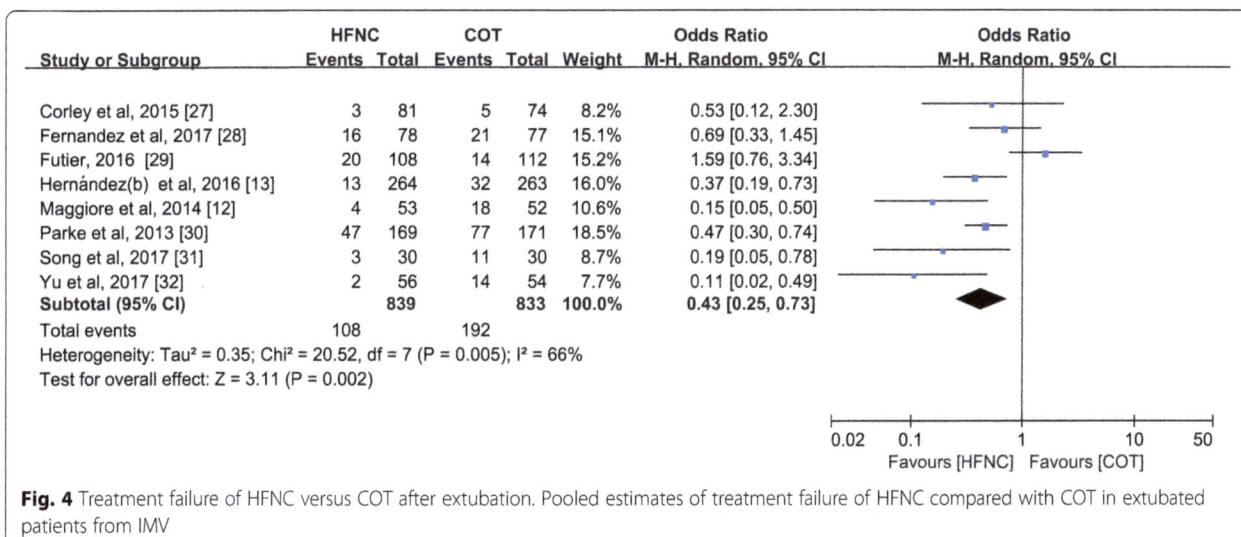

Fig. 4 Treatment failure of HFNC versus COT after extubation. Pooled estimates of treatment failure of HFNC compared with COT in extubated patients from IMV

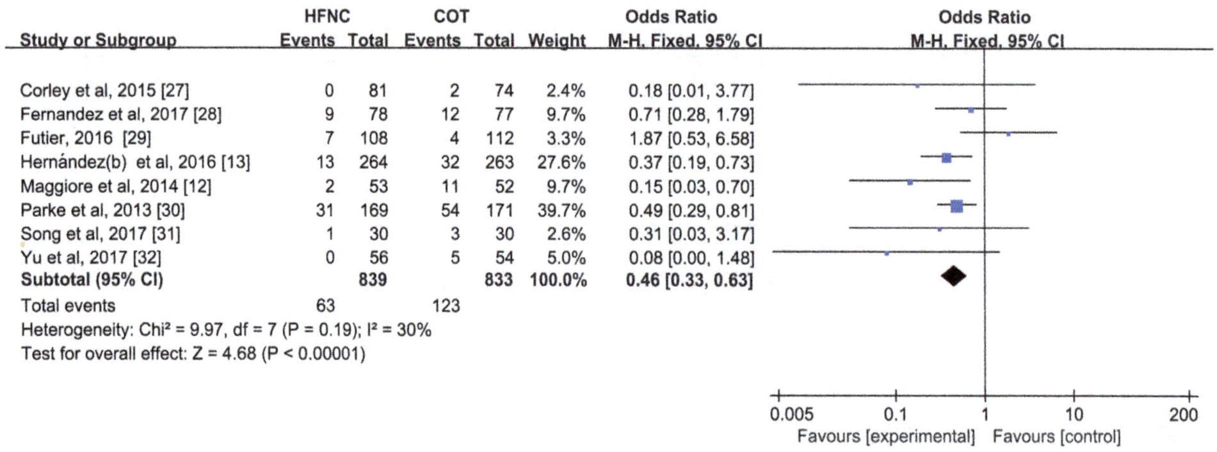

Fig. 5 Reintubation rate of HFNC versus COT after extubation. Pooled estimates of risk of reintubation in patients after extubation supported on HFNC compared with COT

Table 1 Secondary Outcomes

Clinical Outcome	No of Trials (number of patients)	Summary Estimate of Effect (Risk Ratio/Mean Difference with 95% CI)	P-value	I^2 (%)
Trials Comparing HFNC vs. COT as an Initial Support Strategy				
ICU mortality	1(200)[a]	–	–	–
Hospital mortality	2(503)	0.72(0.42–1.25)	0.25	59%
ICU length of stay	–	–	–	–
Hospital length of stay	–	–	–	–
ED length of stay	3(531)[b]	–	–	–
Trials Comparing HFNC vs. COT After Extubation				
ICU mortality	3(787)	0.99(0.47–2.08)	0.97	0%
Hospital mortality	2(683)	0.87(0.47–1.58)	0.64	0%
ICU length of stay	4(710)	3.06(−0.56–6.69)	0.10	0%
Hospital length of stay	1(59)[a]	–	–	–
ED length of stay	–	–	–	–
Trials Comparing HFNC vs. NIV as an Initial Support Strategy				
ICU mortality	1(216)[a]	–	–	–
Hospital mortality	–	–	–	–
ICU length of stay	–	–	–	–
Hospital length of stay	–	–	–	–
ED length of stay	1(204)[a]	–	–	–
Trials Comparing HFNC vs. NIV After Extubation				
ICU mortality	2(1434)	1.20(0.87–1.85)	0.40	0%
Hospital mortality	–	–	–	–
ICU length of stay	1(604)[a]	–	–	–
Hospital length of stay	–	–	–	–
ED length of stay	–	–	–	–

HFNC High flow nasal cannulae, *COT* Conventional oxygen therapy, *ED* Emergency department
[a]only 1 trials was reported, no summary estimate of effect can be combined
[b]3 trials were included, but the data was expressed in different ways (mean/median), no summary estimate of effect can be combined

Table 2 The GRADE Quality Assessment

No of studies	Design	Limitations	Inconsistency	Indirectness	Imprecision	Other considerations	HFNC	COT/NIV	Relative (95% CI)	Absolute	Quality	Importance
Intubation rate of HFNC vs. COT as a primary mode												
5	randomised trials	serious[a]	no serious inconsistency	no serious indirectness	no serious imprecision	reporting bias[b]	46/434 (10.6%)	50/397 (12.6%)	OR 0.74 (0.45 to 1.21)	30 fewer per 1000 (from 65 fewer to 23 more)	⊕⊕OO LOW	CRITICAL
Reintubation rate of HFNC vs. COT after extubation												
8	randomised trials	serious[a]	no serious inconsistency	no serious indirectness	no serious imprecision	reporting bias[b] strong association[c]	63/839 (7.5%)	123/833 (14.8%)	OR 0.47 (0.29 to 0.76)	72 fewer per 1000 (from 31 fewer to 100 fewer)	⊕⊕⊕O MODERATE	CRITICAL
Intubation rate of HFNC vs. NIV as a primary mode												
2	randomised trials	serious[a]	no serious inconsistency	no serious indirectness	no serious imprecision	reporting bias[d]	47/210 (22.4%)	68/210 (32.4%)	OR 0.57 (0.36 to 0.92)	109 fewer per 1000 (from 18 fewer to 173 more)	⊕⊕OO LOW	CRITICAL
Reintubation rate of HFNC vs. NIV after extubation												
2	randomised trials	serious[a]	no serious inconsistency	no serious indirectness	no serious imprecision	reporting bias[d]	118/704 (16.8%)	123/730 (16.8%)	OR 1.00 (0.76 to 1.32)	0 fewer per 1000 (from 35 fewer to 43 more)	⊕⊕OO LOW	CRITICAL
Treatment failure of HFNC vs. COT as a primary mode												
5	randomised trials	serious[a]	no serious inconsistency	no serious indirectness	no serious imprecision	reporting bias[b]	58/434 (13.4%)	71/397 (17.9%)	OR 0.65 (0.43 to 0.98)	55 fewer per 1000 (from 3 fewer to 93 fewer)	⊕⊕OO LOW	CRITICAL
Treatment failure of HFNC vs. COT after extubation												
8	randomised trials	serious[a]	serious inconsistency[e]	no serious indirectness	no serious imprecision	reporting bias[b] strong association[c]	108/893 (12.9%)	192/833 (23%)	OR 0.43 (0.25 to 0.73)	116 fewer per 1000 (from 51 fewer to 161 fewer)	⊕⊕⊕O MODERATE	CRITICAL

GRADE Working Group grades of evidence
High quality: Further research is very unlikely to change our confidence in the estimate of effect
Moderate quality: Further research is likely to have an important impact on our confidence in the estimate of effect and may change the estimate
Low quality: Further research is very likely to have an important impact on our confidence in the estimate of effect and is likely to change the estimate
Very low quality: We are very uncertain about the estimate
CI Confidence interval, OR Odds ratio
[a]Lack of blinding
[b]Funnel plot showed potential publication bias when HFNC vs. COT
[c]OR < 0.5
[d]Funnel plot showed potential publication bias when HFNC vs. NIV
[e]I² = 66%

HFNC reduced intubation rate compared to COT and NIV [39]. Huang et al. had found that HFNC may be benefit to avoid reintubation in critically ill patients with ARF by pooling data of 7 trials (n = 2781) [40]. The most recent review by Zhao et al. included 11 trials (n = 3459) compared HFNC to COT or NIV [41] and found that HFNC reduced intubation rate compared to COT but not to NIV. Our meta-analysis differs from previous meta-analyses in the inclusion criteria utilized, the number of trials and patients included, the outcomes reported, and in summary estimates of treatment effect. We focused on clinical indications for use of HFNC and compared its use to alternative treatments (COT and NIV). Our review represents the largest meta-analysis conducted to date including 18 RCTs and 4251 patients. We found that HFNC (vs. COT) reduced treatment failure when used as an initial support strategy in patients with ARF. Contrary to the findings of Zhao et al. [41], we found that compared to COT, HFNC reduced the rate of treatment failure (low quality) but not intubation rate (low quality evidence). Additionally, we found that HFNC (vs. COT) significantly reduced rates of both extubation failure (moderate quality evidence) and reintubation (moderate quality evidence) when used after extubation. Similar to studies conducted preterm infants, these findings suggests a potential clinical role for HFNC in the post extubation period [42]. Finally, compared to NIV, we found promising preliminary data in 2 trials that HFNC may reduce the rate of intubation when used as an initial support strategy. Taken together these findings support the use of HFNC versus COT as an initial support strategy and after extubation. Notwithstanding, several questions regarding HFNC application remain to be addressed. Further trials are needed to clarify the role for HFNC in different etiologies of ARF and compared to NIV after extubation. Several trials are currently underway to evaluate the effect of HFNC in moderate and severe ARF and in AECOPD (ClinicalTrials.gov: NCT02687074, NCT02439333).

Although HFNC therapy was initially developed for neonatal patients, indications for its use have recently been expanded to include adult patients [6, 43]. Several mechanisms have been postulated to improve oxygenation in patients who are treated with HFNC. First, the high flow rates with HFNC 'washout' carbon dioxide in upper airways and reduce dead space [44]. Second, the peak inspiratory flow of dyspneic patients can be met, and even exceeded, by the administration of high flow gas with HFNC thus reducing the dilution effects of the administered gas with room air [5]. Third, the ability to heated and humidified gas with HFNC facilitates tolerance [45]. Fourth, HFNC may create a small amount of positive pressure in the nasopharynx [46], which may help prevent atelectasis and recruit collapsed alveoli [47]. Patients, especially those with hypoxemic ARF, may benefit from some or all of the purported mechanisms of action associated with HFNC.

Our meta-analysis has several strengths. It is the largest meta-analyses conducted to date and to evaluate HFNC use by clinical indication. It is strengthened by an extensive search, duplicate citation screening and data abstraction, and conduct of a prespecified subgroup analysis. Our meta-analysis also has limitations. First, despite an extensive literature search, we identified only 4 trials [10, 24, 26, 34] comparing HFNC and NIV including 2 initial support strategy trials and 2 trials post-extubation trials. Second, by necessity all trials were deemed to be at high risk of performance bias as the nature of the interventions being applied precluded blinding after treatment allocation. Third, we did not construct funnel plots as fewer than 10 trials were identified for each comparison. Finally, we were not able to pool all data reported for outcomes including ICU and hospital stay, respiratory rate, and PaO₂/FiO₂ ratio due to variability in measuring and reporting of these outcomes.

Conclusions
We found that compared to COT, HFNC significantly reduced treatment failure when used as an initial support strategy and when used after extubation reduced both extubation failure and reintubation rates. In few trials, HFNC reduced intubation rate compared to NIV when used as initial support strategy but did not impact rates of treatment failure and reintubation when used after extubation.

Abbreviations
AECOPD: Acute exacerbation of chronic obstructive pulmonary disease; ARF: Acute respiratory failure; CI: Confidence interval; COT: Conventional oxygen therapy; CPAP: Continuous positive airway pressure; ED: Emergence department; GRADE: The grading of recommendation, assessment, development and evaluation; HFNC: High-flow nasal cannula; ICU: Intensive care unit; IMV: Invasive mechanical ventilation; LOS: Length of stay; MD: Mean difference; NIV: Noninvasive ventilation; OR: Odds ratio; P/F ratio: PaO₂/FiO₂ ratio; RCTs: Randomized controlled trials; Rob: Risk of bias; RR: Respiratory rate

Acknowledgments
We would like to thank Drs. Jiaxi He and Pu Mao, and the fellows of the First Affiliated Hospital of Guangzhou Medical University for editing and proofreading the manuscript.

Funding
The study was supported by National Natural Science Foundation of China (Grant Nos. 81490534 (NZ and HZ), 81770079(YL) and 81370177 (HZ), by National Science and Technology Major Project (No. 2017ZX10204401003), by the Chief Scientist Project of Yangcheng Scholar in Guangzhou (Grant No. 1201541642) and Canadian Institute of Health Research (FDN143285 and CCI132569). Dr. Burns holds a Merit Award from the University of Toronto, (Toronto, Canada).

Authors' contributions

ZX made substantial contributions to the acquisition of data, analysis and interpretation of data and drafting the manuscript. YL made substantial contributions to conception and design and interpretation of data. JZ and XL made substantial contributions to the acquisition of data. XQL and NZ made substantial contributions to conception and design the study. KB and HZ made substantial contributions to conception and design and revised the manuscript. All authors read and approved the final manuscript.

Competing interests

The authors declare that they have no competing interests.

Author details

[1]State Key Laboratory of Respiratory Diseases, National Clinical Research Center for Respiratory Disease, Guangzhou Institute for Respiratory Health, Guangzhou, China. [2]Department of Critical Care Medicine, The First Affiliated Hospital of Guangzhou Medical University, Guangzhou, China. [3]Interdepartmental Division of Critical Care Medicine, University of Toronto, Toronto, ON, Canada. [4]The Keenan Research Centre for Biomedical Science and the Li Ka Shing Knowledge Institute of St. Michael's Hospital, Toronto, ON M5B1W8, Canada. [5]Departments of Anesthesia and Physiology, University of Toronto, Toronto, ON, Canada.

References

1. Azoulay E, Thiery G, Chevret S, Moreau D, Darmon M, Bergeron A, et al. The prognosis of acute respiratory failure in critically ill cancer patients. Medicine. 2004;83(6):360–70.
2. Canet E, Osman D, Lambert J, Guitton C, Heng AE, Argaud L, et al. Acute respiratory failure in kidney transplant recipients: a multicenter study. Crit Care. 2011;15(2):R91.
3. Linko R, Okkonen M, Pettila V, Perttila J, Parviainen I, Ruokonen E, et al. Acute respiratory failure in intensive care units. FINNALI: a prospective cohort study. Intensive Care Med. 2009;35(8):1352–61.
4. O'Driscoll BR, Howard LS, Davison AG. BTS guideline for emergency oxygen use in adult patients. Thorax. 2008;63(Suppl 6):vi1–68.
5. Roca O, Hernandez G, Diaz-Lobato S, Carratala JM, Gutierrez RM, Masclans JR, et al. Current evidence for the effectiveness of heated and humidified high flow nasal cannula supportive therapy in adult patients with respiratory failure. Crit Care. 2016;20(1):109.
6. Papazian L, Corley A, Hess D, Fraser JF, Frat J-P, Guitton C, et al. Use of high-flow nasal cannula oxygenation in ICU adults: a narrative review. Intensive Care Med. 2016;42(9):1336–1349.
7. Costello RW, Liston R, McNicholas WT. Compliance at night with low flow oxygen therapy: a comparison of nasal cannulae and Venturi face masks. Thorax. 1995;50(4):405–6.
8. Cuquemelle E, Pham T, Papon JF, Louis B, Danin PE, Brochard L. Heated and humidified high-flow oxygen therapy reduces discomfort during hypoxemic respiratory failure. Respir Care. 2012;57(10):1571–7.
9. Miguel-Montanes R, Hajage D, Messika J, Bertrand F, Gaudry S, Rafat C, et al. Use of high-flow nasal cannula oxygen therapy to prevent desaturation during tracheal intubation of intensive care patients with mild-to-moderate hypoxemia. Crit Care Med. 2015;43(3):574–83.
10. Stephan F, Barrucand B, Petit P, Rezaiguia-Delclaux S, Medard A, Delannoy B, et al. High-flow nasal oxygen vs noninvasive positive airway pressure in hypoxemic patients after cardiothoracic surgery: a randomized clinical trial. JAMA. 2015;313(23):2331–9.
11. Simon M, Braune S, Frings D, Wiontzek AK, Klose H, Kluge S. High-flow nasal cannula oxygen versus non-invasive ventilation in patients with acute hypoxaemic respiratory failure undergoing flexible bronchoscopy--a prospective randomised trial. Crit Care. 2014;18(6):712.
12. Maggiore SM, Idone FA, Vaschetto R, Festa R, Cataldo A, Antonicelli F, et al. Nasal high-flow versus Venturi mask oxygen therapy after extubation. Effects on oxygenation, comfort, and clinical outcome. Am J Respir Crit Care Med. 2014;190(3):282–8.
13. Hernandez G, Vaquero C, Gonzalez P, Subira C, Frutos-Vivar F, Rialp G, et al. Effect of Postextubation high-flow nasal cannula vs conventional oxygen therapy on reintubation in low-risk patients a randomized clinical trial. JAMA. 2016;315(13):1354–61.
14. Curley GF, Laffy JG, Zhang H, Slutsky AS. Noninvasive respiratory support for acute respiratory failure-high flow nasal cannula oxygen or non-invasive ventilation? J Thorac Dis. 2015;7(7):1092–7.
15. Nishimura M. High-flow nasal cannula oxygen therapy in adults. J Intensive Care. 2015;3(1):15.
16. Levy SD, Alladina JW, Hibbert KA, Harris RS, Bajwa EK, Hess DR. High-flow oxygen therapy and other inhaled therapies in intensive care units. Lancet. 2016;387(10030):1867–78.
17. Demoule A, Rello J. High flow oxygen cannula: the other side of the moon. Intensive Care Med. 2015;41(9):1673–5.
18. Higgins JP, Altman DG, Gotzsche PC, Juni P, Moher D, Oxman AD, et al. The Cochrane Collaboration's tool for assessing risk of bias in randomised trials. BMJ. 2011;343:d5928.
19. Guyatt GH, Oxman AD, Vist GE, Kunz R, Falck-Ytter Y, Alonso-Coello P, et al. GRADE: an emerging consensus on rating quality of evidence and strength of recommendations. BMJ. 2008;336(7650):924–6.
20. Jones PG, Kamona S, Doran O, Sawtell F, Wilsher M. Randomized controlled trial of humidified high-flow nasal oxygen for acute respiratory distress in the emergency department: the HOT-ER study. Respir Care. 2016;61(3):291–9.
21. Lemiale V, Mokart D, Mayaux J, Lambert J, Rabbat A, Demoule A, et al. The effects of a 2-h trial of high-flow oxygen by nasal cannula versus Venturi mask in immunocompromised patients with hypoxemic acute respiratory failure: a multicenter randomized trial. Crit Care. 2015;19(1):380.
22. Bell N, Hutchinson CL, Green TC, Rogan E, Bein KJ, Dinh MM. Randomised control trial of humidified high flow nasal cannulae versus standard oxygen in the emergency department. Emerg Med Australas. 2015;27(6):537–41.
23. Makdee O, Monsomboon A, Surabenjawong U, Praphruetkit N, Chaisirin W, Chakorn T, et al. High-flow nasal cannula versus conventional oxygen therapy in emergency department patients with cardiogenic pulmonary edema: a randomized controlled trial. Ann Emerg Med. 2017;70(4):465–72.e2.
24. Frat JP, Thille AW, Mercat A, Girault C, Ragot S, Perbet S, et al. High-flow oxygen through nasal cannula in acute hypoxemic respiratory failure. N Engl J Med. 2015;372(23):2185–96.
25. Rittayamai N, Tscheikuna J, Praphruetkit N, Kijpinyochai S. Use of high-flow nasal cannula for acute dyspnea and hypoxemia in the emergency department. Respir Care. 2015;60(10):1377–82.
26. Doshi P, Whittle JS, Bublewicz M, Kearney J, Ashe T, Graham R, et al. High-velocity nasal insufflation in the treatment of respiratory failure: a randomized clinical trial. Ann Emerg Med. 2018;72(1):73–83.e5.
27. Corley A, Bull T, Spooner AJ, Barnett AG, Fraser JF. Direct extubation onto high-flow nasal cannulae post-cardiac surgery versus standard treatment in patients with a BMI ≥30: a randomised controlled trial. Intensive Care Med. 2015;41(5):887–94.
28. Fernandez R, Subira C, Frutos-Vivar F, Rialp G, Laborda C, Masclans JR, et al. High-flow nasal cannula to prevent postextubation respiratory failure in high-risk non-hypercapnic patients: a randomized multicenter trial. Ann Intensive Care. 2017;7(1):47.
29. Futier E, Paugam-Burtz C, Godet T, Khoy-Ear L, Rozencwajg S, Delay JM, et al. Effect of early postextubation high-flow nasal cannula vs conventional oxygen therapy on hypoxaemia in patients after major abdominal surgery: a French multicentre randomised controlled trial (OPERA). Intensive Care Med. 2016;42(12):1888–98.
30. Parke R, McGuinness S, Dixon R, Jull A. Open-label, phase II study of routine high-flow nasal oxygen therapy in cardiac surgical patients. Br J Anaesth. 2013;111(6):925–31.
31. Song HZ, Gu JX, Xiu HQ, Cui W, Zhang GS. The value of high-flow nasal cannula oxygen therapy after extubation in patients with acute respiratory failure. Clinics. 2017;72(9):562–7.

32. Yu YT, Qian XZ, Liu CY, Zhu C. Effect of high-flow nasal cannula versus conventional oxygen therapy for patients with thoracoscopic lobectomy after extubation. Can Respir J. 2017;2017:7894631.

33. Ansari BM, Hogan MP, Collier TJ, Baddeley RA, Scarci M, Coonar AS, et al. A randomized controlled trial of high-flow nasal oxygen (Optiflow) as part of an enhanced recovery program after lung resection surgery. Ann Thorac Surg. 2016;101(2):459–64.

34. Hernandez G, Vaquero C, Colinas L, Cuena R, Gonzalez P, Canabal A, et al. Effect of Postextubation high-flow nasal cannula vs noninvasive ventilation on reintubation and Postextubation respiratory failure in high-risk patients: a randomized clinical trial. JAMA. 2016;316(15):1565–74.

35. Maitra S, Som A, Bhattacharjee S, Arora MK, Baidya DK. Comparison of high-flow nasal oxygen therapy with conventional oxygen therapy and noninvasive ventilation in adult patients with acute hypoxemic respiratory failure: a meta-analysis and systematic review. J Crit Care. 2016;35:138–44.

36. Monro-Somerville T, Sim M, Ruddy J, Vilas M, Gillies MA. The effect of high-flow nasal cannula oxygen therapy on mortality and intubation rate in acute respiratory failure: a systematic review and meta-analysis. Crit Care Med. 2017;45(4):e449–e456.

37. Nedel WL, Deutschendorf C, Moraes Rodrigues Filho E. High-flow nasal cannula in critically Ill subjects with or at risk for respiratory failure: a systematic review and meta-analysis. Respir Care. 2017;62(1):123–132.

38. Zhu Y, Yin H, Zhang R, Wei J. High-flow nasal cannula oxygen therapy vs conventional oxygen therapy in cardiac surgical patients: a meta-analysis. J Crit Care. 2016;38:123–8.

39. Ni YN, Luo J, Yu H, Liu D, Liang BM, Liang ZA. The effect of high-flow nasal cannula in reducing the mortality and the rate of endotracheal intubation when used before mechanical ventilation compared with conventional oxygen therapy and noninvasive positive pressure ventilation. A systematic review and meta-analysis. Am J Emerg Med. 2018;36(2):226–33.

40. Huang HW, Sun XM, Shi ZH, Chen GQ, Chen L, Friedrich JO, et al. Effect of high-flow nasal cannula oxygen therapy versus conventional oxygen therapy and noninvasive ventilation on reintubation rate in adult patients after Extubation: a systematic review and meta-analysis of randomized controlled trials. J Intensive Care Med. 2017:885066617705118. https://doi.org/10.1177/0885066617705118.

41. Zhao H, Wang H, Sun F, Lyu S, An Y. High-flow nasal cannula oxygen therapy is superior to conventional oxygen therapy but not to noninvasive mechanical ventilation on intubation rate: a systematic review and meta-analysis. Crit Care. 2017;21(1):184.

42. Wilkinson D, Andersen C, O'Donnell CP, De Paoli AG, Manley BJ. High flow nasal cannula for respiratory support in preterm infants. Cochrane Database Syst Rev. 2016;2:CD006405.

43. Lee JH, Rehder KJ, Williford L, Cheifetz IM, Turner DA. Use of high flow nasal cannula in critically ill infants, children, and adults: a critical review of the literature. Intensive Care Med. 2013;39(2):247–57.

44. Dysart K, Miller TL, Wolfson MR, Shaffer TH. Research in high flow therapy: mechanisms of action. Respir Med. 2009;103(10):1400–5.

45. Chanques G, Constantin JM, Sauter M, Jung B, Sebbane M, Verzilli D, et al. Discomfort associated with underhumidified high-flow oxygen therapy in critically ill patients. Intensive Care Med. 2009;35(6):996–1003.

46. Parke R, McGuinness S, Eccleston M. Nasal high-flow therapy delivers low level positive airway pressure. Br J Anaesth. 2009;103(6):886–90.

47. Suzuki Y, Takasaki Y. Respiratory support with nasal high-flow therapy helps to prevent recurrence of postoperative atelectasis: a case report. J Intensive Care. 2014;2(1):3.

16

Right heart size and function significantly correlate in patients with pulmonary arterial hypertension

Lukas Fischer[1], Nicola Benjamin[1,2], Norbert Blank[3], Benjamin Egenlauf[1,2], Christine Fischer[4], Satenik Harutyunova[1,2], Maria Koegler[1], Hanns-Martin Lorenz[3], Alberto M. Marra[1,2,5], Christian Nagel[1,2,6], Panagiota Xanthouli[1,2], Eduardo Bossone[7] and Ekkehard Grünig[1,2*]

Abstract

Background: The objective of this study was to assess, whether right atrial (RA) and ventricular (RV) size is related to RV pump function at rest and during exercise in patients with pulmonary arterial hypertension (PAH).

Methods: We included 54 patients with invasively diagnosed PAH that had been stable on targeted medication. All patients underwent clinical assessments including right heart catheterization and echocardiography at rest and during exercise. RV output reserve was defined as increase of cardiac index (CI) from rest to peak exercise ($\Delta CI_{exercise}$). Patients were classified according to the median of RA and RV-area. RV pump function and further clinical parameters were compared between groups by student's t-test. Uni- and multivariate Pearson correlation analyses were performed.

Results: Patients with larger RA and/or RV-areas (above a median of 16 and 20cm^2, respectively) showed significantly lower $\Delta CI_{exercise}$, higher mean pulmonary arterial pressure, pulmonary vascular resistance at rest and NT-proBNP levels. Furthermore, patients with higher RV-areas presented with a significantly lower RV stroke volume and pulmonary arterial compliance at peak exercise than patients with smaller RV-size. RV area was identified as the only independent predictor of RV output reserve.

Conclusion: RV and RA areas represent valuable and easily accessible indicators of RV pump function at rest and during exercise. Cardiac output reserve should be considered as an important clinical parameter. Prospective studies are needed for further evaluation.

Keywords: Pulmonary hypertension, Right ventricular output reserve, Pump function, Right ventricular size, Right atrial size

Background

Pulmonary arterial hypertension (PAH) is a complex cardiopulmonary disorder, characterized by progressive changes affecting both the pulmonary vasculature and the right heart [1, 2]. Although the initial pathological changes occur on pulmonary arterioles causing increased pulmonary vascular resistance (PVR), adaptation of right ventricular (RV) pump function is a key determinant of survival [2, 3]. Rising attention is drawn to the concept of RV-arterial coupling, a composite measure of RV pump function and ventricular load [4–6].

Right atrial (RA) [7–9] and RV size have repeatedly been proven of prognostic significance in pulmonary hypertension [2, 10], whereas their impact on RV contractility remains to be determined. Recent studies using magnetic resonance imaging (MRI) have shown, that increased RV-endsystolic or diastolic volumes were significantly related to a worse outcome and reduced RV stroke volume

---
* Correspondence: ekkehard.gruenig@med.uni-heidelberg.de
[1]Centre for Pulmonary Hypertension, Thoraxklinik at Heidelberg University Hospital, Röntgenstrasse 1, D-69126 Heidelberg, Germany
[2]Translational Lung Research Center Heidelberg (TLRC), Member of the German Center for Lung Research (DZL), Heidelberg, Germany
Full list of author information is available at the end of the article

(SV) [11]. In a further study enlargement of RV volumes during follow-up was associated with further clinical signs of disease progression [12].

RV output reserve ($\Delta CI_{exercise}$) defined as increase of cardiac output/cardiac index (CI) during exercise with normal or elevated PVR measured by right heart catheterization (RHC) is an emerging parameter which has shown to be prognostically important in patients with PAH [13, 14]. It solely displays the capacity of the right ventricle to adjust its systolic function to a given level of pulmonary loading[4]. Pulmonary arterial compliance (PAC) reflects the elasticity of the pulmonary arteries. For estimation of pulmonary arterial compliance (or capacitance) the measurement of SV/pulse pressure (cardiac output/heart rate)/(systolicPAP-diastolicPAP) by RHC has been shown to be the most simple and practical method [15, 16].

The objective of the study was to investigate the correlation between right heart size (measured as right atrial and ventricular area by echocardiography) and RV pump function at rest and during exercise (assessed by RHC) and further hemodynamic and clinical parameters. Furthermore, this study aimed to detect correlations and determining factors of RV pump function.

Methods
Patient selection
We retrospectively reviewed all incident (i.e. newly diagnosed) patients aged ≥18 to 80 years with idiopathic, heritable or drug- and toxin-induced or connective tissue disease associated PAH who were diagnosed at the PH-center in Heidelberg between January 1st, 2016 and November 31st, 2016. Inclusion required RHC at rest (confirming PAH, defined as a mean pulmonary arterial pressure ≥25 mmHg, pulmonary arterial wedge pressure ≤15 mmHg and PVR > 3 Wood units [17], and during exercise. Diagnosis of PAH was performed according to the ESC/ERS guidelines [17].

Patients were excluded if they lacked a complete evaluation including medical history, WHO/NYHA functional class assessment, physical examination, electrocardiogram, transthoracic 2D-echocardiography at rest, lung function test, arterial blood gases, 6-min walking distance (6MWD) under standardized conditions [18], laboratory testing including NT-proBNP levels. All examinations were performed at the Thoraxklinik at Heidelberg University Hospital by experienced physicians within 48 h from the right heart catheterization.

Right heart catheterization
The hemodynamic values have been obtained by the charts. The right heart catheterization has been performed in a standardized way in a supine position

using the transjugular access with a triple-lumen 7F-Swan-Ganz thermodilution catheter at rest and during exercise as previously described [19]. Patients had been examined on a variable load supine bicycle ergometer by experienced investigators (CN, BE, SH). Pressures were continuously recorded and averaged over several respiratory cycles during spontaneous breathing, both at rest and during exercise. Cardiac output (CO) was measured by thermodilution at least in triplicate with a variation of less than 10% between the measured values. The zero reference point for pressure recordings was set at ½ of the thoracic diameter below the anterior thorax surface [20]. After the hemodynamic measurement at rest, the supine position was changed to a 45° position. Calibration for exercise measurements were performed as previously described [21]. The exercise test was started with a workload of 25 W. Workload was incrementally increased by 25 W every 2 min to an exercise capacity or symptom limited maximum.

Echocardiography
Resting two dimensional transthoracic echocardiography (TTE) Doppler examinations were performed by experienced cardiac sonographers (EG, CN, BE, SH) with commercially available equipment (Vivid 7, GE Healthcare, Milwaukee, Wisconsin) according to standardized protocol as described previously [9, 22]. TTE measurements were obtained off line from stored DICOM data according to the European Association of Cardiovascular Imaging (EACVI) Guidelines [23]. Specific indices included RA-/RV-area, TAPSE and PASP at rest. For all calculations the mean value of at least 3 measurements was used. PASP was estimated from peak tricuspid regurgitation jet velocities (TRV) according to the equation: PASP = 4 (V) [2] + right atrial pressure, where V is the peak velocity (in m/s) of tricuspid regurgitation jet (TRV) [24]. Right atrial pressure was estimated from characteristics of the inferior vena cava [18]. If it was < 20 mm in diameter and decreased during inspiration we added 5 mmHg, ≥20 mm we added 10 mmHg and 15 mmHg if no decrease of diameter during inspiration occurred.

Cardiopulmonary exercise testing
Patients were examined on a variable load supine bicycle ergometer (model 8420; KHL Corp., Kirkland, Washington) in Heidelberg as described previously [25]. Workload was increased by 25 W every 2 min to an exercise capacity or symptom limited maximum. Peak VO_2 was defined as the highest 30-s average value of oxygen uptake during the last minute of the exercise test.

Ethics statement

The Ethics Committee of the Medical Faculty, University of Heidelberg had no obligation against the conduct of the study (internal number S425/2016). All data were anonymized and the study was conducted in accordance with the amended Declaration of Helsinki.

Statistical methods

Statistical analyses were conducted by two biometricians (CF, NE). Data are described as means ± standard deviations or number and respective percentage. Patients were divided into two groups according to their RV size (larger or smaller RA and/or RV area with value above or below the median of the complete sample). A receiver operating characteristic (ROC) curve analysis for RA and RV area with CI increase below the median of the sample as outcome parameter for further validation of the cut-off values was performed. Quantitative characteristics between the two groups including demographics, hemodynamics and parameters of echocardiography and cardiopulmonary exercise testing were compared by two-sided student's t-tests and nonparametric tests if needed. Frequency distributions were compared by chi-square test or Fisher's exact test. A sensitivity analysis with a threshold of 18 cm^2 for RV area according to the cut-off proposed by the guidelines[17] was performed.

Right heart size (RA and RV area) was compared between patients with higher vs. lower $\Delta CI_{exercise}$ (according to the median of the complete sample).

Differences of the course of CI and SV increase during exercise between patients with smaller vs. larger RA and RV area were analysed with mixed ANOVA. To investigate the associations between clinical parameters, right heart size and output reserve, Pearson's correlation analysis was performed. To identify independent predictors of RV output reserve, multivariate analysis was performed by stepwise forward selection method of logistic regression with the dichotomous variable of the two groups (high or low $\Delta CI_{exercise}$) as outcome variable. Parameters for correlation analysis included demographics, hemodynamics, echocardiographic parameters and measures of cardiopulmonary exercise testing according to clinical significance.

Pulmonary arterial compliance (PAC) was calculated according the formula PAC = SV/ pulse pressure with SV = CO/Heart rate and pulse pressure = sPAP-dPAP. Stroke volume index was calculated with SVI = CI / heart rate.

All tests were two-sided and a pointwise p-value of 0.05 was considered statistically significant. All analyses have been performed using IBM SPSS 23 (SPSS Statistics V23, IBM Corporation, Somers, New York).

Results

Study population (Table 1)

We included 54 patients diagnosed with moderate to severe PAH who fulfilled the inclusion criteria (21 males and 33 females, mean age 53 ± 15 years, 66.7% WHO functional class II, 57.4% double combination therapy; Table 1).

The study cohort presented with a median RA of 16cm^2 and RV of 20 cm^2. ROC curve analysis for RA and RV area with CI increase $< 2.1 \text{ l/min/m}^2$ (median of the sample for CI increase) further supported these proposed cutoff-values of 16cm^2 for RA and 20cm^2 for RV area (Fig. 1). For RV area, 20cm^2 showed a sensitivity of 75% and specificity of 73.1%; an RA area of 16cm^2 presented with a sensitivity of 75% and specificity of 57.7%.

Characteristics of groups with small and large right heart size: According to the median RA and RV area, two subgroups were defined for both RA and RV area: **1) "enlarged right heart size"** (RA $>16 \text{cm}^2$, RV $>20 \text{cm}^2$) and **2) "normal/smaller right heart size"** (RA $\leq 16 \text{cm}^2$, RV $\leq 20 \text{cm}^2$; Table 2).

Both groups did not significantly differ in their demographics (age and BMI), 6MWD, diffusion capacity and peak VO_2 for both RA and RV area. PH-targeted treatment and distribution of combination treatment did also not significantly differ between groups (Table 2).

Patients with enlarged RA- ($n = 21$) and/or RV-area ($n = 24$) had significantly higher mean, systolic and diastolic pulmonary arterial pressures, mean pulmonary vascular resistance, and NT-proBNP levels than patients with normal or smaller right heart size.

Both groups of RA and RV size had well preserved RV function at rest, represented by regular CI and SV, even though PVR and mean pulmonary arterial pressures were elevated in patients with enlarged right heart size. Increase of CI during exercise was significantly smaller in patients with enlarged RA- or RV-areas (Fig. 2a and b). Furthermore, patients with higher RV-area, but not RA-area, presented with a significantly lower SV, SVI and pulmonary arterial compliance at peak exercise than patients with smaller RV-size (Table 2).

SV failed to increase in accordance with the exposed exercise level in patients with large RA- ($p = 0.031$) and/or RV area ($p < 0.001$; Fig. 3). Likewise, SVI was significantly higher in patients with small right heart size, compared to patients with enlarged RA and/or RV area (ANOVA RV $p < 0.001$, RA $p = 0.001$). Furthermore, patients with smaller RV, but not RA, presented with significantly higher peak PAC than patients with RV area above the median (39.5 ± 11.2 ml/mmHg vs. 33.2 ± 15.3 ml/mmHg, $p = 0.027$).

Table 1 Characteristics of the study population

				mean ± SD or n (%)		
Demographics		Age	*(years)*	53	±	14.65
		BMI	*(kg/m²)*	27.9	±	5.69
Gender		male	*n (%)*	21		(38.9)
		female	*n (%)*	33		(61.1)
Diagnosis		IPAH	*n (%)*	31		(57.4)
		HPAH	*n (%)*	8		(14.8)
		APAH	*n (%)*	12		(22.2)
		CTEPH	*n (%)*	3		(5.6)
WHO functional class		I	*n (%)*	1		(1.9)
		II	*n (%)*	36		(66.7)
		III	*n (%)*	17		(31.5)
PAH-targeted medication		Endothelin receptor antagonist		40		(74.1)
		Phosphodiesterase-5-inhibitors		38		(70.4)
		Soluble guanylate cyclase-stimulator		8		(13.0)
		Prostanoids		6		(14.8)
		Calcium channel blockers		2		(03.7)
Combination therapy						
		Mono	*n (%)*	18		(33.3)
		Double	*n (%)*	31		(57.4)
		Triple	*n (%)*	5		(9.3)
RHC	Rest	mPAP	*(mmHg)*	35.5	±	11.69
		sPAP	*(mmHg)*	57.6	±	20.87
		dPAP	*(mmHg)*	23	±	7.87
		PCWP	*(mmHg)*	10	±	3.54
		PVR	*(dyn*sec*cm⁻⁵)*	393.4	±	235.03
		CO	*(l/min)*	5.8	±	1.61
		CI	*(l/min/m²)*	3	±	0.73
		SVI	*(ml/m²)*	41.1	±	10.2
	25 W	Δ CI	*(l/min/m²)*	1.2	±	0.67
	50 W	Δ CI	*(l/min/m²)*	2	±	0.93
	75 W	Δ CI	*(l/min/m²)*	2.6	±	1.15
	Peak	mPAP	*(mmHg)*	56.5	±	15.91
		sPAP	*(mmHg)*	90.2	±	28.36
		dPAP	*(mmHg)*	36.1	±	11.56
		CO	*(l/min)*	10.2	±	3.49
		CI	*(l/min/m²)*	5.3	±	1.59
		SVI	*(ml/m²)*	47.2	±	13.9
Echocardiography		RV area	*(cm²)*	20.1	±	5.59
		RA area	*(cm²)*	16.8	±	6.62
		TAPSE	*(cm)*	2.3	±	0.38
Cardiopulmonary exercise testing (CPET)		peak V'O₂	*(ml/min)*	1126	±	428.88
		peak V'O₂/kg	*(ml/min/kg)*	14.1	±	3.92
		sPAP ₘₐₓ	*(mmHg)*	81.8	±	27.87
		6-MWD	*(m)*	423	±	113.09

Table 1 Characteristics of the study population *(Continued)*

			mean ± SD or n (%)		
Laboratory analysis	NT-proBNP	*(pg/ml)*	470.3	±	856.74
Pulmonary function test (PFT)	DLCOc SB	*(% Soll)*	58.6	±	17.25
	DLCOc VA	*(% Soll)*	70.42	±	20.00

IPAH = idiopathic pulmonary arterial hypertension, *HPAH* = heritable PAH, *APAH* = associated PAH, CTEPH = chronic thromboembolic PH, *RHC* = right heart catheter, *BMI* = Body Mass Index, *RV* = right ventricular, *RA* = right atrial, TAPSE = tricuspid annular plane systolic excursion, VO'_2 = oxygen consumption, *NT-proBNP* = N-terminal pro brain natriuretic peptide, *DLCOc SB* = diffusing capacity transfer factor, *DLCOc / VA* = diffusing capacity transfer coefficient, mPAP = mean pulmonary arterial pressure, *sPAP* = systolic PAP, *dPAP* = diastolic PAP, *PCWP* = pulmonary capillary wedge pressure, *PVR* = pulmonary vascular resistance, CI = Cardiac Index, *SVI* = stroke volume index, *HR* = heart rate, *SV* = stroke volume, Δ = difference

Sensitivity analysis with a threshold of 18 cm^2 for RV area led to the same differences between groups with small and large right heart size. Furthermore, CI increase showed a statistically significant difference for each workload level.

When dichotomising the patient cohort according to RV output reserve (high and low $\Delta CI_{exercise}$) echocardiography showed considerable differences in RV and RA area (p = 0.003 and p = 0.019 respectively; Fig. 4a and b).

Factors associated with right heart size and RV output reserve (Tables 3 and 4)

Univariate analysis of right heart size and output reserve In univariate regression analysis RV and RA area were significantly correlated with NT-proBNP, sPAP, CI during exercise, ΔCI_{Peak} (Fig. 5) and with right heart size (Table 3). RV area additionally significantly correlated with mPAP at rest, CI at rest, PVR at rest and peak mPAP.

$\Delta CI_{exercise}$ significantly positively correlated with age, exercise capacity (6-MWD, peak oxygen consumption, peak oxygen consumption/kg/min), hemodynamics (CO at rest; peak CO and CI during exercise) and lung diffusing capacity (transfer factor DLCOc SB and transfer coefficient DLCOc / VA) (Table 4). A negative correlation was detected between $\Delta CI_{exercise}$ and NT-proBNP, echocardiographic parameters (sPAP, RA area, RV area) and hemodynamics at rest (mPAP, PVR).

Multivariate analysis of output reserve Stepwise forward selection of multivariate logistic regression analysis showed RV area to be the single independent predictor for high or low ΔCI_{Peak} (regression coefficient 0.863, p = 0.027).

Discussion

To the best of our knowledge this is the first study showing that in patents with PAH enlarged RV- or

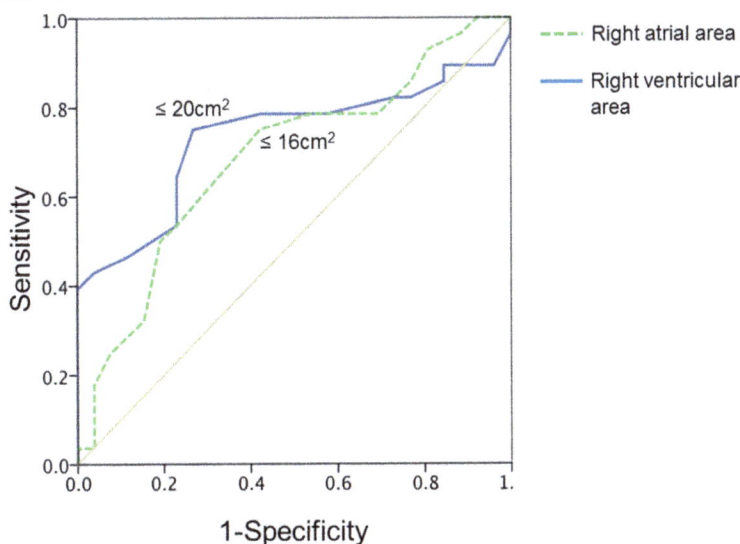

Fig. 1 ROC curve analysis. For RV area, 20cm^2 showed a sensitivity of 75% and specificity of 73.1%; an RA area of 16cm^2 presented with a sensitivity of 75% and specificity of 57.7%

Table 2 Comparison of patients with small and large right heart size

			n	RA area ≤ 16 cm²	n	RA area > 16 cm²	p-value		n	RV area ≤ 20 cm²	n	RV area > 20 cm²	p-value	
Demographics	Age	(years)	33	53.6 ± 14.4	21	52.1 ± 15.3	0.71		30	51.4 ± 13.7	24	55.1 ± 15.8	0.354	
	BMI	(kg/m²)	33	28.3 ± 6.5	21	27.3 ± 4.3	0.537		30	27.5 ± 5.5	24	28.4 ± 6.1	0.591	
	6-MWD	(m)	32	429 ± 124	21	414 ± 97	0.655		30	436 ± 127	23	406 ± 92	0.350	
PAH-targeted medication	ERA			24 (72.7%)		16 (76.2%)	1.0			22 (73.3%)		18 (75%)	1.0	
	PDE5-I			22 (66.7%)		16 (76.2%)	0.549			21 (70%)		17 (70.8%)	1.0	
	sGC stimulator			3 (9.1%)		5 (23.8%)	0.238			3 (10%)		5 (20.8%)	0.443	
	Prostanoids			3 (9.1%)		3 (14.3%)	0.667			2 (6.7%)		4 (16.7%)	0.389	
	Calcium channel blockers			2 (6.1%)		0	0.516			2 (6.7%)		0	0.497	
Combination therapy	Mono	n (%)		13 (39.4%)		5 (23.8%)	0.102			11 (36.7%)		7 (29.2%)	0.414	
	Double	n (%)		17 (51.5%)		14 (66.7%)				17 (56.7%)		14 (58.3%)		
	Triple	n (%)		3 (9.1%)		2 (9.5%)				2 (6.6%)		3 (12.5%)		
Echocardiography	RV area	(cm²)	33	17.3 ± 3.9	21	24.6 ± 4.9	<0.0001 *		30	16.3 ± 3.1	24	25.0 ± 4.0	<0.0001	*
	RA area	(cm²)	33	13.2 ± 2.7	21	22.4 ± 7.1	<0.0001 *		30	13.3 ± 3.2	24	21.1 ± 7.2	<0.0001	*
	sPAP	(mmHg)	33	42 ± 16	21	57 ± 17	0.003 *		30	42 ± 12	24	56 ± 20	0.006	*
	TAPSE	(cm)	33	2.4 ± 0.4	21	2.3 ± 0.4	0.362		30	2.4 ± 0.4	24	2.3 ± 0.4	0.204	
Cardiopulmonary Exercise Testing	peak VO₂	(ml/min)	33	1155 ± 495	21	1080 ± 302	0.536		30	1144 ± 435	24	1103 ± 429	0.730	
	peak VO₂/kg	(ml/min/kg)	33	14.5 ± 4.1	21	13.4 ± 3.7	0.321		30	14.7 ± 3.6	24	13.2 ± 4.2	0.166	
Laboratory analysis	NT-proBNP	(pg/ml)	33	191 ± 231	20	931 ± 1266	0.018 *		30	145 ± 125	23	895 ± 1191	0.006	*
Pulmonary function test	DLCOc SB	(% Soll)	30	58.6 ± 18.6	18	58.6 ± 15.2	0.988		27	60.5 ± 15.3	21	56.2 ± 19.6	0.398	
	DLCOc VA	(% Soll)	30	69.0 ± 21.2	18	72.8 ± 18.1	0.522		27	70.1 ± 19.3	21	70.8 ± 21.3	0.906	
RHC Rest	mPAP	(mmHg)	33	32 ± 10	21	41 ± 13	0.012 *		30	32 ± 9	24	40 ± 13	0.014	*
	sPAP	(mmHg)	33	51 ± 17	21	68 ± 22	0.002 *		30	51 ± 16	24	66 ± 24	0.013	*
	dPAP	(mmHg)	33	21 ± 6	21	26 ± 9	0.032 *		30	21 ± 6	24	26 ± 9	0.018	*
	PAWP	(mmHg)	33	10 ± 3	21	10 ± 4	0.514		30	10 ± 3	24	10 ± 4	0.852	
	PVR	(dyn*sec*cm⁻⁵)	33	335 ± 201	21	486 ± 259	0.03 *		30	311 ± 149	24	496 ± 282	0.006	*
	CI	(l/min/m²)	33	3.08 ± 0.63	21	2.93 ± 0.88	0.470		30	3.19 ± 0.67	24	2.82 ± 0.77	0.062	
	HR	(1/min)	33	74 ± 12	21	76 ± 12	0.480		30	75 ± 10	24	75 ± 13	0.927	
	SV	(ml)	33	79.4 ± 21.2	21	77.1 ± 25.4	0.716		30	80.1 ± 19.0	24	76.4 ± 27.0	0.556	
	SVI	(ml/m²)	33	42.2 ± 8.4	21	39.3 ± 12.6	0.317		30	42.9 ± 8.4	24	38.8 ± 11.9	0.142	
25 W	Δ CI	(l/min/m²)	31	1.4 ± 0.7	20	0.9 ± 0.5	0.008 *		28	1.3 ± 0.7	23	1.0 ± 0.6	0.114	
	HR	(1/min)	31	91 ± 18	20	93 ± 12	0.572		28	91 ± 18	23	93 ± 13	0.623	
	Δ SV	(ml)	31	14.6 ± 20.4	20	6.2 ± 12.3	0.105		28	15.0 ± 21.5	23	6.9 ± 11.5	0.112	

Table 2 Comparison of patients with small and large right heart size (Continued)

			n	RA area ≤ 16 cm²	n	RA area > 16 cm²	p-value		n	RV area ≤ 20 cm²	n	RV area > 20 cm²	p-value	
50 W	ΔCI	(l/min/m²)	31	2.2 ± 1.0	18	1.6 ± 0.7	0.027	*	28	2.28 ± 0.91	21	1.51 ± 0.76	0.003	*
	HR	(1/min)	31	103 ± 17	18	105 ± 17	0.639		28	102 ± 18	21	106 ± 15	0.345	
	ΔSV	(ml)	31	18.0 ± 22.7	18	7.2 ± 13.1	0.041	*	28	21.0 ± 22.5	21	4.7 ± 12.0	0.002	*
75 W	ΔCI	(l/min/m²)	18	2.9 ± 1.2	9	2.0 ± 0.6	0.043	*	16	2.93 ± 1.17	11	2.09 ± 0.96	0.060	
	HR	(1/min)	18	113 ± 16	9	112 ± 12	0.813		16	111 ± 17	11	115 ± 10	0.541	
	ΔSV	(ml)	18	22.2 ± 18.1	9	7.4 ± 18.1	0.045	*	16	25.0 ± 14.2	11	6.0 ± 18.2	0.005	*
Peak	mPAP	(mmHg)	33	54 ± 15	21	61 ± 17	0.115		30	54 ± 15	24	60 ± 17	0.124	
	sPAP	(mmHg)	33	84 ± 26	21	100 ± 30	0.049	*	30	85 ± 25	24	97 ± 31	0.144	
	dPAP	(mmHg)	33	35 ± 12	21	38 ± 11	0.254		30	34 ± 12	24	39 ± 10	0.111	
	CI	(l/min/m²)	33	5.62 ± 1.57	21	4.80 ± 1.52	0.049	*	30	5.92 ± 1.43	24	4.52 ± 1.45	0.001	*
	ΔCI	(l/min/m²)	33	2.54 ± 1.42	21	1.86 ± 0.83	0.033	*	30	2.73 ± 1.34	24	1.7 ± 0.88	0.002	*
	SV	(ml)	33	93.3 ± 26.7	21	86.0 ± 33.8	0.383		30	0.1 ± 0.027	24	0.08 ± 0.029	0.007	*
	PAC	(ml/mmHg)	33	39.0 ± 13.7	21	33.1 ± 12.4	0.108		30	39.5 ± 11.2	24	33.2 ± 15.3	0.027	*
	SVI	(l/m²)	33	49.4 ± 11.5	21	43.7 ± 16.6	0.141		30	53.1 ± 11.1	24	39.8 ± 13.7	<0.001	*

ERA = Endothelin receptor antagonist, PDES-I = Phosphodiesterase-5-inhibitors, sGC stimulator = Soluble guanylate cyclase-stimulator, RHC = right heart catheter, BMI = Body Mass Index, RV = right ventricular, RA = right atrial, TAPSE = tricuspid annular plane systolic excursion, VO2 = oxygen consumption, NT-proBNP = N-terminal pro brain natriuretic peptide, DLCOc SB = diffusion capacity transfer factor, DLCOc / VA = diffusion capacity transfer coefficient, mPAP = mean pulmonary arterial pressure, sPAP = systolic PAP, dPAP = diastolic PAP, PAWP = pulmonary arterial wedge pressure, PVR = pulmonary vascular resistance, CI = Cardiac Index, SVI = stroke volume index, HR = heart rate, SV = stroke volume, Δ = difference

* = significant at level 0.05.; values are given as mean ± standard deviation or n (%)

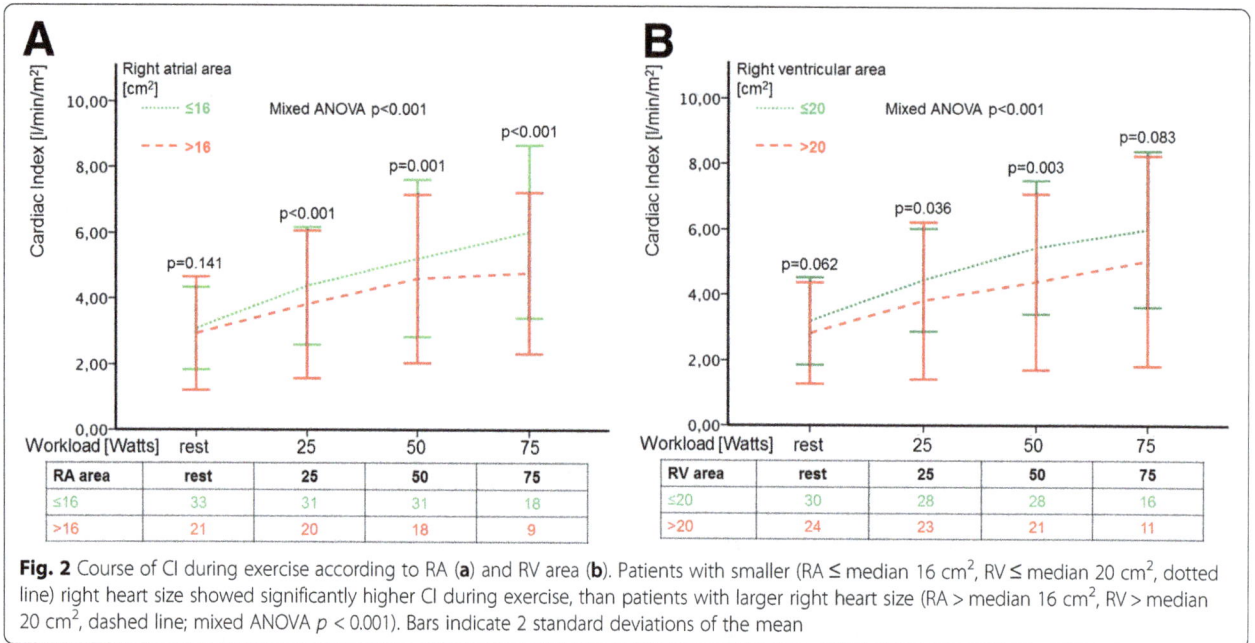

Fig. 2 Course of CI during exercise according to RA (**a**) and RV area (**b**). Patients with smaller (RA ≤ median 16 cm², RV ≤ median 20 cm², dotted line) right heart size showed significantly higher CI during exercise, than patients with larger right heart size (RA > median 16 cm², RV > median 20 cm², dashed line; mixed ANOVA $p < 0.001$). Bars indicate 2 standard deviations of the mean

RA areas (measured by echocardiography) were associated with a significantly reduced RV pump function during exercise (lower $\Delta CI_{exercise}$) measured by right heart catheterization. Furthermore, the study revealed that PAH-patients with larger size of the right heart had higher pulmonary arterial pressures, pulmonary vascular resistance and NT-proBNP levels.

Patients with higher RV-areas presented with a significantly lower stroke volume index and pulmonary arterial compliance at peak exercise than patients with smaller RV-size. RV area was identified as the only independent predictor of RV output reserve (lower $\Delta CI_{exercise}$). Thus, this study gives further evidence that assessing the right heart size by imaging

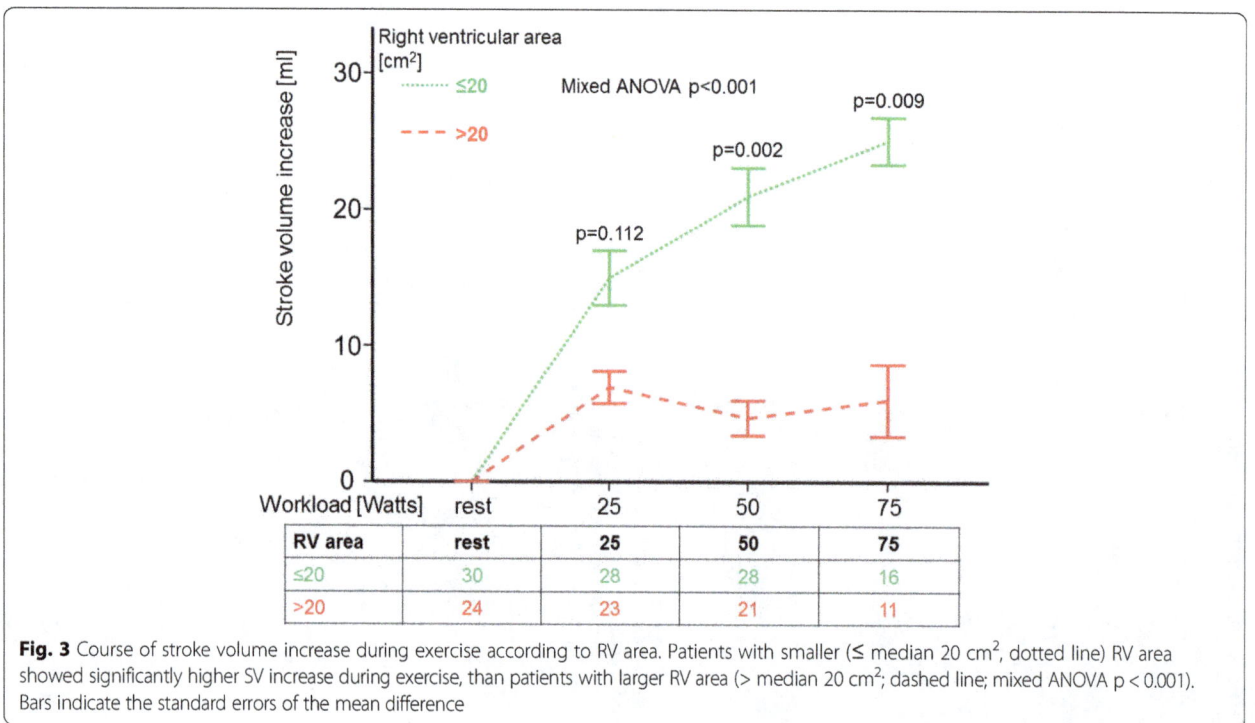

Fig. 3 Course of stroke volume increase during exercise according to RV area. Patients with smaller (≤ median 20 cm², dotted line) RV area showed significantly higher SV increase during exercise, than patients with larger RV area (> median 20 cm²; dashed line; mixed ANOVA p < 0.001). Bars indicate the standard errors of the mean difference

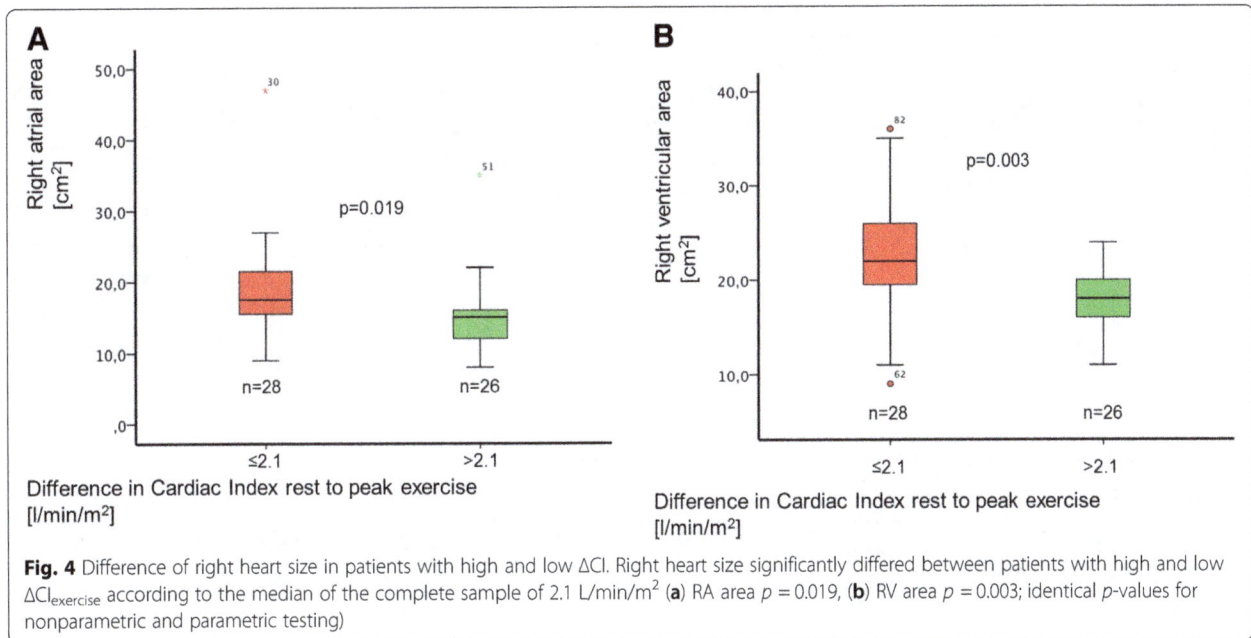

Fig. 4 Difference of right heart size in patients with high and low ΔCI. Right heart size significantly differed between patients with high and low ΔCI$_{exercise}$ according to the median of the complete sample of 2.1 L/min/m^2 (**a**) RA area $p = 0.019$, (**b**) RV area $p = 0.003$; identical p-values for nonparametric and parametric testing)

techniques as echocardiography gives further important clues to RV pump function and cardiopulmonary hemodynamics.

Right heart size, pump function

This study confirms the results of previous studies using MRI which showed that enlarged RV end systolic and end-diastolic volumes were obtained in patients with lower RV stroke volumes [12, 26]. However, in the first previous MRI-study RV volumes were not directly compared with pump function but with survival [26]. Large RV end-diastolic volume and SV at baseline were associated with poorer prognosis. Further dilation of RV with further decrease of SV during follow-up predicted a poor long-term outcome [26]. Most recently these findings have been confirmed by an analysis of the French PAH registry demonstrating that SVI and right atrial pressure were independently associated with death or lung transplantation at first follow-up after initial PAH treatment [27].

Our study demonstrates for the first time a negative relationship between right heart size and RV pump function using 2-D-echocardiography for assessing the RA- and RV-areas in the four chamber view and hemodynamic values from right heart catheterization at rest and during exercise. Patients with enlarged RV area had significantly lower CI and SVI at rest and during exercise. These patients had also higher mean pulmonary arterial pressure, pulmonary vascular resistance at rest and NT-proBNP levels which reflects a more severe disease. The negative impact of RV-enlargement was also demonstrated by a MRI-study

which showed in patients with increasing RV volumes during follow-up a disease progression leading to death or transplantation whereas patients with stable RV volumes remained clinically stable [12]. Changes in RV volumes were even more sensitive parameters for deterioration than the repeated measurement of hemodynamics which remained unchanged [12]. In this study, patients with enlargement of RV volumes had a decline of RV ejection fraction [12]. Two further studies demonstrated a reduction in RV volumes by targeted PAH-therapy, which suggests an improvement of RV pump function [11, 28].

RV output reserve and right heart size

RV output reserve, defined in this study as increase of CI during exercise measured by right heart catheterization, is an emerging parameter which has shown to be of prognostic importance in patients with PH [13, 14]. In this study RV area was identified as the only independent predictor of RV output reserve. This again shows that RV size may reflect the impairment of RV pump function. We hypothesize that increased PAC and reduced increase of RV output during exercise in patients with larger RV and/or RA areas, respectively is due to more severe pulmonary vascular disease. A both reproducible and clinically practical way to evaluate RV output reserve can be performed by invasive measurements[15]. Further prospective studies have to be conducted to evaluate the magnitude of the relation to right heart size and if non/invasive assessment of RA- and RV area or volume are useful for an estimation of RV output reserve.

Table 3 Correlation analysis of right heart size and clinical parameters

	Right atrial area				Right ventricular area		
	n	pearson's R	p-value		n	pearson's R	p-value
Univariate analysis							
Age	54	0.193	0.162		54	- 0.048	0.209
Body mass index	54	0.181	0.190		54	0.733	0.129
6-min walking distance	53	- 0.108	0.441		53	- 0.121	0.387
NT-proBNP	53	0.539	< 0.001	*	53	0.538	< 0.001	*
Echocardiography							
Systolic pulmonary arterial pressure	54	0.307	0.024	*	54	0.567	< 0.001	*
Right atrial area		–			54	0.703	< 0.001	*
Right ventricular area	54	0.703	< 0.001	*		–	
Tricuspid annular plane systolic excursion	54	- 0.128	0.356		54	- 0.082	0.554
Cardiopulmonary exercise testing							
Peak oxygen consumption (V'O$_2$)	54	0.042	0.736		54	0.051	0.713
Peak oxygen consumption/kg (V'O$_2$/kg)	54	- 0.199	0.149		54	- 0.227	0.099
Right heart catheter							
rest							
Mean pulmonary arterial pressure	54	0.176	0.202		54	0.544	< 0.001	*
Cardiac Output	54	- 0.028	0.839		54	- 0.052	0.709
Cardiac Index	54	- 0.209	0.129		54	- 0.281	0.040	*
Pulmonary arterial wedge pressure	54	0.025	0.857		54	- 0.101	0.467
Pulmonary vascular resistance	54	0.175	0.206		54	0.508	< 0.001	*
Stroke volume index	54	−0.244	0.076		54	−0.301	0.027	*
exercise							
Mean pulmonary arterial pressure	54	0.097	0.486		54	0.419	0.002	*
Cardiac Output	54	- 0.177	0.200		54	- 0.223	0.104
Cardiac Index	54	- 0.344	0.011	*	54	- 0.427	0.001	*
Δ CI peak	54	- 0.313	0.021	*	54	- 0.376	0.005	*
Stroke volume index	54	−0.264	0.054		54	−0.407	0.002	*
Lung function / Diffusing capacity							
DLCOc SB	48	- 0.052	0.723		48	- 0.003	0.982
DLCOc /VA	48	0.176	0.231		48	0.137	0.352

CI = Cardiac Index, NT-proBNP = N-terminal pro brain natriuretic peptide, DLCOc SB = diffusion capacity transfer factor, DLCOc /VA = diffusion capacity transfer coefficient
* = significant at level 0.05

Advanced PAH with increased pulmonary load leads to RV dilatation (heterometric adaptation) in order to maintain SV[6]. In this study RV output reserve was significantly linked to RV size.

Study limitations
The retrospective, single-center design of this study with a rather small number of subjects limits the study results. A higher sample size may have led to identification of more independent factors in the multivariate analysis.

Echocardiographic assessments of the right heart are complicated by its complex shape and morphology. Especially in obese patients, patients with chest wall deformities or COPD, the correct assessment of RV size and function becomes a challenging task. In this respect, cardiac MRI becomes particularly appealing, as it does provide a thorough assessment of right heart size and function even in complicated conditions. In our cohort, high quality recordings were used and no comorbidities were interfering the test results. As the determination of RA and RV area is a readily available

Table 4 Uni- and multivariate regression analysis of RV output reserve

Univariate analysis (Δ CI Peak)	n	pearson's R	p-value	
Age	54	0.424	0.001	*
Body mass index	54	0.092	0.506	
6 min walking distance	54	0.278	0.044	*
NT-proBNP	54	- 0.360	0.008	*
Echocardiography				
Systolic pulmonary arterial pressure	54	- 0.462	< 0.001	*
Right atrial area	54	- 0.313	0.021	*
Right ventricular area	54	- 0.376	0.005	*
Tricuspid annular plane systolic excursion	54	0.065	0.64	
Cardiopulmonary exercise testing				
peak oxygen consumption (V'O$_2$)	54	0.466	< 0.001	*
peak oxygen consumption/kg (V'O$_2$/kg)	54	0.380	0.005	*
Right heart catheter				
rest				
mean pulmonary arterial pressure	54	- 0.288	0.035	*
Cardiac Output	54	0.282	0.039	*
Cardiac Index	54	0.223	0.106	
Pulmonary arterial wedge pressure	54	- 0.016	0.906	
pulmonary vascular resistance	54	- 0.366	0.006	*
exercise				
mean pulmonary arterial pressure	54	- 0.073	0.598	
Cardiac Output	54	0.839	< 0.001	*
Cardiac Index	54	0.894	< 0.001	*
Lung function / Diffusing capacity				
DLCOc SB	48	0.361	0.012	*
DLCOc / VA	48	0.342	0.017	*
Multivariate analysis				
Logistic Regression (stepwise forward selection)				
Δ CI exrcise (dichotomous)		Exp (B)		
Right ventricular area	47	0.863	0.027	*
Linear Regression (stepwise forward selection)				
Δ CI Peak (continuous)		pearson's R		
Right ventricular area	47	- 0.360	0.003	*
Age	47	- 0.412	0.001	*

CI = Cardiac Index, NT-proBNP = N-terminal pro brain natriuretic peptide, DLCOc SB = diffusing capacity transfer factor, DLCOc / VA = diffusing capacity transfer coefficient
* = significant at level 0.05, Exp (B) = Regression coefficient

assessment which is practicable in a good quality, its application in clinical practice is more common compared to cardiac MRI. Unfortunately, no MRI data is available for this patient cohort to confirm the hemodynamic data.

Invasive measurements, cardiopulmonary exercise testing and echocardiographic parameters could not be assessed in one single examination. In order to reduce the influence of inter-exam variations, we only included patients that underwent all measures within a time frame of 48 h. The assessment of CI may be complicated by tricuspid insufficiency in patients with PH. Due to the bidirectional blood flow through the tricuspid valve CI may be overestimated in some patients, which may have influenced the results.

The correlation of right heart size and function to TAPSE and other parameters and their prognostic value should be investigated in a larger-scale study.

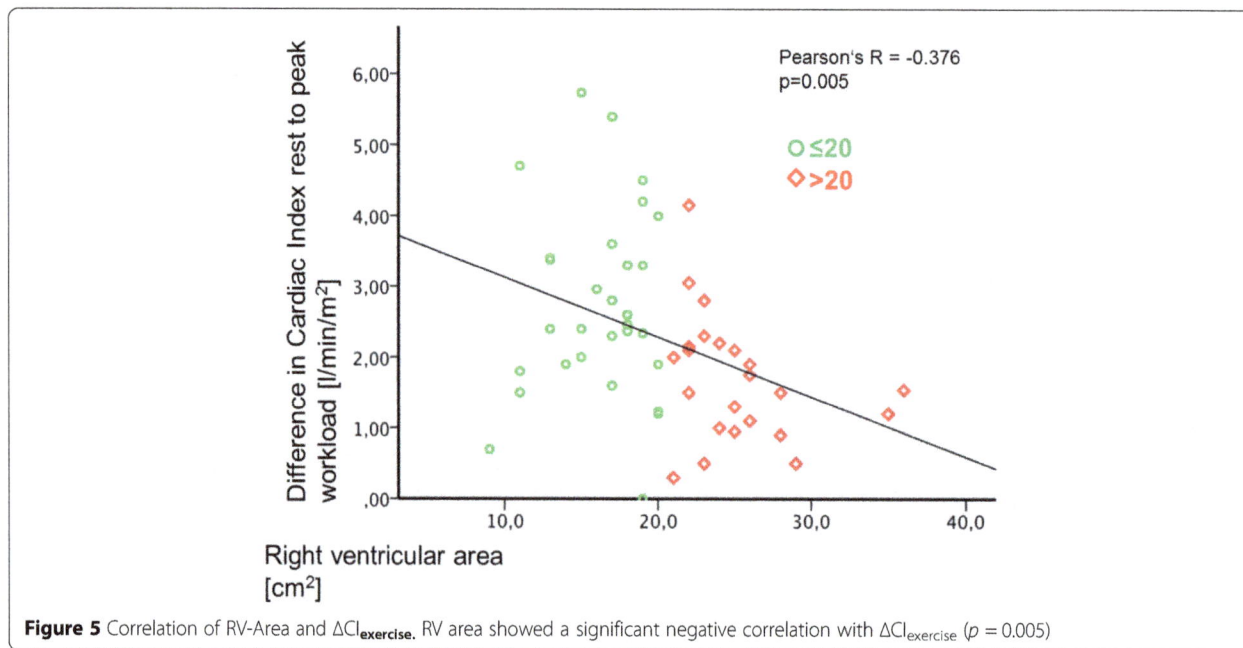

Figure 5 Correlation of RV-Area and $\Delta CI_{exercise}$. RV area showed a significant negative correlation with $\Delta CI_{exercise}$ ($p = 0.005$)

Conclusion

The study shows that assessment of right heart size is important for RV functional characterization and may be helpful since it reflects RV pump function and RV output reserve. RV and RA area by 2-D echocardiography represented a valuable and easily accessible indicator of RV pump function at rest and during exercise. Therefore, these results may be relevant for clinical practice. RV output reserve should be considered as an important clinical parameter. However, prospective studies are needed for further evaluation.

Abbreviations

Δ: Difference; 6MWD: 6-min walking distance; ANOVA: Analysis of variance; APAH: Associated PAH; BMI: Body Mass Index; CI: Cardiac Index; CO: Cardiac Output; CTEPH: Chronic thromboembolic pulmonary hypertension; DLCOc / VA: Diffusing capacity transfer coefficient; DLCOc SB: Diffusing capacity transfer factor; dPAP: Diastolic PAP; Exp (B): Regression coefficient; HPAH: Heritable PAH; HR: Heart rate; IPAH: Idiopathic pulmonary arterial hypertension; mPAP: Mean pulmonary arterial pressure; MRI: Magnetic resonance imaging; NT-proBNP: N-terminal pro brain natriuretic peptide; PAC: Pulmonary arterial compliance; PAH: Pulmonary arterial hypertension; PAP: Pulmonary arterial pressure; PASP: Pulmonary arterial systolic pressure; PCWP: Pulmonary capillary wedge pressure; PH: Pulmonary hypertension; PVR: Pulmonary vascular resistance; RA: Right atrial; RHC: Right heart catheter; RV: Right ventricular; sPAP: Systolic PAP; SV: Stroke volume; SVI: Stroke volume index; TAPSE: Tricuspid annular plane systolic excursion; TRV: Tricuspid regurgitation velocity; TTE: Transthoracic echocardiography; VO'2: Oxygen consumption

Acknowledgements

Not applicable.

Funding

No funding was received for this study.

Authors' contributions

This work was the doctoral thesis of LF. EG, LF, CN, AMM, EB, NB, CF contributed substantially to the study conception and design. EG, LF, CN, BE, SH performed the assessments and patients examinations. LF, MK performed the data collection. NB, CF, LF performed the data analysis. All authors contributed to data interpretation and to the writing of the manuscript. All authors have read and approved the manuscript and agree to be accountable for all aspects of the work in ensuring that questions related to the accuracy or integrity of any part of the work are appropriately investigated and resolved.

Competing interests

LF nothing to disclose. NB received speaker honoraria and travel support from Actelion and Bayer outside the submitted work. BE nothing to disclose. SH received travel support from Actelion and OMT outside the submitted work. MK nothing to disclose. HML received consultancy / speaker fees from: AbbVie, Bristol-Myers Squibb, Roche-Chugai, UCB, MSD, GSK, Sobi, Medac, Novartis, Janssen-Cilag, AstraZeneca, Pfizer, Actelion; speakers bureau: AbbVie, Bristol-Myers Squibb, Roche-Chugai, UCB, MSD, GSK, Sobi, Medac, Novartis, Janssen-Cilag, AstraZeneca, Pfizer, Actelion outside the submitted work. NB received speaker honoraria from Actelion pharmaceuticals. AMM received grants from Italian Helthcare Ministry, grant for young researchers "Ricerca finalizzata 2016 per giovani ricercatori" n. GR-2016-02364727, personal lecture fee from Bayer Healthcare outside the submitted work;. CN reports honoraria for lectures and participation in clinical trials from Actelion, Bayer/MSD, Novartis, speaker honoraria from Boehringer, Astra Zeneca, Berlin Chemie and participation in clinical trials from GSK, United Therapeutics outside the submitted work. CF nothing to disclose. EB nothing to disclose. EG received advisory board member and speaker honoraria from Actelion, Bayer/MSD, GSK, United Therapeutics, Novartis, Pfizer, OrphaSwiss GmbH outside the submitted work.

Author details

[1]Centre for Pulmonary Hypertension, Thoraxklinik at Heidelberg University Hospital, Röntgenstrasse 1, D-69126 Heidelberg, Germany. [2]Translational Lung Research Center Heidelberg (TLRC), Member of the German Center for Lung Research (DZL), Heidelberg, Germany. [3]Department of Rheumatology, University Hospital Heidelberg, Heidelberg, Germany. [4]Institute of Human Genetics, University of Heidelberg, Heidelberg, Germany. [5]IRCCS SDN Research Institute, Naples, Italy. [6]Lung Centre, Klinikum Mittelbaden, Baden-Baden Balg, Baden-Baden, Germany. [7]Heart Department, Cardiology Division, "Cava de' Tirreni and Amalfi Coast" Hospital, University of Salerno, Salerno, Italy.

References

1. D'Alonzo GE, Barst RJ, Ayres SM, et al. Survival in patients with primary pulmonary hypertension. Ann Intern Med. 1991;115(5):343–55.

2. Vonk-Noordegraaf A, Haddad F, Chin KM, et al. Right heart adaptation to pulmonary arterial hypertension: physiology and pathobiology. J Am Coll Cardiol. 2013;62(25):D22–33.

3. Amsallem M, Boulate D, Aymami M, et al. Load adaptability in patients with pulmonary arterial hypertension. Am J Cardiol. 2017;120(5):874–82.

4. Naeije R, Manes A. The right ventricle in pulmonary arterial hypertension. Eur Respir Rev. 2014;23(134):476–87.

5. Vanderpool RR, Pinsky MR, Naeije R, et al. RV-pulmonary arterial coupling predicts outcome in patients referred for pulmonary hypertension. Heart. 2015;101(1):37–43.

6. Vonk Noordegraaf A, Westerhof BE, Westerhof N. The relationship between the right ventricle and its load in pulmonary hypertension. J Am Coll Cardiol. 2017;69(2):236–43.

7. Bustamante-Labarta M, Perrone S, De La Fuente RL, et al. Right atrial size and tricuspid regurgitation severity predict mortality or transplantation in primary pulmonary hypertension. J Am Soc Echocardiogr. 2002;15(10 2):1160–4.

8. Raymond RJ, Hinderliter AL, Willis PW, et al. Echocardiographic predictors of adverse outcomes in primary pulmonary hypertension. J Am Coll Cardiol. 2002;39(7):1214–9.

9. Grunig E, Henn P, D'Andrea A, et al. Reference values for and determinants of right atrial area in healthy adults by 2-dimensional echocardiography. Circ Cardiovasc imaging. 2013;6(1):117–24.

10. Austin C, Alassas K, Burger C, et al. Echocardiographic assessment of estimated right atrial pressure and size predicts mortality in pulmonary arterial hypertension. Chest. 2015;147(1):198–208.

11. van de Veerdonk MC, Huis In TVAE, Marcus JT, et al. Upfront combination therapy reduces right ventricular volumes in pulmonary arterial hypertension. Eur Respir J. 2017;49(6):1700007.

12. van de Veerdonk MC, Marcus JT, Westerhof N, et al. Signs of right ventricular deterioration in clinically stable patients with pulmonary arterial hypertension. Chest. 2015;147(4):1063–71.

13. Blumberg FC, Arzt M, Lange T, Schroll S, Pfeifer M, Wensel R. Impact of right ventricular reserve on exercise capacity and survival in patients with pulmonary hypertension. Eur J Heart Fail. 2013;15(7):771–5.

14. Chaouat A, Sitbon O, Mercy M, et al. Prognostic value of exercise pulmonary haemodynamics in pulmonary arterial hypertension. Eur Respir J. 2014;44(3):704–13.

15. Thenappan T, Prins KW, Pritzker MR, Scandurra J, Volmers K, Weir EK. The critical role of pulmonary arterial compliance in pulmonary hypertension. Ann Am Thorac Soc. 2016;13(2):276–84.

16. Jain P, Rao S, Macdonald P, et al. Diagnostic Performance of Pulmonary Capacitance at Rest and During Exercise in Idiopathic Pulmonary Arterial Hypertension. Heart Lung Circ. 2017. https://doi.org/10.1016/j.hlc.2017.10.019.

17. Galie N, Humbert M, Vachiery JL, et al. 2015 ESC/ERS guidelines for the diagnosis and treatment of pulmonary hypertension: the joint task force for the diagnosis and treatment of pulmonary hypertension of the European Society of Cardiology (ESC) and the European Respiratory Society (ERS): endorsed by: Association for European Paediatric and Congenital Cardiology (AEPC), International Society for Heart and Lung Transplantation (ISHLT). Eur Heart J. 2016;37(1):67–119.

18. Guyatt GH, Pugsley SO, Sullivan MJ, et al. Effect of encouragement on walking test performance. Thorax. 1984;39(11):818–22.

19. Ehlken N, Lichtblau M, Klose H, et al. Exercise training improves peak oxygen consumption and haemodynamics in patients with severe pulmonary arterial hypertension and inoperable chronic thrombo-embolic pulmonary hypertension: a prospective, randomized, controlled trial. Eur Heart J. 2016;37(1):35–44.

20. Kovacs G, Avian A, Olschewski A, Olschewski H. Zero reference level for right heart catheterisation. Eur Respir J. 2013;42(6):1586–94.

21. Kovacs G, Herve P, Barbera JA, et al. An official European Respiratory Society statement: pulmonary haemodynamics during exercise. Eur Respir J. 2017; 50(5):1700578.

22. Grunig E, Weissmann S, Ehlken N, et al. Stress Doppler echocardiography in relatives of patients with idiopathic and familial pulmonary arterial hypertension: results of a multicenter European analysis of pulmonary artery pressure response to exercise and hypoxia. Circulation. 2009;119(13):1747–57.

23. Rudski LG, Lai WW, Afilalo J, et al. Guidelines for the echocardiographic assessment of the right heart in adults: a report from the American Society of Echocardiography endorsed by the European Association of Echocardiography, a registered branch of the European Society of Cardiology, and the Canadian Society of Echocardiography. J Am Soc Echocardiogr. 2010;23(7):685–713 quiz 786-688.

24. Yock PG, Popp RL. Noninvasive estimation of right ventricular systolic pressure by Doppler ultrasound in patients with tricuspid regurgitation. Circulation. 1984;70(4):657–62.

25. Grunig E, Barner A, Bell M, et al. Non-invasive diagnosis of pulmonary hypertension: ESC/ERS guidelines with updated commentary of the Cologne consensus conference 2011. Int J Cardiol. 2011;154(1):S3–12.

26. van Wolferen SA, Marcus JT, Boonstra A, et al. Prognostic value of right ventricular mass, volume, and function in idiopathic pulmonary arterial hypertension. Eur Heart J. 2007;28(10):1250–7.

27. Weatherald J, Boucly A, Chemla D, et al. Prognostic value of follow-up hemodynamic variables after initial Management in Pulmonary Arterial Hypertension. Circulation. 2018;137(7):693–704.

28. Vanderpool RR, Desai AA, Knapp SM, et al. How prostacyclin therapy improves right ventricular function in pulmonary arterial hypertension. Eur Respir J. 2017;50(2):1700764.

Selective activation and proliferation of a quiescent stem cell population in the neuroepithelial body microenvironment

Line Verckist, Isabel Pintelon, Jean-Pierre Timmermans, Inge Brouns and Dirk Adriaensen[*]

Abstract

Background: The microenvironment (ME) of neuroepithelial bodies (NEBs) harbors densely innervated groups of pulmonary neuroendocrine cells that are covered by Clara-like cells (CLCs) and is believed to be important during development and for adult airway epithelial repair after severe injury. Yet, little is known about its potential stem cell characteristics in healthy postnatal lungs.

Methods: Transient mild lung inflammation was induced in mice via a single low-dose intratracheal instillation of lipopolysaccharide (LPS). Bronchoalveolar lavage fluid (BALF), collected 16 h after LPS instillation, was used to challenge the NEB ME in ex vivo lung slices of control mice. Proliferating cells in the NEB ME were identified and quantified following simultaneous LPS instillation and BrdU injection.

Results: The applied LPS protocol induced very mild and transient lung injury. Challenge of lung slices with BALF of LPS-treated mice resulted in selective Ca^{2+}-mediated activation of CLCs in the NEB ME of control mice. Forty-eight hours after LPS challenge, a remarkably selective and significant increase in the number of divided (BrdU-labeled) cells surrounding NEBs was observed in lung sections of LPS-challenged mice. Proliferating cells were identified as CLCs.

Conclusions: A highly reproducible and minimally invasive lung inflammation model was validated for inducing selective activation of a quiescent stem cell population in the NEB ME. The model creates new opportunities for unraveling the cellular mechanisms/pathways regulating silencing, activation, proliferation and differentiation of this unique postnatal airway epithelial stem cell population.

Keywords: Airway epithelium, Neuroepithelial body microenvironment, Stem cell niche, Clara-like cells, Pulmonary neuroendocrine cells, Lipopolysaccharide, Proliferation

Background

The postnatal lung is a conditionally renewing organ with a very low airway epithelial cell turnover in the absence of injury, with less than 1 % of cells dividing at any time point in several species [1, 2]. However, the lungs and airways are capable of rapidly increasing regeneration rate to replace damaged tissue, with local stem and progenitor cells re-entering the cell cycle (for reviews see [3, 4]). Adult stem cells are defined as rare cells present in different niches, with a high proliferative potential and a lifelong ability to self-renew, maintain a variety of cell populations in the steady state and/or replace damaged cells following injury [3, 5, 6].

Neuroepithelial bodies (NEBs) occur in the airway epithelium as densely innervated clusters of pulmonary neuroendocrine cells (PNECs; for review see [7]). In many species (including humans) PNECs are covered by Clara-like cells (CLCs), leaving only thin apical processes of PNECs in contact with the airway lumen. CLCs, PNECs and their extensive innervation together constitute the so-called 'NEB microenvironment (NEB ME)' [8–11]. CLCs have also been referred to as variant Clara cell secretory protein (CCSP)-expressing cells (vCE cells) [12].

The clusters of PNECs release bioactive substances upon stimulation [13–18] and are selectively contacted by mainly vagal afferent nerve terminals [9, 19]. Pulmonary

* Correspondence: dirk.adriaensen@uantwerpen.be
Laboratory of Cell Biology and Histology, Department of Veterinary Sciences, University of Antwerp, Universiteitsplein 1, 2610 Wilrijk, Antwerpen, Belgium

NEBs should therefore be regarded as complex intraepithelial sensory airway receptors, capable of sensing and transducing hypoxic, mechanical, chemical and likely also other stimuli [14, 15, 20](for reviews see [9, 21–23]).

Apart from being airway sensors, NEBs may fulfill some other proposed physiological roles in the airways during fetal and perinatal life [21, 22, 24–26]. The relatively large number of NEBs encountered in the prenatal lung has been explained by their potential role in the regulation of bronchogenesis, as PNECs represent the first cell type that differentiates during embryonic lung development [27]. The possible paracrine regulation of embryonic airway epithelial cell growth by NEBs has been proposed more than 25 years ago based on cell proliferation studies, illustrating that the number of labeled divided cells progressively decreases with increasing distance from NEBs [28].

Throughout the past decade, the NEB ME has been put forward as one of the potential stem cell sources/niches that are dispersed along the epithelial lining of the mammalian respiratory tract [29–32].

The suggested stem cell capacities of the NEB ME in healthy postnatal mouse lungs were recently confirmed using an optimized laser microdissection (LMD) protocol that allows for the selective collection of high quality mRNA samples of the NEB ME [33]. Expression analysis of an extensive panel of genes, selected for their involvement in cell development, proliferation and stem cell signaling, enabled to define a stem cell 'signature' for the NEB ME, an indication that the NEB ME may indeed represent a functional stem cell niche in healthy postnatal mouse airways [33].

Both cell types in the NEB ME, i.e., PNECs and CLCs, have been proposed as potential airway epithelial progenitor cells [12, 34–37]. The observation that NEBs, or at least epithelial cell groups with similar characteristics, show hyperplasia in many airway diseases/disorders [38–40], and seem to play a role as precursors for small cell lung carcinoma (SCLC) [6, 34, 41], evidently suggests a role for PNECs as airway epithelial progenitors. However, the 'stemness' of PNECs is currently questioned since PNECs on their own were not able to restore the airway epithelium after ablation of both Clara cells (CCs) and CLCs [12]. On the other hand, self-renewing and stem cell characteristics have been assigned to CLCs/vCE cells based on lineage-tracing analysis in murine models [12, 42]. During embryonic development, cells surrounding PNECs, i.e., presumptive CLCs, remain undifferentiated [30]. CLCs/vCE cells appear to be resistant to naphthalene ablation because, unlike CCs, they do not express the cytochrome P450 2F2 isozyme [12, 43, 44]. It has been reported that CLCs in postnatal lungs show the capacity to regenerate both CCs

and ciliated cells [45, 46], but that severe epithelial injury is required to activate the stem cell niche for repair [2].

Since the postnatal airway epithelium maintains a very low cell turnover at steady state, experimental damage and the follow-up of epithelial repair processes has typically been used to visualize the proliferative potential of different subsets of airway epithelial cells [1, 47]. A variety of models for severe lung injury and airway epithelial damage have been implemented to activate presumed stem cell niches and study consequent repair throughout the lung epithelium (for reviews see [3, 4, 44, 48, 49]). So far, nearly all information on the postnatal stem cell and regenerative capacities of the NEB ME, and of CLCs in particular, has also been obtained after severe experimental injury of the airway epithelium by naphthalene or genetic modification that fully ablates CCs, and from the consecutive evaluation of epithelial regeneration [12, 35, 37, 50], even in recent publications [43]. Major disadvantages of these methods, however, are the difficulty to distinguish between pathological and potentially physiological events, and the emergence of additional (undesired) hyperplasia of PNECs that apparently compromises the selectivity of activating stem cells for repair.

On the other hand, it has been well documented that all levels of severity of lung injury can be mimicked in animal models involving the application of lipopolysaccharide (LPS; intratracheal [51–53], intranasal [54], intraperitoneal [55]). In mice, intratracheal LPS instillation causes a rapid (few hours) intrapulmonary inflammatory reaction whose course is dependent of the mouse strain, LPS concentration and serotype used [52, 56, 57]. So far, however, the effects of LPS instillation on airway-associated epithelial stem cell niches have not been investigated.

Main goal of the present study was to create a minimally invasive mouse model for activation of the quiescent stem cell niche of the NEB ME. We will show that a single intratracheal instillation of a low dose of LPS –which appears to cause only a very mild and transient injury– is able to do the job. Both morphological, functional and cell proliferation assays are used to detect and quantify the relevant changes in the NEB ME that are induced by LPS challenge.

Methods
Animals
Lung tissue was obtained both from wild type (WT) C57BL/6 J (WT-Bl6) mice, and from a C57BL/6 J based glutamate decarboxylase 67-GFP (GAD67-GFP) mouse strain that harbors GFP fluorescent pulmonary NEBs [58] (The Jackson Laboratory, Charles River, Saint-Germain-sur-l'Arbresle, France). Both male and female mice, mainly at postnatal day (PD) 21, were used. Three-week-old mice have a much smaller lung volume –but a similar number of NEBs–

compared to adults, and hence a higher density of NEBs in lung sections, resulting in more efficient studies. The results were however double-checked for adult mice (8-week-old). The young animals were housed together with their mothers in acrylic cages in an acclimatized room (12/12 h light-dark cycle; 22 ± 3 °C) and were provided with water and food ad libitum. National and international principles of laboratory animal care were followed, and experiments were approved by the local animal ethics committee of the University of Antwerp (ECD 2014–66 and 2017–49). All animals were killed by intraperitoneal (i.p.) injection of an overdose of sodium pentobarbital (Nembutal® 200 mg/kg bodyweight (BW), CEVA Sante Animale, Brussels, Belgium).

LPS instillation

Mice were anesthetized with an i.p. injection of medetomidine (0.25 ml/kg BW; Domitor®, BE-V151742, Orion Pharma, Mechelen, Belgium) and ketamine (17.5 ml/kg BW; Nimatek®, Eurovet, Bladel, The Netherlands) to obtain a light level of surgical anesthesia, subsequently placed on an intubation table (Hallowell EMC, Pittsfield, USA) and intubated with a soft flexible cannula (24G × 3/4"; BD Angiocath; Becton Dickinson; Erembodegem, Belgium) for the intratracheal instillation of 1 mg/kg BW LPS (LPS; *Escherichia coli*; O55:B5; L6529, Sigma, Diegem, Belgium) dissolved in 50 µl of sterile saline (0.9% NaCl; Baxter, Lessen, Belgium). For evaluation of the potential effects of intratracheal instillation itself on the quantified changes in the NEB ME, sham-treated animals received an intratracheal instillation of 50 µl of sterile saline. One hundred µl of air was added to every intratracheal instillation of fluid. After completion of the instillation, anesthesia was reversed by administration of the medetomidine inhibitor atipamezole (2 ml/kg BW; Antisedan®, BE-V153352, Orion Pharma, Mechelen, Belgium) to ameliorate recovery. Animals were euthanized 16 h, 24 h, 48 h, 72 h or 7 days after challenge, as detailed further on.

BrdU injection

As an analog of thymidine, 5-Bromo-2′-deoxyuridine (BrdU) will be incorporated in DNA during the S-phase of cell division. To mark cells that have divided during the experimental window, i.p. injections of BrdU (10 mg/kg; B5002; Sigma, Bornem, Belgium) were given immediately following intratracheal instillation in the treated groups, and at the same time point in untreated matched control mice. BrdU injections were repeated at 24 h and 48 h post-instillation. After recovery, animals were returned to their mothers until the day of euthanasia, 24 h, 48 h or 72 h after LPS challenge or any of the other treatments. Additionally, a few mice received BrdU at time points 0 h and 24 h but were sacrificed 7 days following LPS instillation. The lungs were then processed for cryosectioning and immunostaining (see further on).

Plethysmography

Lung function parameters were measured using an unrestrained mouse Whole-Body Plethysmograph (VENT2; EMKA Technologies; Paris, France). Expiratory time (Te), relaxation time (RT), end-inspiratory pause (EIP) and tidal volume (TV) were evaluated at different time points (1 h, 2 h, 4 h, 6 h, 8 h, 12 h) after start of the experiment (LPS instillation, sham treatment, untreated controls; WT-Bl6; $n = 4$ for each group).

Bronchoalveolar lavage

Sixteen hours after LPS or sham instillation, WT-Bl6 mice (n = 4 for each group) were euthanized and exsanguinated. Untreated WT-Bl6 mice (n = 4) served as an additional control. Bronchoalveolar lavage fluid (BALF) was collected by instillation and suction of a salt solution (2×1 ml; 0.9% NaCl) in the lungs via a tracheal cannula. BALF was stored at 4 °C until further use. In accordance with literature [59], the time point of 16 h after LPS treatment was chosen to allow the animals to recover completely from the anesthetics and still be able to detect effects from a combination of early and late phase mediators in the BALF. The collected BALF was first centrifuged (12 min, 150G), the cell-free supernatant fluid was removed and used as a stimulus solution for the NEB ME in lung slices in live cell imaging (LCI) experiments (see below). The cell pellet was used to prepare cytospin slides for evaluation of the cells that are present in the pulmonary air spaces. The pellet was resuspended to an end concentration of about 10^6 cells/ml in phosphate-buffered saline (PBS; 0.01 M, pH 7.4), containing 5% bovine serum albumin (BSA; B4287, Sigma). 150 µl of this mixture was centrifuged (5 min, 800G) to generate cytospin preparations (Shandon Cytospin 3 Cytocentrifuge, Fisher Scientific, Erembodegem, Belgium) of BALF cells. After air-drying, the slides were fixed and stained using a fast routine blood cell staining method (Diff-Quick; DQ-ST, MICROPTIC, Barcelona, Spain), and mounted in Entellan (Merck; Overijse, Belgium). Cell types in the BALF cytospins were morphologically characterized under a light microscope and compared between LPS-challenged, sham-treated and untreated controls. Data were used only for general interpretation of the inflammatory effect of instillation, and no further quantification was performed.

Preparation of live lung slices

Live lung slices were prepared as previously published [60]. In short, WT-Bl6 mice ($n = 3$) were euthanized and the lung tissue was stabilized by slowly instilling a 2% agarose solution (37 °C, low-melt agarose, A4018, Sigma) via a tracheal cannula. After inflation, lungs were dissected and transferred to an ice-cold physiological solution. Precision-cut lung slices (120 µm thick) were sectioned using a vibratome (Microm HM650 V; Microm International, Walldorf, Germany) and 6–8 slices per animal were subsequently kept in the cold physiological solution until further manipulation within the next few hours (maximally 6 h).

Live cell imaging

As previously reported in detail [8], different cell types in the NEB ME and in the surrounding airway epithelium, such as PNECs, CLCs, CCs and ciliated cells, can be identified in live lung vibratome slices after staining with the fluorescent dye 4-Di-2-ASP (Molecular Probes D-289, Fisher Scientific) and loading with the Ca^{2+} indicator Fluo-4 AM (Molecular Probes F-14202; Fisher Scientific). In short, lung slices were consecutively incubated for 4 min in 4 μM 4-Di-2-ASP in Dulbecco's modified Eagle's medium/F-12 (DMEM-F-12; Gibco, Fisher Scientific) at 37 °C, rinsed, and incubated for 1 h at room temperature in 10 μM Fluo-4 AM. For experimental LCI purposes, the lung slices were submerged in a tissue bath (2 ml) mounted on the microscope stage, continuously perfused with physiological solution by a gravity-fed system (flow rate of 0.5 ml/min). Perfusion was paused when BALF was manually pipetted onto the lung slice in the tissue bath. Physiological solution containing a high extracellular potassium concentration ($[K^+]_o$) was prepared by equimolar substitution of KCl for NaCl [8].

High-resolution LCI was performed as extensively described before [8, 13, 60]. In short, a microlens-enhanced dual spinning disk confocal system (Ultra-VIEW ERS; PerkinElmer, Zaventem, Belgium), equipped with an argon-krypton laser was used. Time-lapse images of changes in Fluo-4 fluorescence (excitation max. 494 nm; emission max. 516 nm) were recorded (2 images/s; 488-nm laser excitation; bandpass 500–560 emission filter) and analyzed off-line by Volocity 2 software (Improvision, Coventry, UK). Regions of interest were manually drawn around identified cell groups of interest, and the fluorescence intensity was plotted against time. Changes in Fluo-4 fluorescence should be interpreted as relative changes in the intracellular Ca^{2+} concentration ($[Ca^{2+}]_i$). All graphs presented are representative of multiple experiments performed under the respective conditions.

Immunohistochemical staining of lung cryosections for the evaluation of cell division

All mice included in the LPS challenge experiments, including sham-treated and untreated controls, were processed for cryosectioning and immunostaining as detailed below. Mice were euthanized and the lungs were transcardially perfused with physiological solution and subsequently filled with 4% paraformaldehyde (PF)

via a tracheal cannula. Lungs, trachea, esophagus and heart were dissected *en bloc*, deaerated in a mild vacuum, and immersion-fixed in the same fixative for 30 min. After rinsing in PBS, tissues were stored overnight in 20% sucrose (in PBS; 4 °C), and mounted in Tissue-Tek O.C.T. (4583; Sakura Finetek Europe, Zoeterwoude, The Netherlands). Consecutive cryostat sections (20 μm thick; Leica CM1950, Diegem, Belgium) of the whole tissue blocks were thaw-mounted on poly-L-lysine-coated microscope slides following a strict pattern (see further on), dried at 37 °C (2 h) and kept at − 80 °C until further use.

Immunohistochemical incubations were performed at room temperature in a closed humidified container. All primary and secondary antisera were diluted in PBS containing 10% normal horse serum and 0.1% BSA (PBS*). Before incubation with the primary antisera, cryostat sections were permeabilized for 1 h with PBS* containing 1% Triton X-100. Sections were then incubated overnight with a combination of the primary antibodies listed in Table 1. For visualization of the immunolabeling, sections were further incubated for 4 h with secondary antibodies (Table 2).

After a final wash in PBS, the sections were mounted in Citifluor (19,470; Ted Pella, Redding, CA).

For each animal, a few cryosections were routinely stained with hematoxylin and eosin (H&E), dehydrated in a graded series of ethanol and xylene, and mounted in Entellan. Lung sections were evaluated under a light microscope for the histological evaluation of epithelial damage, interstitial inflammation, edema and leukocyte recruitment, as characteristics of pulmonary inflammation and lung injury [61].

A bright-field/epifluorescence microscope (Zeiss Axiophot, Carl Zeiss, Jena, Germany) was used to image the H&E-stained lung cryosections and DiffQuick stained BALF cytospins, and to quickly screen the immunostaining results. All fluorescence images were obtained using a microlens-enhanced dual spinning disk confocal microscope (UltraVIEW VoX; PerkinElmer) equipped with 488 nm, 561 nm and 640 nm diode lasers for excitation of

Table 1 List of primary antisera used for immunohistochemistry

Primary Antisera Antigen	Host	Mc/Pc	Source
Bromo deoxyuridine (BrdU)	Rat	Mc	Abcam ab6326, Cambridge, UK
Calcitonin gene-related peptide (CGRP)	Rabbit	Pc	Sigma C3866, Bornem, Belgium
CGRP	Goat	Pc	Abcam ab36001
Urine protein 1 (UP1)/Clara cell secretory protein (CCSP)	Rabbit	Pc	Abcam ab40873

Table 2 List of secondary antisera used for immunohistochemistry

Secondary Antisera Antigen	Source	Dilution
Cy™5-conjugated Fab fragments of goat anti-rabbit IgG	Jackson ImmunoResearch 111–117-003, West Grove, PA, USA	1/2000
Cy™3-conjugated donkey anti-rat IgG	Jackson ImmunoResearch 712–165-153	1/1000
FITC-conjugated donkey anti-goat IgG	Jackson ImmunoResearch 705–095-147	1/500
Cy™5-conjugated donkey anti-rabbit IgG	Jackson ImmunoResearch 711–175-152	1/500

FITC/GFP, Cy3 and Cy5. Images were acquired and processed using Volocity 6.3.1 software (PerkinElmer).

Data acquisition, quantification and statistics

Quantification of the BrdU-positive cells was performed by manually counting the fluorescent nuclei in the areas of interest. Lung cryosections (20 μm-thick) were collected and selected in a reproducible manner. Per slide, two sections were mounted in such a way that the distance between both sections is 200 μm. In short, ten consecutive sections were mounted on different slides, after which the following 10 sections were mounted in the same order on these slides. The next 20 consecutive sections were collected on 10 new slides, and so on until the lung tissue was completely cut. Then, a first slide for staining was selected based on the presence of airway branches and presumably NEBs. Starting from this slide, six more were taken every 10 slides, thereby avoiding the possibility that more than one section of the same NEB ME could be found and/or counted in the selected slides when immunostained for BrdU and some reference markers. As such, for every mouse in the different treatment groups (LPS-treated, sham treated and untreated control), between 60 and 100 NEBs were visualized under the microscope, by their GFP fluorescence in GAD67-GFP mice or CGRP immunostaining in WT-Bl6 mice, and the PNECs and BrdU-positive cells in the NEB ME were counted.

For each animal in all of the experimental groups, the mean number of BrdU-positive cells per NEB ME was calculated and the data were statistically compared between the different treatment groups, using a nonparametric Kruskal-Wallis test followed by Dunn's multiple comparisons test. Data are represented as (mean ± SEM).

Potential differences in the number of BrdU-positive cells between the two mouse strains were statistically evaluated using the unpaired t-test for each treatment group, after checking normal distribution of the counts.

Results

Evaluation of the pulmonary effects of low dose LPS challenge

Although the recorded plethysmographic data did not qualify for quantification, due to individual variation inherent to the use of unrestrained young mice, some of the observations were of importance for the presented study. Apart from clear but variable differences in the measurements of TE, RT, EIP and TV between untreated controls and LPS-challenged (and to a lesser extent also sham-treated) mice during the first 2 to 6 h, plethysmography could no longer distinguish LPS-challenged from untreated animals 8 h or longer after treatment (data not shown).

To assess possible inflammatory changes in the airway environment, BALF was collected from the same animals that had been monitored by plethysmography (16 h after instillation of LPS or saline and untreated), and processed for the generation of cytospin preparations. While BALF of healthy control animals showed macrophage-like cells only (Fig. 1a), the majority of leukocytes in the LPS-treated mice appeared to be neutrophils (Fig. 1c, d). Neutrophils were also seen in BALF of the sham-treated mice (Fig. 1b), but clearly to a lesser extent than after LPS challenge.

The applied single low-dose intratracheal LPS challenge did not cause obvious histological changes in the airway epithelium or alveolar areas in H&E-stained lung sections (Fig. 2).

An important element for the interpretation of the following experimental data is that this combined approach (plethysmography, evaluation of the collected BALF; lung histology), supports the idea that the applied single low dose of intratracheal LPS induces a mild and transient inflammation.

Application of BALF from LPS-challenged mice to the NEB ME of healthy control mice

Apart from detecting/recording $[Ca^{2+}]_i$ fluctuations in the NEB ME, freshly cut live lung slices co-loaded with 4-Di-2-Asp and Fluo-4, also allowed to differentiate between all cell types in the NEB ME and the surrounding airway epithelium (for detailed explanation see [8]). In short, very small and moderately fluorescent grouped NEB cells are encircled by a virtually non-fluorescent rim that harbors much larger CLCs, and are further surrounded by intermingled strongly fluorescent polygonal ciliated cells and large rounded unstained CCs (Fig. 3b).

To allow fast evaluation of the effect of LPS-induced inflammatory mediators on the NEB ME, BALF that had been collected from mice 16 h after intratracheal instillation of LPS, was applied to lung slices of healthy control mice in the course of the LCI experiments.

BALF of LPS-treated mice was seen to induce a reversible and reproducible $[Ca^{2+}]_i$ rise, selectively in CLCs

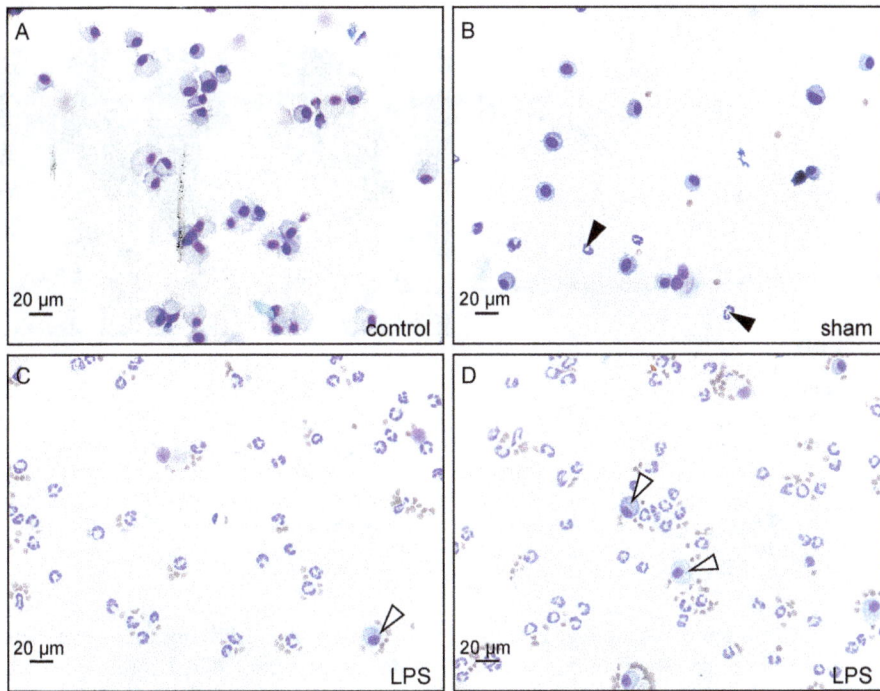

Fig. 1 Representative images, with similar cell densities, of Diff-Quick-stained cytospin preparations of BALF collected from mice that received no instillation (untreated healthy control animal; **a**), 16 h after an intratracheal instillation with 0.9% NaCl (sham-treatment; **b**), or with LPS (**c, d**). Cell densities of the cytospin preparations were 'normalized' between the experimental groups and are therefore unrelated to the initial cell numbers in the BALF. **a** BALF of a healthy control mouse contains virtually no other cells than macrophages (acentric oval nuclei and bluish cytoplasm). **b** Some neutrophils (segmented nuclei and unstained cytoplasm; *arrowheads*) appear to be infiltrated in the airways after a sham instillation but macrophages still constitute the majority of cells in this sample. **c, d** Massive neutrophil influx is seen as a response to the LPS instillation, and consequently a relatively low number of macrophages (*open arrowheads*). Note that the preparations of treated animals also harbor some red blood cells (small brownish dots)

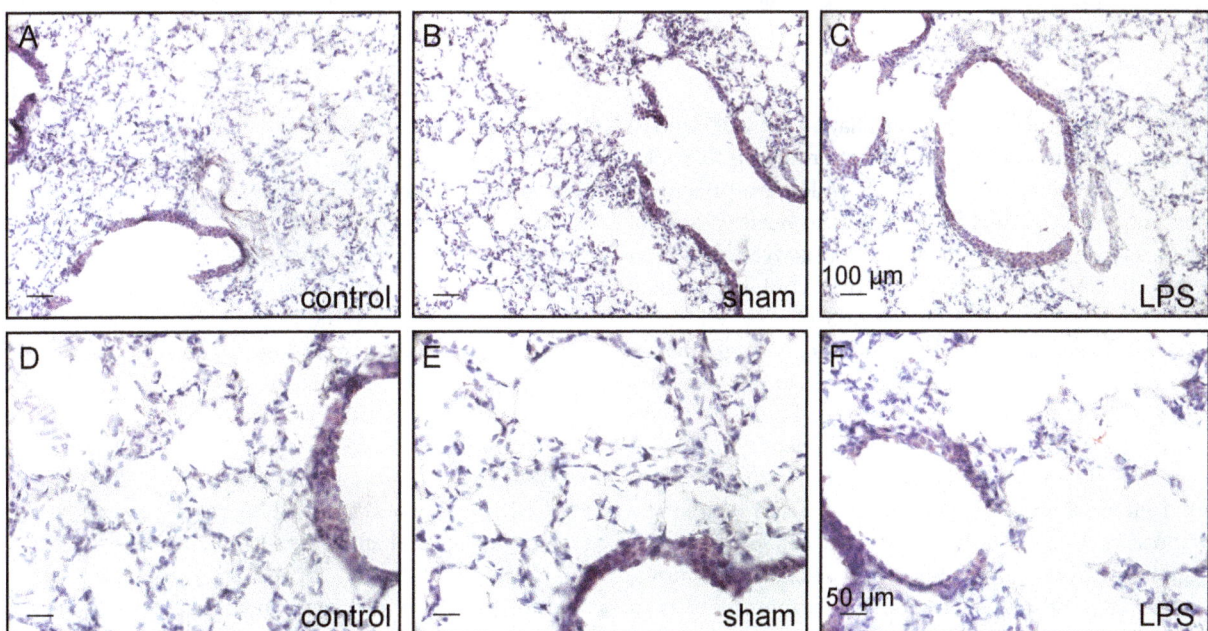

Fig. 2 Representative images of HE-stained lung cryosections from untreated control (**a, d**), and 48 h after intratracheal instillation with 0.9% NaCl (sham-treatment; **b, e**), or with LPS (**c, f**). Note that lung morphology shows no clear histological differences between the groups

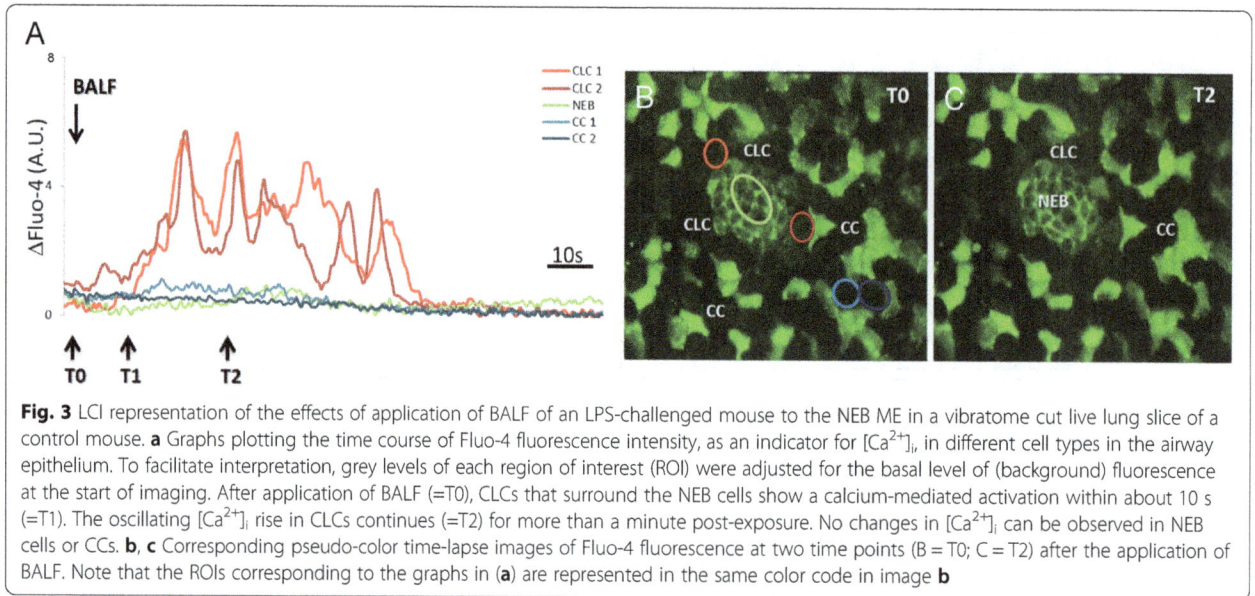

Fig. 3 LCI representation of the effects of application of BALF of an LPS-challenged mouse to the NEB ME in a vibratome cut live lung slice of a control mouse. **a** Graphs plotting the time course of Fluo-4 fluorescence intensity, as an indicator for $[Ca^{2+}]_i$, in different cell types in the airway epithelium. To facilitate interpretation, grey levels of each region of interest (ROI) were adjusted for the basal level of (background) fluorescence at the start of imaging. After application of BALF (=T0), CLCs that surround the NEB cells show a calcium-mediated activation within about 10 s (=T1). The oscillating $[Ca^{2+}]_i$ rise in CLCs continues (=T2) for more than a minute post-exposure. No changes in $[Ca^{2+}]_i$ can be observed in NEB cells or CCs. **b, c** Corresponding pseudo-color time-lapse images of Fluo-4 fluorescence at two time points (B = T0; C = T2) after the application of BALF. Note that the ROIs corresponding to the graphs in (**a**) are represented in the same color code in image **b**

of the NEB ME (Fig. 3). CLCs appeared to react within about 10 s after administration of BALF and revealed $[Ca^{2+}]_i$ oscillations for about a minute. On the other hand, NEB cells, CCs and ciliated cells did not show a $[Ca^{2+}]_i$ rise. Comparable challenge of lung slices with LPS (15 µg/ml in physiological solution) or with BALF of sham and untreated control mice did not induce a $[Ca^{2+}]_i$ rise in any cell type in the NEB ME or airway epithelium, while the physiological responsiveness of the lung slices could be confirmed by the typical fast and reversible $[Ca^{2+}]_i$ increase in NEB cells and a slightly delayed $[Ca^{2+}]_i$ rise in CLCs, following a 5-s application of 50 mM K^+ (not shown) [8].

Effects of a single intratracheal instillation with LPS and the resulting transient mild inflammation on the NEB ME
The above observation that CLCs– which are presumed quiescent airway epithelial stem cells in healthy control mice – show a calcium-mediated activation upon short-term application of BALF that contains soluble mediators from the airways of LPS-challenged mice, raised the question as to what the effects might be on CLCs that experience long-term exposure to these mediators in airways of LPS-treated mice. To follow up on the hypothesis that activation of quiescent (non-dividing) stem cells might be linked to proliferation, the potential effect of intratracheal administration of a single low dose of LPS on airway epithelial cell proliferation in general, and on the NEB ME in particular, was monitored using simultaneous BrdU incorporation as a marker for cells that divide during the experimental window. Three experimental groups were included: untreated control mice, mice receiving an intratracheal

instillation with LPS, and mice with an intratracheal instillation of a 0.9% NaCl solution (= sham control).

In cryosections of the lungs of untreated healthy 3-week-old WT-Bl6 mice, hardly any divided cells were discerned in control airway epithelium (CAE) within the investigated time windows (24, 48 (Fig. 4a) or 72 h) as confirmed by BrdU labeling. The very rare divided epithelial cells appeared to be randomly distributed. The majority of cells with BrdU-labeled nuclei in the airways of these untreated controls were found subepithelially (Fig. 4a). As a positive control, BrdU incorporation was evaluated in sections of a piece of small intestine that was additionally collected from each mouse. A large number of divided (BrdU-labeled) epithelial cells was invariably observed in crypts of the intestinal villi (Fig. 4b).

Forty-eight hours after a single intratracheal instillation with low-dose LPS, a considerable number of divided (BrdU-positive) epithelial cells was detected, typically clustered in distinct areas of the airway epithelium of WT-Bl6 mice (Fig. 5a).

In sham-treated WT-Bl6 mice, BrdU-positive cells also appeared to be more numerous at specific locations in the airway epithelium (Fig. 5c) than in untreated controls, although the increase was less pronounced than that seen in LPS-treated mice.

Double immunostaining of the BrdU-labeled sections for CGRP, as a marker for NEBs, revealed that the great majority of divided airway epithelial cells were located in the NEB ME following LPS challenge (Fig. 5b, d).

All of the above data were obtained using 3-week-old mice, but a similar selective cell proliferation (BrdU positive nuclei) in the NEB ME was observed in LPS-challenged adult mice (not shown).

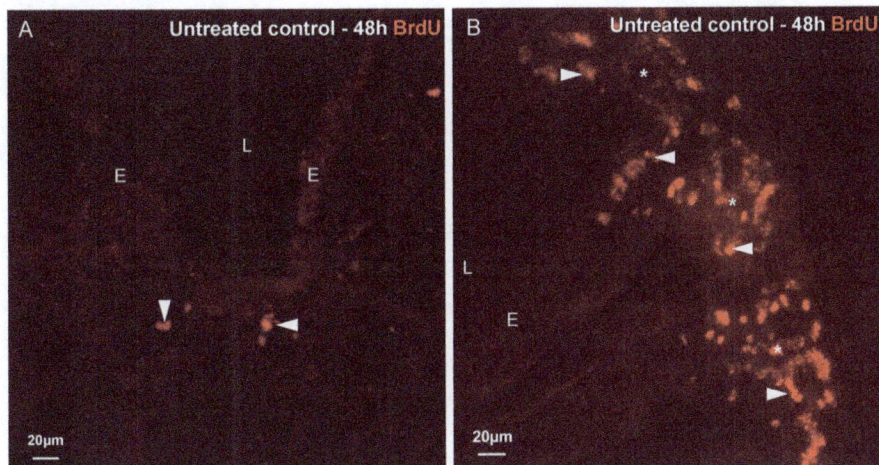

Fig. 4 Immunostaining for BrdU (*red* Cy3 fluorescence) in cryosections of an intrapulmonary airway (**a**) and small intestine (**b**) of the same mouse that received no treatment, except for the BrdU injections (i.p.), 48 h and 24 h prior to sacrifice. **a** The airway epithelium rarely harbors divided BrdU-positive cells. The majority of BrdU-labeled nuclei (*arrowheads*) are located in subepithelial layers. **b** In the crypts (*asterisks*) and the basal parts of the villus epithelium of the small intestine, a large number of BrdU-labeled nuclei (*arrowheads*)– i.e., originating from cells that have divided during the 48 h experimental window– can be observed. *L: airway lumen, E: airway epithelium*

Given the apparent close link between NEBs and divided (BrdU-labeled) epithelial cells in the airways of LPS-challenged mice, the use of GAD67-GFP mice that harbor intrinsically GFP-fluorescent NEBs [58] would offer considerable advantages for further quantification. Therefore, we verified whether similar results could be obtained in WT-Bl6 and GAD67-GFP mice. Comparable to what was seen using WT-Bl6 mice with CGRP as a NEB marker (Figs. 5a, b and 6a, b), LPS-treated GAD67-GFP mice also showed BrdU-labeled (divided) airway epithelial cells that were selectively grouped around GFP-fluorescent NEBs (Fig. 6c, d).

Both in healthy controls, sham-treated and LPS-challenged mice, the numbers of CGRP- or GFP-positive PNECs with BrdU-positive nuclei were very low after 48 h exposure.

Since the majority of proliferating (BrdU-labeled) airway epithelial cells in LPS-treated mice was located in the NEB ME, closely surrounding NEB cells, and because BALF of LPS-challenged mice was seen to selectively activate CLCs in the NEB ME, we further investigated whether BrdU-positive cells co-label with markers for CCs/CLCs.

Characterization of the cell type(s) that typically divide in the NEB ME following LPS challenge

To further confirm the identity of BrdU-labeled cells in the NEB ME as CLCs, lung sections (48 h after LPS instillation) were additionally immunostained for CCSP, a marker of both CCs and CLCs surrounding NEB cells. CCSP was used due to the lack of a selective marker for CLCs in postnatal lungs and revealed that cells with BrdU-labeled nuclei in the NEB ME invariably co-stained for CCSP (Fig. 7c), confirming that mainly CLCs were concerned.

Selection of the most relevant time window to study cell proliferation in the NEB ME following LPS challenge

Because single intratracheal instillation of LPS appeared to specifically induce cell division (BrdU incorporation) in the NEB ME in a 48 h time window, we next evaluated whether this was the most relevant time point for visualization/quantification of cell proliferation in the NEB ME. To this end, three time windows were included in a pilot experiment; lungs were collected 24 h, 48 h and 72 h after LPS challenge. Our preliminary data revealed BrdU-labeled airway epithelial cells in the NEB ME already after 24 h, although the effect appeared to be much more prominent 48 h after LPS challenge (Figs. 5a,b, 6 and 7). After 72 h, some of the BrdU-labeled epithelial cells were located a few cells away from NEBs, making this time window somewhat less selective for the NEB ME.

Interestingly, 7 days after LPS challenge, BrdU-positive nuclei could still be detected in CCSP-positive CLCs in the NEB ME, similar to what was seen after 48 h, but also in CCSP-labeled CCs in the surrounding airway epithelium (Fig. 8).

Because the NEB ME is the main area of interest for the present investigation, and considering the observed calcium-mediated activation of CLCs, the time window of 48 h BrdU incorporation after LPS challenge was chosen for further quantification of cell proliferation in the NEB ME.

Quantitative analysis of BrdU-labeled cells in the NEB ME after LPS treatment

Evaluation of potential differences between WT-Bl6 and GAD67-GFP mice

Cell division was quantified in a 48 h time window using WT-Bl6 and GAD67-GFP mice that had been injected

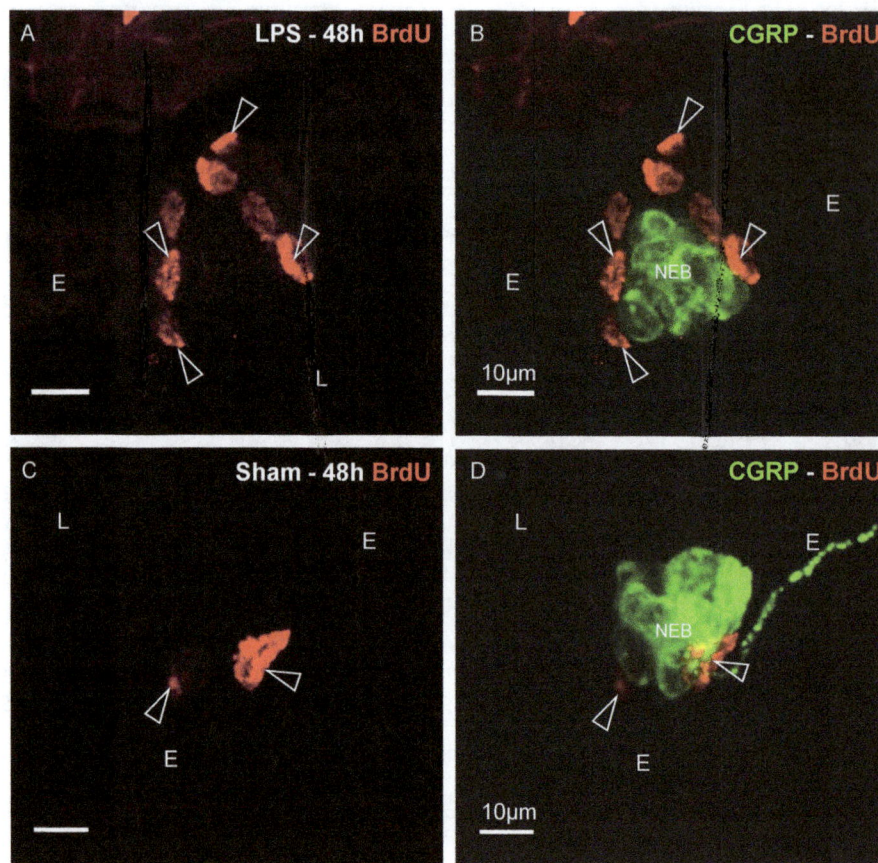

Fig. 5 Immunostaining for BrdU (*red* Cy3 fluorescence) and CGRP (*green* FITC fluorescence) in intrapulmonary airways 48 h after an intratracheal LPS (**a, b**) or sham instillation (**c, d**) in WT-Bl6 mice. **a** After LPS challenge, clustered BrdU-positive (divided) cells are observed in the epithelial layer (*open arrowheads*). **b** Additional CGRP immunostaining reveals that the intraepithelial BrdU-labeled cells are typically grouped around NEBs. **c, d** After a sham instillation, intraepithelial BrdU-positive cells also appear to be located in the neighborhood of NEBs (*open arrowhead*), but are less numerous than after LPS treatment. *L: airway lumen, E: airway epithelium*

with BrdU at time point zero and after 24 h. Three groups were included, i.e., mice receiving a single intratracheal injection with either LPS or 0.9% NaCl at time point zero, and untreated control mice.

To avoid that unlikely variations in cell proliferation between WT-Bl6 mice and GAD67-GFP mice would hamper the interpretation of observed differences, both mouse strains were included in the quantifications.

The significance of possible variations between GAD67-GFP ($n = 5$) and WT-Bl6 (n = 5) mice was evaluated by means of a nonparametric t-test on the percentages of NEBs that showed BrdU-positive cells for the two treatment groups (LPS-challenged WT-Bl6: $72.2 \pm 4.4\%$ vs. LPS-challenged GAD67-GFP mice: $61.9 \pm 2.1\%$, $p = 0.1$; sham-treated WT-Bl6: $23.2 \pm 2.6\%$ vs. sham-treated GAD67-GFP mice: $19.3 \pm 3.5\%$, $p = 0.4$) and on the mean number of BrdU-positive cells per activated NEB ME (LPS-challenged WT-Bl6: 3.45 ± 0.37 vs. LPS-challenged GAD67-GFP mice: 3.30 ± 0.26, $p = 0.1$; sham-treated WT-Bl6: 1.54 ± 0.53 vs. sham-treated GAD67-GFP

mice: 1.78 ± 0.07, $p = 0.4$). Consequently, data for the two strains could be pooled for further quantification of the potential differences between the experimental groups.

Correlation between the number of BrdU-labeled cells and the number of PNECs in NEBs

To examine whether the size (number of PNECs) of NEBs is important for the number of divided cells in the NEB ME, the number of BrdU-positive cells was plotted out against the number of PNECs for each counted NEB of all animals in the treatment groups. Although the mean number of PNECs per NEB (10.8 ± 0.6 for LPS-treated animals vs. 11.3 ± 1.0 for sham-treated) was, as expected, not significantly different for both groups (unpaired t-test; $p > 0.66$), the mean number of BrdU-positive cells per NEB ME (0.5 ± 0.1 for sham-treated vs. 2.1 ± 0.3 for LPS-treated mice) was significantly higher ($p < 0.0005$) in the LPS-challenged mice (Fig. 9).

Overall, larger NEBs (more PNECs) appeared to harbor in their ME a modestly higher number of cells that

Selective activation and proliferation of a quiescent stem cell population in the neuroepithelial...

179

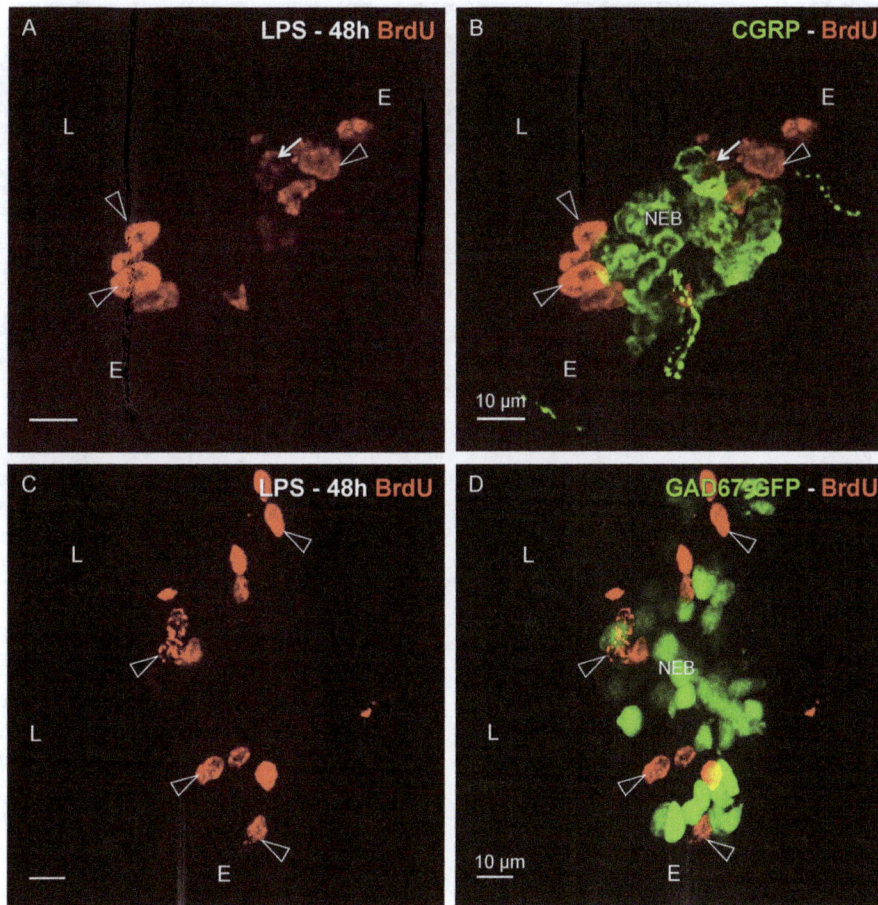

Fig. 6 Comparison of the distribution of BrdU-labeled (*red* Cy3 fluorescence) airway epithelial cells 48 h after LPS challenge of WT-Bl6 (**a**, **b**) and GAD67-GFP mice (**c**, **d**). **a**, **c** Clustered BrdU-positive nuclei (*open arrowheads*) can be observed at distinct locations in the airway epithelium. Combination with CGRP immunostaining (**b**; *green* FITC fluorescence) for WT-Bl6 mice, or visualization of GFP-fluorescent NEB cells (**d**) in GAD67-GFP mice, reveals that the majority of divided cells that have incorporated BrdU are found in the immediate neighborhood of NEBs. No obvious differences can be seen between WT-Bl6 and GAD67-GFP mice. Note that only very occasionally, a BrdU-positive nucleus can be seen in a NEB cell (*arrow*; **a**, **b**). *L: airway lumen, E: airway epithelium*

have divided during a 48 h time window, although only a small non-significant positive trend in the correlation between the number of PNECs and the number of divided cells in the NEB ME was observed for the complete set of quantified NEBs in both treatment groups (sham-treated: $r = 0.20$; LPS-treated mice: $r = 0.31$; Fig. 9).

Further quantifications were therefore carried out without additional analysis of the number of PNECs in each NEB.

Percentage of NEBs that harbor divided cells in their ME

Extensive quantification of BrdU-labeled (divided) cells in the NEB ME in the airways of LPS-challenged, sham-treated and untreated controls revealed clear differences between the experimental groups (Fig. 10). Mice that received an intratracheal LPS instillation harbored a significantly higher mean percentage (Non-parametric Kruskal-Wallis test) of

NEBs with BrdU-positive cells in their ME ($72.2 \pm 2.4\%$), as compared to sham-treated animals ($23.2 \pm 2.6\%$) and untreated control mice ($9.2 \pm 2.4\%$).

Number of divided cells per NEB ME

A closer look at the number of BrdU-stained cells (framed areas in Fig. 10; Table 3) did not show clustering of divided cells in the NEB ME in untreated control mice (mean number of BrdU-positive cells for all NEBs with divided cells: 1.14 ± 0.3 BrdU-positive cells/NEB ME; total of 10.5 BrdU-positive cells/100 NEBs). In the sham experiments, relatively more NEBs showed divided cells in their ME, but similar to the untreated controls they were mainly observed as solitary BrdU-stained cells (mean number: 1.51 ± 0.26 BrdU-positive cells/NEB ME; total of 35 BrdU-positive cells/100 NEBs). However, clustering of divided cells in the NEB ME was seen after LPS treatment, with 40% of the NEBs harboring three to

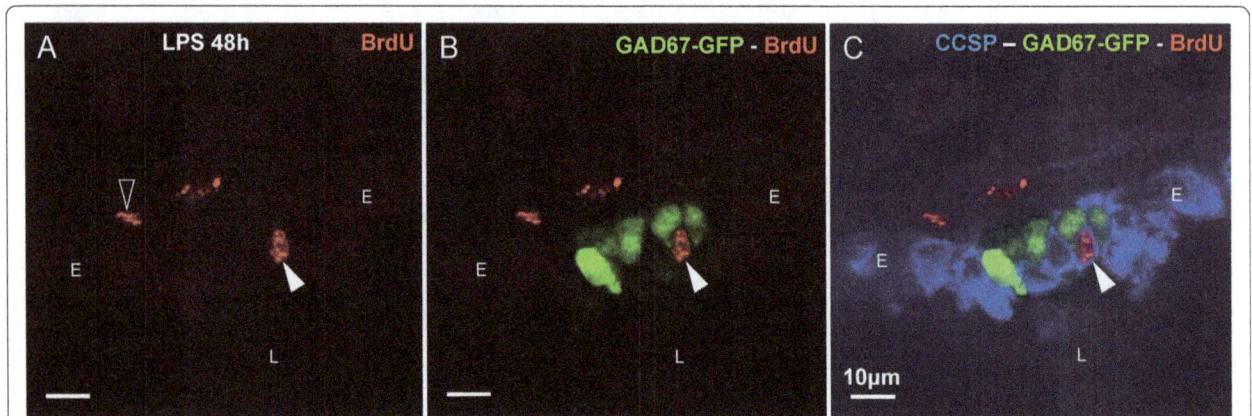

Fig. 7 Single confocal optical section of the airway epithelium in a cryosection of the lungs of a GAD67-GFP mouse 48 h after challenge with LPS. **a** BrdU-positive nucleus (*arrowhead; red* Cy3 fluorescence) in the airway epithelium, and some subepithelial BrdU staining (*open arrowhead*). **b** Combination with GAD67-GFP fluorescence (*green*), marking PNECs in the NEB ME. **c** Image of the three channels. In the same section, CCs/ CLCs are immunostained for the Clara cell-specific protein CCSP (*blue* pseudo-color of Cy5 fluorescence), and are seen to surround GFP-labeled NEB cells. Note that the divided epithelial cell (BrdU-labeled nucleus; *arrowhead*) is located adjacent to the PNECs and co-stained with CCSP, and can therefore be identified as a CLC. *L: airway lumen, E: airway epithelium*

eight BrdU-stained cells and 10% of the NEBs even nine or more (mean number: 3.55 ± 0.6 BrdU-positive cells/ NEB ME; total of 256.3 BrdU-positive cells/100 NEBs).

Overall (Fig. 10 and Table 3), quantitative analysis revealed that the NEB MEs in untreated controls typically display a very low number of BrdU-positive airway epithelial cells, indicating that virtually no cells have divided

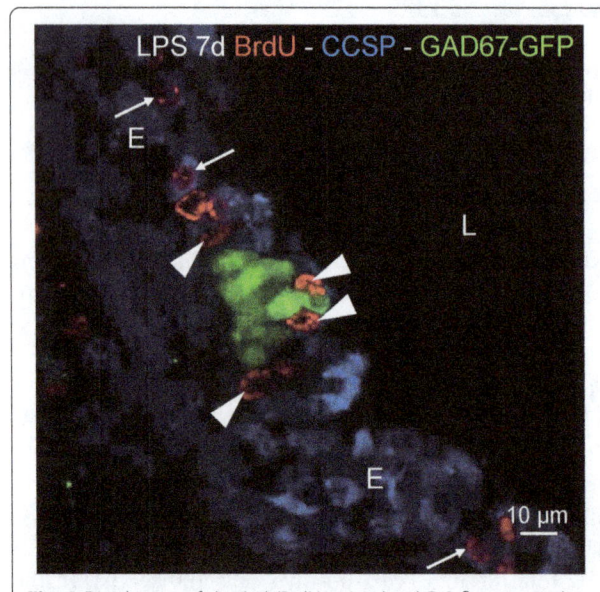

Fig. 8 Distribution of divided (BrdU-stained; *red* Cy3 fluorescence) airway epithelial cells seven days after LPS challenge. Similar to the 48 h time window, several CCSP-immunostained (*blue* pseudo-color of Cy5 fluorescence), BrdU-positive nuclei (*arrowheads*) can be observed specifically surrounding GAD67-GFP fluorescent (*green*) PNECs in the NEB ME. Note, however, the additional presence of CCSP-stained BrdU-labeled CCs in the surrounding airway epithelium (*open arrowheads*). *L: airway lumen, E: airway epithelium*

during the 48 h experimental window. The manipulation of intratracheal instillation (0.9% NaCl; sham-control) on its own appeared to induce a limited but enhanced cell division in the NEB ME, whereas the percentage of NEBs with BrdU-stained cells in the NEB ME and the total number of divided cells were remarkably higher after LPS instillation.

Subdivision of BrdU-labeled cell types in the NEB ME

For a limited number of experiments (n = 3 GAD67-GFP mice per group), all BrdU-labeled cells of each NEB ME were individually identified– as CLCs or PNECs– and counted (data shown in Fig. 11). Clearly, the number of divided PNECs was very limited compared to that of CLCs in the NEB ME. Moreover, the mean number of BrdU-labeled PNECs was not significantly different between the three experimental groups (Kruskal-Wallis; $p = 0.25$).

These additional data further confirmed the significantly higher number of divided CLCs in the LPS-treated group (Kruskal-Wallis; $p = 0.01$).

Discussion

Despite having a very low cellular turnover rate in healthy conditions, the lung and airway epithelium are capable of responding quickly to acute injury, due to the presence of a restricted set of quiescent stem cells that are able to re-enter the cell cycle [4]. Detailed knowledge of the molecular characteristics, silencing and activation pathways of these specific types of stem cells will be essential for a good understanding of the possibilities for lung regeneration after injury. It is, however, very challenging to study rare cell populations with potential but 'dormant' stem cell characteristics in healthy lungs.

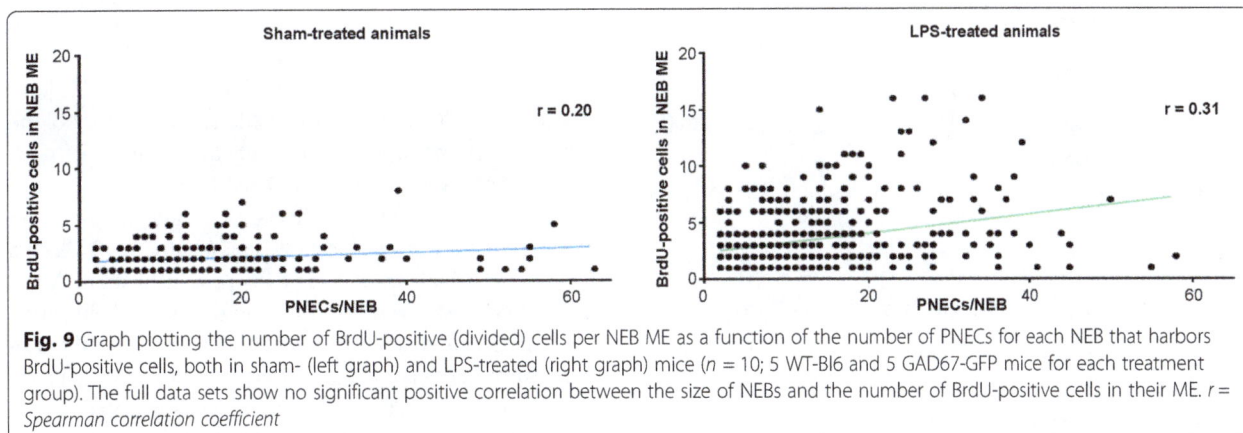

Fig. 9 Graph plotting the number of BrdU-positive (divided) cells per NEB ME as a function of the number of PNECs for each NEB that harbors BrdU-positive cells, both in sham- (left graph) and LPS-treated (right graph) mice (*n* = 10; 5 WT-Bl6 and 5 GAD67-GFP mice for each treatment group). The full data sets show no significant positive correlation between the size of NEBs and the number of BrdU-positive cells in their ME. *r* = *Spearman correlation coefficient*

Subject of the present study are poorly studied potential airway stem cells that are selectively located in the pulmonary NEB ME. We developed a highly reproducible and minimally invasive model for transient lung inflammation, based on a single low-dose intratracheal LPS instillation.

The bacterial endotoxin LPS is commonly used to induce a pulmonary inflammatory response because it is easy to administer and it tends to result in a reproducible lung injury (for review see [57]). According to literature data, intratracheal instillation with doses of 0.2 mg LPS/kg BW or less may be regarded as physiological [52], whereas 5 mg LPS/kg BW results in a moderate reversible lung injury [62, 63], which prompted us to apply 1 mg LPS/kg BW in the presented model.

Unrestrained whole-body plethysmography revealed that respiratory functions –selected parameters were Te, RT, EIP and TV– were compromised during the first two to six hours following a single low-dose LPS challenge, but also that these physiological parameters returned to the level of untreated control mice within 8 h after treatment.

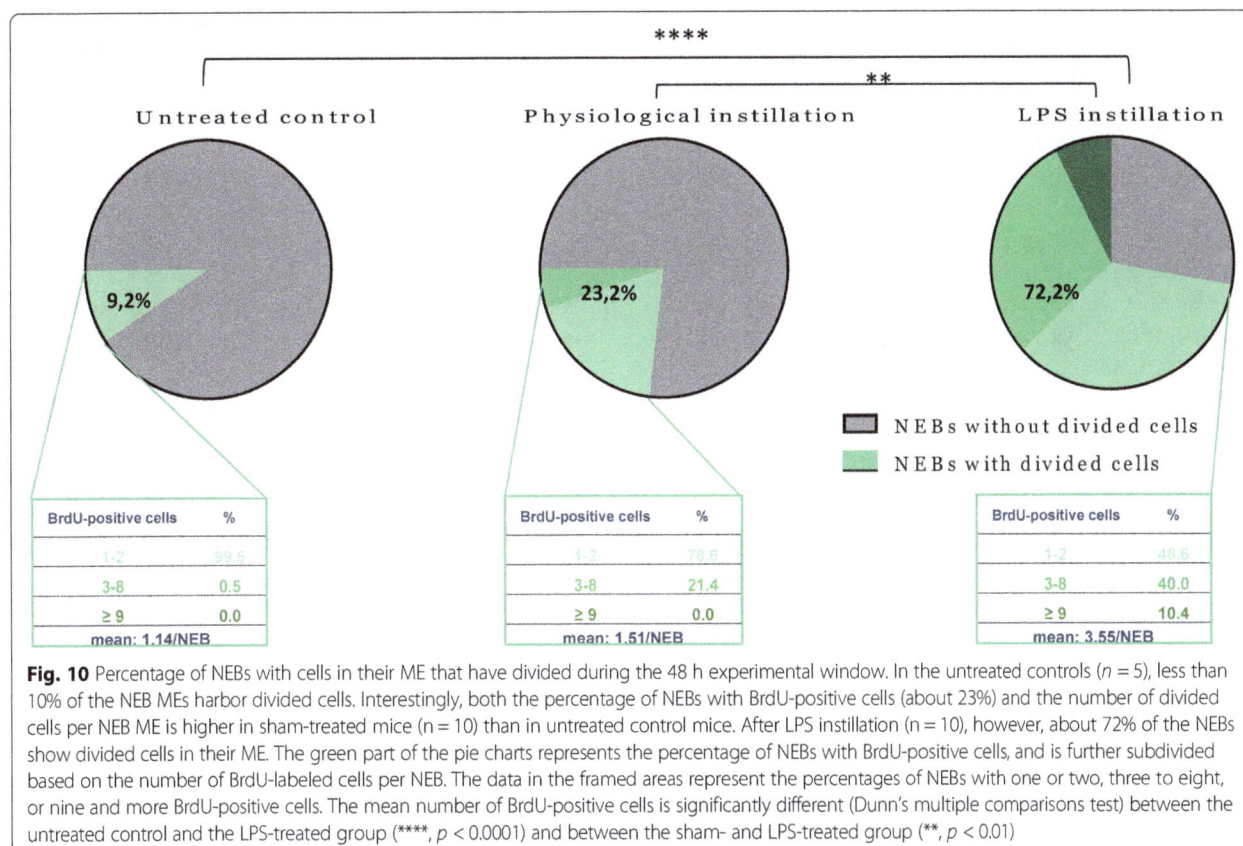

Fig. 10 Percentage of NEBs with cells in their ME that have divided during the 48 h experimental window. In the untreated controls (*n* = 5), less than 10% of the NEB MEs harbor divided cells. Interestingly, both the percentage of NEBs with BrdU-positive cells (about 23%) and the number of divided cells per NEB ME is higher in sham-treated mice (n = 10) than in untreated control mice. After LPS instillation (n = 10), however, about 72% of the NEBs show divided cells in their ME. The green part of the pie charts represents the percentage of NEBs with BrdU-positive cells, and is further subdivided based on the number of BrdU-labeled cells per NEB. The data in the framed areas represent the percentages of NEBs with one or two, three to eight, or nine and more BrdU-positive cells. The mean number of BrdU-positive cells is significantly different (Dunn's multiple comparisons test) between the untreated control and the LPS-treated group (****, *p* < 0.0001) and between the sham- and LPS-treated group (**, *p* < 0.01)

Table 3 Representation of the total number of BrdU-positive cells in the NEB ME

Untreated control					
Total number of BrdU+ cells	11	8	11	9	0
NEB ME with ≤2 BrdU+ cells	6	6	6	7	0
≥2 BrdU+ cells ≥9 BrdU+ cells	1 0	1 0	0 0	0 0	0 0
Sham-treated					
Total number of BrdU+ cells	16	61	54	21	15
NEB ME with ≤2 BrdU+ cells	10	21	25	10	9
≥2 BrdU+ cells ≥9 BrdU+ cells	0 0	9 0	4 0	1 0	0 0
LPS-treated					
Total number of BrdU+ cells	187	316	135	130	190
NEB ME with ≤2 BrdU+ cells	13	33	32	30	49
≥2 BrdU+ cells ≥9 BrdU+ cells	4 20	36 6	21 0	9 2	20 1

The table includes both the total numbers of BrdU-positive cells in the NEB ME per mouse (n = 5; GAD67-GFP mice) for each experimental group, and a separation of NEB MEs in different subgroups, i.e., NEB ME with 'mainly' single (two or less) BrdU-labeled cells and NEB ME with higher numbers of divided cells (three to eight, or nine and more)

Cytospin preparations of BALF, collected 16 h after LPS treatment, showed many neutrophils, indicative of an inflammatory reaction. This observation is in line with literature data showing that intratracheal LPS exposure resulted in a pulmonary infiltration of neutrophils as early as 4 h after challenge [51]. At the time point of evaluation of cell division, i.e., 48 h after LPS instillation, the morphology of the airway epithelium could not be distinguished from that in untreated control mice, as shown in H&E-stained lung cryostat sections.

It can be concluded that the intratracheal LPS challenge used in the present study does initiate an early influx of neutrophils, reminiscent of airway inflammation, but that the resulting injury is very mild and transient. The latter aspect is in contrast to the severe lung injury models that so far have been used in the majority of studies dealing with the activation of dedicated airway epithelial stem cell niches [44, 57], and will be discussed further on.

Cell-free BALF has been reported to harbor elevated cyto- and chemokine levels in the early phase (4 h–24 h hours) after intratracheal LPS instillation [52]. In the later phase (24-48 h post-instillation) these cytokine concentrations normalize, although the number of neutrophils remains elevated for at least 72 h [52].

To evaluate the potential effects of soluble mediators in BALF on healthy mouse airway epithelium, we collected BALF of LPS-challenged mice 16 h post-instillation. Acute short-term application of this BALF to the airway epithelium, and in particular to the NEB ME, in ex vivo lung slices of control mice in the course of LCI experiments, revealed a reversible and reproducible selective calcium-mediated activation of CLCs, but not of NEB cells, CCs or ciliated cells. Since administration of BALF of control mice (sham-treated and untreated), or of an LPS-containing solution, in our settings failed to mimic the activation of CLCs, it is reasonable to assume that one of the soluble inflammatory mediators released by activated macrophages and/or infiltrated neutrophils in the BALF may trigger the observed calcium-mediated activation of CLCs. So far, the identity of the molecule that is responsible for activation of the CLCs remains unknown and needs further investigation, which was not the focus of the present study.

Logically assuming that the NEB MEs in LPS-challenged mice are continuously exposed to bronchoalveolar lining fluid that harbors the same mediators as BALF, the presented study was designed to find out what could be the effect on CLCs as a potential quiescent stem cell population.

Mainly during fetal and early postnatal life, stem cell characteristics have been ascribed to CLCs [12, 30, 64–67]. Lineage-tracing models suggest that CLCs have the capacity to self-renew [12, 42]. Clara cell-like precursors appear to generate both Clara and ciliated cells during development and repair, driven by Notch signaling [45, 46], and have been suggested to contribute to homeostasis of the intrapulmonary airway epithelium [35, 42].

Full depletion of progenitor CCs and lineage tracing have resulted in the identification of a rare label-retaining

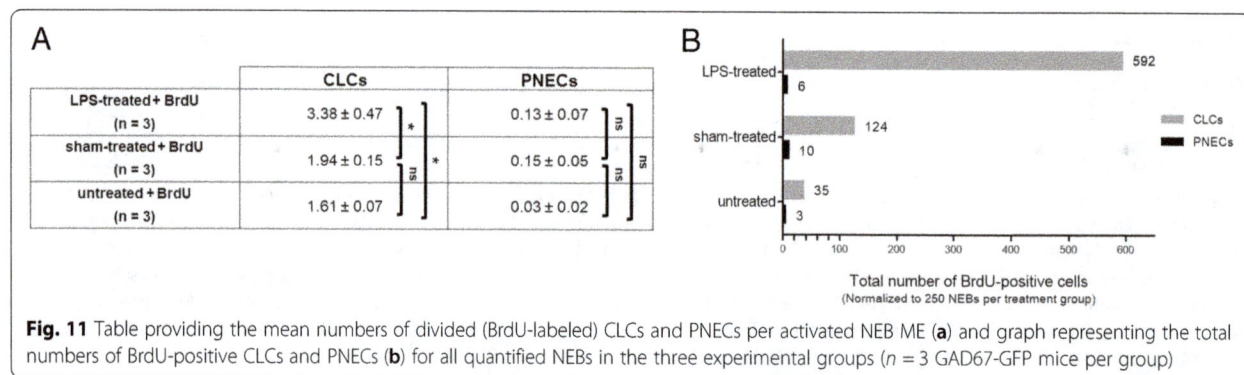

Fig. 11 Table providing the mean numbers of divided (BrdU-labeled) CLCs and PNECs per activated NEB ME (**a**) and graph representing the total numbers of BrdU-positive CLCs and PNECs (**b**) for all quantified NEBs in the three experimental groups (n = 3 GAD67-GFP mice per group)

and self-renewing subpopulation of CCs in the NEB ME [68], referred to as CLCs in the present study, which behave as airway epithelial stem cells and/or are critical for stem cell maintenance [12]. Both regeneration and tumor formation may be directed by CCs or at least subpopulations of CCs with progenitor or stem cell characteristics [50, 69–71].

Until now, it has been believed that severe injury is required to activate dedicated airway epithelial stem cell niches –such as the NEB ME– for repair, while replacement of epithelial cells after mild injury (including homeostasis) is thought to be managed by the large pool of general CCs [2]. Interestingly, we show here that mild injury under the right conditions definitely can result in the selective activation of silent CLCs in the NEB ME and not of general CCs.

Our observation (both from LCI and cell proliferation studies) of the activation of dedicated airway epithelial stem cells, in the apparent absence of damage, suggests that early mediators of the induced inflammation may be directly involved in activating the stem cells. This idea is supported by recent publications pointing out the emerging role of neutrophils in repair after lung injury, highlighting the essential contribution of neutrophils – which can transmigrate into the airspaces within minutes after the initial insult– in both early injury and repair (for review see [72]).

Incorporation of the thymidine analogue BrdU in DNA during the S-phase of cell division is a commonly used method to follow cell proliferation in a selected experimental time window [73, 74]. In the present study, BrdU incorporation for 48 h and subsequent BrdU immunostaining in cryostat sections, revealed that cell division was very rare in airway epithelium of untreated control mice, while a large number of BrdU-positive (divided) cells were present in the epithelium of small intestinal villi. These observations are in accordance with literature reports for rodents, with an estimated life time of about 4 days for enterocytes in the small intestine, whereas the turnover time of postnatal airway epithelium is more than 100 days [47]. Although some differences in proliferation of airway epithelial cells –probably due to health and pathogen status, strain and age of individual animals– have been reported (for review see [75]), cell division remains remarkably low in the absence of injury [4].

In our experimental setting, combined LPS challenge and BrdU incorporation resulted in a strongly enhanced proliferation of epithelial cells, the majority of which are typically grouped around NEB cells 48 h after LPS challenge. At that time point, the number of divided cells in the NEB ME was found to be 24.6 fold higher in LPS-treated mice than in untreated controls (256.3 vs. 10.4 BrdU-positive cells/100 NEBs), with some NEBs showing up to 24 divided cells in their ME niche. Quantification of the divided cells for each NEB ME and comparison between the LPS-treated and untreated control group showed that LPS challenge induced a highly significant proliferation of cells surrounding the NEBs, i.e., more than 72% of all counted NEBs harbored divided cells in their ME after 48 h as opposed to less than 10% in control mice. Double staining for CCSP, a marker for CCs and CLCs, as well as the location of the proliferated cell type were used to identify the majority of divided cells in the NEB ME as CLCs. The observation that CCSP-positive, BrdU-retaining CLCs were still found in the NEB ME 7 days after LPS challenge, in addition to the presence of CCSP-positive BrdU-labeled CCs dispersed in the airway epithelium surrounding NEBs, strongly implicates CLCs in the NEB ME as a population of self-renewing stem cells.

Although the adopted single low-dose intratracheal LPS challenge mouse model was shown to cause only mild and transient inflammation, it did induce a prominent selective proliferation of CLCs in the NEB ME.

No significant correlation was found between the size of NEBs (number of PNECs) and the number of BrdU-positive (divided) CLCs in the NEB ME following LPS challenge. The observed trend that larger NEBs harbored slightly more divided CLCs might simply be explained by the fact that the absolute number of CLCs is higher around large groups of PNECs.

In sham-treated mice (intratracheal instillation with saline), divided cells were also observed in an elevated percentage of NEBs (more than 23%), compared to untreated animals (less than 10%), but the total number of BrdU-positive cells was still limited compared to that observed following LPS challenge. Plethysmography showed that respiratory parameters did initially also change in sham-treated animals, but that they restored faster than in LPS-treated animals. Whereas BALF of untreated control mice harbored macrophages only, BALF of sham mice additionally contained neutrophils, but clearly less than BALF of LPS-instilled mice. Although the number of divided airway epithelial cells in sham-treated mice is small compared to that seen after LPS in our experiments, the preferential location of BrdU-labeled cells surrounding PNECs in the NEB ME is interestingly similar to the selective CLC proliferation seen after LPS treatment and suggestive of a joint mechanism of action, possibly involving early neutrophil mediators as discussed above.

Apart from CLCs (vCE cells), PNECs in the NEB ME have also been put forward as a cell type with potential airway epithelial stem cell characteristics [34, 35], although this hypothesis is still the subject of controversy.

The classic view that PNECs are terminally differentiated [76, 77], is challenged by the notion that repair of severe airway injury is associated with hyperplasia of PNECs [35]. Chemically or genetically induced full depletion of CCs revealed a typical proliferation of PNECs [36, 70]. Although at least subpopulations of PNEC-like progenitors are believed to give rise to CCs and even to alveolar epithelial cells during early development [30, 78, 79], most studies suggest that PNECs are not able to restore adult airway epithelium after ablation of all types of CCs [12]. Elimination of PNECs prior to CC depletion seems to have no apparent consequence for CC regeneration [34], but the same study reports that to some extent PNECs may contribute to CCs and ciliated cells following severe lung injury.

The presented data (LPS treatment; 48 h experimental window) show a very low number of divided PNECs in the NEB ME, which is not significantly different between LPS-challenged, sham and untreated control mice. In contrast to the well-illustrated proliferation of endocrine cells (PNECs) in addition to CLCs/vCE cells in several studies that are based on a full depletion of CCs [12, 35, 70], our LPS-based transient mild injury model for the selective proliferation of CLCs offers the important advantage that PNECs in the NEB ME are not affected by the procedure. The latter is in agreement with our observation that soluble mediators in BALF of LPS-challenged mice result in a calcium-mediated activation of CLCs but not of PNECs in the NEB ME in lung slices of control mice.

Certainly, PNECs can secrete regulatory factors –e.g. gastrin-releasing peptide (bombesin) and CGRP, potential epithelial cell mitogens [80]– that may support and regulate airway epithelial cell renewal/proliferation and differentiation. PNECs, however, are not only able to produce, store and secrete a variety of bioactive substances –some of which may directly influence CLCs [13]– but also to monitor calcium-mediated events in surrounding CLCs [14], and may therefore be involved in creating a niche to maintain the stem cell characteristics of CLCs.

Conclusion

Based on a single low-dose intratracheal LPS instillation, a highly reproducible and minimally invasive lung inflammation model was generated and validated for inducing selective activation of a quiescent airway stem cell population –the so-called CLCs/vCE cells– in the NEB ME.

Important advantages compared to earlier models, which were mainly based on full ablation of CCs, are the absence of both severe epithelial injury and additional proliferation of endocrine cells (PNECs).

The fact that CLCs in the NEB ME can be activated from a silent to a dividing stem cell population in the absence of severe airway epithelial damage creates new opportunities for unraveling the cellular mechanisms/

pathways regulating silencing, activation, proliferation and differentiation of this unique postnatal airway epithelial stem cell population.

The presented data are supportive of potentially important selective roles of the postnatal airway stem cell niche of the NEB ME, and enable the identification of pathways that should allow uncoupling of essential repair mechanisms from severe lung injury and inflammation.

Abbreviations

$[Ca^{2+}]_i$: Intracellular calcium concentration; $[K^+]_o$: Extracellular potassium concentration; 4-Di-2-ASP: 4-(4-diethylaminostyryl)-N-methylpyridinium iodide; BALF: Bronchoalveolar lavage fluid; BrdU: 5-bromo-2'-deoxyuridine; BSA: Bovine serum albumin; BW: Bodyweight; CAE: Control airway epithelium; CC: Clara cell; CCSP: Clara cell secretory protein; CGRP: Calcitonin gene-related peptide; CLC: Clara-like cell; DMEM-F-12: Dulbecco's modified Eagle's medium/F-12; EIP: End-inspiratory pause; GAD67: Glutamic acid decarboxylase 67; H&E: Hematoxylin and eosin; i.p.: Intraperitoneal; LCI: Live cell imaging; LMD: Laser microdissection; LPS: Lipopolysaccharide; Mc: Monoclonal; ME: Microenvironment; NEB ME: Neuroepithelial body microenvironment; NEB: Neuroepithelial body; PBS: Phosphate-buffered saline; Pc: Polyclonal; PD: Postnatal day; PF: Paraformaldehyde; PNEC: Pulmonary neuroendocrine cell; ROI: Region of interest; RT: Relaxation time; SCLC: Small cell lung carcinoma; SEM: Standard error of means; Te: Expiratory time; TV: Tidal volume; UP1: Urine protein 1; vCE: Variant CCSP-expressing; WT-Bl6: Wild type C57BL/6 J

Acknowledgements

The authors wish to thank Dominique De Rijck, Robrecht Lembrechts, Carmen Rottiers, Francis Terloo, Elien Theuns, Sofie Thys and Danny Vindevogel for their assistance.

Funding

This study was financially supported by a GOA BOF 2015 grant (No. 30729) of the University of Antwerp.

Authors' contributions

LV developed and carried out the experiments and prepared the manuscript. DA and IB designed the experiments, supervised the analysis and edited the manuscript. All authors regularly discussed the experiments and data, commented on the text, and read and approved the submitted manuscript.

Competing interests

The authors declare that they have no competing interests.

References

1.   Thurlbeck WM. Postnatal growth and development of the lung. Am Rev Respir Dis. 1975;111:803–44.

2. Giangreco A, Arwert EN, Rosewell IR, Snyder J, Watt FM, Stripp BR. Stem cells are dispensable for lung homeostasis but restore airways after injury. Proc Natl Acad Sci U S A. 2009;106:9286–91.

3. Bertoncello I, McQualter JL. Lung stem cells: do they exist? Respirology. 2013;18:587–95.

4. Stabler CT, Morrisey EE. Developmental pathways in lung regeneration. Cell Tissue Res. 2017;367:677–85.

5. Bishop AE. Pulmonary epithelial stem cells. Cell Prolif. 2004;37:89–96.

6. Rock JR, Hogan BL. Epithelial progenitor cells in lung development, maintenance, repair, and disease. Annu Rev Cell Dev Biol. 2011;27:493–512.

7. Adriaensen D, Scheuermann DW. Neuroendocrine cells and nerves of the lung. Anat Rec. 1993;236:70–86.

8. De Proost I, Pintelon I, Brouns I, Kroese AB, Riccardi D, Kemp PJ, Timmermans JP, Adriaensen D. Functional live cell imaging of the pulmonary neuroepithelial body microenvironment. Am J Respir Cell Mol Biol. 2008;39:180–9.

9. Brouns I, Pintelon I, Timmermans JP, Adriaensen D. Novel insights in the neurochemistry and function of pulmonary sensory receptors. Adv Anat Embryol Cell Biol. 2012;211:1–115.

10. Haller CJ. A scanning and transmission electron-microscopic study of the development of the surface-structure of neuroepithelial bodies in the mouse lung. Micron. 1994;25:527–38.

11. Stahlman MT, Gray ME. Ontogeny of neuroendocrine cells in human-fetal lung 1. An electron-microscopic study. Lab Investig. 1984;51:449–63.

12. Hong KU, Reynolds SD, Giangreco A, Hurley CM, Stripp BR. Clara cell secretory protein-expressing cells of the airway neuroepithelial body microenvironment include a label-retaining subset and are critical for epithelial renewal after progenitor cell depletion. Am J Respir Cell Mol Biol. 2001;24:671–81.

13. De Proost I, Pintelon I, Wilkinson WJ, Goethals S, Brouns I, Van Nassauw L, Riccardi D, Timmermans JP, Kemp PJ, Adriaensen D. Purinergic signaling in the pulmonary neuroepithelial body microenvironment unraveled by live cell imaging. FASEB J. 2009;23:1153–60.

14. Lembrechts R, Brouns I, Schnorbusch K, Pintelon I, Kemp PJ, Timmermans JP, Riccardi D, Adriaensen D. Functional expression of the multimodal extracellular calcium-sensing receptor in pulmonary neuroendocrine cells. J Cell Sci. 2013;126:4490–501.

15. Lembrechts R, Brouns I, Schnorbusch K, Pintelon I, Timmermans JP, Adriaensen D. Neuroepithelial bodies as mechanotransducers in the intrapulmonary airway epithelium: involvement of TRPC5. Am J Respir Cell Mol Biol. 2012;47:315–23.

16. Pan J, Yeger H, Cutz E. Innervation of pulmonary neuroendocrine cells and neuroepithelial bodies in developing rabbit lung. J Histochem Cytochem. 2004;52:379–89.

17. Cutz E, Chan W, Track NS. Bombesin, calcitonin and leu-enkephalin immunoreactivity in endocrine cells of human lung. Experientia. 1981;37:765–7.

18. Gallego R, Garcia-Caballero T, Roson E, Beiras A. Neuroendocrine cells of the human lung express substance-P-like immunoreactivity. Acta Anat (Basel). 1990;139:278–82.

19. Brouns I, Oztay F, Pintelon I, De Proost I, Lembrechts R, Timmermans JP, Adriaensen D. Neurochemical pattern of the complex innervation of neuroepithelial bodies in mouse lungs. Histochem Cell Biol. 2009;131:55–74.

20. Pan J, Copland I, Post M, Yeger H, Cutz E. Mechanical stretch-induced serotonin release from pulmonary neuroendocrine cells: implications for lung development. Am J Physiol Lung Cell Mol Physiol. 2006;290:L185–93.

21. Adriaensen D, Brouns I, Van Genechten J, Timmermans JP. Functional morphology of pulmonary neuroepithelial bodies: extremely complex airway receptors. Anat Rec. 2003;270:25–40.

22. Linnoila RI. Functional facets of the pulmonary neuroendocrine system. Lab Investig. 2006;86:425–44.

23. Cutz E, Jackson A. Neuroepithelial bodies as airway oxygen sensors. Respir Physiol. 1999;115:201–14.

24. Cutz E, Yeger H, Pan J, Ito T. Pulmonary neuroendocrine cell system in health and disease. Curr Respir Med Rev. 2008;4:174–86.

25. Sorokin SP, Hoyt RF. On the supposed function of neuroepithelial bodies in adult mammalian lungs. News Physiol Sci. 1990;5:89–95.

26. Sorokin SP, Hoyt RF Jr, Shaffer MJ. Ontogeny of neuroepithelial bodies: correlations with mitogenesis and innervation. Microsc Res Tech. 1997;37:43–61.

27. Van Lommel A. Pulmonary neuroendocrine cells (PNEC) and neuroepithelial bodies (NEB): chemoreceptors and regulators of lung development. Paediatr Respir Rev. 2001;2:171–6.

28. Hoyt RF, Sorokin SP, Mcdowell EM, Mcnelly NA. Neuroepithelial bodies and growth of the airway epithelium in developing hamster lung. Anat Rec. 1993;236:15–24.

29. Li F, He J, Wei J, Cho WC, Liu X. Diversity of epithelial stem cell types in adult lung. Stem Cells Int. 2015;2015:728307.

30. Guha A, Vasconcelos M, Cai Y, Yoneda M, Hinds A, Qian J, Li G, Dickel L, Johnson JE, Kimura S, et al. Neuroepithelial body microenvironment is a niche for a distinct subset of Clara-like precursors in the developing airways. Proc Natl Acad Sci U S A. 2012;109:12592–7.

31. Rawlins EL, Okubo T, Que J, Xue Y, Clark C, Luo X, Hogan BL. Epithelial stem/progenitor cells in lung postnatal growth, maintenance and repair. Cold Spring Harb Symp Quant Biol. 2008;73:291–5.

32. Asselin-Labat ML, Filby CE. Adult lung stem cells and their contribution to lung tumourigenesis. Open Biol. 2012;2:120094.

33. Verckist L, Lembrechts R, Thys S, Pintelon I, Timmermans JP, Brouns I, Adriaensen D. Selective gene expression analysis of the neuroepithelial body microenvironment in postnatal lungs with special interest for potential stem cell characteristics. Respir Res. 2017;18:87.

34. Song H, Yao E, Lin C, Gacayan R, Chen MH, Chuang PT. Functional characterization of pulmonary neuroendocrine cells in lung development, injury, and tumorigenesis. Proc Natl Acad Sci U S A. 2012;109:17531–6.

35. Reynolds SD, Giangreco A, Power JHT, Stripp BR. Neuroepithelial bodies of pulmonary airways serve as a reservoir of progenitor cells capable of epithelial regeneration. Am J Pathol. 2000;156:269–78.

36. Peake JL, Reynolds SD, Stripp BR, Stephens KE, Pinkerton KE. Alteration of pulmonary neuroendocrine cells during epithelial repair of naphthalene-induced airway injury. Am J Pathol. 2000;156:279–86.

37. Giangreco A, Reynolds SD, Stripp BR. Terminal bronchioles harbor a unique airway stem cell population that localizes to the bronchoalveolar duct junction. Am J Pathol. 2002;161:173–82.

38. Davies SJ, Gosney JR, Hansell DM, Wells AU, du Bois RM, Burke MM, Sheppard MN, Nicholson AG. Diffuse idiopathic pulmonary neuroendocrine cell hyperplasia: an under-recognised spectrum of disease. Thorax. 2007;62:248–52.

39. Pan J, Yeger H, Ratcliffe P, Bishop T, Cutz E. Hyperplasia of pulmonary neuroendocrine bodies (NEB) in lungs of prolyl hydroxylase −1(PHD-1) deficient mice. Adv Exp Med Biol. 2012;758:149–55.

40. Naizhen X, Linnoila RI, Kimura S. Co-expression of Achaete-Scute Homologue-1 and calcitonin gene-related peptide during NNK-induced pulmonary neuroendocrine hyperplasia and carcinogenesis in hamsters. J Cancer. 2016;7:2124–31.

41. Sutherland KD, Proost N, Brouns I, Adriaensen D, Song JY, Berns A. Cell of origin of small cell lung cancer: inactivation of Trp53 and Rb1 in distinct cell types of adult mouse lung. Cancer Cell. 2011;19:754–64.

42. Rawlins EL, Okubo T, Xue Y, Brass DM, Auten RL, Hasegawa H, Wang F, Hogan BL. The role of Scgb1a1+ Clara cells in the long-term maintenance and repair of lung airway, but not alveolar, epithelium. Cell Stem Cell. 2009; 4:525–34.

43. Guha A, Deshpande A, Jain A, Sebastiani P, Cardoso WV. Uroplakin 3a+ cells are a distinctive population of epithelial progenitors that contribute to airway maintenance and post-injury repair. Cell Rep. 2017;19:246–54.

44. Vaughan AE, Chapman HA. Regenerative activity of the lung after epithelial injury. Biochim Biophys Acta. 2013;1832:922–30.

45. Xing Y, Li A, Borok Z, Li C, Minoo P. NOTCH1 is required for regeneration of Clara cells during repair of airway injury. Stem Cells. 2012;30:946–55.

46. Collins BJ, Kleeberger W, Ball DW. Notch in lung development and lung cancer. Semin Cancer Biol. 2004;14:357–64.

47. Blenkinsopp WK. Proliferation of respiratory tract epithelium in the rat. Exp Cell Res. 1967;46:144–54.

48. Wansleeben C, Barkauskas CE, Rock JR, Hogan BL. Stem cells of the adult lung: their development and role in homeostasis, regeneration, and disease. Wiley Interdiscip Rev Dev Biol. 2013;2:131–48.

49. Lynch TJ, Engelhardt JF. Progenitor cells in proximal airway epithelial development and regeneration. Cell Biochem. 2014;115:1637–45.

50. Stripp BR, Maxson K, Mera R, Singh G. Plasticity of airway cell proliferation and gene expression after acute naphthalene injury. Am J Phys. 1995;269: L791–9.

51. Starcher B, Williams I. A method for intratracheal instillation of endotoxin into the lungs of mice. Lab Anim. 1989;23:234–40.

52. Vernooy JHJD, Dentener MA, van Suylen RJ, Buurman WA, Wouters EFM. Intratracheal instillation of lipopolysaccharide in mice induces apoptosis in bronchial epithelial cells. Am J Respir Cell Mol Biol. 2001;24:569–76.

53. Zhang Y, Xu T, Pan Z, Ge X, Sun C, Lu C, Chen H, Xiao Z, Zhang B, Dai Y, Liang G. Shikonin inhibits myeloid differentiation protein 2 to prevent LPS-induced acute lung injury. Br J Pharmacol. 2018;175:840–54.

54. Nelson AJ, Roy SK, Warren K, Janike K, Thiele GM, Mikuls TR, Romberger DJ, Wang D, Swanson B, Poole JA. Sex differences impact the lung-bone inflammatory response to repetitive inhalant lipopolysaccharide exposures in mice. J Immunotoxicol. 2018;15:73–81.

55. Fodor RS, Georgescu AM, Cioc AD, Grigorescu BL, Cotoi OS, Fodor P, Copotoiu SM, Azamfirei L. Time- and dose-dependent severity of lung injury in a rat model of sepsis. Romanian J Morphol Embryol. 2015;56:1329–37.

56. Alm AS, Li K, Chen H, Wang D, Andersson R, Wang X. Variation of lipopolysaccharide-induced acute lung injury in eight strains of mice. Respir Physiol Neurobiol. 2010;171:157–64.

57. Matute-Bello G, Frevert CW, Martin TR. Animal models of acute lung injury. Am J Physiol Lung Cell Mol Physiol. 2008;295:L379–99.

58. Schnorbusch K, Lembrechts R, Pintelon I, Timmermans JP, Brouns I, Adriaensen D. GABAergic signaling in the pulmonary neuroepithelial body microenvironment: functional imaging in GAD67-GFP mice. Histochem Cell Biol. 2013;140:549–66.

59. Stapleton CM, Jaradat M, Dixon D, Kang HS, Kim SC, Liao G, Carey MA, Cristiano J, Moorman MP, Jetten AM. Enhanced susceptibility of staggerer (RORalphasg/sg) mice to lipopolysaccharide-induced lung inflammation. Am J Physiol Lung Cell Mol Physiol. 2005;289:L144–52.

60. Pintelon I, De Proost I, Brouns I, Van Herck H, Van Genechten J, Van Meir F, Timmermans JP, Adriaensen D. Selective visualisation of neuroepithelial bodies in vibratome slices of living lung by 4-Di-2-ASP in various animal species. Cell Tissue Res. 2005;321:21–33.

61. Matute-Bello G, Downey G, Moore BB, Groshong SD, Matthay MA, Slutsky AS, Kuebler WM. Acute lung injury in animals study G: an official American Thoracic Society workshop report: features and measurements of experimental acute lung injury in animals. Am J Respir Cell Mol Biol. 2011;44:725–38.

62. Chang YW, Tseng CP, Lee CH, Hwang TL, Chen YL, Su MT, Chong KY, Lan YW, Wu CC, Chen KJ, et al. Beta-Nitrostyrene derivatives attenuate LPS-mediated acute lung injury via the inhibition of neutrophil-platelet interactions and NET release. Am J Physiol Lung Cell Mol Physiol. 2018;314:L654–69.

63. Jiang Z, Chen Z, Li L, Zhou W, Zhu L. Lack of SOCS3 increases LPS-induced murine acute lung injury through modulation of Ly6C(+) macrophages. Respir Res. 2017;18:217.

64. Snyder JC, Teisanu RM, Stripp BR. Endogenous lung stem cells and contribution to disease. J Pathol. 2009;217:254–64.

65. Roomans GM. Tissue engineering and the use of stem/progenitor cells for airway epithelium repair. Eur Cell Mater. 2010;19:284–99.

66. Kratz JR, Yagui-Beltran A, Jablons DM. Cancer stem cells in lung tumorigenesis. Ann Thorac Surg. 2010;89:S2090–5.

67. Sullivan JP, Minna JD, Shay JW. Evidence for self-renewing lung cancer stem cells and their implications in tumor initiation, progression, and targeted therapy. Cancer Metastasis Rev. 2010;29:61–72.

68. Reynolds SD, Malkinson AM. Clara cell: progenitor for the bronchiolar epithelium. Int J Biochem Cell Biol. 2010;42:1–4.

69. Plopper CG, Suverkropp C, Morin D, Nishio S, Buckpitt A. Relationship of cytochrome-P-450 activity to Clara cell cytotoxicity. 1. Histopathologic comparison of the respiratory-tract of mice, rats and hamsters after parenteral administration of naphthalene. J Pharmacol Exp Ther. 1992;261:353–63.

70. Reynolds SD, Hong KU, Giangreco A, Mango GW, Guron C, Morimoto Y, Stripp BR. Conditional Clara cell ablation reveals a self-renewing progenitor function of pulmonary neuroendocrine cells. Am J Physiol Lung Cell Mol Physiol. 2000;278:1256–63.

71. Crosby LM, Waters CM. Epithelial repair mechanisms in the lung. Am J Physiol Lung Cell Mol Physiol. 2010;298:L715–31.

72. Blazquez-Prieto J, Lopez-Alonso I, Huidobro C, Albaiceta GM. The emerging role of neutrophils in repair after acute lung injury. Am J Respir Cell Mol Biol. 2018;59:289–94.

73. Taupin P. BrdU immunohistochemistry for studying adult neurogenesis: paradigms, pitfalls, limitations, and validation. Brain Res Rev. 2007;53:198–214.

74. Kameyama H, Kudoh S, Udaka N, Kagayama M, Hassan W, Hasegawa K, Niimori-Kita K, Ito T. BrdU label retaining cells in mouse terminal bronchioles. Histol Histopathol. 2014;29:659–68.

75. Rawlins EL, Hogan BL. Epithelial stem cells of the lung: privileged few or opportunities for many? Development. 2006;133:2455–65.

76. Gosney JR. Pulmonary neuroendocrine cell system in pediatric and adult lung disease. Microsc Res Tech. 1997;37:107–13.

77. Hoyt RF Jr, McNelly NA, Sorokin SP. Dynamics of neuroepithelial body (NEB) formation in developing hamster lung: light microscopic autoradiography after 3H-thymidine labeling in vivo. Anat Rec. 1990;227:340–50.

78. Li Y, Linnoila RI. Multidirectional differentiation of Achaete-Scute homologue-1-defined progenitors in lung development and injury repair. Am J Respir Cell Mol Biol. 2012;47:768–75.

79. Khoor A, Gray ME, Singh G, Stahlman MT. Ontogeny of Clara cell-specific protein and its mRNA: their association with neuroepithelial bodies in human fetal lung and in bronchopulmonary dysplasia. J Histochem Cytochem. 1996;44:1429–38.

80. Cutz E, Yeger H, Pan J. Pulmonary neuroendocrine cell system in pediatric lung disease-recent advances. Pediatr Dev Pathol. 2007;10:419–35.

cGMP interacts with tropomyosin and downregulates actin-tropomyosin-myosin complex interaction

Lihui Zou[1†], Junhua Zhang[1†], Jingli Han[1], Wenqing Li[1], Fei Su[2], Xiaomao Xu[3], Zhenguo Zhai[4*] and Fei Xiao[1*]

Abstract

Background: The nitric oxide-soluble guanylate cyclase-cyclic guanosine monophosphate (NO-sGC-cGMP) signaling pathway, plays a critical role in the pathogenesis of pulmonary arterial hypertension (PAH); however, its exact molecular mechanism remains undefined.

Methods: Biotin-cGMP pull-down assay was performed to search for proteins regulated by cGMP. The interaction between cGMP and tropomyosin was analyzed with antibody dependent pull-down in vivo. Tropomyosin fragments were constructed to explore the tropomyosin-cGMP binding sites. The expression level and subcellular localization of tropomyosin were detected with Real-time PCR, Western blot and immunofluorescence assay after the 8-Br-cGMP treatment. Finally, isothermal titration calorimetry (ITC) was utilized to detect the binding affinity of actin-tropomyosin-myosin in the existence of cGMP-tropomyosin interaction.

Results: cGMP interacted with tropomyosin. Isoform 4 of *TPM1* gene was identified as the only isoform expressed in the human pulmonary artery smooth muscle cells (HPASMCs). The region of 68-208aa of tropomyosin was necessary for the interaction between tropomyosin and cGMP. The expression level and subcellular localization of tropomyosin showed no change after the stimulation of NO-sGC-cGMP pathway. However, cGMP-tropomyosin interaction decreased the affinity of tropomyosin to actin.

Conclusions: We elucidate the downstream signal pathway of NO-sGC-cGMP. This work will contribute to the detection of innovative targeted agents and provide novel insights into the development of new therapies for PAH.

Keywords: Cyclic guanosine monophosphate, Tropomyosin, Actin, Myosin, Interaction

Background

PAH is a serious yet poorly understood disease characterized by elevated pulmonary artery pressure and vascular resistance and may ultimately result in right heart failure and death. The burden of small pulmonary arteries increases due to the contraction of vascular smooth muscle cells, which plays a crucial role in regulating of pulmonary vascular resistance and in the development of PAH [1]. However, the regulatory mechanism of the contraction of intrapulmonary arteries is poorly understood, and further investigations, especially those on molecular biomarkers, are essential for decoding the underlying pathogenic mechanism of PAH.

The NO-sGC-cGMP pathway is closely associated with PAH. cGMP exerts its biological activity mainly via three main groups of down-stream targets: cGMP-dependent protein kinases, cGMP-gated cation channels, and phosphodiesterases. Malfunctions in NO production, sGC activity, and cGMP degradation cause pulmonary arterial vasodilatation through abnormal vascular smooth muscle cell proliferation and platelet aggregation [2].

Our previous study found that the activation of NO-sGC-cGMP pathway led to abnormal expression of multiple genes including SERPINB2, MMP1, GREM1, and IL8 [3]. We have demonstrated that SERPINB2, also known as PAI-2, suppresses the proliferation and

* Correspondence: zhaizhenguo2011@126.com; xiaofei3965@bjhmoh.cn
[†]Lihui Zou and Junhua Zhang contributed equally to this work.
[4]Department of Respiratory and Critical Care Medicine, China-Japan Friendship Hospital, Beijing 100029, People's Republic of China
[1]The MOH Key Laboratory of Geriatrics, Beijing Hospital, National Center of Gerontology, Beijing 100730, People's Republic of China
Full list of author information is available at the end of the article

migration of cultured HPASMCs and speeds their apoptosis [4]. The mRNA level of PAI-2 in peripheral blood cells of PAH patients was significantly decreased and the expression of PAI-2 was up-regulated by sGC activator. PAI-2 can be used as a potential biomarker for vascular remodeling of PAH [5]. MMP1 encodes matrix metalloprotease-1, a member of the matrix metalloprotease (MMP) family, which are the major proteases involved in tissue remodelling of the extracellular matrix by degrading all types of matrix components. Therefore, NO-sGC-cGMP pathway may assuage or reverse the vascular remodeling in PAH by regulating genes including PAI-2 and MMP1.

However, besides these downstream-regulated genes, little is known about the interaction proteins of cGMP. As a second messenger in cells, cGMP hardly acts as isolated species while performing its functions in vivo. In our current study, we performed the Biotin-cGMP pull-down assay to search for the proteins interacted and regulated by cGMP with a human pulmonary artery smooth muscle cell line. Fortunately, we found that cGMP interacted with tropomyosin, a key factor that regulates smooth muscle contraction. Tropomyosin regulated the productive interaction between myosins and actin by shifting its position on the actin filament. The isothermal titration calorimetry (ITC) assay was then utilized to explore the fast actin-tropomyosin-myosin complex alteration after the activation of NO-sGC-cGMP pathway. We demonstrated that actin-tropomyosin-myosin interaction was downregulated in the existence of cGMP-tropomyosin interaction competition and caused the down-regulation of muscle contraction. All these findings demonstrate the functional interaction between cGMP and tropomyosin, which is involved in the regulation of muscle contraction.

Methods
Cell culture and treatment
HPASMCs (ScienCell Research Laboratories, Carlsbad, USA), identified by immuefluorescent antibodies to α-smooth muscle actin and desmin, were isolated from human pulmonary arteries [6]. Smooth muscle cell medium (ScienCell Research Laboratories, Carlsbad, USA) supplemented with 2% fetal bovine serum and 1% smooth muscle cell growth supplement was utilized. HPASMCs were then maintained at 37 °C humidified atmosphere of 5% carbondioxide. P3 ~ P5 cells were used for experiments. The exponentially growing HPASMCs were treated with 100 μM of 8-Br-cGMP (Sigma–Aldrich Corp., St. Louis, USA) for 24 h.

Biotin-cGMP pull-down assay
10 μM of Biotin-cGMP and the negative control Biotin (Biolog life science institute, Bremen, Germany) were nurtured in a mix of whole HPASMC cell lysates at 4 °C

for 6 h with gentle rotation. Biotin-cGMP fusion protein and Biotin protein were then attached to 100 μl of streptavidin magnetic beads at 4 °C for 6 h. After being gently washed by lysis buffer for 3–5 times gently to reduce nonspecific binding, beads were incubated with 50 μl of glycine elution buffer (100 mM, PH 2.5) for 10 min. Then, 10 μl of NH_4HCO_3 neutralization buffer was added to each elution collection tube to neutralize the pH of the contents upon elution. The elution fractions were boiled in sodium dodecyl sulphate-polyacrylamide gel electrophoresis (SDS–PAGE) loading buffer and analyzed by silver staining method or immune blotting analysis. After having been excised, protein bands were subjected to in-gel trypsin digestion and analysed by mass spectrometry.

RNA extraction, reverse transcription, and real-time PCR
Total RNAs were extracted from HPASMCs with Trizol reagent (Invitrogen Life Technologies, Carlsberg, USA), following the manufacturer's protocol (Invitrogen). The reverse transcription was performed with the total RNAs (2 μg) and the Moloney Murine Leukemia Virus reverse transcription kit (Invitrogen Life Technologies, Carlsberg, USA).

Real-time PCR was performed to quantify *TPM1* gene, and expression of the internal control gene *ACTIN* was determined by iQ5 Multicolor Real-time PCR Detection System (Bio-Rad Laboratories, Hercules, CA, USA). The PCR reaction used 9.9 μl of distilled water, 12.5 μl of 2X SYBR® Premix Ex TaqTMII, 0.8 μl each for primers, and 1 μl of DNA template, constructing a total volume of 25 μl. The two-step PCR protocol was performed using SYBR® Premix Ex TaqTM II (Takara Biotech Co., Dalian, China) following the manufacturer's instruction. It included one cycle of 95 °C for 30 s, 40 cycles of 95 °C for 5 s, and 60 °C for 30 s. Each reaction was run in triplicate. The Ct values for relative quantification of gene expression were used to determine the *TPM1* expression levels. The PCR primers for *TPM1* were as follows: 5'-GCTG CAGAGGATAAGTACTC-3' (forward), 5'-CATGTTGT TTAACTCCAGT-3' (reverse); *β-ACTIN* 5'-GGCGGCA CCACCATGTACCCT-3' (forward), 5'-AGGGGCCGGA CTCGTCATACT -3' (reverse). The PCR primers for *TPM1* gene isoforms were as follows: Primer 1: 5'- CGGT CGCCCCCTTGGGAAAG -3' (forward), 5'- GCTTGTC GGAAAGGACCTTGATCTC -3' (reverse); Primer 2: 5'- AGTGAGAGAGGCATGAAAGTC -3' (forward), 5'- A ATTTAGTTACTGACCTCTCCGCA -3' (reverse); Primer 3: 5'- CGGGCTGAGTTTGCGGAGAGG -3' (forward), 5'- AAGGAATGGAAGTCTCGGAAGA -3' (reverse).

Protein isolation and Western blot
Cells were collected and rinsed with PBS solution, and the protein was extracted by using the protein lysis buffer (including 1% NP-40, 1 μg/ml aprotinin, 1 μg/ml

leupeptin, and 100 μg/ml PMSF). The protein concentration was assessed with a Bio-Rad DC Protein Assay (Bio-Rad, Hercules, USA). Then, 50 μg of proteins were used for sodium dodecyl sulphate-polyacrylamide gel electrophoresis. Subsequently, the proteins were transferred to nitrocellulose membranes by electro blotting (Millipore Corp., Boston, USA). Membranes were blocked in 5% milk, washed with PBST (PBS with 0.1% Tween), and incubated with 1:1000 anti-tropomyosin antibody (cell signaling technology, Danvers, USA) at 4 °C for 12 h and 0.4 μg/ml anti-actin antibody (ZSBIO, Beijing, China) at 4 °C for 1 h. After the washing and incubation with 0.08 μg/ml horseradish peroxidase-conjugated anti-IgG antibody (ZSBIO, Beijing, China) at 4 °C for 1 h in 5% milk, the membranes were washed for three times and subjected to the enhanced chemiluminescent reagents (Millipore Corp., Boston, USA) for the distinction of protein bands.

Immunofluorescence assay
Cells were grown and treated with 8-Br-cGMP on cover slips. Cultured cells were affixed with methanol at room temperature for 20 min. After being washed with PBS

for three times, cover slips were blocked for 60 min in BSA blocking buffer, then incubated with diluted primary antibody at room temperature for 2 h. Cells were rinsed in PBS three times (for 5 min each), then incubated with diluted fluorochrome-conjugated secondary antibody (ZSBIO, Beijing, China) at room temperature for 1 h in dark. After stained with DAPI and stored with mounting medium, the samples were examined under confocal microscope.

Isothermal titration calorimetry assay
Interaction analysis among actin, myosin, and tropomyosin were performed at 298 K (degree kelvin) with a MicroCal Isothermal Titration Calorimeter ITC200 instrument (Malvern, England). The investigations were performed according to a strictly standardized protocol [7–9]. The highly purified proteins were prepared by Sephadex G-50 column with automated protein separation chromatography system (Jinhua Inc., Shanghai, China). Typically, the syringe was filled with 60 μL of protein solution at a concentration of 0.05 μM that subsequently titrated into a 300 μL protein with the concentration of 0.005 μM in the cell. There were twenty

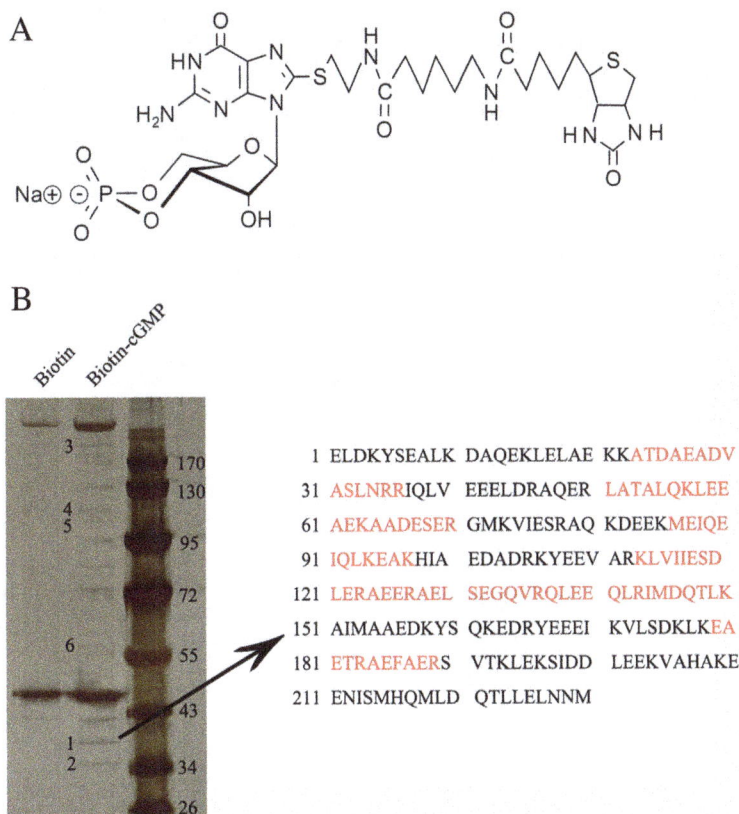

Fig. 1 cGMP directly interacts with tropomyosin. (**a**) The chemical structural formula of 8-[Biotin]-AET-cGMP. Biotin is connected to the 8-position of cyclic GMP via a 11 atom spacer. (**b**) Characterization of interaction proteins with cGMP in vitro. Cell extractions from HPASMCs were pulled down with the biotin-cGMP, subjected to SDS–PAGE and visualized by silver staining. The bands associated with cGMP were pointed out by the numbers (bands 1–6) and identified by mass spectrometry. The peptides of the band 1 belong to tropomyosin are indicated by red letters

injections of 2 μL each with a spacing of 120 s between injections employed to allow the system to reach the equilibrium. Heat generated by titrant dilution was tested by a control experiment, titrating into buffer alone, in uniform arragements. On the basis of a self-sufficient binding sites model, the MicroCal-Origin 7.0 software was applied to fit the integrated heat data of the titrations by a non-linear least-squares minimization algorithm.

The fitting parameters were ΔH (reaction enthalpy change in cal mol^{-1}), ΔS (the changes in entropyin cal mol^{-1}), K (the inverse of equilibrium binding constant in M^{-1}), and N (molar ratio of the proteins in the complex). Δ H value is equal to the constant pressure heat of reaction. The positive value of Δ H means heat absorption and the negative value represents heat release. Entropy is a measure of system disorder. ΔS associates with the change in the amount of substance before and after reaction in the system.Gibbs free energy (ΔG) had a relationship with ΔH that was ΔG = ΔH-TΔS = -RTlnKa ($R = 8.314$ J mol^{-1} K^{-1}, $T = 298.15$ K), which was applied to calculate the reaction energy eventually. All the ΔG obtained by calculation testified the spontaneous reactions in our experiments.

Statistical analysis

All data attained in triplicate independent experiments were assessed via SPSS statistics 20.0 and GraphPad prism 5 (GraphPad software, Inc., La Jolla, USA). Data are showed as mean ± SD. Statistical comparisons were carried out with the student t test for investigating two-group data. A P value of < 0.05 was considered statistically significant

Results

cGMP directly interacted with tropomyosin

Biotin-cGMP is a cGMP analog that has similar properties with cGMP (Fig. 1a). The bands characteristic to cGMP are presented in Fig. 1b. Compared with the negative control biotin, six bands were uniquely associated with cGMP (line 2). The protein bands associated with cGMP were then extracted, digested with trypsin and analysed by mass spectrometry. The result showed that 5 peptides of the band 1 belonged to the protein tropomyosin, which was involved in the regulatory system of actin-myosin interaction. The other bands corresponded to the protein keratin and some uncharacterized proteins with protein scores less than 66, suggesting the observed match was a random event.

Isoform 4 was expressed in the HPASMCs

In order to determine which isoform was expressed in the HPASMCs, we performed three PCR using primers designed on the basis of the three difference sequences (Fig. 2). The products of PCR were cloned into pGEM®-T expression vector and sequenced, which was found to be in full compliance with isoform 4. The partial base sequences were shown in Fig. 2. The sequencing results also

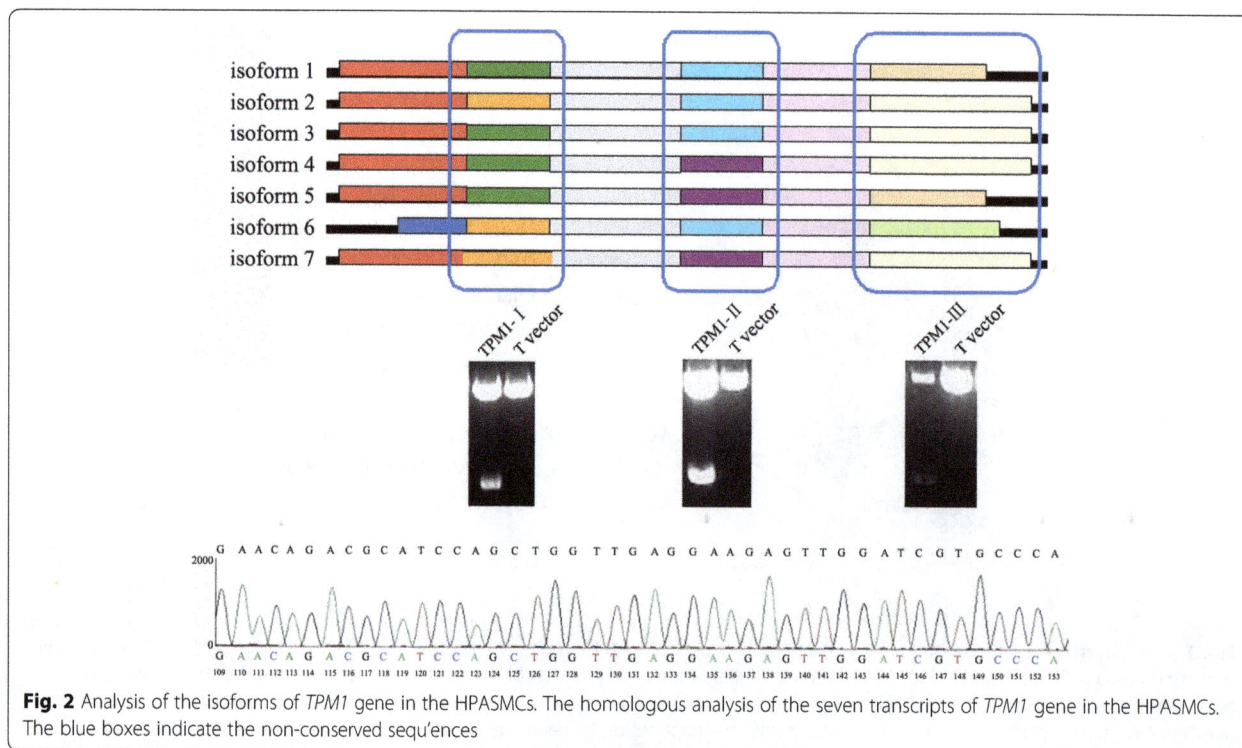

Fig. 2 Analysis of the isoforms of *TPM1* gene in the HPASMCs. The homologous analysis of the seven transcripts of *TPM1* gene in the HPASMCs. The blue boxes indicate the non-conserved sequ'ences

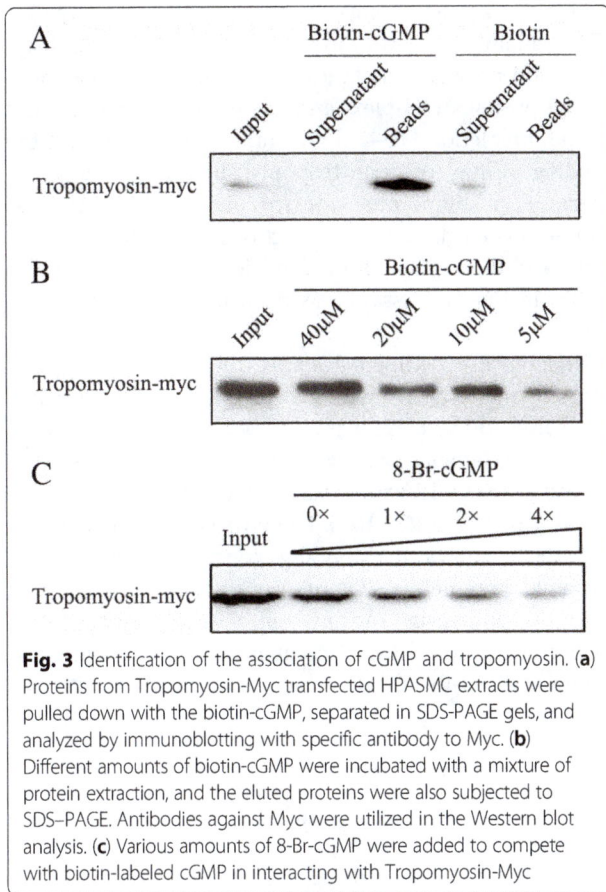

Fig. 3 Identification of the association of cGMP and tropomyosin. (**a**) Proteins from Tropomyosin-Myc transfected HPASMC extracts were pulled down with the biotin-cGMP, separated in SDS-PAGE gels, and analyzed by immunoblotting with specific antibody to Myc. (**b**) Different amounts of biotin-cGMP were incubated with a mixture of protein extraction, and the eluted proteins were also subjected to SDS–PAGE. Antibodies against Myc were utilized in the Western blot analysis. (**c**) Various amounts of 8-Br-cGMP were added to compete with biotin-labeled cGMP in interacting with Tropomyosin-Myc

indicated that isoform 4 was the only isoform expressed in the HPASMCs.

cGMP specifically bound to tropomyosin

To further confirm the interaction between cGMP and tropomyosin in vivo, antibody dependent pull-down was performed. Isoform 4 of *TPM1* gene was amplified and cloned into pcDNA3.1(–)-cMyc vector, then transfected into cultured HPASMCs. The biotinylated cGMP and the biotin alone were both incubated with HPASMC cell lysates. Tropomyosin-Myc was validated with antibody against Myc in the biotin-cGMP pull-down protein complexes, but not in the biotin pull-down protein complexes (Fig. 3a). Meanwhile, the interaction between cGMP and tropomyosin was alterable in the existence of different amounts of biotin-cGMP (Fig. 3b). Furthermore, competition assay was performed to detect the specificity of cGMP and tropomyosin interaction. The interaction between cGMP and tropomyosin was competed by 8-Br-cGMP (non-biotinylated cGMP) in a dose-related manner (Fig. 3c).

Region of 68-208aa was necessary for the interaction between tropomyosin and cGMP

To explore the binding sites of tropomyosin interacted with cGMP, tropomyosin fragments (aa 1–284, aa 68–284, aa 142–284, aa 209–284, aa 1–208, aa 1–141, and aa 1–67, respectively named as wild type, N-mutation 1,

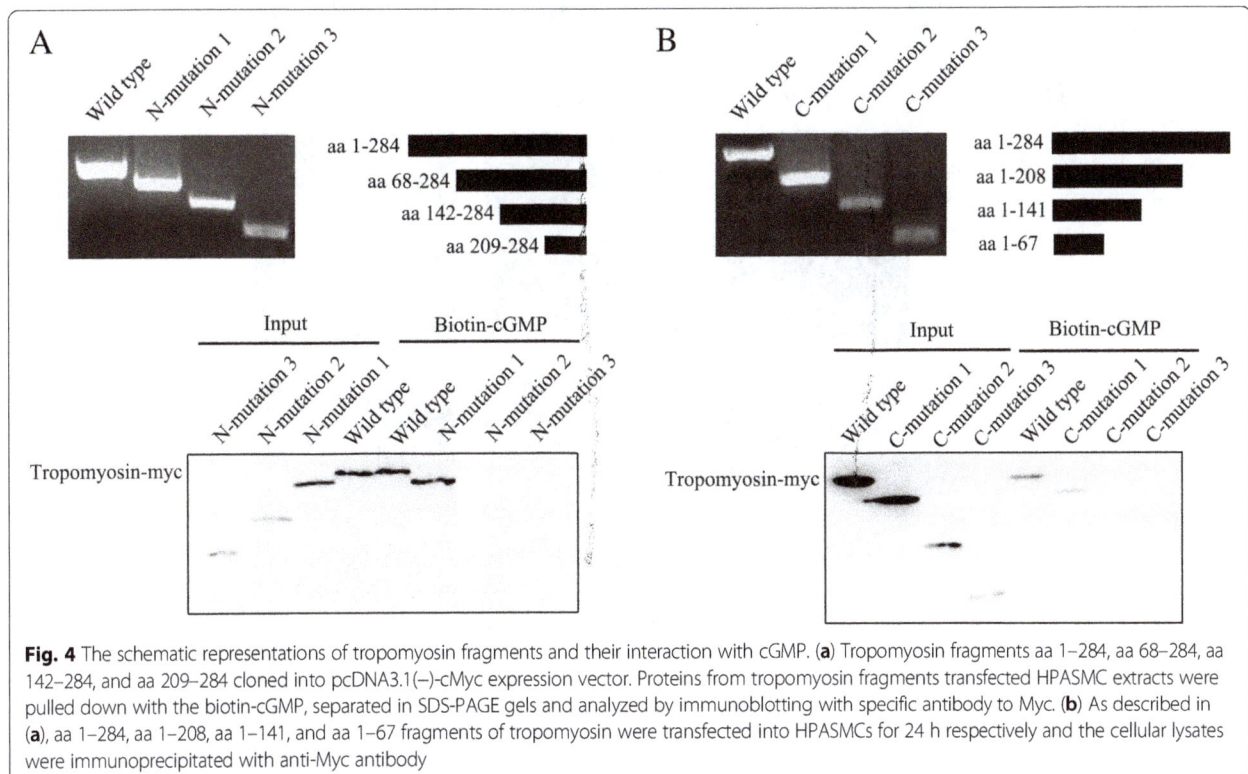

Fig. 4 The schematic representations of tropomyosin fragments and their interaction with cGMP. (**a**) Tropomyosin fragments aa 1–284, aa 68–284, aa 142–284, and aa 209–284 cloned into pcDNA3.1(–)-cMyc expression vector. Proteins from tropomyosin fragments transfected HPASMC extracts were pulled down with the biotin-cGMP, separated in SDS-PAGE gels and analyzed by immunoblotting with specific antibody to Myc. (**b**) As described in (**a**), aa 1–284, aa 1–208, aa 1–141, and aa 1–67 fragments of tropomyosin were transfected into HPASMCs for 24 h respectively and the cellular lysates were immunoprecipitated with anti-Myc antibody

N-mutation 2, N-mutation 3, C-mutation 1, C-mutation 2, and C-mutation 3) were inserted into pcDNA3.1(–)-c-Myc vector and then transfected into cultured HPASMCs. These vectors could express Myc-fused protein in cells. Antibody-dependent pull-down was repeated. As shown in Fig. 4a and b, wild type, N-mutation 1, and C-mutation 1 were detected in the immunocomplexes. In contrast, N-mutation 2, N-mutation 3, C-mutation 2, and C-mutation 3 were absent from the immunocomplexes with antibodies against Myc. Collectively, these results indicated that there was a cGMP binding site at aa 68–208 of the tropomyosin protein.

cGMP had no effect on TPM1 expression and subcellular localization

HPASMCs were induced by 8-Br-cGMP (100 μM), TPM1 expression was not significantly dysregulated after 8-Br-cGMP induction compared to the control cells (Fig. 5a, b, and c). cGMP has no effect on tropomyosin subcellular localization after 8-Br-cGMP induction compared to the control cells (Fig. 5d).

Analysis of actin-tropomyosin-myosin interactions by ITC

ITC is mainly applied to explore molecular binding reactions and provides the binding constant, the molar ratio of the proteins complex, and the enthalpy change (ΔH) of the interaction [10–12]. We utilized ITC to detect the binding affinity of actin-tropomyosin-myosin. However, there were numerous non-specific binding activities caused by electrostatic interactions in each assay. To minimize this, the sodium chloride concentration of the buffer in the ITC assays was decreased from 50 mM to 5 mM.

Under the experimental status, the binding affinity of tropomyosin to actin-myosin was significantly up-regulated compared to the control group (Fig. 6a and b). However, the binding affinity was significantly down-regulated after adding 8-Br-cGMP, with K value changed from $(4.60 \times 10^5 \pm 7.84 \times 10^4)$ to $(3.45 \times 10^5 \pm 4.34 \times 10^4)$ (Fig. 6b and c).

Table 1 shows the binding constants and thermodynamic parameters. There was a stronger affinity of actin, tropomyosin and myosin without treatment of 8-Br-cGMP proved by ΔG compared to the experimental group with 8-Br-cGMP, which is consistent with the

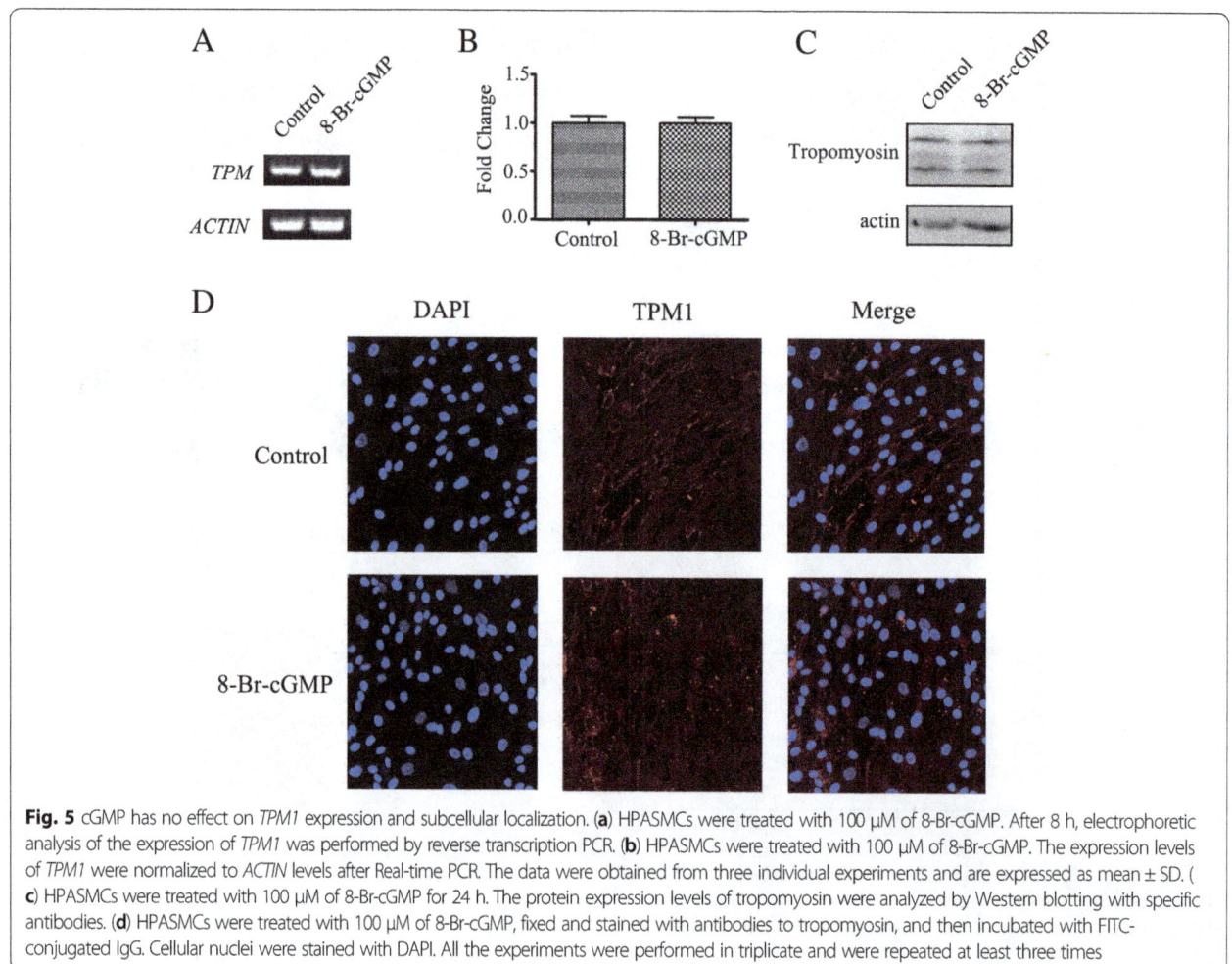

Fig. 5 cGMP has no effect on TPM1 expression and subcellular localization. (**a**) HPASMCs were treated with 100 μM of 8-Br-cGMP. After 8 h, electrophoretic analysis of the expression of TPM1 was performed by reverse transcription PCR. (**b**) HPASMCs were treated with 100 μM of 8-Br-cGMP. The expression levels of TPM1 were normalized to ACTIN levels after Real-time PCR. The data were obtained from three individual experiments and are expressed as mean ± SD. (**c**) HPASMCs were treated with 100 μM of 8-Br-cGMP for 24 h. The protein expression levels of tropomyosin were analyzed by Western blotting with specific antibodies. (**d**) HPASMCs were treated with 100 μM of 8-Br-cGMP, fixed and stained with antibodies to tropomyosin, and then incubated with FITC-conjugated IgG. Cellular nuclei were stained with DAPI. All the experiments were performed in triplicate and were repeated at least three times

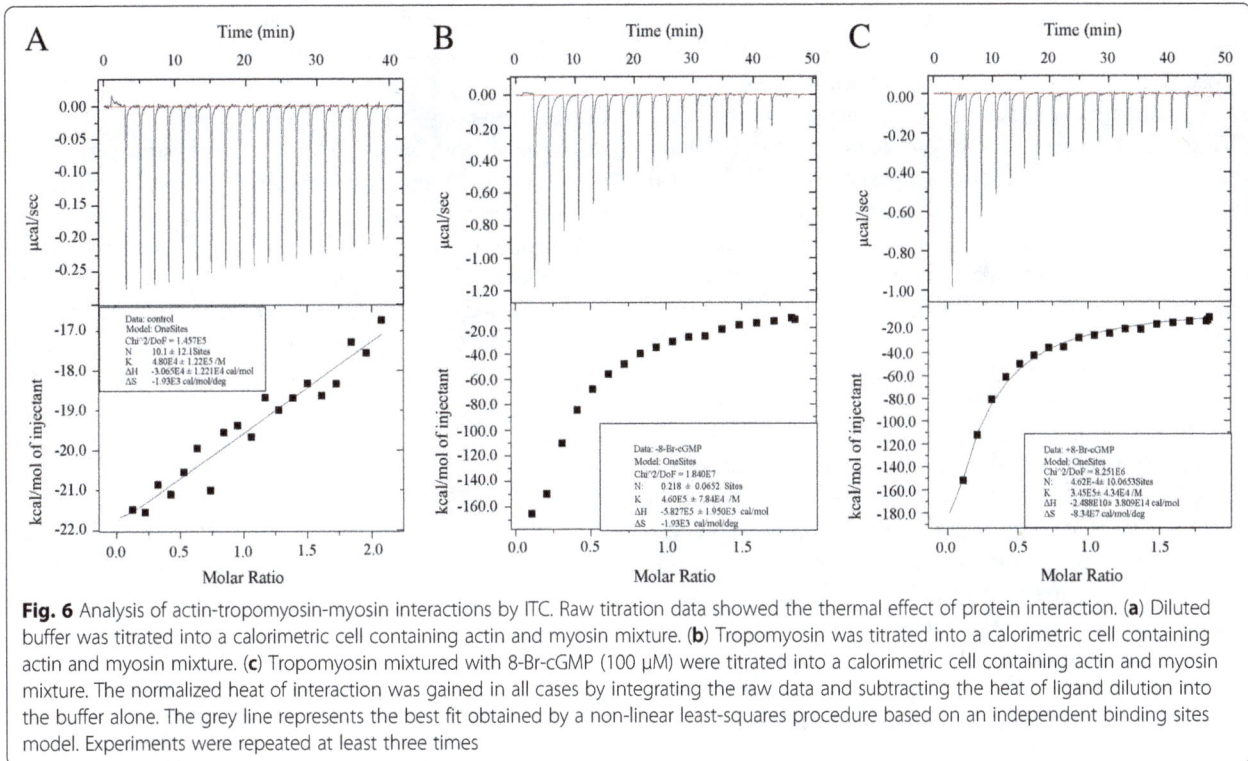

Fig. 6 Analysis of actin-tropomyosin-myosin interactions by ITC. Raw titration data showed the thermal effect of protein interaction. (**a**) Diluted buffer was titrated into a calorimetric cell containing actin and myosin mixture. (**b**) Tropomyosin was titrated into a calorimetric cell containing actin and myosin mixture. (**c**) Tropomyosin mixtured with 8-Br-cGMP (100 μM) were titrated into a calorimetric cell containing actin and myosin mixture. The normalized heat of interaction was gained in all cases by integrating the raw data and subtracting the heat of ligand dilution into the buffer alone. The grey line represents the best fit obtained by a non-linear least-squares procedure based on an independent binding sites model. Experiments were repeated at least three times

meaning of another parameter K value. Significant difference was found between the experimental group without 8-Br-cGMP and the group with 8-Br-cGMP ($P < 0.05$), suggesting a distinct obstruction of the formation of actin-tropomyosin-myosin complex.

Discussion

Smooth muscle cell is the most important regulator of the blood vessel contraction in the body. Smooth muscle contraction can be caused by several physiochemical agents. The ectopic regulation of NO production, sGC activity and cGMP degradation contributes to the development of pulmonary vasorelaxation, which is closely related to the effect of smooth muscle cell. Riociguat (BAY 63–2521), the sGC stimulator, has a dual effect on PAH by promoting pulmonary vasorelaxation and reducing fibrosis [13]. However, the molecular mechanism by which NO-sGC-cGMP pathway causes pulmonary vasorelaxation remains undefined.

In this study, by performing Biotin-cGMP pull-down assay and ITC analysis, we found that cGMP interacted with tropomyosin, which lead to the structural and

functional alterations in the actin-tropomyosin-myosin complex. Tropomyosin, as a coiled-coil molecule which associates head-to-tail to form super-helical polymers, has 284 aa in length with a molecular mass of about 33 kDa [14]. Mammals utilize *TPM1*, *TPM2*, *TPM3*, and *TPM4* to express more than 40 tropomyosin isoforms by alternative splicing [15]. The functions of isoforms are variables determined by the timing and tissue specificity of gene expression, mRNA, and protein localization. For example, tropomyosin 4 [16] expression is enhanced and tropomyosin 1 [17] expression is altered in smooth muscle cells shifting from a contractile to a synthetic phenotype. Tropomyosin 6 is a relatively late marker for smooth muscle maturation in both mice and human beings [18]. Thus, the diverse functions of tropomyosin isoforms have offered an impressive mechanism to illustrate the variation of actin-myosin interaction in different intracellular compartments [19]. We performed PCR using primers designed based on the non-conserved sequences and found that isoform 4 was the only isoform expressed in our HPASMCs.

Table 1 Binding constants and thermodynamic parameters of actin-tropomyosin-myosin systems detected with ITC

Interaction	T	K(/mol)	ΔH (kcal/mol)	ΔS(kcal/mol)	ΔG(kcal/mol)
Control/Actin+Myosin	298.15	$4.80 \times 10^4 \pm 1.22 \times 10^5$	-30.70 ± 12.20	-0.08	-30.70 ± 12.20
Tropomyosin/Actin+Myosin	298.15	$4.60 \times 10^5 \pm 7.84 \times 10^4$	$-5.83 \times 10^5 \pm 1.95 \times 10^5$	-1.93	$-5.82 \times 10^5 \pm 1.95 \times 10^5$
Tropomyosin/Actin+Myosin+ 8-Br-cGMP	298.15	$3.45 \times 10^5 \pm 4.34 \times 10^4$	$-2.49 \times 10^7 \pm 3.81 \times 10^{11}$	-8.34×10^4	$-3.43 \times 10^4 \pm 3.81 \times 10^{11}$

It is becoming increasingly clear that muscle contraction is controlled by the sliding filament mechanism, whose central feature is the interplay of myosin with actin filaments [20]. The heads of myosin in the thick filament bind to actin in the thin filament (made of actin and tropomyosin) as induced by some physiochemical signals. Tropomyosin plays a crucial role in the regulating the interaction between actin and myosin and altering the sliding of myosin filaments, thus serving as a regulator of muscle contraction [21].

In our current study, we demonstrated that there was an interaction between cGMP and tropomyosin, and the cGMP binding site was aa 68–208 of the tropomyosin protein. According to the 3-D protein structure from the Protein Data Bank (PDB, https://www.rcsb.org/), aa 98–233 of tropomyosin is the key fragment that regulates the interaction between myosin and actin. Thus, cGMP and tropomyosin interaction may compete to the binding site of tropomyosin and actin, finally leading to the decrease of the interaction between myosin and actin. This was in accordance with the "steric blocking mechanism" that the migration of tropomyosin into the center of the filament groove increases the interaction between the myosin head and actin [20].

Furthermore, smooth muscle contraction is set up in motion by the discharge of Ca^{2+} [22–24]. ATPase is also needed during the contraction [25]. Therefore, Ca^{2+} and ATPase can be added to the mixure for ITC assay, permitting the myosin head to interact with the actin filament and cause contraction.

We also found in our study that, although cGMP interacted with tropomyosin, it had no effect on tropomyosin expression and subcellular localization. The expression of tropomyosin can be regulated by other factors; for example, miR-21 can down-regulate *TPM1* to inhibit tumor growth, and thus miR-21 functions as an oncogene [26]. Another second messenger cAMP also negatively regulates the mRNA level of tropomyosin in cultured rat vascular smooth muscle cells [27]. We assume that there are two main ways of tropomyosin to exert its functions: one way is the activated pathway, in which expression and localization are adjusted by unique signals or modifications; and the other way is the physical interaction, i.e. tropomyosin exerts crucial functions via its interactions with other critical cellular proteins.

This preliminary study clearly demonstrated an interaction of cGMP with tropomyosin, although we still have no data on cGMP-tropomyosin interaction in vivo. In addition to investigations on the pulmonary artery pressure after the increase of cGMP level in tropomyosin 1 knock-out mice, and hPASMC contraction after cGMP increase and TPM1 knockdown, we also will detect the cGMP-tropomyosin interaction in PAH mice. Also, the structure of cGMP and actin-tropomyosin-myosin complex need be further defined with methods such as x-ray diffraction and electron microscopy.

Conclusions

In summary, our study delineated a physical interaction between cGMP and tropomyosin, that might contribute to the alterations of the structure and function of the actin-tropomyosin-myosin complex and finally bridge the suppressive effect of pulmonary vasorelaxation. These findings shed new light on molecular mechanism by which NO-sGC-cGMP pathway acts as a down-regulation factor of muscle contraction in the pathogenesis of PAH.

Abbreviations
HPASMC: Human pulmonary artery smooth muscle cell;; ITC: Isothermal titration calorimetry; NO-sGC-cGMP: Nitric oxide-soluble guanylate cyclase-cyclic guanosine monophosphate; PAH: Pulmonary arterial hypertension

Funding
This work was supported in part by Grant 7172193 from the Beijing Natural Science Foundation, Grant 2017ZX09304026 from the National Science and Technology Major Project for Significant New Drugs Creation, Grant 81571384 from the National Natural Science Foundation of China, Grant BJ-2018-137 from the Beijing Hospital Nova Project.

Authors' contributions
FX and ZZ contributed to the design of the project. JZ, JH and WL performed ITC assay and data analysis. FS and XX performed pull down assay. LZ performed experiments and data analysis, and wrote the manuscript. All authors read and approved the final manuscript.

Competing interests
The authors declare that they have no competing interests.

Author details
[1]The MOH Key Laboratory of Geriatrics, Beijing Hospital, National Center of Gerontology, Beijing 100730, People's Republic of China. [2]Department of Pathology, Beijing Hospital, National Center of Gerontology, Beijing 100730, People's Republic of China. [3]Department of Respiratory and Critical Care Medicine, Beijing Hospital, National Center of Gerontology, Beijing 100730, People's Republic of China. [4]Department of Respiratory and Critical Care Medicine, China-Japan Friendship Hospital, Beijing 100029, People's Republic of China.

References
1. Schermuly RT, Ghofrani HA, Wilkins MR, Grimminger F. Mechanisms of disease: pulmonary arterial hypertension. Nat Rev Cardiol. 2011;8(8):443–55.
2. Baliga RS, Macallister RJ, Hobbs AJ. Vasoactive peptides and the pathogenesis of pulmonary hypertension: role and potential therapeutic application. Handb Exp Pharmacol. 2013;218:477–511.

3. Zou L, Xu X, Zhai Z, Yang T, Jin J, Xiao F. Identification of downstream target genes regulated by the nitric oxide-soluble guanylate cyclase-cyclic guanosine monophosphate signal pathway in pulmonary hypertension. J Int Med Res. 2016;44(3):508–19.

4. Zhang S, Zou L, Yang T, Yang Y, Zhai Z, Xiao F. The sGC activator inhibits the proliferation and migration, promotes the apoptosis of human pulmonary arterial smooth muscle cells via the up regulation of plasminogen activator inhibitor-2. Exp Cell Res. 2015;332(2):278–87.

5. Zou L, Zhang S, Xu X, Xiao F, Zhai Z. Expression of PAI-2 mRNA in peripheral blood leucocytes and regulation by sGC activator in pulmonary hypertension. Zhonghua Yi Xue Za Zhi. 2016;96(16):1247–51.

6. Wang G, Liu X, Meng L, Liu S, Wang L, Li J. Up-regulated lipocalin-2 in pulmonary hypertension involving in pulmonary artery SMC resistance to apoptosis. Int J Biol Sci. 2014;10(7):798–806.

7. Wylie T, Garg R, Ridley AJ, Conte MR. Analysis of the interaction of Plexin-B1 and Plexin-B2 with Rnd family proteins. PLoS One. 2017;12(10):e0185899.

8. Sun Q, He J, Yang H, Li S, Zhao L, Li H. Analysis of binding properties and interaction of thiabendazole and its metabolite with human serum albumin via multiple spectroscopic methods. Food Chem. 2017;233:190–6.

9. Hands-Taylor KL, Martino L, Tata R, Babon JJ, Bui TT, Drake AF. Heterodimerization of the human RNase P/MRP subunits Rpp20 and Rpp25 is a prerequisite for interaction with the P3 arm of RNase MRP RNA. Nucleic Acids Res. 2010;38(12):4052–66.

10. Rajarathnam K, Rosgen J. Isothermal titration calorimetry of membrane proteins - progress and challenges. Biochim Biophys Acta. 2014;1838(1 Pt A):69–77.

11. Pierce MM, Raman CS, Nall BT. Isothermal titration calorimetry of protein-protein interactions. Methods. 1999;19(2):213–21.

12. Loh W, Brinatti C, Tam KC. Use of isothermal titration calorimetry to study surfactant aggregation in colloidal systems. Biochim Biophys Acta. 2016; 1860(5):999–1016.

13. Stasch JP, Pacher P, Evgenov OV. Soluble guanylate cyclase as an emerging therapeutic target in cardiopulmonary disease. Circulation. 2011;123(20):2263–73.

14. Ruiz-Opazo N, Nadal-Ginard B. Alpha-tropomyosin gene organization. Alternative splicing of duplicated isotype-specific exons accounts for the production of smooth and striated muscle isoforms. J Biol Chem. 1987; 262(10):4755–65.

15. Gunning P, O'Neill G, Hardeman E. Tropomyosin-based regulation of the actin cytoskeleton in time and space. Physiol Rev. 2008;88(1):1–35.

16. Abouhamed M, Reichenberg S, Robenek H, Plenz G. Tropomyosin 4 expression is enhanced in dedifferentiating smooth muscle cells in vitro and during atherogenesis. Eur J Cell Biol. 2003;82(9):473–82.

17. Girjes AA, Keriakous D, Cockerill GW, Hayward IP, Campbell GR, Campbell JH. Cloning of a differentially expressed tropomyosin isoform from cultured rabbit aortic smooth muscle cells. Int J Biochem Cell Biol. 2002;34(5):505–15.

18. Vrhovski B, McKay K, Schevzov G, Gunning PW, Weinberger RP. Smooth muscle-specific alpha tropomyosin is a marker of fully differentiated smooth muscle in lung. J Histochem Cytochem. 2005;53(7):875–83.

19. Gunning PW, Schevzov G, Kee AJ, Hardeman EC. Tropomyosin isoforms: divining rods for actin cytoskeleton function. Trends Cell Biol. 2005;15(6):333–41.

20. Behrmann E, Muller M, Penczek PA, Mannherz HG, Manstein DJ, Raunser S. Structure of the rigor actin-tropomyosin-myosin complex. Cell. 2012;150(2): 327–38.

21. Parry DA, Squire JM. Structural role of tropomyosin in muscle regulation: analysis of the x-ray diffraction patterns from relaxed and contracting muscles. J Mol Biol. 1973;75(1):33–55.

22. Ueda K, Kimura-Sakiyama C, Aihara T, Miki M, Arata T. Calcium-dependent interaction sites of tropomyosin on reconstituted muscle thin filaments with bound myosin heads as studied by site-directed spin-labeling. Biophys J. 2013;105(10):2366–73.

23. Gergely J. Molecular switches in troponin. Adv Exp Med Biol. 1998;453:169–76.

24. Li MX, Wang X, Sykes BD. Structural based insights into the role of troponin in cardiac muscle pathophysiology. J Muscle Res Cell Motil. 2004;25(7):559–79.

25. Sweeney HL, Houdusse A. Structural and functional insights into the myosin motor mechanism. Annu Rev Biophys. 2010;39:539–57.

26. Zhu S, Si ML, Wu H, Mo YY. MicroRNA-21 targets the tumor suppressor gene tropomyosin 1 (TPM1). J Biol Chem. 2007;282(19):14328–36.

27. Ohara O, Nakano T, Teraoka H, Arita H. cAMP negatively regulates mRNA levels of actin and tropomyosin in rat cultured vascular smooth muscle cells. J Biochem. 1991;109(6):834–9.

19

Long-term outcomes following first short-term clinically important deterioration in COPD

Ian P. Naya[1]* (iD), Lee Tombs[2], Hana Muellerova[1], Christopher Compton[1] and Paul W. Jones[1]

Abstract

Background: Chronic obstructive pulmonary disease (COPD) is characterized by varying trajectories of decline. Information regarding the prognostic value of preventing short-term clinically important deterioration (CID) in lung function, health status, or first moderate/severe exacerbation as a composite endpoint of worsening is needed. We evaluated post hoc the link between early CID and long-term adverse outcomes.

Methods: CID was defined as ≥100 mL decrease in forced expiratory volume in 1 s (FEV_1), ≥4-unit increase in St George's Respiratory Questionnaire (SGRQ) score from baseline, and/or a moderate/severe exacerbation during enrollment in two 3-year studies. Presence of CID was assessed at 6 months for the principal analysis (TORCH) and 12 months for the confirmatory analysis (ECLIPSE). Association between presence (+) or absence (-) of CID and long-term deterioration in FEV_1, SGRQ, future risk of exacerbations, and all-cause mortality was assessed.

Results: In total, 2870 (54%; TORCH) and 1442 (73%; ECLIPSE) patients were CID+. At 36 months, in TORCH, CID+ patients (vs CID-) had sustained clinically significant worsening of FEV_1 (- 117 mL; 95% confidence interval [CI]: - 134, - 100 mL; $P < 0.001$) and SGRQ score (+ 6.42 units; 95% CI: 5.40, 7.45; $P < 0.001$), and had higher risk of exacerbations (hazard ratio [HR]: 1.61 [95% CI: 1.50, 1.72]; $P < 0.001$) and all-cause mortality (HR: 1.41 [95% CI: 1.15, 1.72]; $P < 0.001$). Similar risks post-CID were observed in ECLIPSE.

Conclusions: A CID within 6–12 months of follow-up was consistently associated with increased long-term risk of exacerbations and all-cause mortality, and predicted sustained meaningful loss in FEV_1 and health status amongst survivors.

Trial registration: NCT00268216; NCT00292552.

Keywords: Clinically important deterioration, Composite measures, COPD, Mortality

Introduction

The heterogeneous and progressive nature of chronic obstructive pulmonary disease (COPD) has prompted interest in developing reliable measurements of its progression beyond mean decline rates in forced expiratory volume in 1 s (FEV_1) [1–3]. Improvement in FEV_1 is regularly assessed in clinical trials and has been shown to correlate with improvements in symptoms, health status [4, 5], and reductions in exacerbation rates [6, 7]. However, FEV_1 alone is not sufficient to evaluate the longitudinal changes in the severity of COPD at an individual level [8], and other outcomes are required to monitor disease activity [9].

Recently, a composite measure of deterioration has been developed, comprising: lung function (≥100 mL decline in FEV_1), health status (≥4-unit increase in St George's Respiratory Questionnaire [SGRQ]), and the incidence of a moderate/severe exacerbation [10]. The thresholds for FEV_1 and SGRQ were chosen as the accepted minimum clinically important differences (MCID) for these outcomes [11, 12]. The occurrence of one or more of these events was considered a clinically important deterioration (CID). Several short-term COPD studies have employed this endpoint as an a priori and post hoc measure of instability [10, 13–18]. In short-term trials, incremental gains in the

* Correspondence: ian.p.naya@gsk.com
[1]Respiratory Medicine, GSK, Brentford, Middlesex, UK
Full list of author information is available at the end of the article

prevention of short-term CID have been shown when comparing mono- and dual-bronchodilator therapy with placebo, between dual- and mono-bronchodilator therapy, and with dual-bronchodilator or triple therapy versus ICS/LABA therapy [10, 13–18]; however, the relationship between short-term CID and long-term outcome is unknown.

Management of COPD has moved towards a patient-centered approach, with regular monitoring of the adequacy of care, with the goal of matching appropriate therapy to patients who will benefit most effectively from them [3]. Understanding the association between short-term disease worsening and long-term outcomes would help physicians to better personalize pharmacological treatment at an early stage of a patient's disease.

This post hoc analysis used data from a 3-year interventional study (TOwards a Revolution in COPD Health [TORCH]) [19] and a 3-year observational study (Evaluation of COPD Longitudinally to Identify Predictive Surrogate End-points [ECLIPSE]) [8, 20] to assess whether worsening of COPD, as measured by the presence of any component of the composite CID during the first 6 to 12 months, was a predictor of poor medium-to long-term outcome after a further 30 to 24 months of follow-up, respectively. Analysis of the TORCH data constituted the principal analysis as the presence of CID could be assessed earlier, at 6 months. In the ECLIPSE study CID could only be assessed at 12 months, and so was used as a confirmatory analysis to see if the prognostic findings of the TORCH study could be replicated.

Methods
Study design and treatments
The TORCH study (SCO30003, NCT00268216) was a double-blind, placebo-controlled, randomized study that assessed spirometric values, health status, frequency of exacerbations, and mortality in patients randomized to fluticasone propionate/salmeterol (FP/SAL) 500/50 µg, FP 500 µg, SAL 50 µg, or placebo [19]. The ECLIPSE study (SCO104960, NCT00292552) was a large, observational, longitudinal study of patients with moderate-to-very-severe COPD aimed at defining COPD phenotypes and identifying biomarkers to help predict disease progression [8, 20]. Detailed methodologies for both studies have been previously published [8, 19–21]. Both studies were conducted in accordance with the Declaration of Helsinki and good clinical practice guidelines, and approved by the relevant ethics review committees. All participants gave written informed consent.

Patients
Patients with a diagnosis of COPD in the TORCH study were aged 40–80 years, current or former smokers with ≥10 smoking pack-years, had a pre-bronchodilator

$FEV_1 < 60\%$ of predicted value and a pre-bronchodilator FEV_1/forced vital capacity (FVC) ratio ≤ 0.70. Exclusion criteria included a diagnosis of asthma or respiratory disorders other than COPD, lung-volume reduction or lung transplant surgery, and receiving long-term oral corticosteroid therapy.

In the ECLIPSE study patients were aged 40–75 years, with baseline post-bronchodilator $FEV_1 < 80\%$ of predicted value, baseline post-bronchodilator FEV_1/FVC ≤0.70, and ≥ 10 smoking pack-years. Exclusion criteria included known respiratory disorders other than COPD, history of other significant inflammatory disease, COPD exacerbation ≤4 weeks prior to enrollment, and prior lung surgery.

Outcomes and assessments
Assessment of post-bronchodilator FEV_1, and SGRQ score, was performed at 24, 48, 72, 96, 120, and 156 weeks post-treatment in the TORCH study [19]. In the ECLIPSE study, post-bronchodilator FEV_1 was assessed at 3, 6, 12, 18, 24, 30, and 36 months after treatment, COPD-specific version of the SGRQ (SGRQ-C) was assessed annually, and exacerbations were assessed throughout the study. All-cause mortality and the frequency of moderate or severe exacerbations were assessed in both studies.

Composite CID was defined as any one of the following component events: (i) decrease of ≥100 mL from baseline in post-bronchodilator FEV_1 [11]; (ii) increase of ≥4 units in SGRQ score from baseline [12]; (iii) incidence of a moderate/severe exacerbation (acute worsening of COPD requiring oral corticosteroids, antibiotics, emergency department treatment, or hospitalization).

Patients were categorized into two subgroups: (i) those who met ≥1 CID criteria within the first 6 months (TORCH) after enrollment (CID+), and (ii) those who did not (CID-). In the confirmatory analysis using ECLIPSE data, patient subgroups with (CID+) and without (CID-) a composite CID were defined within the first 12 months of enrollment. CID2+ and CID3+ patients were individuals with two or all three CID component deteriorations occurring at the assessment time, respectively.

Outcomes were assessed by CID status (CID+ or CID-) in a combined analysis, irrespective of which treatment patients were randomized to in the TORCH study.

Statistical analysis
Since this was an analysis of the effect of changes in clinical outcomes (irrespective of treatment), analyses of TORCH study data were performed on the full intent-to-treat (ITT) population, with all treatment groups combined. Mean changes from baseline in post-bronchodilator FEV_1 or SGRQ scores were compared (CID+ group vs CID- group) using a repeated

measures model (least squares [LS] mean) including covariates of post-bronchodilator FEV_1 deterioration status at Week 24, smoking status, geographical region, baseline FEV_1 or SGRQ, time in weeks, week-by-baseline, and week-by-deterioration status at Week 24. Time to first moderate/severe or severe exacerbation and mortality in the 130 weeks after Week 24 were analyzed using Cox proportional hazards model with covariates of deterioration status at Week 24, smoking status at screening, and geographical region. Hazard ratios (HR) and confidence intervals (CI) were derived for the CID+ versus CID- group.

All comers were included in the ECLIPSE study data analysis, irrespective of physician choice of management. Statistical comparisons in LS mean change from baseline in post-bronchodilator FEV_1 or SGRQ score for the CID+ versus CID- group were obtained from a repeated measures model including covariates of deterioration status at Month 12, smoking status at screening, geographical region, age, gender, baseline post-bronchodilator FEV_1 or SGRQ, week, week-by-baseline, and week-by-deterioration status at Month 12. For the composite endpoint, FEV_1 and SGRQ data were only used from common time points. Time to first moderate/severe or severe exacerbation and mortality in the 24 months after Month 12 were analyzed using Cox proportional hazards model with covariates of deterioration status at 12 months, smoking status at screening, geographical region, sex, and age. HRs and CIs were derived for CID+ versus CID- group.

In both studies, baseline and demographic data were generated using descriptive statistics, presented as mean (standard deviation [SD]) and n values (%).

Results
Patients
In the TORCH study, the ITT population included 2870 patients in the CID+ group and 2422 patients in the CID- group (Fig. 1). The most and least common cause of CID in the first 6 months was exacerbation (33%) and deterioration in SGRQ (17%), respectively (Fig. 1). Demographics and baseline characteristics were generally similar in the CID+ and CID- groups, although the proportion of female patients, patients with ≥2 previous exacerbations, and patients receiving inhaled corticosteroids (ICS) in the 12 months prior to the run-in period was greater in the CID+ compared with the CID- group (Table 1).

The ECLIPSE study comprised 1442 patients in the CID+ group and 531 patients in the CID- group (Additional file 1: Figure S1; online data supplement). Demographics and baseline characteristics were generally similar in the CID+ and CID- groups, with the differences following the same pattern as for the TORCH study (Additional file 2: Table S1; online data supplement).

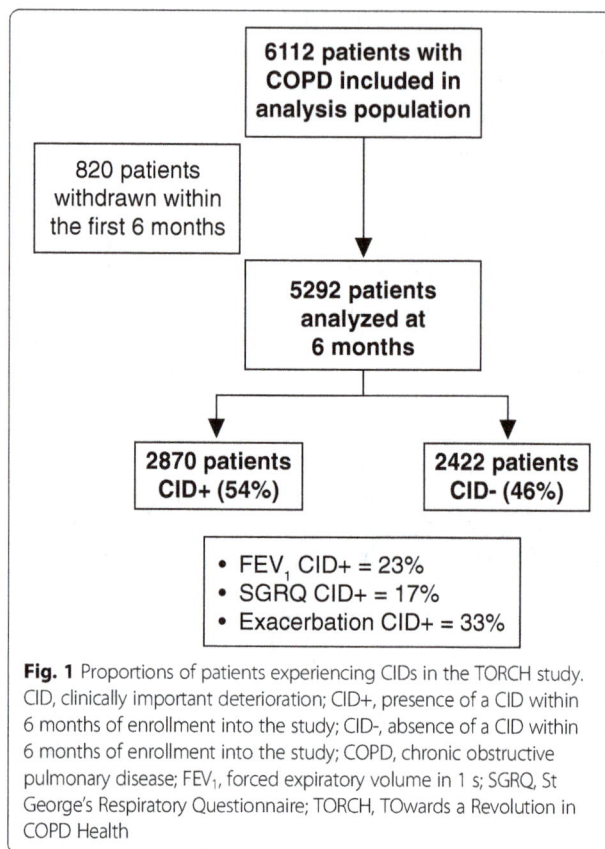

Fig. 1 Proportions of patients experiencing CIDs in the TORCH study. CID, clinically important deterioration; CID+, presence of a CID within 6 months of enrollment into the study; CID-, absence of a CID within 6 months of enrollment into the study; COPD, chronic obstructive pulmonary disease; FEV_1, forced expiratory volume in 1 s; SGRQ, St George's Respiratory Questionnaire; TORCH, TOwards a Revolution in COPD Health

Changes in lung function and health status over time based on CID status (TORCH study)
Post-bronchodilator FEV_1 decreased in both CID groups at a similar rate from Week 24 to the end of follow up (Fig. 2a). Patients free of all CID events (CID- group) had an improvement in FEV_1 at 24 weeks that returned to baseline at 156 weeks (Fig. 2a). By contrast, patients in the CID+ group showed a modest mean deterioration in FEV_1 at Week 24, which was clinically important at 156 weeks (between-group difference: - 117 mL, 95% CI: -134, - 100; $P < 0.001$; Fig. 2a). At the 3-year time point, the odds of a deficit in lung function of ≥100 mL or ≥ 200 mL from baseline were approximately two-fold higher in the CID+ compared with the CID- group (Table 2).

Patients in the CID- group had clear improvement in health status at Week 24, with a decrease in SGRQ score from baseline of approximately 8 units; Fig. 2b. In the CID+ group, patients showed an increase from baseline in SGRQ score of 1.33 units (representing a worsening health status) at Week 24 (Fig. 2b). At study end, the difference in SGRQ score in the CID+ versus CID- group remained above the MCID (+ 6.42 units, 95% CI: 5.40, 7.45; $P < 0.001$; Fig. 2b). Patients in the CID+ group had greater odds of having a ≥ 4-unit and ≥ 8-unit worsening in SGRQ score from baseline at 36 months compared with those in the CID- group (Table 2).

Table 1 Patient demographics and baseline characteristics (TORCH study; ITT population)

	CID+ population (N = 2870)	CID- population (N = 2422)	Total (N = 5292)
Age (years), mean (SD)	64.7 (8.2)	65.1 (8.4)	64.9 (8.3)
Male, n (%)	2151 (75)	1895 (78)	4046 (76)
BMI, kg/m², mean (SD)	25.3 (5.3)	25.5 (5.2)	25.4 (5.2)
Current smoker at screening, n (%)	1277 (44)	1072 (44)	2349 (44)
Post-bronchodilator % predicted FEV$_1$, mean (SD)	44.7 (13.8)	44.8 (12.8)	44.7 (13.4)
Patients receiving ICS in the 12 months prior to the run-in period, n (%)	1455 (51)	1037 (43)	2492 (47)
Previous exacerbations, n (%)			
0	1122 (39)	1164 (48)	2286 (43)
1	711 (25)	617 (25)	1328 (25)
≥ 2	1037 (36)	641 (26)	1678 (32)

BMI body mass index, *CID* clinically important deterioration, *CID+* presence of a CID within 6 months of enrollment into the study, *CID-* absence of a CID within 6 months of enrollment into the study, *ICS* inhaled corticosteroid, *ITT* intent-to-treat, *SD* standard deviation, *TORCH* TOwards a Revolution in COPD Health

Future risk of exacerbations and all-cause mortality based on CID status (TORCH study)

Patients in the CID+ group had a significantly higher risk of exacerbations compared with patients in the CID- group. This pattern was observed for both moderate/severe exacerbations (HR [CID+ vs CID-]: 1.61; 95% CI: 1.50, 1.72; P < 0.001; Fig. 3a) and severe exacerbations requiring hospitalization (HR [CID+ vs CID-]: 1.55; 95% CI: 1.38, 1.73; P < 0.001; Fig. 3b). Median time to first moderate-to-severe exacerbation in the CID- group was 520 days compared with 265 days in the CID+ group. Patients in the CID+ group had a 41% increased risk of all-cause mortality compared with those in the CID- group (HR [CID+ vs CID-]: 1.41; 95% CI: 1.15, 1.72%; P < 0.001; Fig. 3c; Table 2).

Comparison of CID type and frequency with all-cause mortality (TORCH study)

Worsening of each component of the CID was associated with increased mortality risk by a broadly similar magnitude (19–29%) compared with absence of that CID event type; however, this was only statistically significant for the exacerbations and SGRQ components (Fig. 4). Freedom from all CIDs was associated with lower mortality risk than freedom from just one CID component alone (SGRQ or exacerbations or FEV$_1$), indicating that each CID component contributed to the overall mortality risk. However, as so few patients had multiple types of CID events in the first 6-months, there remains some uncertainty in defining a CID-dose effect (Fig. 4).

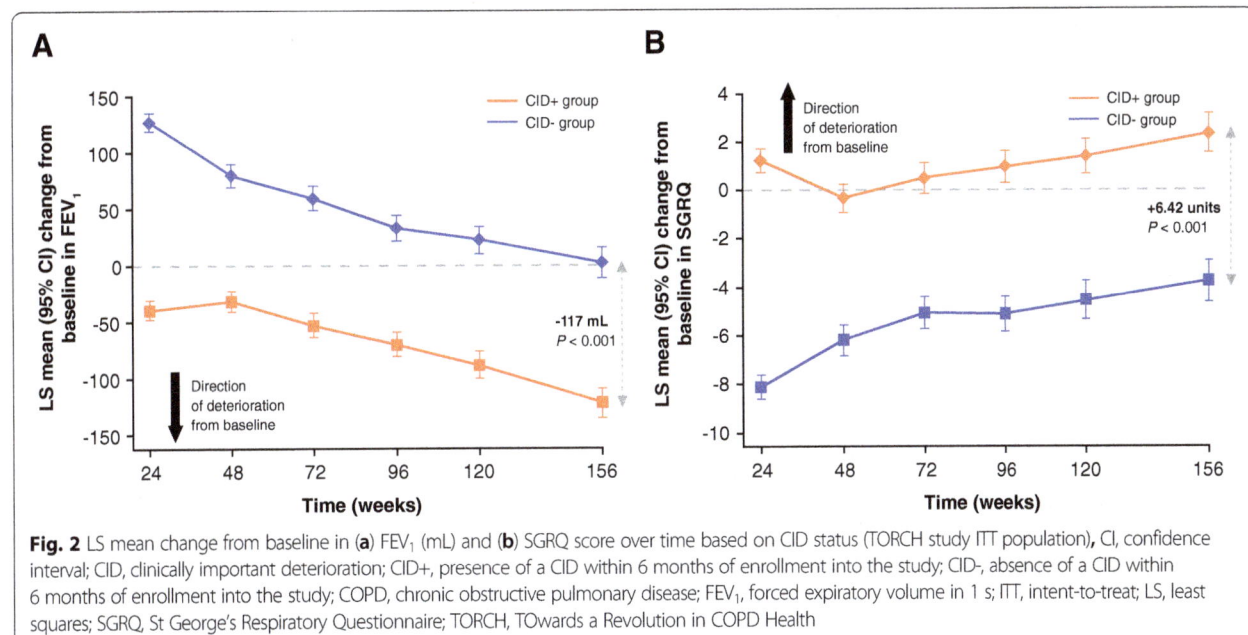

Fig. 2 LS mean change from baseline in (**a**) FEV$_1$ (mL) and (**b**) SGRQ score over time based on CID status (TORCH study ITT population), CI, confidence interval; CID, clinically important deterioration; CID+, presence of a CID within 6 months of enrollment into the study; CID-, absence of a CID within 6 months of enrollment into the study; COPD, chronic obstructive pulmonary disease; FEV$_1$, forced expiratory volume in 1 s; ITT, intent-to-treat; LS, least squares; SGRQ, St George's Respiratory Questionnaire; TORCH, TOwards a Revolution in COPD Health

Table 2 Odds/Risk of long-term adverse outcomes based on CIDs in the first 6 months of the TORCH study (ITT population)

Outcome	CID+ population (N = 2870)	CID- population (N = 2422)	CID+ vs CID-, OR (95% CI)
≥100 mL decrease in FEV$_1$[a], n (%)	2004 (70)	1296 (54)	2.00 (1.78, 2.24)*
≥200 mL decrease in FEV$_1$[a], n (%)	1696 (59)	1018 (42)	1.97 (1.77, 2.20)*
≥4-unit increase in SGRQ[a], n (%)	1516 (67)	930 (53)	1.82 (1.60, 2.07)*
≥8-unit increase in SGRQ[a], n (%)	1342 (59)	827 (47)	1.65 (1.45, 1.88)*
Moderate-to-severe COPD exacerbation[b], n (%)	2082 (73)	1450 (60)	1.61[c] (1.50, 1.72)*
Hospitalization events[b], n (%)	797 (28)	491 (20)	1.55[c] (1.38, 1.73)*
Risk (HR) of all-cause mortality[b], n (%)	237 (8)	160 (7)	1.41[c] (1.15, 1.72)*

*P < 0.001, [a]risk of deterioration at 36-months assessed from the pre-randomization period; [b]risk of a new exacerbation or all-cause death assessed from Week 24; [c]data report HR (95% CI)

CID clinically important deterioration, CID+ presence of a CID within 6 months of enrollment into the study, CID- absence of a CID within 6 months of enrollment into the study, FEV$_1$ forced expiratory volume in 1 s, HR hazard ratio, ITT intent-to-treat, OR odds ratio, SGRQ St George's Respiratory Questionnaire, TORCH TOwards a Revolution in COPD Health

Predictions of long-term outcomes based on individual component deteriorations (TORCH study)

Individual CID event types within the first 6 months were associated with a greater risk of deterioration in that outcome at 3 years. For example, the change from baseline in FEV$_1$ after 36 months was - 193 mL (95% CI: -213, - 172) for patients who had an FEV$_1$ CID event in the first 6 months, compared with - 51 mL (95% CI: -74, - 27) and - 38 mL (95% CI: -57, - 20) for patients with a SGRQ and exacerbation CID event in the first 6 months, respectively (Additional file 2: Table S2; online data supplement). Similarly, SGRQ and exacerbation CID events led to the greatest risk of future deteriorations in health status and exacerbations, respectively (Additional file 2: Table S2; online data supplement).

FEV$_1$ CID events or exacerbation CID events by 6 months had similar long-term impacts on health status at 36 months (+ 3.56 units [95% CI: 2.31, 4.80] and + 3.70 units [95% CI: 2.56, 4.83], respectively; Additional file 2: Table S2; online data supplement).

Analysis of the ECLIPSE study data

In the ECLIPSE study, changes in FEV$_1$ and SGRQ between the CID+ and CID- groups were similar to those observed in the TORCH study (Fig. 5a and Fig. 5b, respectively). At study end, the difference in mean change from baseline in FEV$_1$ was - 115 mL (95% CI: -141, - 89; P < 0.001) and the difference in mean change from baseline SGRQ was + 4.67 units (95% CI: 3.32, 6.02; P < 0.001).

Compared with patients in the CID- group, those in the CID+ group had a significantly higher risk of moderate/severe exacerbations (HR: 2.54; 95% CI: 2.20, 2.93; P < 0.001; Table 3; Fig. 6a), exacerbations requiring hospitalization (HR: 2.81; 95% CI: 2.17, 3.63; P < 0.001; Table 3; Fig. 6b), and all-cause mortality (HR: 1.59; 95% CI: 1.04, 2.41; P = 0.031; Table 3; Fig. 6c).

Discussion

This exploratory analysis evaluated whether CID status (a composite measure of early deterioration in COPD),

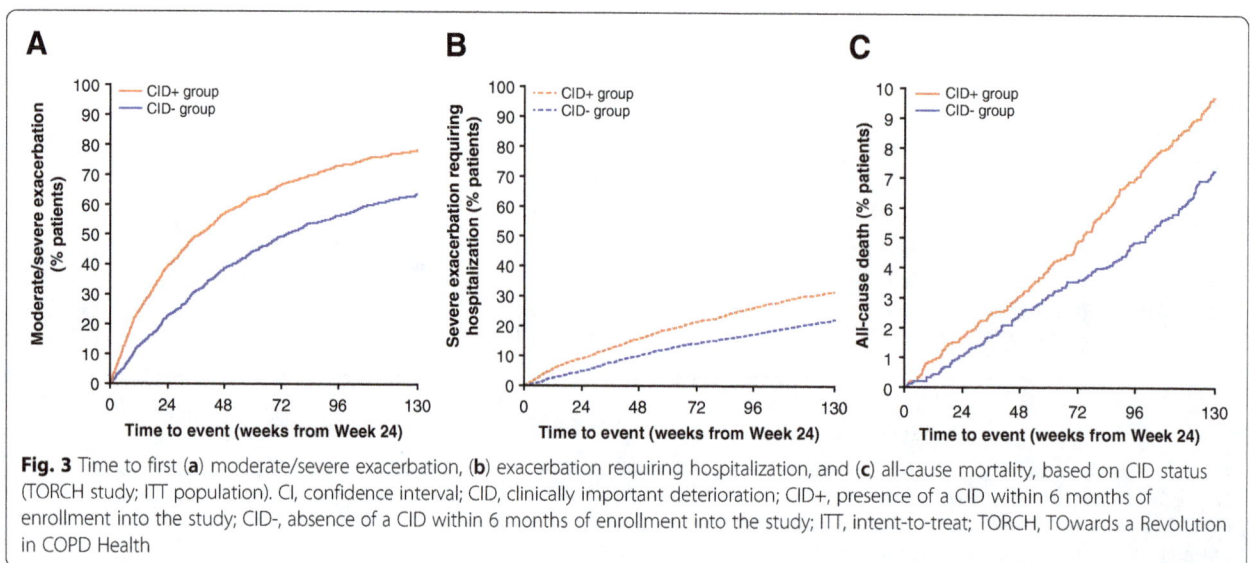

Fig. 3 Time to first (**a**) moderate/severe exacerbation, (**b**) exacerbation requiring hospitalization, and (**c**) all-cause mortality, based on CID status (TORCH study; ITT population). CI, confidence interval; CID, clinically important deterioration; CID+, presence of a CID within 6 months of enrollment into the study; CID-, absence of a CID within 6 months of enrollment into the study; ITT, intent-to-treat; TORCH, TOwards a Revolution in COPD Health

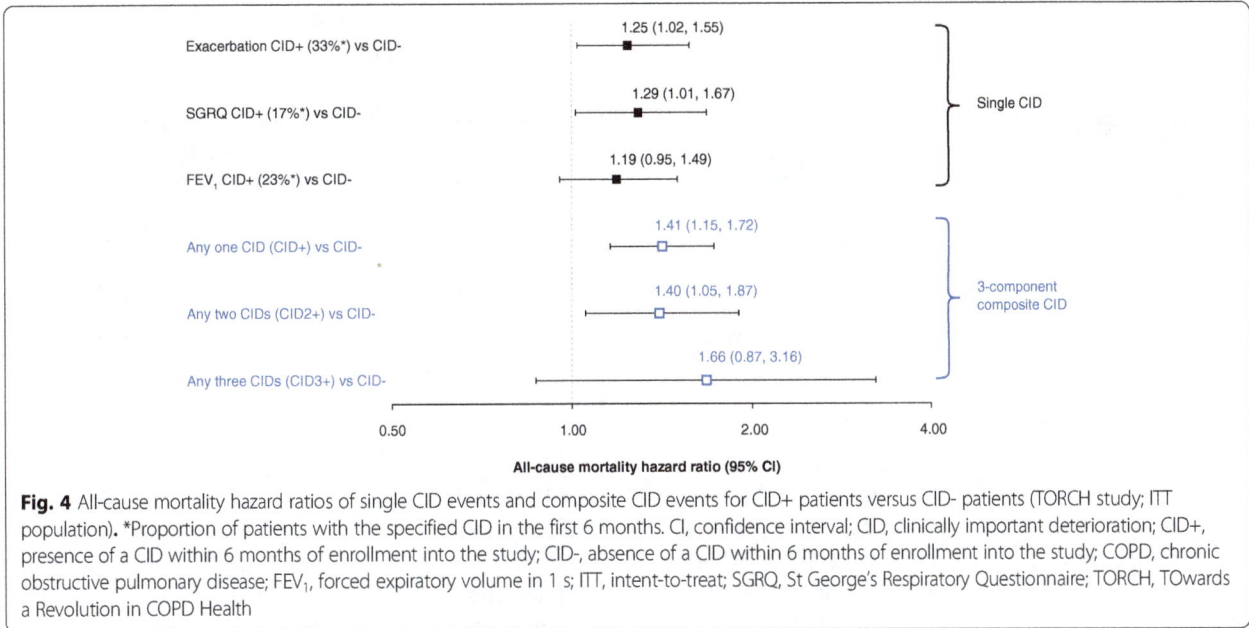

Fig. 4 All-cause mortality hazard ratios of single CID events and composite CID events for CID+ patients versus CID- patients (TORCH study; ITT population). *Proportion of patients with the specified CID in the first 6 months. CI, confidence interval; CID, clinically important deterioration; CID+, presence of a CID within 6 months of enrollment into the study; CID-, absence of a CID within 6 months of enrollment into the study; COPD, chronic obstructive pulmonary disease; FEV$_1$, forced expiratory volume in 1 s; ITT, intent-to-treat; SGRQ, St George's Respiratory Questionnaire; TORCH, TOwards a Revolution in COPD Health

assessed after the first 6 months of observation, could be used to predict a range of medium- to long-term patient outcomes after 3 years of follow-up. Patients who experienced a CID event in the first 6–12 months were found, in two separate 3-year studies (TORCH and ECLIPSE), to have consistently worse long-term outcomes, including sustained and important loss of FEV$_1$ and health status, and a greater risk of exacerbation and mortality, compared with more stable patients free of short-term CID events [11, 12].

Disease progression in COPD is not confined to decline in FEV$_1$. Medium-term deterioration in patients with COPD has been reported in terms of SGRQ score [22], six-minute walking distance [23] and daily physical activity [24]. The correlation between changes in these different measures of severity is not strong, as reported, for example, between FEV$_1$ and SGRQ [4, 25], exacerbations and FEV$_1$ [26] and physical activity, FEV$_1$ and SGRQ [24]. As no single measure appears to capture all aspects of worsening COPD reliably in all patients, there is a strong argument for a new composite measure.

A composite CID assessment of multifactorial deterioration within 6 months of randomization in the TORCH study was shown to predict an increase in the

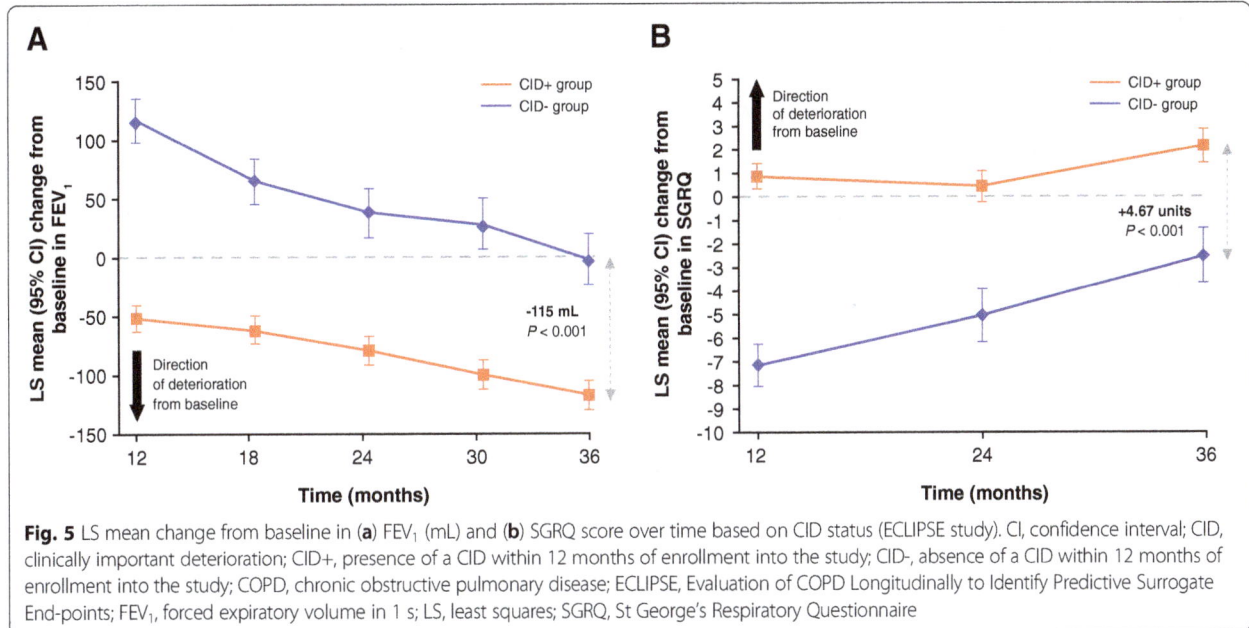

Fig. 5 LS mean change from baseline in (**a**) FEV$_1$ (mL) and (**b**) SGRQ score over time based on CID status (ECLIPSE study). CI, confidence interval; CID, clinically important deterioration; CID+, presence of a CID within 12 months of enrollment into the study; CID-, absence of a CID within 12 months of enrollment into the study; COPD, chronic obstructive pulmonary disease; ECLIPSE, Evaluation of COPD Longitudinally to Identify Predictive Surrogate End-points; FEV$_1$, forced expiratory volume in 1 s; LS, least squares; SGRQ, St George's Respiratory Questionnaire

Table 3 Risk of long-term adverse outcomes based on CIDs in the first 12 months of the ECLIPSE study

Outcome within 130 weeks of follow-up	CID+ population (N = 1442)	CID- population (N = 531)	CID+ vs CID-, HR (95% CI)
Moderate/severe COPD exacerbation, n (%)	1082 (75)	232 (44)	2.54 (2.20, 2.93)*
Hospitalization events, n (%)	454 (31)	66 (12)	2.81 (2.17, 3.63)*
Risk (HR) of all-cause mortality, n (%)	121 (8)	27 (5)	1.59 (1.04, 2.41)†

*$P < 0.001$; †$P = 0.031$

CID clinically important deterioration, CID+ presence of a CID within 6 months of enrollment into the study, CID- absence of a CID within 6 months of enrollment into the study, ECLIPSE Evaluation of COPD Longitudinally to Identify Predictive Surrogate End-points, FEV₁ forced expiratory volume in 1 s, HR hazard ratio, ITT intent-to-treat, SGRQ St George's Respiratory Questionnaire

risk of mortality to a greater extent than any single component of deterioration (eg, exacerbations). Patients free of any CID component within the first 6 months of the TORCH study had the lowest mortality risk, even compared with those experiencing only one CID component. Therefore, it would appear short-term deterioration assessed by a composite CID may predict all-cause mortality, long term. This has also been shown in a post hoc analysis of the Understanding Potential Long-Term Impacts on Function with Tiotropium (UPLIFT; NCT00144339) study, which used the same definition of CID as that presented here [27]. Furthermore, a recent analysis focused on the subgroup of patients who received the most intensified treatment in the TORCH study (FP/SAL 500/50 μg) showed similar levels of sustained loss in lung function and health status, and similarly increased risk of exacerbation and all-cause mortality in CID+ versus CID- patients compared with those presented here [28], indicating that the predictive power of on-treatment CID is not influenced by that same treatment after the CID event. Additionally, the presence of a composite CID was able to predict an increased risk of deterioration in all of the three CID domains at 3 years, supporting our rationale for using a combined measure of short-term deterioration,

rather than a single measure. The predictive power of CID status in each study was evident (at 6 months in TORCH and 12 months in the ECLIPSE study). In both studies, after 36 months, the difference in change from baseline between the CID+ and CID- groups for both FEV₁ and SGRQ score was statistically significant and exceeded the MCID for those outcome measures [11, 12]. Importantly, CID status also predicted all-cause mortality in both studies; an outcome that did not form part of the composite measure.

Although the cumulative 3-year outcomes were worse for the CID+ than the CID- group, the subsequent rate of further decline in the CID measures, beyond the assessment period (6 months for TORCH and 12 months for ECLIPSE), was similar for the two groups. Minimal recovery was observed following an initial CID, indicating that these events could signify permanent loss in health status and lung function.

Guidelines advocate regular monitoring of the adequacy of COPD care in individual patients looking at exacerbations, symptom and lung function to prevent disease progression [3]. However, no formal framework for such monitoring has been advocated. We believe indicators of increased disease activity based on a lack of favorable treatment response across the CID event types may have utility and prognostic value. The composite

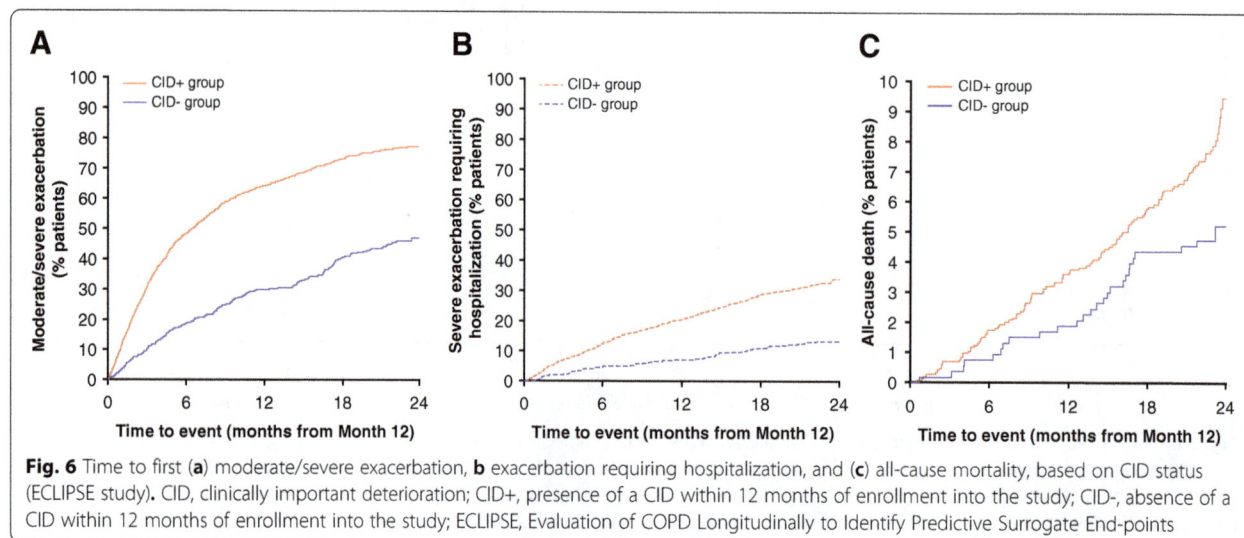

Fig. 6 Time to first (**a**) moderate/severe exacerbation, **b** exacerbation requiring hospitalization, and (**c**) all-cause mortality, based on CID status (ECLIPSE study). CID, clinically important deterioration; CID+, presence of a CID within 12 months of enrollment into the study; CID-, absence of a CID within 12 months of enrollment into the study; ECLIPSE, Evaluation of COPD Longitudinally to Identify Predictive Surrogate End-points

CID presented in this exploratory analysis appears to be a potential tool to identify increased disease activity and predict poor long-term outcome in patients with COPD based on short-term deterioration on treatment [10, 16]. While other researchers have suggested that a lack of stability in lung function or health status could predict increased future risk in COPD [6, 29], to our knowledge, the use of a prognostic composite endpoint of treatment response containing lung function, health status, and exacerbation frequency, has not previously been reported. This composite CID captures the heterogeneous nature of COPD by incorporating relatively short-term clinical measures of these three different COPD outcomes. Using a three-component composite measure of deterioration in COPD ensures that variability in a patient's response to therapy and potential for deterioration is fully captured. In concordance with this view, a recent composite CID analysis, highlighted little or no statistical concordance between the different component measures of deterioration, utilized in a 1-year exacerbation study [13].

Limitations of this analysis included its post hoc nature and the greater number of patients in the CID+ group versus the CID- group with a baseline history of exacerbations and who received ICS prior to the study in both trials, which could influence their likelihood of having an exacerbation CID. This difference did not impact long-term outcomes post-CID in this study, with prognostic findings in previous analyses of TORCH also demonstrating similar results across all treatment arms [28, 30, 31]. The CID concept developed here is in some respects opportunistic as it utilizes outcome measures available in existing clinical trial data sets. However, it includes three domains of COPD progression that can be measured relatively easily in large numbers of patients, unlike exercise capacity and daily physical activity which are more difficult to measure. Another potential limitation concerns two of the measures that form the composite CID endpoint. The complexity of post-bronchodilator rather than pre-bronchodilator FEV_1 measurement, and use of the long and complicated SGRQ rather than the simpler COPD Assessment Test (CAT), which also has an MCID [32, 33], will restrict their use to clinical trials. However, whilst the TORCH study focused on post-bronchodilator FEV_1, our analysis of the ECLIPSE study data used both post- and pre-bronchodilator FEV_1 values in the CID assessment, providing concordant findings (data not shown). Furthermore, this analysis was a test of principle and prospective studies will confirm the use of these measurements and test whether use of other outcomes, like CAT, might be more applicable to routine practice, or may replace SGRQ in assessing deterioration in health status [17, 34, 35].

Another aspect of this analysis determined by the primary trial datasets was the time and frequency at which data for all three components was available. The earliest assessment of a CID was dictated by the availability of data at 6 and 12 months in the TORCH and ECLIPSE studies, respectively. It remains unclear whether short-term assessment of a CID could be made earlier than assessed in either of these studies. It is possible that using more frequent CID assessments of FEV_1 and health status, rather than a single time point assessment as employed here, can provide more accurate prognostic assessments of mortality risk for each of these individual component event types, as suggested in a recent post hoc analysis of the UPLIFT trial [36]. As prognostic assessments in several landmark studies have identified concordant increased risk of exacerbations requiring hospitalization and mortality post CID in populations not enriched for exacerbation risk [27, 36, 37], we propose future prospective studies designed to monitor CID events in a broader symptomatic patient cohort with regular 3 monthly visits could have similar or greater predictive ability. This will be of importance to test whether less severely affected patients who are at high risk of poor medium-term outcomes can be identified and more optimally treated. These questions are being investigated prospectively in ongoing studies.

This analysis tested the predictive validity of the CID, an event-based, categorical measure of a patient's state. Previous analyses have tested the utility of CID as a measure of treatment efficacy and the benefit of escalation in therapy from mono- to dual-bronchodilation, dual-bronchodilation compared with ICS/LABA and triple therapy versus ICS/LABA therapy [10, 13–18]. All three components of the CID may find application in clinical trials, however perhaps its greatest potential may lie in predicting long-term response to treatment. Currently this requires the use of trials that are typically of 3 years' duration that may introduce bias due to differential dropout of patients with more severe disease [38]. A validated surrogate marker of medium-term outcome, such as CID status, may allow shorter term trials to test disease modification or more reliably identify candidate treatments for long-term trials.

Conclusions

The results of this retrospective analysis of two 3-year COPD studies demonstrate that short-term deterioration assessed using a composite CID endpoint had prognostic value in identifying patients with increased future risk of a sustained loss of lung function and health status, and importantly increased incidence of exacerbations requiring hospitalization and all-cause mortality. This concept of evaluating short-term changes across multiple endpoints may be a useful tool for physicians in identifying patients at greater risk of worsening of COPD and in designing trials to test treatments that may mitigate that risk.

Abbreviations

BMI: Body mass index; CAT: COPD Assessment Test; CI: Confidence intervals; CID: Clinically important deterioration; COPD: Chronic obstructive pulmonary disease; ECLIPSE: Evaluation of COPD Longitudinally to Identify Predictive Surrogate End-points; FEV_1: Forced expiratory volume in 1 s; FP: Fluticasone propionate; FVC: Forced vital capacity; HR: Hazard ratio; ICS: Inhaled corticosteroids; ITT: Intent-to-treat; LABA: Long-acting β adrenoceptor agonists; LS: Least squares; MCID: Minimum clinically important difference; OR: Odds ratio; SAL: Salmeterol; SD: Standard deviation; SGRQ: St George's respiratory questionnaire; TORCH: Towards a Revolution in COPD Health; UPLIFT: Understanding Potential Long-Term Impacts on Function with Tiotropium

Acknowledgements

Editorial support in the form of preparation of the first draft based on input from all authors, and collation and incorporation of author feedback to develop subsequent drafts was provided by Matthew Robinson, DPhil, of Fishawack Indicia Ltd., UK, and was funded by GSK.

Funding

This study was funded by GlaxoSmithKline (GSK) SCO30003 [NCT00268216] and SCO104960 [NCT00292552]). The funders of the study had a role in study design, data analysis, data interpretation, and writing of the report.

Patient consent

Not applicable.

Data sharing

Anonymized individual participant data and study documents can be requested for further research from www.clinicalstudydatarequest.com.

Authors' contributions

IPN, LT, and HM contributed to the study concept and design and were involved in data analysis and interpretation. CC and PWJ were involved in data analysis and interpretation. All authors were involved in preparation and review of the manuscript and approved the final version to be submitted. All authors agree to be accountable for all aspects of the work.

Competing interests

IPN, HM, CC, and PWJ are employees of GSK and hold GSK stocks/shares. LT is a contingent worker at GSK.

Author details

[1]Respiratory Medicine, GSK, Brentford, Middlesex, UK. [2]Precise Approach Ltd, Contingent worker on assignment at GSK, Uxbridge, Middlesex, UK.

References

1. Casanova C, Aguirre-Jaime A, de Torres JP, Pinto-Plata V, Baz R, Marin JM, et al. Longitudinal assessment in COPD patients: multidimensional variability and outcomes. Eur Respir J. 2014;43:745–53.

2. Celli BR, Cote CG, Marin JM, Casanova C, Montes de Oca M, Mendez RA, et al. The body-mass index, airflow obstruction, dyspnea, and exercise capacity index in chronic obstructive pulmonary disease. N Engl J Med. 2004;350:1005–12.

3. GOLD. Global strategy for the diagnosis, management, and prevention of chronic obstructive pulmonary disease. Updated 2018. http://goldcopd.org. Accessed 21 May 2018.

4. Jones PW, Donohue JF, Nedelman J, Pascoe S, Pinault G, Lassen C. Correlating changes in lung function with patient outcomes in chronic obstructive pulmonary disease: a pooled analysis. Respir Res. 2011;12:161.

5. Westwood M, Bourbeau J, Jones PW, Cerulli A, Capkun-Niggli G, Worthy G. Relationship between FEV1 change and patient-reported outcomes in randomised trials of inhaled bronchodilators for stable COPD: a systematic review. Respir Res. 2011;12:40.

6. Calverley PM, Postma DS, Anzueto AR, Make BJ, Eriksson G, Peterson S, et al. Early response to inhaled bronchodilators and corticosteroids as a predictor of 12-month treatment responder status and COPD exacerbations. Int J Chron Obstruct Pulmon Dis. 2016;11:381–90.

7. Martin AL, Marvel J, Fahrbach K, Cadarette SM, Wilcox TK, Donohue JF. The association of lung function and St. George's respiratory questionnaire with exacerbations in COPD: a systematic literature review and regression analysis. Respir Res. 2016;17:40.

8. Agusti A, Calverley PM, Celli B, Coxson HO, Edwards LD, Lomas DA, et al. Characterisation of COPD heterogeneity in the ECLIPSE cohort. Respir Res. 2010;11:122.

9. Oga T, Tsukino M, Hajiro T, Ikeda A, Koyama H, Mishima M, et al. Multidimensional analyses of long-term clinical courses of asthma and chronic obstructive pulmonary disease. Allergol Int. 2010;59:257–65.

10. Singh D, Maleki-Yazdi MR, Tombs L, Iqbal A, Fahy WA, Naya I. Prevention of clinically important deteriorations in COPD with umeclidinium/vilanterol. Int J Chron Obstruct Pulmon Dis. 2016;11:1413–24.

11. Donohue JF. Minimal clinically important differences in COPD lung function. COPD. 2005;2:111–24.

12. Jones PW. St. George's respiratory questionnaire: MCID. COPD. 2005;2:75–9.

13. Anzueto AR, Kostikas K, Mezzi K, Shen S, Larbig M, Patalano F, et al. Indacaterol/glycopyrronium versus salmeterol/fluticasone in the prevention of clinically important deterioration in COPD: results from the FLAME study. Respir Res. 2018;19:121.

14. Anzueto AR, Vogelmeier CF, Kostikas K, Mezzi K, Fucile S, Bader G, et al. The effect of indacaterol/glycopyrronium versus tiotropium or salmeterol/fluticasone on the prevention of clinically important deterioration in COPD. Int J Chron Obstruct Pulmon Dis. 2017;12:1325–37.

15. Buhl R, McGarvey L, Korn S, Ferguson GT, Gronke L, Hallmann C, et al. Benefits of tiotropium + olodaterol over tiotropium at delaying clinically significant events in patients with COPD classified as GOLD B. Am J Respir Crit Care Med. 2016;193:A6779.

16. Maleki-Yazdi MR, Singh D, Anzueto A, Tombs L, Fahy WA, Naya I. Assessing short-term deterioration in maintenance-naive patients with COPD receiving umeclidinium/vilanterol and tiotropium: a pooled analysis of three randomized trials. Adv Ther. 2016;33(12):2188–99.

17. Naya I, Compton C, Ismaila A, Birk R, Brealey N, Tabberer M, et al. Preventing clinically important deterioration with single-inhaler triple therapy in COPD. ERJ Open Res. 2018; In press.

18. Naya I, Tombs L, Lipson D, Compton C. Preventing clinically important deterioration of COPD with addition of umeclidinium to inhaled corticosteroid/long-acting β2-agonist therapy:an integrated post hoc analysis. Adv Ther. 2018; In press.

19. Calverley PM, Anderson JA, Celli B, Ferguson GT, Jenkins C, Jones PW, et al. Salmeterol and fluticasone propionate and survival in chronic obstructive pulmonary disease. N Engl J Med. 2007;356:775–89.

20. Vestbo J, Anderson W, Coxson HO, Crim C, Dawber F, Edwards L, et al. Evaluation of COPD longitudinally to identify predictive surrogate end-points (ECLIPSE). Eur Respir J. 2008;31:869–73.

21. Vestbo J. The TORCH (towards a revolution in COPD health) survival study protocol. Eur Respir J. 2004;24:206–10.

22. Spencer S, Calverley PM, Sherwood Burge P, Jones PW, Disease ISGISiOL. Health status deterioration in patients with chronic obstructive pulmonary disease. Am J Respir Crit Care Med. 2001;163:122–8.

23. Oga T, Nishimura K, Tsukino M, Sato S, Hajiro T, Mishima M. Exercise capacity deterioration in patients with COPD: longitudinal evaluation over 5 years. Chest. 2005;128:62–9.

24. Waschki B, Kirsten AM, Holz O, Mueller KC, Schaper M, Sack AL, et al. Disease progression and changes in physical activity in patients with chronic obstructive pulmonary disease. Am J Respir Crit Care Med. 2015;192:295–306.

25. Nagai K, Makita H, Suzuki M, Shimizu K, Konno S, Ito YM, et al. Differential changes in quality of life components over 5 years in chronic obstructive pulmonary disease patients. Int J Chron Obstruct Pulmon Dis. 2015;10:745–57.

26. Celli BR, Thomas NE, Anderson JA, Ferguson GT, Jenkins CR, Jones PW, et al. Effect of pharmacotherapy on rate of decline of lung function in chronic obstructive pulmonary disease: results from the TORCH study. Am J Respir Crit Care Med. 2008;178:332–8.

27. Han MK, Halpin DMG, Martinez FJ, Miravitlles M, Singh D, de la Hoz A, et al. A composite endpoint of clinically important deterioration in chronic obstructive pulmonary disease and its association with increased mortality: a post hoc analysis of the UPLIFT study. Am J Respir Crit Care Med. 2018; 197:A4245.

28. Naya I, Driessen MT, Paly V, Gunsoy N, Risebrough N, Briggs A, et al. Long-term consequences of clinically important deterioration in patients with chronic obstructive pulmonary disease treated with twice-daily inhaled corticosteroid/long-acting β2-agonist therapy: results from the TORCH study. Am J Respir Crit Care Med. 2018;197:A3042.

29. Wilke S, Jones PW, Mullerova H, Vestbo J, Tal-Singer R, Franssen FM, et al. One-year change in health status and subsequent outcomes in COPD. Thorax. 2015;70:420–5.

30. Naya I, Tombs L, Jones P. Short-term clinically important deterioration predicts long-term clinical outcome in COPD patients: a post-hoc analysis of the TORCH trial. Thorax. 2015;70:A34–5.

31. Naya I, Tombs L, Jones P. Combination therapy with inhaled salmeterol plus fluticasone propionate is more effective than salmeterol alone in reducing the risk of clinically important deterioration in COPD: a post-hoc analysis of the TORCH trial. Thorax. 2015;70:A136–A37.

32. Jones PW, Harding G, Berry P, Wiklund I, Chen WH, Kline Leidy N. Development and first validation of the COPD assessment test. Eur Respir J. 2009;34:648–54.

33. Kon SS, Canavan JL, Jones SE, Nolan CM, Clark AL, Dickson MJ, et al. Minimum clinically important difference for the COPD assessment test: a prospective analysis. Lancet Respir Med. 2014;2:195–203.

34. Lipson DA, Barnacle H, Birk R, Brealey N, Locantore N, Lomas DA, et al. FULFIL trial: once-daily triple therapy for patients with chronic obstructive pulmonary disease. Am J Respir Crit Care Med. 2017;196:438–46.

35. Lipson DA, Barnhart F, Brealey N, Brooks J, Criner GJ, Day NC, et al. Once-daily single-inhaler triple versus dual therapy in patients with COPD. N Engl J Med. 2018;378:1671–80.

36. Rabe KF, Halpin D, Martinez F, Singh D, Han MK, Zehendner CM, et al. Relative timing of clinically important deterioration and related long-term outcomes in copd: a post hoc analysis of the uplift study. Pneumologie. 2018;72:86–7.

37. Naya I, Tombs L, Mullerova H, Compton C, Jones P. Long-term outcome following first clinically important deterioration in COPD. Eur Respir J. 2016; 48:PA304.

38. Vestbo J, Anderson JA, Calverley PM, Celli B, Ferguson GT, Jenkins C, et al. Bias due to withdrawal in long-term randomised trials in COPD: evidence from the TORCH study. Clin Respir J. 2011;5:44–9.

20

Influence of viral infection on the relationships between airway cytokines and lung function in asthmatic children

Toby C. Lewis[1,4,6], Ediri E. Metitiri[1], Graciela B. Mentz[6], Xiaodan Ren[4], Ashley R. Carpenter[1], Adam M. Goldsmith[1], Kyra E. Wicklund[1,5], Breanna N. Eder[1], Adam T. Comstock[1], Jeannette M. Ricci[1], Sean R. Brennan[1], Ginger L. Washington[1], Kendall B. Owens[1], Bhramar Mukherjee[3], Thomas G. Robins[4], Stuart A. Batterman[4], Marc B. Hershenson[1,2]* and the Community Action Against Asthma Steering Committee

Abstract

Background: Few longitudinal studies examine inflammation and lung function in asthma. We sought to determine the cytokines that reduce airflow, and the influence of respiratory viral infections on these relationships.

Methods: Children underwent home collections of nasal lavage during scheduled surveillance periods and self-reported respiratory illnesses. We studied 53 children for one year, analyzing 392 surveillance samples and 203 samples from 85 respiratory illnesses. Generalized estimated equations were used to evaluate associations between nasal lavage biomarkers (7 mRNAs, 10 proteins), lung function and viral infection.

Results: As anticipated, viral infection was associated with increased cytokines and reduced FVC and FEV_1. However, we found frequent and strong interactions between biomarkers and virus on lung function. For example, in the absence of viral infection, CXCL10 mRNA, MDA5 mRNA, CXCL10, IL-4, IL-13, CCL4, CCL5, CCL20 and CCL24 were negatively associated with FVC. In contrast, during infection, the opposite relationship was frequently found, with IL-4, IL-13, CCL5, CCL20 and CCL24 levels associated with less severe reductions in both FVC and FEV_1.

Conclusions: In asthmatic children, airflow obstruction is driven by specific pro-inflammatory cytokines. In the absence of viral infection, higher cytokine levels are associated with decreasing lung function. However, with infection, there is a reversal in this relationship, with cytokine abundance associated with reduced lung function decline. While nasal samples may not reflect lower airway responses, these data suggest that some aspects of the inflammatory response may be protective against viral infection. This study may have ramifications for the treatment of viral-induced asthma exacerbations.

Keywords: Asthma, Chemokine, Children, Cytokine, FEV_1, FVC, Rhinovirus, Urban, Viral

Background

Geographic areas with high concentrations of low-income and minority ethnicity residents have high levels of asthma morbidity and mortality [1–3]. The factors leading to loss of asthma control and asthma exacerbations are complex.

Previous studies have identified atopy, inadequate treatment, respiratory viral infections and environmental exposures as important drivers of asthma morbidity [4–7].

The effects of real-world respiratory viral infections on airway inflammation remain largely undefined. We [8] and others [9–12] have examined the innate immune response of children with asthma to natural colds. We found that nasal aspirate cytokine levels significantly increased in children with asthma. In addition, we found that a subset of cytokines (IFN-γ, CXCL8, CCL2, CCL4, CCL5, and CCL20) correlated

* Correspondence: mhershen@umich.edu
[1]Departments of Pediatrics and Communicable Diseases, University of Michigan Medical School, 1150 W. Medical Center Dr., Building MSRB2, Room 3570B, Ann Arbor, MI 48109-5688, USA
[2]Molecular and Integrative Physiology, University of Michigan Medical School, Ann Arbor, USA
Full list of author information is available at the end of the article

with self-reported respiratory tract symptoms. However, we did not examine the influences of viral infection or nasal cytokines on airway function. Further, by limiting comparisons to samples taken during virus-negative well periods and viral-induced exacerbations, we ignored the potential effects of subacute viral infection. Finally, our cross-sectional study did not allow us to examine patterns of variables over time, which could provide more consistent information about the cytokines that drive lung function changes in chronic asthma.

The current study is drawn from an observational cohort of asthmatic school age children from Detroit who were concurrently enrolled in investigations examining the relationship between near-roadway exposures on asthma outcomes [13]. In addition to collecting measures of asthma health, we collected nasal lavage for detection of viral infection and measurement of respiratory tract cytokines and other biomarkers, and performed spirometry to assess lung function. We sought to determine the cytokines that drive reduced airflow, together with the influence of viral infections on these relationships. We hypothesized that children with greater respiratory tract inflammation would demonstrate worse airway function, and that viral infections would increase inflammation and negatively impact asthma symptoms and airway function. While our hypothesis was generally correct, we found that, in the presence of viral infection, higher levels of cytokines were associated with reduced lung function decline.

Methods
Study design and screening questionnaire
This study was conducted by Community Action Against Asthma (CAAA), a community-based participatory research (CBPR) partnership. School-age children with known or probable asthma were recruited using a screening questionnaire [14] distributed at community venues and through door-to-door recruitment in neighborhoods near highways. The questionnaire included demographic information, eight symptom questions, and if their child had ever been diagnosed by a medical care provider with any of the following conditions: asthma, bronchitis, bronchiolitis, reactive airways disease, pneumonia, or asthmatic bronchitis. In addition, parents were asked whether their child had taken prescription medication for any of these conditions in the last 12 months and, if so, whether they were taking these medications on a daily basis. Classification of asthma severity was based on symptom frequency and reported inhaled steroid use (Additional file 1: Table S1). This study was approved by the University of Michigan Medical School Institutional Review Board (IRBMED) (ID# HUM00018442) and conducted according to CBPR principles under the auspices of the CAAA Steering Committee.

Data and sample collection
Fifty-three children participated in a two-week surveillance assessment period of health status each season from fall 2010 to summer 2011. During each two-week surveillance period, staff obtained spirometry, symptom reports and nasal lavage samples during three home visits. Respiratory symptoms were assessed using a modification of a previously developed respiratory symptom score [15] which assessed fever, cough, sore throat, nasal symptoms, wheezing, difficulty breathing and interference with usual activities (see Additional file 1: Table S2). Families were given a calendar and a simple respiratory symptom scale to mark the level of their symptoms.

From winter 2010 to summer 2011, measurements were repeated during a one-week period whenever the child experienced a symptomatic respiratory illness as defined by a symptom score of two or higher (referred to as a "sick period"). We intentionally set a low symptom threshold in order to maximize sensitivity to detect viral illnesses. Families contacted a central phone number when the child became ill. Staff would tally the symptom score over the phone and when symptoms reached the appropriate threshold, would begin a "sick period" assessment within 48 h of the phone call (median time to first sample was 72 h after the development of symptoms). Staff also conducted weekly telephone calls to identify illnesses in progress that families may not have called in to report, and would initiate a "sick period" collection if family reported that the child had current symptoms.

Spirometry
Using protocols that we developed and successfully utilized in large-scale community-based asthma studies [7], staff conducted spirometry to assess lung function during home visits, using the EasyOne spirometer (NDD, Andover, MA). Additional details on spirometric procedures are described in Additional file 1.

Nasal lavage
Nasal lavage samples were collected three times during a two-week surveillance period or three times during a one-week sick period by the field staff. Two squirts of isotonic 0.65% sodium chloride (estimated to be < 1 ml per nostril, B.F. Ascher, Lenexa, KS) were instilled into the child's nostrils Subjects then blew their nose into a zippered plastic bag, and three ml of M4RT viral transport medium (Remel, Lenexa, KS) was added. After collection, samples were double bagged, placed in a transport cooler at 0 °C, conveyed to a local laboratory (Henry Ford Health System Epidemiology Lab) for preliminary processing and freezing to − 70 °C, and subsequently transported to Ann Arbor on dry ice.

Detection of respiratory viruses

Whole nasal lavage samples were homogenized using a hand held homogenizer (Thermo Fisher Scientific, Waltham, MA). Nucleic acids were extracted using TRIzol-LS (ThermoFisher, Waltham, MA), chloroform and an RNeasy Mini Kit (Qiagen, Valencia, CA). Samples were analyzed for viral nucleic acid by multiplex PCR using the Seeplex RV-15 ACE detection kit (Seegene, Concord, CA). This kit detects human adenovirus, bocavirus 1–4, coronaviruses 229E/NL63 and OC43, enterovirus, influenza A and B, metapneumovirus, parainfluenza viruses 1–4, RSV A and B and rhinovirus A, B and C. For surveillance samples, all specimens were analyzed for virus; for sick samples, specimens from the same sick week were pooled prior to analysis (samples from sick periods were not pooled for cytokine or viral copy number determination, see below).

Nasal lavage mRNA and protein expression

All nasal lavage samples were analyzed for mRNA and protein. cDNA was synthesized from total RNA by Taqman reverse transcriptase kit (Qiagen). DNA was digested with DNase I (Qiagen). CXCL8, CXCL10, IRF7, RIG-I, MDA5, TLR3 and IFN-λ1 mRNA expression were measured by qPCR. Specific primers and probes spanning exon-exon junctions (intron splice-sites) were used to prevent amplification of genomic DNA (Additional file 1: Table S3, Online Repository). Expression levels were normalized to GAPDH using the ΔΔCt method. Reactions with a cycle number higher than 35 were not included in the analysis. CXCL8, CXCL10, CCL2, CCL4, CCL5, CCL20, CCL24, IL-4, IL-13 and soluble ICAM-1 (sICAM) protein levels were determined by multiplex immune assay (Affymetrix, Santa Clara, CA). Minimum detection levels for the proteins assayed are provided in the Additional file 1: Table S4. Biomarkers were chosen based on previous studies showing elevations after RV infection, our interest in examining biomarkers we had not previously studied, difficulty of detecting some biomarkers or cytokines in the nasal aspirate fluid, cost and availability.

Statistical analysis

Assessment of the distribution of spirometric data and nasal lavage biomarkers was conducted using means, medians, histograms and QQ plots (data not shown). Because of strong right skewedness, biomarker values were natural log transformed for subsequent analyses. The effects of viral infection on group median nasal lavage mRNA and protein expression were analyzed by the Wilcoxon Median Test. We chose to use a non-parametric test because the transformed cytokine distributions were still slightly skewed, with a number of zero values and high outliers which we did not exclude from the analysis. In addition, because we divided subjects and samples by asthma

severity, we had a small sample size for some measures. Finally, in the case of TLR3 and IFN-λ1 mRNAs, which were detected in only 35 and 11% of the samples, data were analyzed as binary variables by Fisher's exact test.

For our primary analyses, we evaluated the strength of association between mean respiratory tract inflammatory responses and pulmonary function using generalized estimating equations (GEE) with an exchangeable correlation structure using the identity link in the case of continuous outcomes and the log link for binary ones (SAS, Cary, NC). This design allowed us to test the influence of cytokine on lung function with and without virus. GEE was used rather than logistic or Poisson models because of the longitudinal nature of the data and the repeated observations for each child [16, 17]. The GEE procedure can be used for small populations [18]. All individual samples (virus-negative and virus-positive "surveillance samples," virus-negative and virus-positive "sick samples") were included in the analysis. We adjusted for covariates including age, gender, ethnicity/race, smoker in the home, caregiver educational attainment, self-reported atopy, caregiver depressive symptom score, season and whether the sample was from a surveillance or sick period. Family income, baseline asthma severity, medication use and proximity to high-traffic highways were evaluated but not included in final models as they were not significant predictors or were collinear with other covariates in the model. In a secondary analysis, linear plots of lung function and cytokine level when virus was either absent or present were generated. Additional details on statistical analysis are described in Additional file 1.

Results

Study participants

Fifty-three children between 5 and 12 years-old were enrolled. Subjects predominantly self-identified as African-American (Table 1). The majority was reported by their parent/caregiver to be atopic, exposed to tobacco smoke and live in a household with an income ≤ $15,000. Most children reported symptoms or medication use consistent with mild intermittent or mild persistent asthma, but one-quarter had moderate-to-severe persistent disease. At enrollment, one-quarter of the subjects were taking inhaled corticosteroids or used them within the last year. Group mean FVC, FEV_1 and PEF during the first surveillance period were in the range of normal, but FEV_1/FVC ratio and FEF_{25-75} were reduced (Table 2). It should be noted that, although all children met initial criteria for participation, only 47 of 53 children performed acceptable expiratory maneuvers for spirometric analysis.

Participant respiratory illnesses

From September 2010 to August 2011, 392 surveillance samples were collected, 105 (26%) of which were positive

Table 1 Participant baseline characteristics ($n = 53$)

Age in years, mean (SD)	9.7 (2.1)
Female gender, n (%)	23 (43.4)
Race, Non-Hispanic African-American, n (%)	46 (86.8)
Household income ≤ $15,000, n (%)	30 (56.6)
Caregiver years of education ≤12, n (%)	30 (56.6)
Caregiver depression CESD score, mean (SD)	8.8 (5.1)
Smoker in household, n (%)	36 (67.9)
Asthma severity, N (%)	
Moderate or severe persistent	14 (26.4)
Mild persistent	27 (50.9)
Mild intermittent	12 (22.6)
Atopy (self-reported), yes (%)	38 (71.7)
Any asthma medication use in last 12 months, n (%)	
Inhaled corticosteroids	12 (22.6)
Short acting bronchodilator only	21 (39.6)
No asthma medication	20 (37.7)
Asthma control test (ACT) score, mean (SD)	20.0 (4.2)

Table 3 Participant viral infections

	N	% of total
Surveillance collection ($N = 410$)		
No virus	288	70.2
Virus	94	22.9
Rhinovirus		
Single infections	46	11.2
Multiple infections	4	1.0
Non-rhinovirus		
Single infections[a]	39	9.5
Multiple infections	5	1.2
Cold collection (number of pooled samples = 92)		
No virus	55	60.0
Virus	28	30.4
Rhinovirus		
Single infections	20	21.7
Multiple infections	2	2.2
Non-rhinovirus		
Single infections[b]	6	6.5
Multiple infections	0	0.0

[a]Coronavirus 229E/NL63 (9), RSV A (8), coronavirus OC43 (5), RSV B (4), influenza A (4), influenza B (3), adenovirus (2), metapneumovirus (2), parainfluenza 2 (2)
[b]Influenza A (2), influenza B, coronavirus 229E/NL63, parainfluenza 2, RSV B

for one or more viruses. From December 2010 to August 2011, there were 85 self-reported respiratory illnesses, for which 233 samples were collected. Analysis of pooled samples for each illness showed that 30 (35%) of these illnesses were positive for at least one virus. RV was detected in 54 out of 105 (51%) of the virus-positive surveillance samples and 23 out of 30 (77%) of virus-positive sick illnesses (Table 3).

Effects of viral infection on lung function

We examined the influence of asthma severity on the lung function response to viral infection. When we divided subjects into mild intermittent, mild persistent and moderate-to-severe persistent asthma, we found that subjects with moderate-to-severe persistent asthma experienced significant ($p < 0.05$) reductions in FVC and FEV_1 after viral infection (Fig. 1). Changes in FEV_1/FVC ($p = 0.08$) and FEF_{25-75} ($p = 0.09$) did not reach statistical significance.

Table 2 Baseline surveillance valid health measures

	N	Median (Range)
Symptom Score	53	2.3 (0, 27)
Lung function (% of predicted)	N	Mean (SD)
FVC	43	98.5 (17.0)
FEV_1	43	90.3 (18.3)
FEV_1/FVC ratio	43	79.3 (6.6)
FEF_{25-75}	42	70.8 (21.9)
PEF	42	91.3 (19.1)

Effects of viral infection on nasal lavage biomarkers

All nasal samples were analyzed for mRNA expression of CXCL8, CXCL10, IFN-λ1, TLR3, MDA5, RIG-I and IRF7. Samples were also analyzed for CXCL8, CXCL10, IL-4, IL-13, sICAM-1, CCL2, CCL4, CCL5, CCL20 and CCL24 protein. The median individual surveillance and sick period samples analyzed per subject was 7 (range, 1–12) and 3 (range, 2–15), respectively. MDA-5, RIG-I, IRF7, CXCL10 and CXCL8 mRNA were detected in the 73–99% of the samples, whereas TLR3 and IFN-λ1 mRNA were detected in 35 and 11% of the samples, respectively.

The effect of viral infection on group median cytokine data are shown in Table 4. Viral infections were associated with significantly increased mRNA expression of CXCL10, RIG-I and MDA5 and protein expression of all biomarkers tested. In addition, viral infections were associated with an increase in the percentage of samples with detectable TLR3 and IFN-λ1 mRNA. Responses to RV and non-RV infections were generally similar, except for TLR3 mRNA and CXCL8 protein, which were not increased in non-RV infections (data not shown).

Next, we examined the influence of asthma severity on the cytokine responses to viral infection. In subjects with moderate-to-severe persistent asthma, viral infection was associated with significant increases in mRNA expression of CXCL10 and MDA5 (Fig. 2). Viral infection was also associated with increased mRNA expression of CXCL10 in

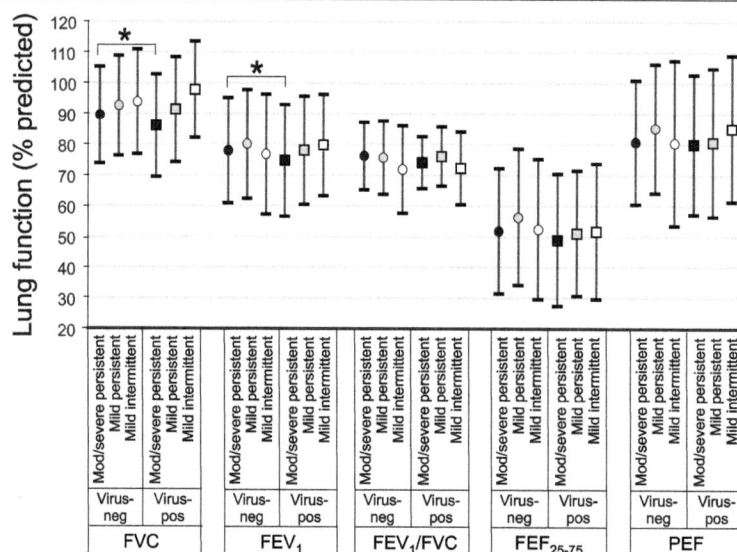

Fig. 1 Effect of viral infection on spirometry in subjects with moderate-to-severe persistent (black symbols), mild persistent (grey symbols) and mild intermittent asthma (white symbols). FVC, FEV1, FEF25–75 and PEF are shown (mean ± SD). GEE models were used for pairwise comparison of the means (*$p < 0.05$)

Table 4 Effect of viral infection on nasal lavage mRNA and protein expression

	Virus-negative			Virus-positive			
mRNA	N	Median	IQR	N	Median	IQR	p-value
CXCL8	404	4.68	(2.15, 9.71)	174	5.01	(2.45, 10.78)	0.54
CXCL10	404	0.001	(0.00, 0.01)	174	0.0098	(0.001, 0.06)	< 0.01
IRF7	404	0.06	(0.02, 0.14)	174	0.06	(0.02, 0.14)	0.99
RIG-I	404	0.01	(0.00, 0.03)	174	0.02	(0.00, 0.05)	0.04
MDA5	404	0.01	(0.00, 0.03)	174	0.02	(0.01, 0.07)	< 0.01
Binary	N	Detected (%)		N	Detected (%)		p-value
TLR3	404	132/404 (32.7)		174	69 (39.7)		0.11
IFN-λ1	404	30/404 (7.4)		174	33 (19.0)		< 0.01
Protein	N	Median	IQR	N	Median	IQR	p-value
CXCL8	433	177.00	(71.5, 431.6)	172	253.35	(97.25, 868.9)	< 0.01
CXCL10	429	397.90	(213.9, 656.2)	171	703.20	(419.5, 1553.5)	< 0.01
IL-4	436	15.60	(4.9, 51.65)	175	31.10	(9.3, 75.2)	< 0.01
IL-13	428	4.60	(0.0, 27.1)	167	18.80	(0.0, 37.8)	< 0.01
sICAM1	431	293.20	(100.8, 643.6)	170	560.20	(207.6, 1219.2)	< 0.01
CCL2	433	71.40	(26.9, 132.9)	170	103.70	(40.3, 219.6)	< 0.01
CCL4	426	300.9	(40.3, 1261.9)	170	1198.65	(163.0, 3050.6)	< 0.01
CCL5	433	5.00	(0.0, 18.1)	174	9.55	(0.0, 27.4)	< 0.01
CCL20	439	290.3	(78.0, 651.1)	178	580.0	(186.1, 1184.5)	< 0.01
CCL24	434	4.47	(1.06, 14.24)	175	9.16	(2.56, 21.06)	< 0.01

Levels of mRNA expression are normalized to GAPDH. Group median data are shown except for TLR3 and IFN-λ1 mRNA, for which results were analyzed as binary variables. Samples were divided into virus-negative and virus positive. Differences were analyzed by the Wilcoxon Median Test except for TLR3 and IFN-λ1 which were analyzed by Fisher's exact test

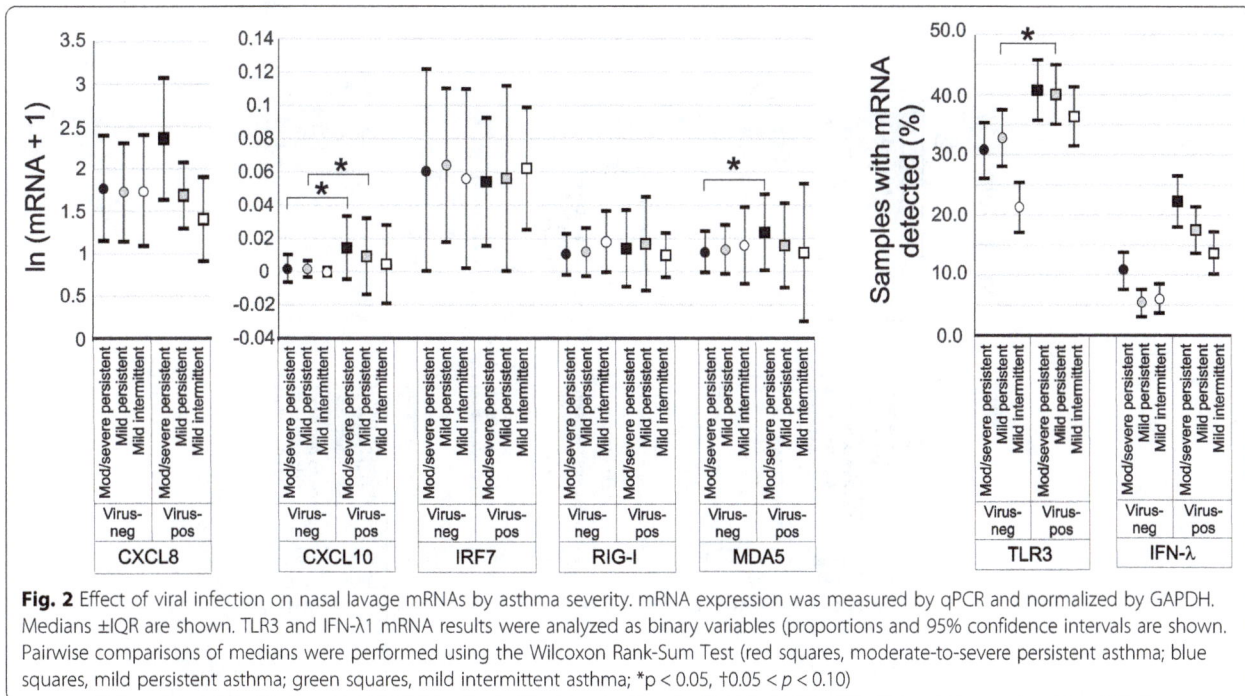

Fig. 2 Effect of viral infection on nasal lavage mRNAs by asthma severity. mRNA expression was measured by qPCR and normalized by GAPDH. Medians ±IQR are shown. TLR3 and IFN-λ1 mRNA results were analyzed as binary variables (proportions and 95% confidence intervals are shown. Pairwise comparisons of medians were performed using the Wilcoxon Rank-Sum Test (red squares, moderate-to-severe persistent asthma; blue squares, mild persistent asthma; green squares, mild intermittent asthma; *p < 0.05, †0.05 < p < 0.10)

subjects with mild persistent asthma. Viral infection was associated with an increase in the number of samples with detectable TLR3 mRNA expression in subjects with mild persistent asthma. Finally, compared to other virus-positive groups, the number of IFN-λ1 mRNA-positive samples tended to be higher in infected subjects with moderate-to-severe asthma ($p = 0.09$).

In moderate-to-severe persistent asthmatics, viral infection was associated with increased protein abundance of CXCL10, IL-4, sICAM-1, CCL2, CCL20 and CCL24 (Fig. 3). In mild persistent asthmatics, viral infection was associated with increased protein abundance of CXCL10, sICAM-1, CCL2, CCL4, CCL5, CCL20 and CCL24. Virus-positive samples from subjects with mild intermittent asthma showed no significant increases in protein expression.

Associations of nasal lavage biomarker, viral infection and lung function

Next, we evaluated the strength of association between respiratory tract inflammatory responses and pulmonary function using GEE, including an interaction term between viral presence and inflammatory marker. Most unexpectedly, we found frequent and strong interactions between biomarkers and virus on lung function. For FVC, statistically significant interactions between viral infection and inflammation were seen for CXCL10 mRNA, TLR3 mRNA, IL-4, IL-13, CCL5, CCL20 and CCL24 (Additional file 1: Table S5). The interaction between viral infection and CCL4 approached statistical significance. In contrast, CXCL10 protein showed a negative association with FVC independently of infection.

Figure 4 shows the graphical relationships between nasal lavage biomarker levels and FVC in the absence and presence of viral infection. (Panels for the binary variables TLR3 and IFN-λ mRNA are not shown.) In the absence of virus, there were significant negative associations between biomarker and FVC for CXCL10 mRNA, MDA5 mRNA, CXCL10, IL-4, IL-13, CCL4, CCL5, CCL20 and CCL24. In the presence of virus, there were significant positive associations between biomarker and FVC for IL-4, IL-13, CCL5, CCL20 and CCL24.

Longitudinal analysis also showed a significant influence of viral infection on the associations between biomarkers and FEV_1 (Additional file 1: Table S6). For FEV_1, statistically significant interactions between viral infection and inflammation were seen for CXCL10 and TLR3 mRNA, IL-4 and CCL24 levels. Interactions with CCL4 and CCL5 approached statstsical significance. CXCL10 protein levels had negative associations with FEV_1, independent of viral infection. Again, these patterns are discerned graphically (Fig. 5). In the absence of virus, there were significant negative associations between biomarker and FEV_1 for CXCL10, RIG-I and MDA5 mRNA. In the presence of virus, there were significant positive associations between biomarker and FEV_1 for MDA5 mRNA, IL-4, IL-13, sICAM-1, CCL2, CCL5, CCL20 and CCL24.

The influence of viral infection on the relationships between nasal lavage biomarkers and FEV_1/FVC, FEF_{25-75} and PEF are fully described in this article's Online Repository (Additional file 1: Tables S7-S9). For these lung function parameters there was less of an effect of viral infection on cytokine level. For FEV_1/FVC, FEF_{25-75} and

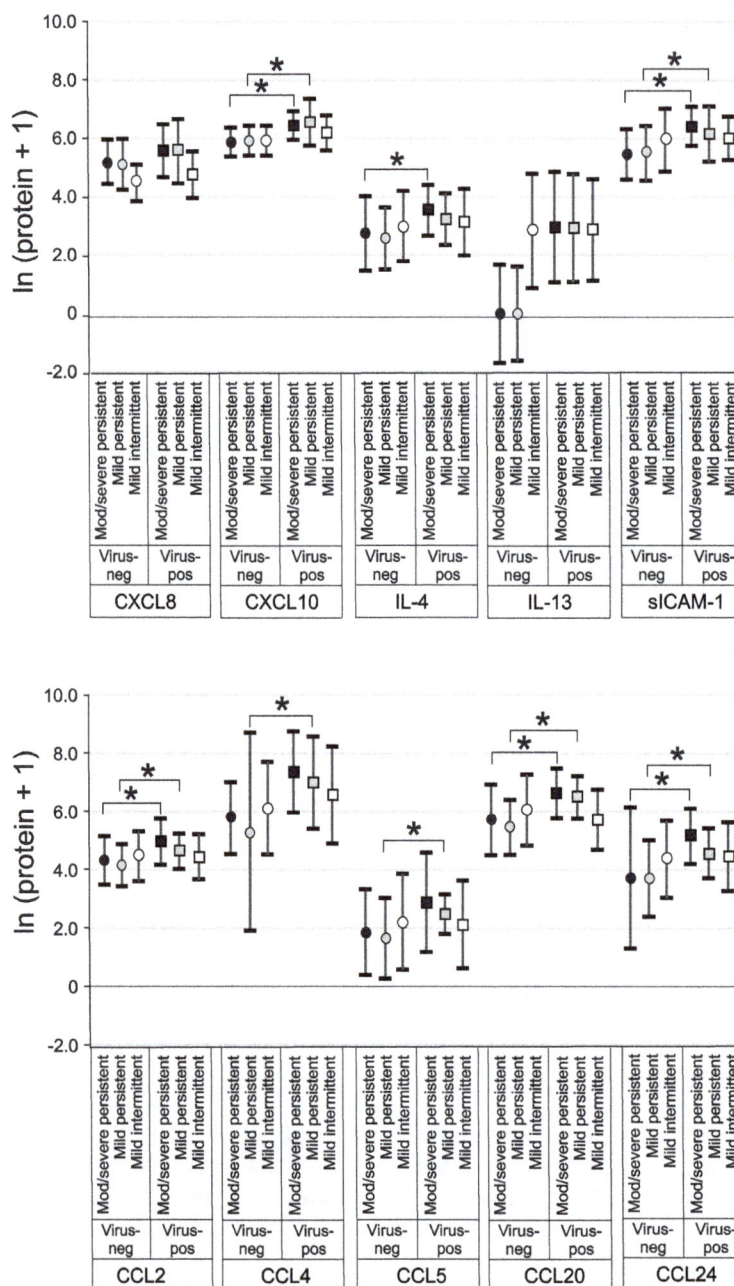

Fig. 3 Effects of viral infection on nasal lavage cytokine concentrations by asthma severity (median ± IQR). Cytokines were measured by multiplex immune assay. Pairwise comparisons of medians were performed using the Wilcoxon Rank-Sum Test (black symbols, moderate-to-severe persistent asthma; grey symbols, mild persistent asthma; white symbols, mild intermittent asthma; *p < 0.05)

PEF, statistically significant interactions between viral infection and inflammation were seen for CXCL10 mRNA. For PEF, interactions between viral infection and RIG-I and TLR3 mRNA were also seen. RIG-I mRNA had a negative association with FEV_1/FVC independent of viral infection. CXCL8 mRNA and protein levels had a negative association with FEF_{25-75} independent of viral infection. RIG-I and MDA5 mRNA had negative associations with PEF independent of viral infection. Finally,

viral infection was strongly associated with significant reductions in FEF_{25-75}.

Discussion

Previous studies have shown increased abundance of airway cytokines following both natural [8–12, 19, 20] and experimental [21, 22] colds. In this report, we examine the interactive effects of viral infection and airway cytokines on lung function in patients with

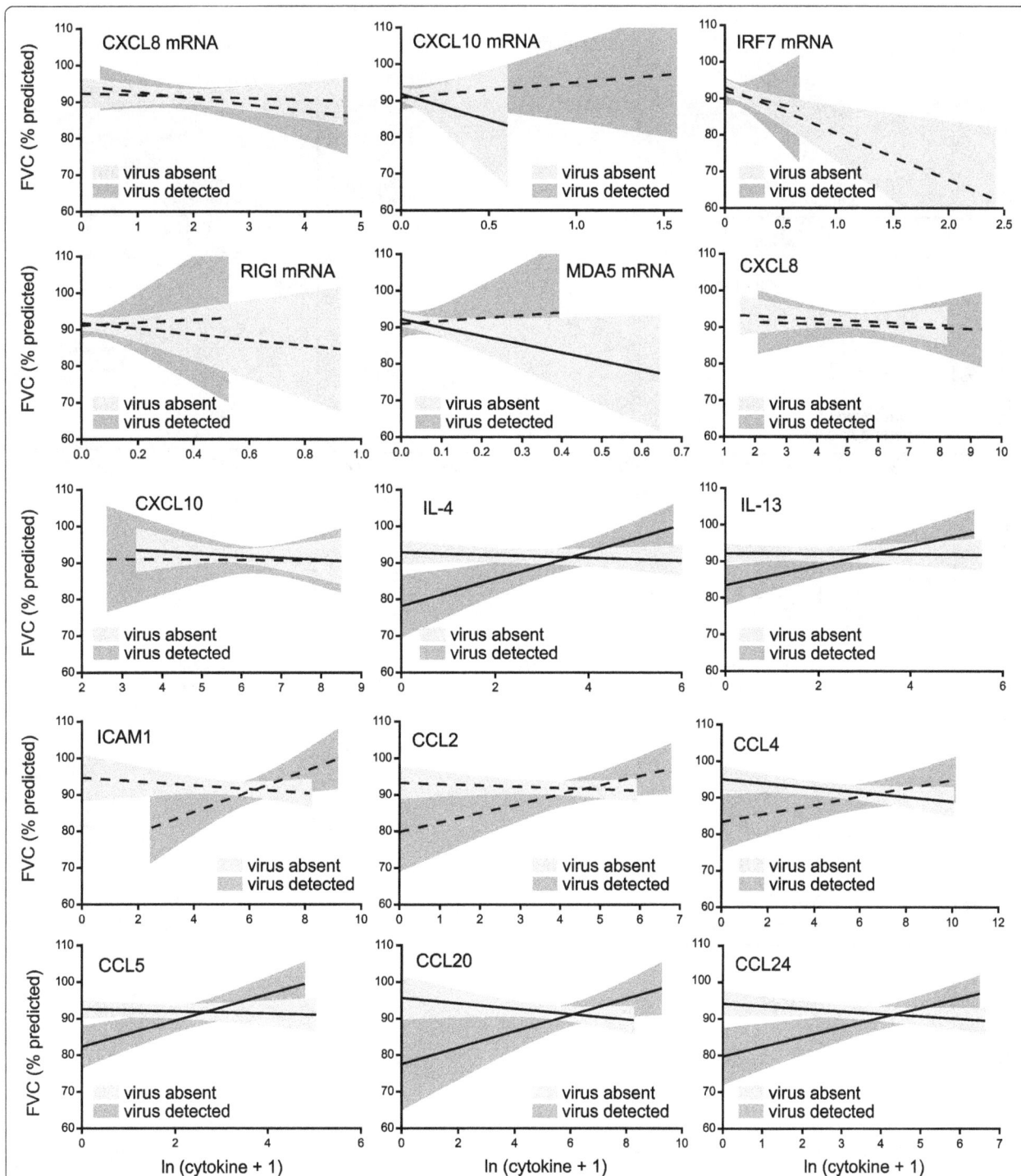

Fig. 4 Effect of viral infection on the relationships between log-transformed nasal lavage biomarker levels and percent predicted FVC. In the absence of virus, we found negative associations between biomarker level and FVC (unadjusted 95% confidence intervals are shown in light grey, solid lines indicate a statistically significant association between cytokine and FVC by GEE; dashed lines indicate no statistically significant association). However, in the presence of virus, increasing levels of biomarker had a positive effect on FVC (unadjusted 95% confidence intervals are shown in dark grey; solid lines indicate a statistically significant association). For clarity individual data points are not shown here, but may be found in Additional file 2: Figure S1

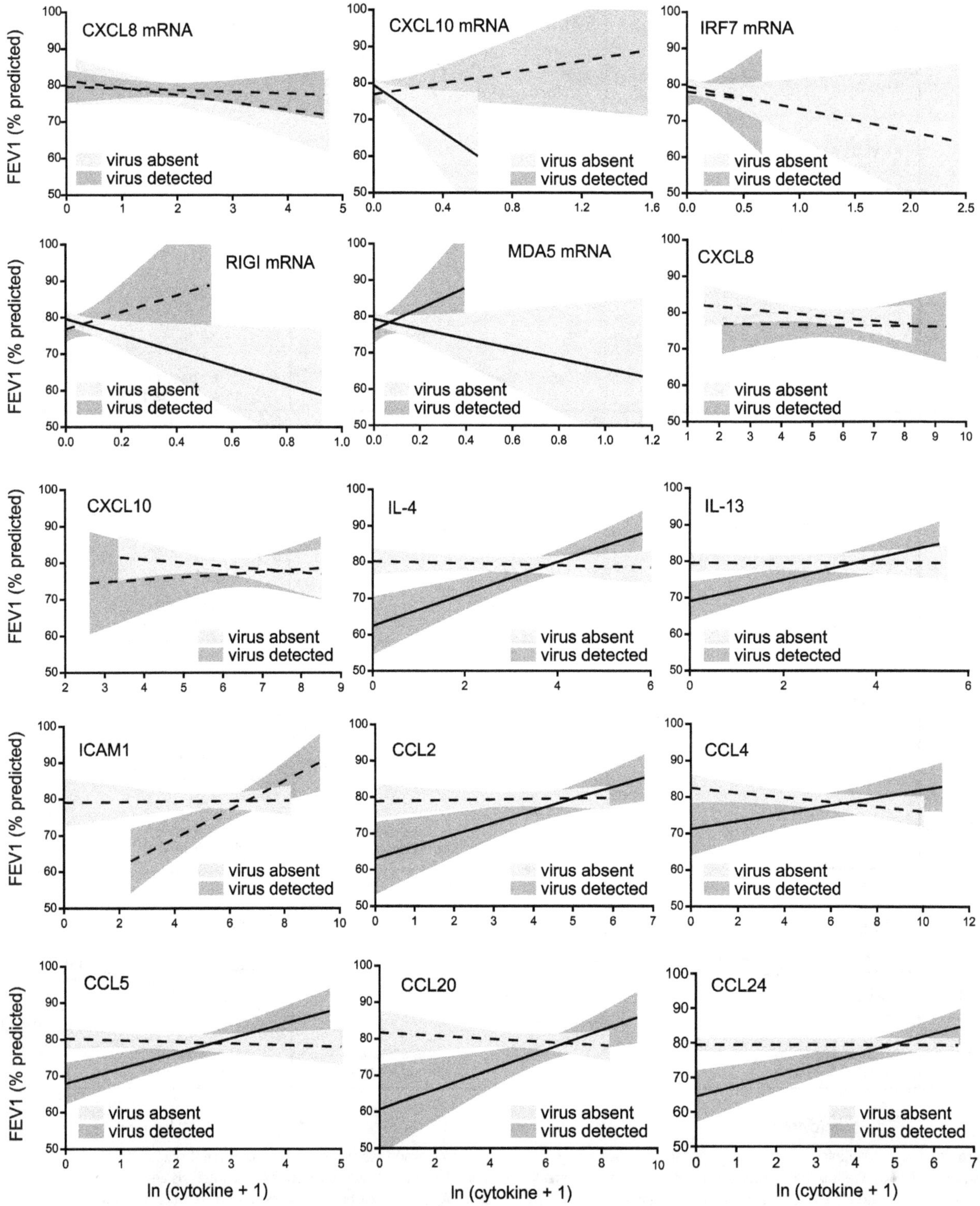

Fig. 5 Effect of viral infection on the relationships between log-transformed nasal lavage biomarker levels and percent predicted FEV1. In the absence of virus, we found negative associations between biomarker level and FEV1 (95% confidence intervals are shown in light grey, with solid lines indicating a significant association between cytokine and FEV1 by GEE; dashed lines indicate no statistically significant association). In the presence of virus, increasing levels of biomarker had a positive effect on FEV1 (95% confidence intervals are shown in dark grey; solid lines indicate a statistically significant association). For clarity individual data points are not shown here, but may be found in Additional file 3: Figure S2

asthma. We anticipated that, in the absence of virus, children with greater airway inflammation would demonstrate worse airway function. Consistent with this, in the absence of viral infection, several nasal lavage biomarkers correlated negatively with lung function. For example, CXCL10 mRNA, MDA5 mRNA, CXCL10, IL-4, IL-13, CCL4, CCL5, CCL20 and CCL24 were each negatively associated with FVC. We also expected that viral infections would increase inflammation and negatively impact airway function. Accordingly, we found that viral infection had independent positive associations with nearly all nasal lavage biomarkers and, in subjects with moderate-to-severe persistent asthma, negative influences on FVC and FEV_1. However, we found many cases in which there was a significant interactive effect between viral infection and lung function, in that the simultaneous presence of viral infection and high cytokine levels was associated with less severe reductions in lung function. Among other associations, in the presence of a virus, IL-4, IL-13, CCL5, CCL20 and CCL24 each positively correlated with both FVC and FEV_1. Thus, whereas airway inflammation is associated with reduced lung function in the absence of viral infection, cytokine expression is associated with a diminution of lung function deficits caused by viral infection.

Cytokines promote proliferation and chemotaxis of phagocytes and granulocytes expressing antiviral substances including granule proteins, antimicrobial peptides, proteolytic enzymes and reactive oxygen species, consistent with a protective function. On the other hand, an exuberant response to RV, a virus that infects relatively few airway cells [23, 24] and possesses minimal cytotoxic effects compared to influenza or adenovirus [25], could be maladaptive. In a mouse model of RV infection, CXCR2 [26] and TLR2 [27] null mice both show reduced airway inflammation and responsiveness but no change in viral load, suggesting that cytokines mediate RV-induced tissue injury. However, in the present study, we show that, in the context of respiratory viral infection, higher expression of pro-inflammatory cytokines is associated with less severe reductions in lung function. This study may have ramifications for the treatment of viral-induced asthma exacerbations. For example, treatments aimed at reducing the expression of specific pro-inflammatory cytokines may reduce symptoms but also attenuate the potential protective effects of these cytokines on lung function. Indeed, a recent multicenter study of children admitted to the emergency department for asthma exacerabtions showed that viral detection was associated with failure of management with oral corticosteroids and inhaled bronchodilators [28].

As noted above, we also obtained important information regarding the influence of airway cytokines on lung function in the absence of viral infection. IL-4, IL-13 and other type 2 cytokines have long been known to be drivers of allergic asthma [29, 30], and many studies have shown increased chemokine levels in the airways of patients with asthma compared to controls [31–39]. In our longitudinal study, we found that, in the absence of viral infection, CXCL10, IL-4, IL-13, CCL4, CCL5, CCL20 and CCL24 were each negatively associated with FVC. We also found that CXCL10 mRNA MDA5 mRNA and IFN-λ1 mRNA were each negatively associated with FVC and FEV_1. mRNA expression of CXCL10 and MDA5 are each known to be induced by IFN-γ, a type 1 cytokine [40, 41]. While we did not measure IFN-γ, these data suggest a potential negative influence of this cytokine on lung function in urban children with chronic asthma in the uninfected state. Levels of bronchoalveolar IFN-γ, a canonical type 1 cytokine, were recently associated with severe asthma [42]. Exhaled breath IFN-γ was noted to be a significant indicator of childhood asthma severity, as measured by FEV_1 [43].

We were initially surprised that airway cytokines correlated with FVC more strongly than pulmonary function parameters. However, FVC has previously been noted to negatively correlate with outdoor and indoor environmental exposures in children [44–47] and adults [48]. FVC in children has also been negatively correlated with various biomarkers including airway macrophage carbon content [45], exhaled breath malondialdehyde [46] and sputum dipalmitoylphosphatidylcholine [49].

We also obtained new information on the influence of asthma severity on the response to viral infection. Virus-induced induction of airway cytokines was not decreased in children with moderate-to-severe persistent asthma compared to subjects less severe disease, and in many cases viral-induced increases in cytokine level were significant in subjects with persistent asthma but not subjects with intermittent asthma. While there were significant overlapping ranges between the asthma severity groups, these data, obtained from asthmatic subjects experiencing natural colds, do not support the concept that patients with severe asthma have deficient antiviral responses [50–52]. On the other hand, our data are consistent with a recent study showing that, following experimental RV infection, subjects with allergic asthma show greater levels of nasal and bronchial cytokines, chemokines and IFNs compared to control subjects [53]. In addition, the absence of a reduction in viral-induced mRNA or protein expression in children with moderate-to-severe persistent asthma demonstrates that the positive associations we found between nasal lavage cytokine level and lung function are not due to increased cytokine production in subjects with better lung function.

There are several limitations to our study. First, we used nasal lavage to sample the respiratory tract of children with asthma. This method allowed repeated collection of samples from children as young as 5 years-old in a relatively non-invasive manner. While previous studies have shown that gene expression among asthmatic children is altered similarly in nasal and bronchial airways [53, 54], measurements of nasal lavage cannot actually represent the airway biology, and we did not validate our method by comparing our results with lower respiratory tract specimens such as sputum, breath condensate or bronchoalveolar lavage. Second, we studied a relatively small number of children ($n = 53$). Third, we found that 26.1% of surveillance samples were positive for virus, compared to 33.7% of self-reported respiratory illnesses. Thus, subjects were only slightly more likely to have a virus during self-reported sick periods than during surveillance sample collection. We believe the low viral detection rate during symptomatic episodes can be explained by the fact that samples from symptomatic illnesses were not collected in the fall and instead were only collected from January to August, when rhinovirus infections are less prevalent. Cold-like illnesses were unlikely to represent false-negative viral infections, as they were unaccompanied by increases in nasal aspirate MDA5, a double-stranded RNA pattern recognition receptor which was increased in virus-positive samples and has been shown to be induced following RV infection [55]. Nor were cold-like illnesses associated with reduced pulmonary function. Also, the symptom threshold for "sick" sample collection was quite low (2 or more). The reasoning behind this was to increase the likelihood of capturing viral illnesses for study. We also offered a $50 financial reimbursement for each sick period assessment which served to offset the family time and effort needed to participate in sick assessment/nasal secretion collection. These design elements contributed to a low viral detection rate. For example, a symptom score of two could be achieved simply with a runny and stuffy nose, which could easily represent allergic rhinitis rather than a cold. Fourth, despite extensive training and coaching in spirometry, many expiratory maneuvers were excluded due to inadequate data quality. We have evaluated the impact of our data cleaning procedures and found no systematic exclusion of children compared to the overall study population, and thus feel these procedures are unlikely to introduce selection bias. Fifth, the current analysis evaluates associations between biomarker levels, viral detection, and spirometry obtained on the same day, and does not evaluate for the possibility of lagged effects. Sixth, some of our assessments, such as medication use, asthma severity, and atopy, were based on self-report and were not independently validated, leaving open the possibility of measurement error. Seventh, our data from urban children with asthma may not be generalizable to other groups of asthmatic children. As we have shown previously [14], these children tend to be undertreated, as reflected by the number of subjects who were not taking medication (and therefore labeled as

"intermittent asthmatics"). Urban children with asthma who are not treated with inhaled steroids may be more susceptible to viral-induced reductions in airway function than suburban children [56, 57]. Eighth, we did not take into account bacterial colonization in our study. Bacterial colonization could alter the response to rhinovirus infection [58].

Finally, while we found that proximity to high-traffic highways was not a significant predictor of lung function or the relationship between viral exposure and lung function, we have not yet formally examined the effect of specific exposures. Detroit has a history of elevated air pollution and nonattainment of the ozone and particulate matter standards [59]. We previously examined relationships between lung function and ambient levels of ozone and particulate matter in a longitudinal cohort study of school-age children with asthma in Detroit [7]. In a two-pollutant model including PM_{10} and O_3, there was an association between O_3 exposure and diurnal variation of FEV_1 1 day after exposure in children without self-reported cold symptoms and a larger odds ratio for children with cold symptoms. It is therefore conceivable that specific pollutants could have intensified the effects of viral infection on lung function.

Conclusions

We conclude that in urban children with asthma, in the absence of respiratory virus, selected nasal lavage cytokines are significantly associated with reduced lung function. These data firmly establish the link between airway inflammation and asthma severity in a longitudinal cohort of children with stable asthma. However, in the presence of viral infection, there is a reversal in the relationship between nasal cytokines and clinical outcome, with higher levels correlating with less severe reductions in lung function. While nasal samples may not reflect lower airway responses, these data suggest that some aspects of the inflammatory response may be protective against viral infection. This study provides new insight into the host response to respiratory viral infections, and may have ramifications for the treatment of viral-induced asthma exacerbations.

Acknowledgements

Community Action Against Asthma (CAAA) is a community-based participatory research partnership that consists of the following organizations: Arab American Center for Community and Social Services, Community Health and Social Services Center Inc., Detroit Hispanic Development Corporation, Detroiters Working for Environmental Justice, Eastside Community Network, Friends of

Parkside, Southwest Detroit Environmental Vision, and faculty from the University of Michigan School of Medicine and the School of Public Health and a community asthma activist. CAAA is an affiliated partnership of the Detroit Community-Academic Urban Research Center. The authors thank Henry Ford Health System Epidemiology Lab for their collaboration, including initial processing and storage of nasal lavage samples, Ricardo de Majo for database design and technical assistance with encrypted data transfer, and Lucas Carlton for quality assessment of spirometry.

Funding
This work was supported by National Institutes of Health grants ES016769 (TCL), ES014677 (TGR), HL081420 (MBH) and AI114220 (TCL and MBH), and Environmental Protection Agency grant EPA-G2008-STAR-B1 (SAB).

Authors' contributions
TCL and MBH conceived and designed the study, analyzed and interpreted data, and drafted and revised the manuscript for important intellectual content. EEM analyzed samples and interpreted data. GBM developed the statistical strategy and analyzed data. XR and KEW analyzed and interpreted the data. ARC and BNE obtained informed consent and collected samples. AMG, ATC, JMR, SRB, GLW and KBO analyzed samples. BM developed the statistical strategy. TGR and SAB designed the study. All authors read and approved the final manuscript.

Competing interests
The authors declare that they have no competing interests.

Author details
[1]Departments of Pediatrics and Communicable Diseases, University of Michigan Medical School, 1150 W. Medical Center Dr., Building MSRB2, Room 3570B, Ann Arbor, MI 48109-5688, USA. [2]Molecular and Integrative Physiology, University of Michigan Medical School, Ann Arbor, USA. [3]Departments of Biostatistics, University of Michigan School of Public Health, University of Michigan, Ann Arbor, MI 48109, USA. [4]Environmental Health Sciences, University of Michigan School of Public Health, University of Michigan, Ann Arbor, MI 48109, USA. [5]Epidemiology, University of Michigan School of Public Health, University of Michigan, Ann Arbor, MI 48109, USA. [6]Health Behavior/Health Education, University of Michigan School of Public Health, University of Michigan, Ann Arbor, MI 48109, USA.

References
1. Carr W, Zeitel L, Weiss K. Variations in asthma hospitalizations and deaths in New York City. Am J Public Health. 1992;82:59–65.
2. Gottlieb DJ, Beiser AS, O'Connor GT. Poverty, race, and medication use are correlates of asthma hospitalization rates. A small area analysis in Boston. Chest. 1995;108:28–35.
3. Akinbami LJ, Moorman JE, Liu X. Asthma prevalence, health care use, and mortality: United States, 2005-2009. Natl Health Stat Report. 2011;12:1–14.
4. Rosenstreich DL, Eggleston P, Kattan M, Baker D, Slavin RG, Gergen P, Mitchell H, McNiff-Mortimer K, Lynn H, Ownby D, Malveaux F. The role of cockroach allergy and exposure to cockroach allergen in causing morbidity among inner-city children with asthma. N Engl J Med. 1997;336:1356–63.
5. Eggleston PA, Malveaux FJ, Butz AM, Huss K, Thompson L, Kolodner K, Rand CS. Medications used by children with asthma living in the inner city. Pediatrics. 1998;101:349–54.
6. Gergen PJ, Mitchell H, Lynn H. Understanding the seasonal pattern of childhood asthma: results from the national cooperative inner-city asthma study (NCICAS). J Pediatr. 2002;141:631–6.
7. Lewis TC, Robins TG, Dvonch JT, Keeler GJ, Yip FY, Mentz GB, Lin X, Parker EA, Israel BA, Gonzalez L, Hill Y. Air pollution-associated changes in lung function among asthmatic children in Detroit. Environ Health Perspect. 2005;113:1068–75.
8. Lewis TC, Henderson TA, Carpenter AR, Ramirez IA, McHenry CL, Goldsmith AM, Ren X, Mentz GB, Mukherjee B, Robins TG, Joiner TA, Mohammad LS, Nguyen ER, Burns MA, Burke DT, Hershenson MB. Nasal cytokine responses to natural colds in asthmatic children. Clin Exp Allergy. 2012;42:1734–44.
9. Pizzichini MM, Pizzichini E, Efthimiadis A, Chauhan AJ, Johnston SL, Hussack P, Mahony J, Dolovich J, Hargreave FE. Asthma and natural colds. Inflammatory indices in induced sputum: a feasibility study. Am J Respir Crit Care Med. 1998;158:1178–84.
10. Teran LM, Seminario MC, Shute JK, Papi A, Compton SJ, Low JL, Gleich GJ, Johnston SL. RANTES, macrophage-inhibitory protein 1α, and the eosinophil product major basic protein are released into upper respiratory secretions during virus-induced asthma exacerbations in children. J Infect Dis. 1999;179:677–81.
11. Grissell TV, Powell H, Shafren DR, Boyle MJ, Hensley MJ, Jones PD, Whitehead BF, Gibson PG. IL-10 gene expression in acute virus-induced asthma. Am J Respir Crit Care Med. 2005;172:433–9.
12. Santiago J, Hernandez-Cruz JL, Manjarrez-Zavala ME, Montes-Vizuet R, Rosete-Olvera DP, Tapia-Diaz AM, Zepeda-Peney H, Teran LM. Role of monocyte chemotactic protein-3 and -4 in children with virus exacerbation of asthma. Eur Respir J. 2008;32:1243–942.
13. Vette A, Burke J, Norris G, Landis M, Batterman S, Breen M, Isakov V, Lewis T, Gilmour MI, Kamal A, Hammond D, Vedantham R, Bereznicki S, Tian N, Croghan C. The near-road exposures and effects of urban air pollutants study (NEXUS): study design and methods. Science Total Environ. 2013;448:38–47.
14. Lewis T, Robins T, Joseph C, Parker E, Israel B, Rowe Z, Edgren K, Salinas M, Martinez M, Brown R. Identification of gaps in the diagnosis and treatment of childhood asthma using a community-based participatory research approach. J Urban Health. 2004;81:472–88.
15. Lemanske RF, Jackson DJ, Gangnon RE, Evans MD, Li Z, Shult PA, Kirk CJ, Reisdorf E, Roberg KA, Anderson EL, Carlson-Dakes KT, Adler KJ, Gilbertson-White S, Pappas TE, Dasilva DF, Tisler CJ, Gern JE. Rhinovirus illnesses during infancy predict subsequent childhood wheezing. J Allergy Clin Immunol. 2005;116:571–7.
16. Liang K-Y, Zeger SL. Longitudinal data analysis using generalized linear models. Biometrika. 1986;73:13–22.
17. Ballinger GA. Using generalized estimating equations for longitudinal data analysis. Organ Res Methods. 2004;7:127–50.
18. Ma Y, Mazumdar M, Memtsoudis SG. Beyond repeated-measures analysis of variance: advanced statistical methods for the analysis of longitudinal data in anesthesia research. Reg Anesth Pain Med. 2012;37:99–105.
19. Miller EK, Hernandez JZ, Wimmenauer V, Shepherd BE, Hijano D, Libster R, Serra ME, Bhat N, Batalle JP, Mohamed Y, Reynaldi A, Rodriguez A, Otello M, Pisapia N, Bugna J, Bellabarba M, Kraft D, Coviello S, Ferolla FM, Chen A, London SJ, Siberry GK, Williams JV, Polack FP. A mechanistic role for type III IFN-λ1 in asthma exacerbations mediated by human rhinoviruses. Am J Respir Crit Care Med. 2012;185:508–16.
20. Manthei DM, Schwantes EA, Mathur SK, Guadarrama AG, Kelly EA, Gern JE, Jarjour NN, Denlinger LC. Nasal lavage VEGF and TNF-α levels during a natural cold predict asthma exacerbations. Clin Exp Allergy. 2014;44:1484–93.
21. Message SD, Laza-Stanca V, Mallia P, Parker HL, Zhu J, Kebadze T, Contoli M, Sanderson G, Kon OM, Papi A, Jeffery PK, Stanciu LA, Johnston SL. Rhinovirus-induced lower respiratory illness is increased in asthma and related to virus load and Th1/2 cytokine and IL-10 production. Proc Natl Acad Sci U S A. 2008;105:13562–7.
22. Adura PT, Reed E, Macintyre J, del Rosario A, Roberts J, Pestridge R, Beegan R, Boxall CB, Xiao C, Kebadze T, Aniscenko J, Cornelius V, Gern JE, Monk PD, Johnston SL, Djukanović R. Experimental rhinovirus 16 infection in moderate asthmatics on inhaled corticosteroids. Eur Respir J. 2014;43:1186–9.
23. Arruda E, Boyle TR, Winther B, Pevear DC, Gwaltney JM, Hayden FG. Localization of human rhinovirus replication in the upper respiratory tract by in situ hybridization. J Infect Dis. 1995;171:1329–33.

24. Mosser AG, Brockman-Schneider R, Amineva S, Burchell L, Sedgwick JB, Busse WW, Gern JE. Similar frequency of rhinovirus-infectible cells in upper and lower airway epithelium. J Infect Dis. 2002;185:734–43.

25. Winther B, Gwaltney JM, Hendley JO. Respiratory virus infection of monolayer cultures of human nasal epithelial cells. Am Rev Respir Dis. 1990;141:839–45.

26. Nagarkar DR, Wang Q, Shim J, Zhao Y, Tsai WC, Lukacs NW, Sajjan U, Hershenson MB. CXCR2 is required for neutrophilic airway inflammation and hyperresponsiveness in a mouse model of human rhinovirus infection. J Immunol. 2009;183:6698–707.

27. Han M, Chung Y, Young Hong J, Rajput C, Lei J, Hinde JL, Chen Q, Weng SP, Bentley JK, Hershenson MB. Toll-like receptor 2–expressing macrophages are required and sufficient for rhinovirus-induced airway inflammation. J Allergy Clin Immunol. 2016;138:1619–30.

28. Ducharme FM, Zemek R, Chauhan BF, Gravel J, Chalut D, Poonai N, Guertin MC, Quach C, Blondeau L, Laberge S, Network. DrgotPERiCP: factors associated with failure of emergency department management in children with acute moderate or severe asthma: a prospective, multicentre, cohort study. Lancet Respir Med. 2016;4:990–8.

29. Robinson DS, Hamid Q, Ying S, Tsicopoulos A, Barkans J, Bentley AM, Corrigan C, Durham SR, Kay AB. Predominant TH2-like bronchoalveolar T-lymphocyte population in atopic asthma. N Engl J Med. 1992;326:298–304.

30. Woodruff PG, Modrek B, Choy DF, Jia G, Abbas AR, Ellwanger A, Arron JR, Koth LL, Fahy JV. T-helper type 2–driven inflammation defines major subphenotypes of asthma. Am J Respir Crit Care Med. 2009;180:388–95.

31. Alam R, York J, Boyars M, Stafford S, Grant JA, Lee J, Forsythe P, Sim T, Ida N. Increased MCP-1, RANTES, and MIP-1alpha in bronchoalveolar lavage fluid of allergic asthmatic patients. Am J Respir Crit Care Med. 1996;153:1398–404.

32. Holgate ST, Bodey KS, Janezic A, Frew AJ, Kaplan AP, Teran LM. Release of RANTES, MIP-1α , and MCP-1 into asthmatic airways following endobronchial allergen challenge. Am J Respir Crit Care Med2. 1997;156: 1377–83.

33. Tillie-Leblond I, Hammad H, Desurmont S, Pugin J, Wallaert B, Tonnel A-B, Gosset P. CC chemokines and interleukin-5 in bronchial lavage fluid from patients with status asthmaticus. Am J Respir Crit Care Med. 2000;162:586–92.

34. Ravensberg AJ, Ricciardolo FLM, van Schadewijk A, Rabe KF, Sterk PJ, Hiemstra PS, Mauad T. Eotaxin-2 and eotaxin-3 expression is associated with persistent eosinophilic bronchial inflammation in patients with asthma after allergen challenge. J Allergy Clin Immunol. 2005;115:779–85.

35. Dent G, Hadjicharalambous C, Yoshikawa T, Handy RLC, Powell J, Anderson IK, Louis R, Davies DE, Djukanovic R. Contribution of eotaxin-1 to eosinophil chemotactic activity of moderate and severe asthmatic sputum. Am J Respir Crit Care Med. 2004;169:1110–7.

36. Ko FWS, Lau CYK, Leung TF, Wong GWK, Lam CWK, Lai CKW, Hui DSC. Exhaled breath condensate levels of eotaxin and macrophage-derived chemokine in stable adult asthma patients. Clin Exp Allergy. 2006;36:44–51.

37. Fitzpatrick AM, Higgins M, Holguin F, Brown LAS, Teague WG. The molecular phenotype of severe asthma in children. J Allergy Clin Immunol. 2010;125:851–7 e818.

38. Hastie AT, Moore WC, Meyers DA, Vestal PL, Li H, Peters SP, Bleecker ER. Analyses of asthma severity phenotypes and inflammatory proteins in subjects stratified by sputum granulocytes. J Allergy Clin Immunol. 2010;125: 1028–36 e1013.

39. Robroeks CMHHT, Rijkers GT, Jöbsis Q, Hendriks HJE, Damoiseaux JGMC, Zimmermann LJI, Van Schayck OP, Dompeling E. Increased cytokines, chemokines and soluble adhesion molecules in exhaled breath condensate of asthmatic children. Clin Exp Allergy. 2010;40:77–84.

40. Narumi S, Hamilton TA. Inducible expression of murine IP-10 mRNA varies with the state of macrophage inflammatory activity. J Immunol. 1991;146:3038–44.

41. Kang DC, Gopalkrishnan RV, Wu Q, Jankowsky E, Pyle AM, Fisher PB. mda-5: an interferon-inducible putative RNA helicase with double-stranded RNA-dependent ATPase activity and melanoma growth-suppressive properties. Proc Natl Acad Sci U S A. 2002;99:637–42.

42. Raundhal M, Morse C, Khare A, Oriss TB, Milosevic J, Trudeau J, Huff R, Pilewski J, Holguin F, Kolls J, Wenzel S, Ray P, Ray A. High IFN-γ and low SLPI mark severe asthma in mice and humans. J Clin Invest. 2015;125:3037–50.

43. Robroeks CMHHT, Van De Kant KDG, Jöbsis Q, Hendriks HJE, Van Gent R, Wouters EFM, Damoiseaux JGMC, Bast A, Wodzig WKWH, Dompeling E. Exhaled nitric oxide and biomarkers in exhaled breath condensate indicate the presence, severity and control of childhood asthma. Clin Exp Allergy. 2007;37:1303–11.

44. Koenig JQ, Mar TF, Allen RW, Jansen K, Lumley T, Sullivan JH, Trenga CA, Larson T, Liu LJ. Pulmonary effects of indoor- and outdoor-generated particles in children with asthma. Environ Health Perspect. 2005;113:499–503.

45. Kulkarni N, Pierse N, Rushton L, Grigg J. Carbon in airway macrophages and lung function in children. N Engl J Med. 2006;355:21–30.

46. Romieu I, Barraza-Villarreal A, Escamilla-Nuñez C, Almstrand A-C, Diaz-Sanchez D, Sly PD, Olin A-C. Exhaled breath malondialdehyde as a marker of effect of exposure to air pollution in children with asthma. J Allergy Clin Immunol. 2008;121:903–9 e906.

47. Barone-Adesi F, Dent JE, Dajnak D, Beevers S, Anderson HR, Kelly FJ, Cook DG, Whincup PH. Long-term exposure to primary traffic pollutants and lung function in children: cross-sectional study and meta-analysis. PLoS One. 2015;10:e0142565.

48. Kunzli N, Ackermann-Liebrich U, Brandli O, Tschopp J, Schindler C, Leuenberger P. Clinically "small" effects of air pollution on FVC have a large public health impact. Swiss study on air pollution and lung disease in adults (SAPALDIA) - team. Eur Respir J. 2000;15:131–6.

49. Shaheen MA, Mahmoud MA, Abdel Aziz MM, El Morsy HI, Abdel Khalik KA. Sputum dipalmitoylphosphatidylcholine level as a novel airway inflammatory marker in asthmatic children. Clin Respir J. 2009;3:95–101.

50. Wark PA, Johnston SL, Bucchieri F, Powell R, Puddicombe S, Laza-Stanca V, Holgate ST, Davies DE. Asthmatic bronchial epithelial cells have a deficient innate immune response to infection with rhinovirus. J Exp Med. 2005;201:937–47.

51. Contoli M, Message SD, Laza-Stanca V, Edwards MR, Wark PA, Bartlett NW, Kebadze T, Mallia P, Stanciu LA, Parker HL, Slater L, Lewis-Antes A, Kon OM, Holgate ST, Davies DE, Kotenko SV, Papi A, Johnston SL. Role of deficient type III interferon-lambda production in asthma exacerbations. Nat Med. 2006;12:1023–6.

52. Sykes A, Macintyre J, Edwards MR, del Rosario A, Haas J, Gielen V, Kon OM, McHale M, Johnston SL. Rhinovirus-induced interferon production is not deficient in well controlled asthma. Thorax. 2014;69:240–6.

53. Hansel TT, Tunstall T, Trujillo-Torralbo M-B, Shamji B, del-Rosario A, Dhariwal J, Kirk PDW, Stumpf MPH, Koopmann J, Telcian A, Aniscenko J, Gogsadze L, Bakhsoliani E, Stanciu L, Bartlett N, Edwards M, Walton R, Mallia P, Hunt TM, Hunt TL, Hunt DG, Westwick J, Edwards M, Kon OM, Jackson DJ, Johnston SL. A comprehensive evaluation of nasal and bronchial cytokines and chemokines following experimental rhinovirus infection in allergic asthma: increased interferons (IFN-γ and IFN-λ) and type 2 inflammation (IL-5 and IL-13). EBioMed. 2017;19:128–38.

54. Poole A, Urbanek C, Eng C, Schageman J, Jacobson S, O'Connor BP, Galanter JM, Gignoux CR, Roth LA, Kumar R, Lutz S, Liu AH, Fingerlin TE, Setterquist RA, Burchard EG, Rodriguez-Santana J, Seibold MA. Dissecting childhood asthma with nasal transcriptomics distinguishes subphenotypes of disease. J Allergy Clin Immunol. 2014;133:670–8 e612.

55. Wang Q, Nagarkar DR, Bowman ER, Schneider D, Gosangi B, Lei J, Zhao Y, McHenry CL, Burgens RV, Miller DJ, Sajjan U, Hershenson MB. Role of double-stranded rna pattern recognition receptors in rhinovirus-induced airway epithelial cell responses. J Immunol. 2009; 183:6989–97.

56. Liu L, Poon R, Chen L, Frescura A-M, Montuschi P, Ciabattoni G, Wheeler A, Dales R. Acute effects of air pollution on pulmonary function, airway inflammation, and oxidative stress in asthmatic children. Environ Health Perspect. 2009;117:668–74.

57. Delfino RJ, Zeiger RS, Seltzer JM, Street DH, McLaren CE. Association of asthma symptoms with peak particulate air pollution and effect modification by anti-inflammatory medication use. Environ Health Perspect. 2002;110:A607–17.

58. Kloepfer KM, Lee WM, Pappas TE, Kang TJ, Vrtis RF, Evans MD, Gangnon RE, Bochkov YA, Jackson DJ, Lemanske RF Jr, Gern JE. Detection of pathogenic bacteria during rhinovirus infection is associated with increased respiratory symptoms and asthma exacerbations. J Allergy Clin Immunol. 2014;133: 1301–7 e1303.

59. Keeler Gerald J, Dvonch T, Yip Fuyuen Y, Parker Edith A, Isreal Barbara A, Marsik Frank J, Morishita M, Barres James A, Robins Thomas G, Brakefield-Caldwell W, Sam M. Assessment of personal and community-level exposures to particulate matter among children with asthma in Detroit, Michigan, as part of community action against asthma (CAAA). Environ Health Perspect. 2002;110:173–81.

21

Quantitative CT analysis using functional imaging is superior in describing disease progression in idiopathic pulmonary fibrosis compared to forced vital capacity

J. Clukers[1]*[†] iD, M. Lanclus[2]*[†], B. Mignot[2], C. Van Holsbeke[2], J. Roseman[2], S. Porter[3], E. Gorina[3], E. Kouchakji[3], K. E. Lipson[3], W. De Backer[1,2] and J. De Backer[2]

Abstract

Background: Idiopathic pulmonary fibrosis (IPF) is chronic fibrosing pneumonia with an unpredictable natural disease history. Functional respiratory imaging (FRI) has potential to better characterize this disease. The aim of this study was to identify FRI parameters, which predict FVC decline in patients with IPF.

Methods: An IPF-cohort (treated with pamrevlumab for 48 weeks) was retrospectively studied using FRI. Serial CT's were compared from 66 subjects. Post-hoc analysis was performed using FRI, FVC and mixed effects models.

Results: Lung volumes, determined by FRI, correlated with FVC (lower lung volumes with lower FVC) ($R^2 = 0.61$, $p < 0.001$). A negative correlation was observed between specific image based airway radius (siRADaw) at total lung capacity (TLC) and FVC ($R^2 = 0.18$, $p < 0.001$). Changes in FVC correlated significantly with changes in lung volumes ($R^2 = 0.18$, $p < 0.001$) and siRADaw ($R^2 = 0.15$, $p = 0.002$) at week 24 and 48, with siRADaw being more sensitive to change than FVC. Loss in lobe volumes ($R^2 = 0.33$, $p < 0.001$), increasing fibrotic tissue ($R^2 = 0.33$, $p < 0.001$) and airway radius ($R^2 = 0.28$, $p < 0.001$) at TLC correlated with changes in FVC but these changes already occur in the lower lobes when FVC is still considered normal.

Conclusion: This study indicates that FRI is a superior tool than FVC in capturing of early and clinically relevant, disease progression in a regional manner.

Keywords: Functional respiratory imaging is superior in describing disease in IPF

Background

Idiopathic pulmonary fibrosis (IPF) is a fatal, chronic fibrosing interstitial pneumonia with a variable and unpredictable natural history [1–3]. Diagnosing IPF at an early stage enables more effective treatment and improvement of the long-term clinical outcome of this progressive debilitating disease [4–6]. Predicting prognosis is an important part of IPF management, but it remains difficult in individual patients with the current standard

---
* Correspondence: johan.clukers@student.uantwerpen.be; maarten.lanclus@fluidda.com
[†]J. Clukers and M. Lanclus contributed equally to this work.
[1]Faculty of Medicine & Health Sciences, University of Antwerp (UAntwerpen), Universiteitsplein 1, 2610 Antwerpen, Belgium
[2]FluidDA nv, Groeningenlei 132, 2550 Kontich, Belgium
Full list of author information is available at the end of the article

investigations as forced vital capacity (FVC) and high resolution computed tomography (HRCT) [7, 8].

FVC best predicts disease progression and mortality [9, 10]. It therefore serves as a primary endpoint in IPF, although it's not a proven surrogate for mortality [11, 12]. A 2–6% change in predicted FVC has been proposed as the minimal clinical important difference [9], and where 10% decline in absolute FVC correlated well with mortality [10]. Due to weak signal-to-noise ratios [13], FVC is not able to pick up small changes in progressing fibrosis in these patients. In future studies, where patients are treated with (combination of) antifibrotic drugs, its use as a clinical endpoint is less compelling since FVC decline is impacted by this therapy [14–16].

The disease stage, as measured by HRCT, has been correlated to lung function measurements [17, 18]. In recent years quantitative computer-derived CT (qCT) variables have been studied in IPF, and have been shown to be superior predictors of mortality compared to any visually scored CT parameter (e.g. extent of fibrosis) [19, 20]. Despite these advances in the field, no radiological marker is widely accepted as a biomarker in IPF [21].

Functional respiratory imaging (FRI) is a post-processing technology that utilizes multi-slice HRCT scans and computational fluid dynamics (CFD) to assess the overall lung health and function in a regional manner by quantifying endpoints as airway volume and resistance [22, 23]. FRI is considered a more sensitive method for observing changes in airway volume and resistance than classical lung function tests (e.g. forced expiratory volume in 1 s) [23–25]. This image-based method can also be used to provide a comprehensive assessment of airway tree changes [24, 26] (Fig. 1). Therefore FRI has the potential to better characterize disease, provide more accurate information in treatment follow-up of a patient in clinical practice and to predict and evaluate therapeutic interventions in many respiratory conditions. Comparable qCT methods to FRI have been used, in IPF and other fibrotic lung disease, as (treatment) endpoint [27–29].

The use of FRI and other qCT measurements may thus allow better monitoring of disease progression and response to treatment, improving our understanding of this disease.

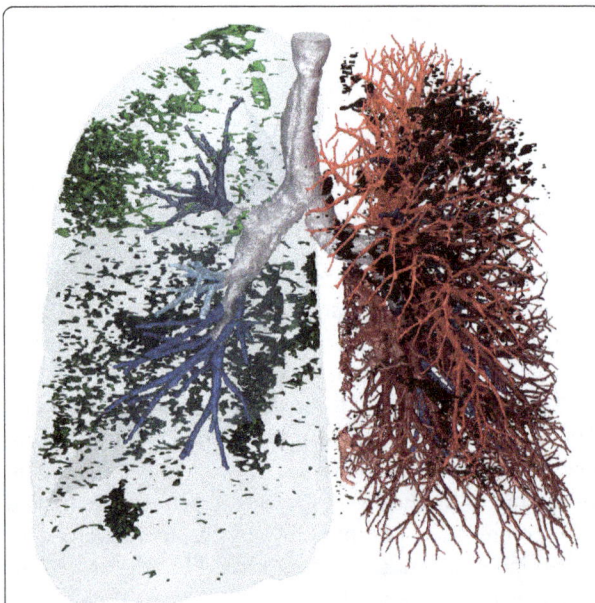

Fig. 1 Functional Respiratory Imaging provides visualisation and quantification of airway volumes (depicted in blue), lobe volumes, fibrosis (depicted in green), emphysema (depicted in black) and blood vessel volumes (depicted in red)

Methods
Study design
The aim of this study was to identify FRI parameters, which predict FVC decline in patients with IPF. We retrospectively studied data from a Phase 2 open-label, dose-escalation study to evaluate the safety and efficacy of an anti-CTGF monoclonal antibody, pamrevlumab (FG-3019), for treatment of IPF. In the Phase 2 study, conducted by FibroGen, Inc., diagnosis of IPF was based on a usual interstitial pneumonia (UIP)-pattern on HRCT or a possible UIP-pattern with a UIP-pattern on surgical lung biopsy, as per applicable diagnostic guidelines at the time (2011) [2]. HRCT scans, with a breath hold at inspiration and used as outcome measure in the original study protocol, were taken at baseline, 24 weeks and 48 weeks after treatment commenced (n = 89 enrolled; 67 completed treatment; 66 full data set). The trial was composed of two dose cohorts. In the first, patients had been diagnosed with IPF within 5 years of trial inclusion with FVC ≥ 45% predicted and DL_{CO} ≥ 30% predicted and participants had to show disease progression in the last year (FVC decline ≥10%, HRCT worsening, and/or other objective changes). In the second cohort, the minimum FVC % predicted was raised to 55%. For all subjects, baseline HRCT had to indicate 10–50% reticular fibrosis and no more than 25% honeycombing. This study was performed in accordance with the Declaration of Helsinki. (www.ClinicalTrials.gov number NCT01262001) (Raghu Eur Respir J 2016; 47: 1481–1491) [29]. The investigators initiated this study in consultation with FibroGen, Inc. for use of the original HRCT data.

Methods and analysis
Post-hoc analysis of this patient cohort was performed using FRI and mixed effects (regression) models on all available data in the data set, to understand change from baseline at week 24 and at week 48 for all patients in FRI parameters relative to FVC in terms of disease progression. Detailed explanation of this technique can be found in Additional file 1 and the FRI manual [30]. Subjects in this study had complete CT scans at baseline, week 24 weeks and week 48 weeks. FRI parameters were determined for the whole lung (all lobes), for the lower lung zones (right and left lower lobes) and for the upper lung zones (right upper and middle lobe; left upper lobe). Typical FRI parameters that were included were: specific image-based airway radius (siRADaw), percentage of fibrotic tissue at total lung capacity (TLC) and predicted lobe volume at TLC. In addition, sample size calculations were conducted to demonstrate sensitivity to change for each measurement (PFT or FRI parameter), from

Table 1 Patient characteristics

Number of subjects		89
Age [y] (range)		68 (47–82)
Male, n (%)		71 (79.8)
Time from IPF diagnosis, n (%)	< 1 year	34 (38.2)
	1–3 years	33 (37.1)
	> 3 years	22 (24.7)
FVC [L] (range)		2.52 (1.32–5.51)
FVC [% predicted] (range)		65.9 (42.6–111.7)

baseline to week 48. Sample sizes were obtained for a power goal of 80%, a significance level of 0.05 and two-tailed. These were based on the effect sizes calculated on the mean and standard deviation of the within subject differences between week 48 and baseline.

Results

Patient characteristics are shown in Table 1. Subjects were predominately male with a mean FVC < 80% predicted.

On univariate analysis, good correlation between lung volume based on FRI assessment and FVC was demonstrated ($R^2 = 0.61$, $p < 0.001$) (Fig. 2). A negative correlation between specific airway radius and FVC was demonstrated at TLC ($R^2 = 0.18$, $p < 0.001$) (Fig. 2). At TLC, FVC decline correlated significantly with lung volume decline ($R^2 = 0.18$, $p < 0.001$) and increase in specific airway radius ($R^2 = 0.15$, $p = 0.002$) (Fig. 3) both at TLC. The lower lobes were most affected (Fig. 4). Importantly, a decline in FVC was not observed until a 40–50% loss of lower lobe volume was measured.

In more advanced disease (i.e. lower FVC) there was a negative correlation with fibrotic tissue (Fig. 5). Again,

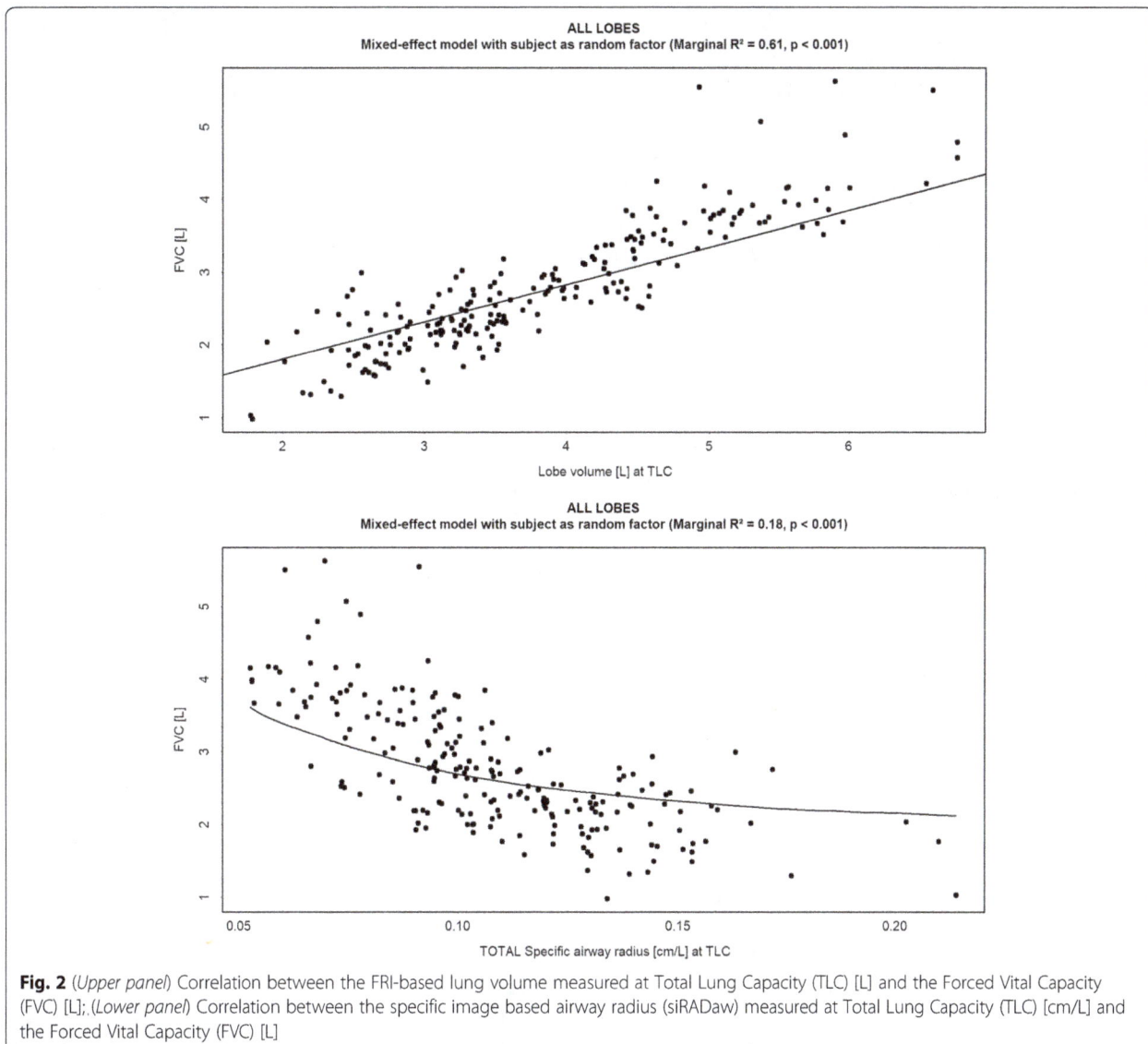

Fig. 2 (*Upper panel*) Correlation between the FRI-based lung volume measured at Total Lung Capacity (TLC) [L] and the Forced Vital Capacity (FVC) [L]; (*Lower panel*) Correlation between the specific image based airway radius (siRADaw) measured at Total Lung Capacity (TLC) [cm/L] and the Forced Vital Capacity (FVC) [L]

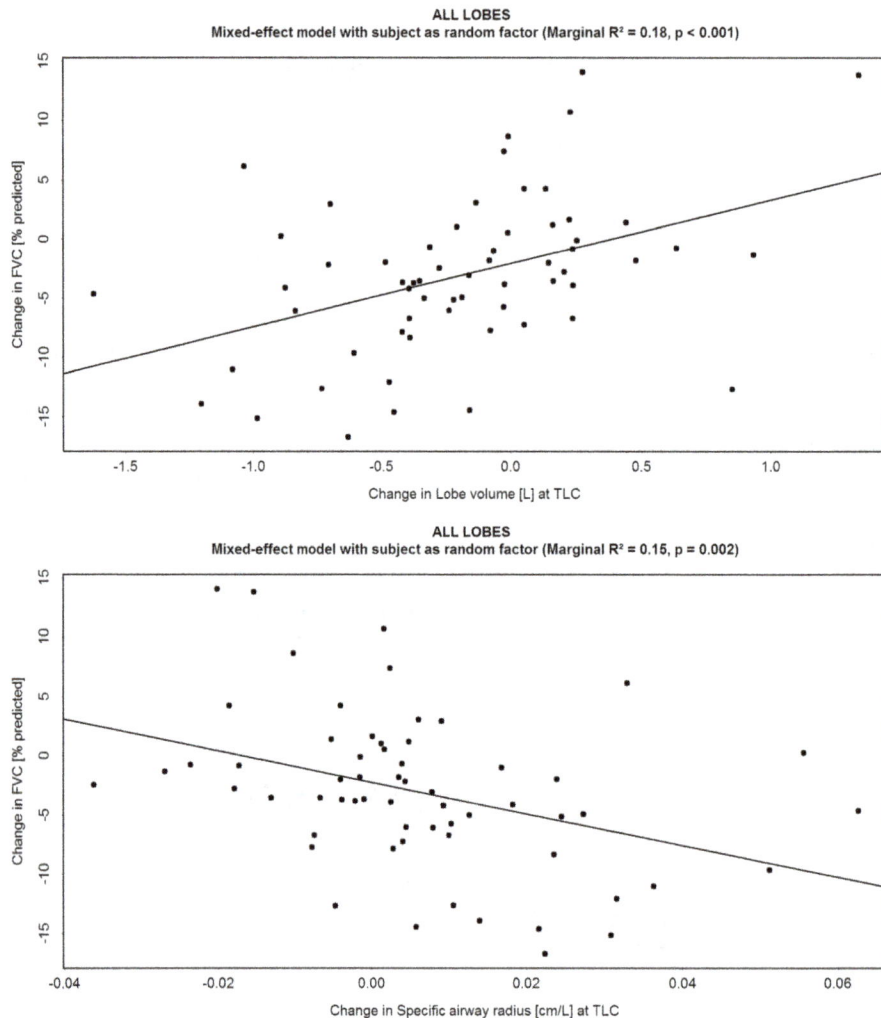

Fig. 3 (*Upper panel*) Correlation between the change in lung volume measured at Total Lung Capacity (TLC) [L] and the change in Forced Vital Capacity (FVC) [% predicted]; (*Lower panel*) Correlation between the change in specific image based airway radius (siRADaw) measured at Total Lung Capacity (TLC) [cm/L] and change in FVC (% predicted)

the same observation can be made that the lower lobes are more diseased.

Airway radius (expressed as siRADaw) increased with FVC decline (Fig. 6). This effect was more pronounced in the lower lobes. In contrast to observations made in the lobe volumes, there was a trend of divergence (regression lines) for a lower FVC, indicating that more pronounced disease correlated with larger airways relative to the total lung volume.

Airway radius (siRADaw) also correlates positively with fibrotic tissue ($R^2 = 0.31$, $p < 0.001$) (Fig. 7), i.e. airways enlarge, calculated in respect to the total lung volumes, with progressive disease.

Sample size calculations based on FRI parameters measured for the lower lobes were more sensitive in detecting change after 48 weeks (FVC: $N = 43$, effect size dz. = 0.437; lower lobe volumes: $N = 42$, effect size dz. =

0.443; lower lobe fibrosis: $N = 28$, effect size dz. = 0.549; lower lobe specific airway radius: $N = 38$, effect size dz. = 0.467). Moreover, when only considering patients with an FVC > 75% predicted at baseline, siRADaw lowered the required patient number from 101 to 13 patients (effect size dz. = 0.281 to 0.847) in demonstrating a significant change after 48 weeks. When assessing the changes after 24 weeks in this subgroup a sample size of 428 (effect size dz. = 0.136) was required when considering FVC as endpoint and 26 patients (effect size dz. = 0.572) for siRADaw endpoint. Dz stands for standardised difference scores, a technique typically used in within subject designs.

Discussion

Our data shows a correlation between declining FVC with the FRI determined parameters: declining lung volumes, increasing fibrotic tissue and increase in the specific airway radius. For these three FRI parameters, the lower lobes are more affected even at the mild stage of the disease, keeping with early reports on IPF [31, 32].

IPF is a heterogeneous and unpredictable disease. The use of FVC is widespread in clinical research and practice, although the drawbacks and shortcomings of this test are well known [9, 10, 33, 34]. The use of qCT, as a new biomarker of disease characterisation, shows great potential in resolving the issue with FVC. Current qCT methods have focused on the lung parenchyma and pulmonary vessels. Many of these methods have great difficulty separating honeycombing from traction bronchiectasis and emphysema. Consequently, objective quantification of traction bronchiectasis severity, which has been reported as an important predictor of mortality in IPF, has been challenging [19–21, 35, 36].

FRI also captures lower lobe disease (50 to 60% predicted lobe volume) before any decline can be seen in FVC (100% predicted) [1, 2]. An explanation for this finding could be in the fact that FVC is patient effort dependent and is the sum total of everything that happens in the both lungs. The upper lobes likely compensate for the volume loss of the lower lobes. FVC remains fairly stable – or at least progresses slowly – until an FVC $\pm 75\%$ predicted (Fig. 4) at which point the upper lobes also show progressive loss in volume and a more pronounced decline in FVC (convergence of the regression lines for the upper and lower lobes). This places the significant but weak correlations between FRI and FVC in perspective; that is, FRI already reveals disease related information not (yet) captured by the conventional lung function test. Similar correlations on (semi)-qCT for simultaneous changes in fibrosis

and FVC have been reported [35, 37] with this exception that our data differentiates between upper and lower lobes and quantifies the loss of lobe volumes.

To the best of our knowledge we report, for the first time, the use of an automated method for quantification of traction bronchiectasis, overcoming the problems with semi-quantitative methods, which are inherently subjective and liable to significant interobserver variability. The airways are capturing disease signal that cannot solely be explained by the extent of disease itself. This is in keeping with a previous visual score study [38].

The observation that, progressive disease correlated with an increase in siRADaw (i.e. airway volumes), could likely be explained as a combination of two processes: traction bronchiectasis and the intra-pulmonary pressure re-distribution due to increased stiffness (resistance) of alveolar region.

In a CT scan taken at TLC during a breath hold, the intra-thoracic pressure tends to redistribute due to the stiffness of the alveolar region and subsequently dilates the central and distal airways as illustrated in Fig. 8. The relative enlargement of the airways is maintained and possibly exacerbated by traction bronchiectasis. The latter entails an increase in airway luminal dimensions due to the traction exerted by the fibrosis on the airway wall, as well as bronchiolar proliferation, both resembling disease progression in IPF [39].

HRCT findings of traction bronchiectasis correlate well with histopathology of fibroblast foci: profusion of fibroblastic foci is strikingly related to the severity of traction bronchiectasis [40, 41]. Traction bronchiectasis shows to be a clear indicator of mortality and remains a significant predictor of a poor outcome, independent of

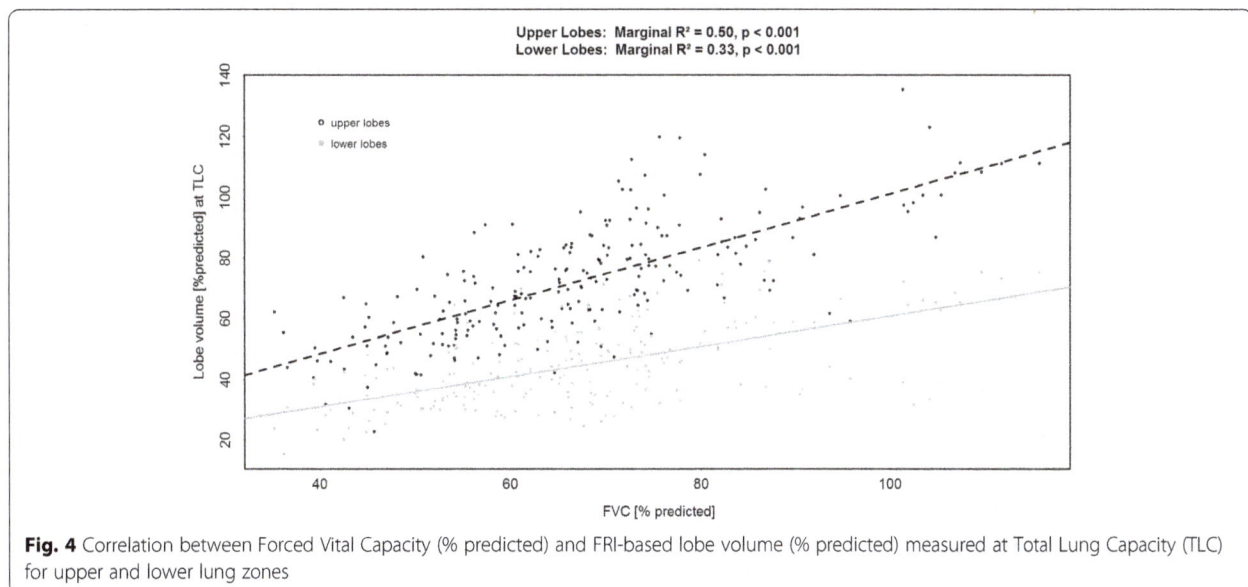

Fig. 4 Correlation between Forced Vital Capacity (% predicted) and FRI-based lobe volume (% predicted) measured at Total Lung Capacity (TLC) for upper and lower lung zones

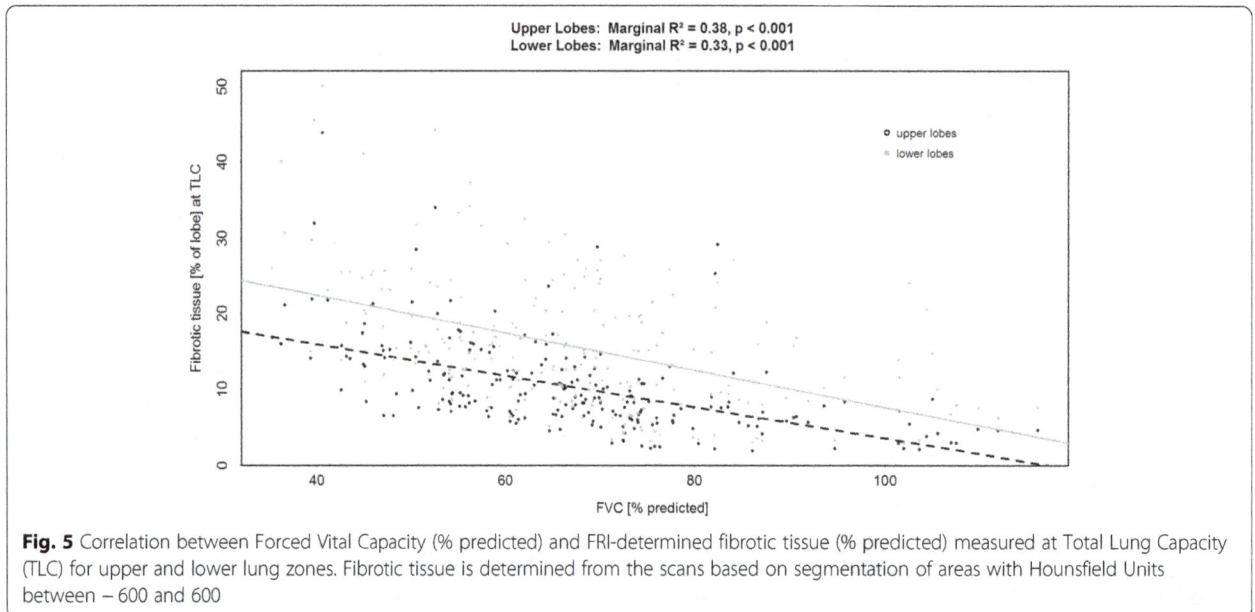

Fig. 5 Correlation between Forced Vital Capacity (% predicted) and FRI-determined fibrotic tissue (% predicted) measured at Total Lung Capacity (TLC) for upper and lower lung zones. Fibrotic tissue is determined from the scans based on segmentation of areas with Hounsfield Units between − 600 and 600

other associated parenchymal interstitial lung disease patterns [38, 42, 43]. Patients, recruited from the INPULSIS trials with possible UIP pattern on HRCT (i.e. traction bronchiectasis and no honeycombing), show to have the same grade of disease progression as a response to treatment with nintedanib in comparison to patients with definite UIP pattern (i.e. honeycombing) [44].

The specific airway radius may have a greater potential in predicting disease severity and progression than FRI-based lobe volumes alone, because of the increasing difference between the upper and lower lung zones in more advanced disease. Furthermore, siRADaw shows greater sensitivity for detecting change, especially in

what are considered mildly diseased patients with an FVC > 75% predicted. Other IPF patient cohorts with mild disease eventually show progression [45, 46], thus regional information in IPF is clinically relevant and can be accurately captured using FRI.

Many patients with a FVC > 75% predicted demonstrated FRI characteristics associated with progressively declining FVC. This is an argument for the fact that early or asymptomatic disease is not detected by classical PFT measurements (i.e. FVC). Consequently, quantifying regional information about lung structures may reduce sample sizes needed to detect decline and treatment effect in IPF studies with new therapeutic options. Prospective

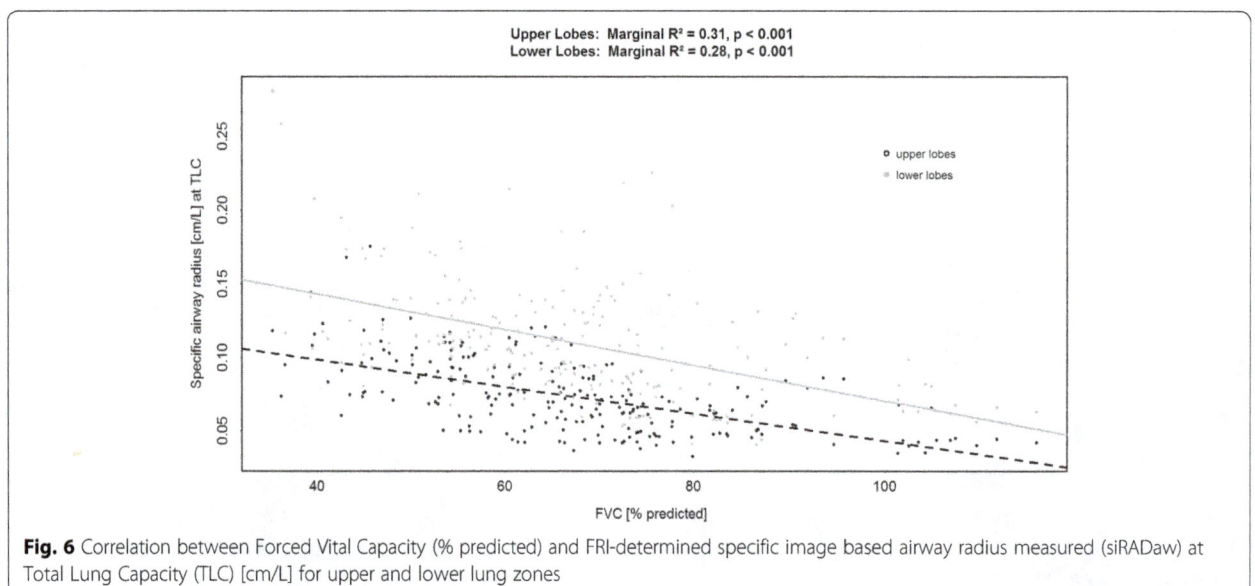

Fig. 6 Correlation between Forced Vital Capacity (% predicted) and FRI-determined specific image based airway radius measured (siRADaw) at Total Lung Capacity (TLC) [cm/L] for upper and lower lung zones

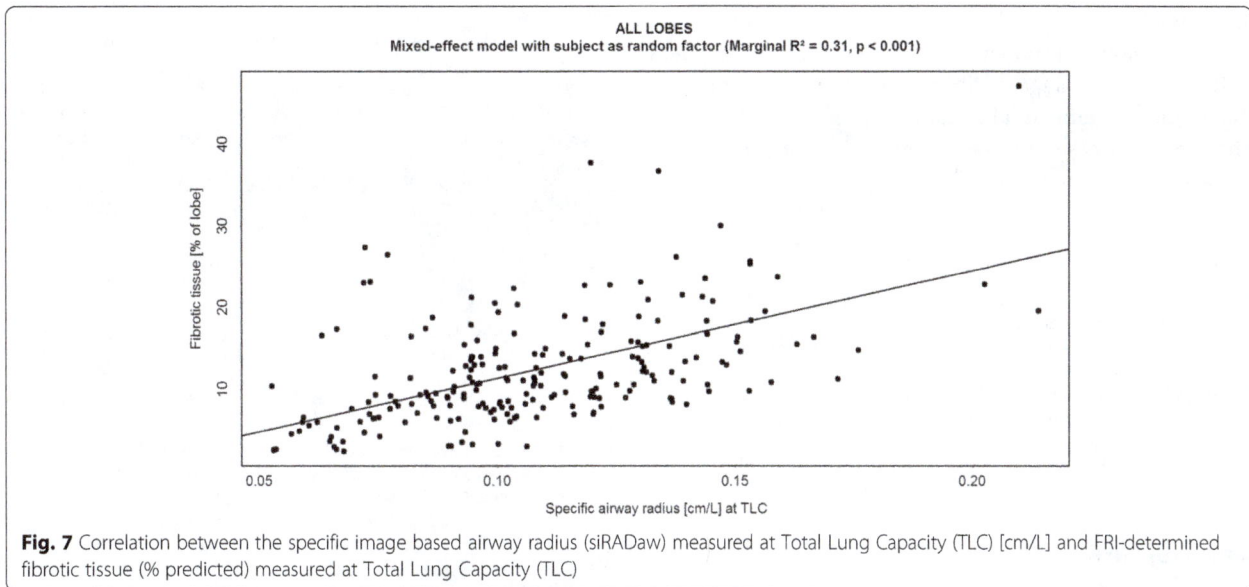

Fig. 7 Correlation between the specific image based airway radius (siRADaw) measured at Total Lung Capacity (TLC) [cm/L] and FRI-determined fibrotic tissue (% predicted) measured at Total Lung Capacity (TLC)

validation of FRI use in IPF is warranted to, reliably, stratify patients in clinical trials as well as predicting outcome in individuals.

We acknowledge the fact that we didn't compare our FRI measurements to a gold standard, although IPF clinical trial design has struggled the last decades to find a primary clinical endpoint (FVC or a qCT measurement) that can be routinely used with adequate precision [47, 48].

The correlation between decline in FVC and progressive reticular fibrosis (after 48 weeks) was also established in the original study cohort by a qCT method [29], as by another recent study [49]. This does

demonstrate the utility and relevance of our qCT method (FRI) and accompanying results.

All patients studied in this trial were treated with a novel investigational drug (pamrevlumab) and no placebo arm was included in this study. The mixed effects model used in the statistical analysis of the data, however ensured that disease progression could be captured by using all available measurement points while correcting for multiple measurements per patient, thereby mitigating the potentially confounding effect of the treatment. The progression itself could potentially be influenced by a treatment effect so this IPF cohort does not represent natural disease progression.

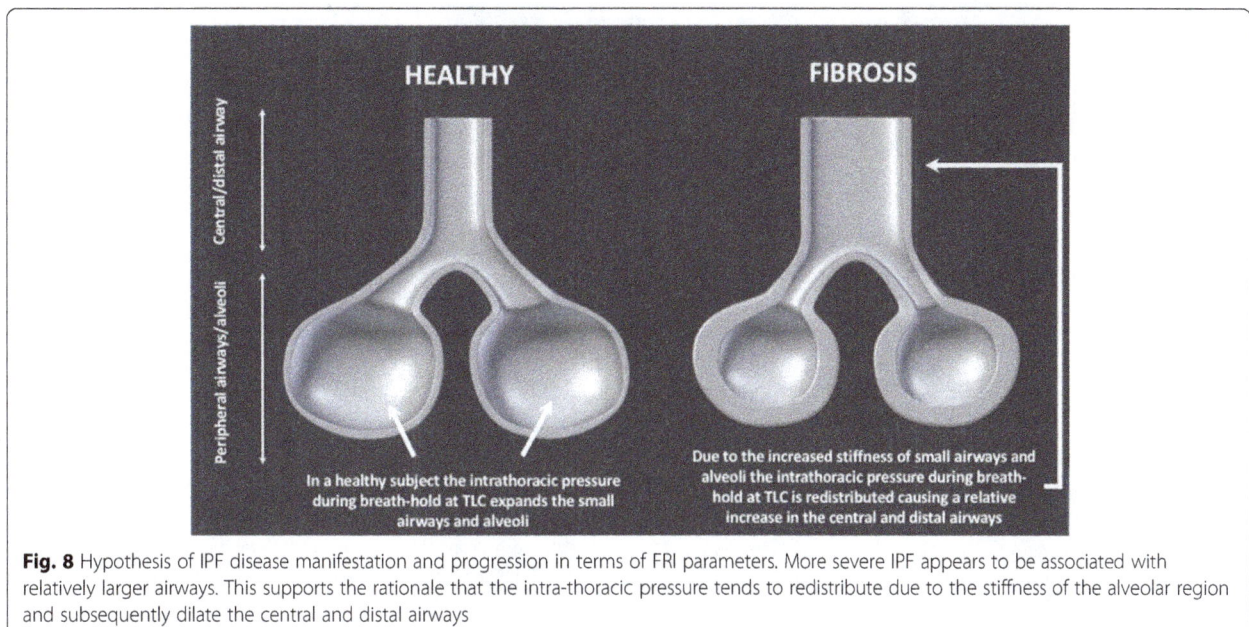

Fig. 8 Hypothesis of IPF disease manifestation and progression in terms of FRI parameters. More severe IPF appears to be associated with relatively larger airways. This supports the rationale that the intra-thoracic pressure tends to redistribute due to the stiffness of the alveolar region and subsequently dilate the central and distal airways

Conclusion

In conclusion, in patients with IPF, FRI parameters (siRADaw, percentage of fibrotic tissue at TLC and predicted lobe volume at TLC) allow monitoring of regional changes in disease and may capture disease progression in patients with preserved FVC.

Abbreviations

(HR)CT: (High resolution) computed tomography; CFD: Computational fluid dynamics; FRI: Functional respiratory imaging; FVC: Forced vital capacity; IPF: Idiopathic pulmonary fibrosis; iVlobe: Imaging lobar volume; PFT: Pulmonary function test; qCT: Quantitative computer derived computed tomography; siRADaw: Specific image based airway radius; TLC: Total lung capacity; UIP: Usual interstitial pneumonia

Acknowledgements
Not applicable.

Funding
Not applicable.

Authors' contributions

Conception and design: JC, ML, WDB, JDB. Analysis and interpretation: JC, ML, BM, CVH, WDB, JDB. Drafting the manuscript for important intellectual content: JC, ML, BM, CVH, JR, SP, EG, EK, KL, WDB, JDB. All authors read and approved the final manuscript.

Competing interests

- Dr. J. Clukers has nothing to disclose.
- Dr. M. Lanclus has nothing to disclose.
- Dr. B. Mignot reports personal fees from FLUIDDA nv, outside the submitted work.
- Dr. C. Van Holsbeke reports personal fees from FLUIDDA nv, outside the submitted work.
- Dr. J. Roseman has nothing to disclose.
- Dr. S. Porter reports personal fees from FibroGen, Inc., during the conduct of the study; personal fees from FibroGen, Inc., outside the submitted work. Dr. Porter has a pending patent US. 9,480,449 issued to FibroGen, Inc.
- Dr. E. Gorina reports personal fees from FibroGen, Inc., during the conduct of the study; personal fees from FibroGen, Inc., outside the submitted work.
- Dr. E. Kouchakji reports other from FibroGen, Inc., outside the submitted work.
- Dr. K. E. Lipson reports personal fees and other from FibroGen, Inc., outside the submitted work; In addition, Dr. Lipson has a patent US 9,587,016 issued to FibroGen, Inc.
- Dr. W. De Backer has nothing to disclose.
- Dr. J. De Backer reports to be founder and CEO of FLUIDDA nv, a company that actively develops and markets part of the technology described in this paper.

Author details

[1]Faculty of Medicine & Health Sciences, University of Antwerp (UAntwerpen), Universiteitsplein 1, 2610 Antwerpen, Belgium. [2]FluidDA nv, Groeningenlei 132, 2550 Kontich, Belgium. [3]FibroGen Inc., 409 Illinois Street, San Francisco, CA 94158, USA.

References

1. Kolb M, Collard HR. Staging of idiopathic pulmonary fibrosis: past, present and future. Eur Respir Rev. 2014;23:220–4.
2. Raghu G, Collard HR, Egan JJ, Martinez FJ, Behr J, Brown KK, et al. An official ATS/ERS/JRS/ALAT statement: idiopathic pulmonary fibrosis: evidence-based guidelines for diagnosis and management. Am J Respir Crit Care Med. 2011; 183:788–824.
3. Selman M, Carrillo G, Estrada A, Mejia M, Becerril C, Cisneros J, et al. Accelerated variant of idiopathic pulmonary fibrosis: clinical behavior and gene expression pattern. PLoS One. 2007;2:e482.
4. Cottin V, Richeldi L. Neglected evidence in idiopathic pulmonary fibrosis and the importance of early diagnosis and treatment. Eur Respir Rev. 2014; 23:106–10.
5. Kolb M, Richeldi L, Behr J, Maher TM, Tang W, Stowasser S, et al. Nintedanib in patients with idiopathic pulmonary fibrosis and preserved lung volume. Thorax. 2017;72:340–6.
6. Cicchitto G, Sanguinetti CM. Idiopathic pulmonary fibrosis: the need for early diagnosis. Multidiscip Respir Med. 2013;8:53.
7. Ley B, Bradford WZ, Weycker D, Vittinghoff E, du Bois RM, Collard HR. Unified baseline and longitudinal mortality prediction in idiopathic pulmonary fibrosis. Eur Respir J. 2015;45:1374–81.
8. Martinez FJ, Collard HR, Pardo A, Raghu G, Richeldi L, Selman M, et al. Idiopathic pulmonary fibrosis. Nature Reviews Disease Primers. 2017;3:17074.
9. du Bois RM, Weycker D, Albera C, Bradford WZ, Costabel U, Kartashov A, et al. Forced vital capacity in patients with idiopathic pulmonary fibrosis: test properties and minimal clinically important difference. Am J Respir Crit Care Med. 2011;184:1382–9.
10. Latsi PI, du Bois RM, Nicholson AG, Colby TV, Bisirtzoglou D, Nikolakopoulou A, et al. Fibrotic idiopathic interstitial pneumonia: the prognostic value of longitudinal functional trends. Am J Respir Crit Care Med. 2003;168:531–7.
11. Albera C. Challenges in idiopathic pulmonary fibrosis trials: the point on end-points. Eur Respir Rev. 2011;20:195–200.
12. Raghu G, Collard HR, Anstrom KJ, Flaherty KR, Fleming TR, King TE Jr, et al. Idiopathic pulmonary fibrosis: clinically meaningful primary endpoints in phase 3 clinical trials. Am J Respir Crit Care Med. 2012;185:1044–8.
13. Pellegrino R, Viegi G, Brusasco V, Crapo RO, Burgos F, Casaburi R, et al. Interpretative strategies for lung function tests. Eur Respir J. 2005;26:948–68.
14. King TE Jr, Bradford WZ, Castro-Bernardini S, Fagan EA, Glaspole I, Glassberg MK, et al. A phase 3 trial of pirfenidone in patients with idiopathic pulmonary fibrosis. N Engl J Med. 2014;370:2083–92.
15. Noble PW, Albera C, Bradford WZ, Costabel U, Glassberg MK, Kardatzke D, et al. Pirfenidone in patients with idiopathic pulmonary fibrosis (CAPACITY): two randomised trials. Lancet. 2011;377:1760–9.
16. Richeldi L, du Bois RM, Raghu G, Azuma A, Brown KK, Costabel U, et al. Efficacy and safety of nintedanib in idiopathic pulmonary fibrosis. N Engl J Med. 2014;370:2071–82.
17. Lopes AJ, Capone D, Mogami R, Cunha DL, Melo PL, Jansen JM. Correlation of tomographic findings with pulmonary function parameters in nonsmoking patients with idiopathic pulmonary fibrosis. J Bras Pneumol. 2007;33:671–8.
18. Jacob J, Bartholmai BJ, Rajagopalan S, Kokosi M, Nair A, Karwoski R, et al. Automated quantitative computed tomography versus visual computed tomography scoring in idiopathic pulmonary fibrosis: validation against pulmonary function. J Thorac Imaging. 2016;31:304–11.
19. Jacob J, Bartholmai BJ, Rajagopalan S, Kokosi M, Nair A, Karwoski R, et al. Mortality prediction in idiopathic pulmonary fibrosis: evaluation of computer-based CT analysis with conventional severity measures. Eur Respir J. 2017;49:1.
20. Yoon RG, Seo JB, Kim N, Lee HJ, Lee SM, Lee YK, et al. Quantitative assessment of change in regional disease patterns on serial HRCT of fibrotic interstitial pneumonia with texture-based automated quantification system. Eur Radiol. 2013;23:692–701.
21. Robbie H, Daccord C, Chua F, Devaraj A. Evaluating disease severity in idiopathic pulmonary fibrosis. Eur Respir Rev. 2017;26. https://doi.org/10.1183/16000617.0051-2017.
22. De Backer J, Vos W, Vinchurkar S, Van Holsbeke C, Poli G, Claes R, et al. The effects of extrafine beclometasone/formoterol (BDP/F) on lung function, dyspnea, hyperinflation, and airway geometry in COPD patients: novel insight using functional respiratory imaging. J Aerosol Med Pulm Drug Deliv. 2015;28:88–99.

23. De Backer JW, Vos WG, Vinchurkar SC, Claes R, Drollmann A, Wulfrank D, et al. Validation of computational fluid dynamics in CT-based airway models with SPECT/CT. Radiology. 2010;257:854–62.

24. De Backer LA, Vos W, De Backer J, Van Holsbeke C, Vinchurkar S, De Backer W. The acute effect of budesonide/formoterol in COPD: a multi-slice computed tomography and lung function study. Eur Respir J. 2012;40:298–305.

25. De Backer LA, Vos WG, Salgado R, De Backer JW, Devolder A, Verhulst SL, et al. Functional imaging using computer methods to compare the effect of salbutamol and ipratropium bromide in patient-specific airway models of COPD. Int J Chron Obstruct Pulmon Dis. 2011;6:637–46.

26. De Backer J, Van Holsbeke C, Vos W, Vinchurkar S, Dorinsky P, Rebello J, et al. Assessment of lung deposition and analysis of the effect of fluticasone/salmeterol hydrofluoroalkane (HFA) pressurized metered dose inhaler (pMDI) in stable persistent asthma patients using functional respiratory imaging. Expert Rev Respir Med. 2016;10:927–33.

27. Kim HJ, Brown MS, Chong D, Gjertson DW, Lu P, Kim HJ, et al. Comparison of the quantitative CT imaging biomarkers of idiopathic pulmonary fibrosis at baseline and early change with an interval of 7 months. Acad Radiol. 2015;22:70–80.

28. Kim HJ, Brown MS, Elashoff R, Li G, Gjertson DW, Lynch DA, et al. Quantitative texture-based assessment of one-year changes in fibrotic reticular patterns on HRCT in scleroderma lung disease treated with oral cyclophosphamide. Eur Radiol. 2011;21:2455–65.

29. Raghu G, Scholand MB, de Andrade J, Lancaster L, Mageto Y, Goldin J, et al. FG-3019 anti-connective tissue growth factor monoclonal antibody: results of an open-label clinical trial in idiopathic pulmonary fibrosis. Eur Respir J. 2016;47:1481–91.

30. De Backer J, De Backer W. Introduction to functional respiratory imaging: a novel approach to assess lung health. Kontich: FLUIDDA nv; 2017.

31. Hunninghake GW, Zimmerman MB, Schwartz DA, King TE Jr, Lynch J, Hegele R, et al. Utility of a lung biopsy for the diagnosis of idiopathic pulmonary fibrosis. Am J Respir Crit Care Med. 2001;164:193–6.

32. Raghu G, Mageto YN, Lockhart D, Schmidt RA, Wood DE, Godwin JD. The accuracy of the clinical diagnosis of new-onset idiopathic pulmonary fibrosis and other interstitial lung disease: a prospective study. Chest. 1999;116:1168–74.

33. Richeldi L, Ryerson CJ, Lee JS, Wolters PJ, Koth LL, Ley B, et al. Relative versus absolute change in forced vital capacity in idiopathic pulmonary fibrosis. Thorax. 2012;67:407–11.

34. Wells AU. Forced vital capacity as a primary end point in idiopathic pulmonary fibrosis treatment trials: making a silk purse from a sow's ear. Thorax. 2013;68:309–10.

35. Jacob J, Bartholmai BJ, Rajagopalan S, Kokosi M, Egashira R, Brun AL, et al. Serial automated quantitative CT analysis in idiopathic pulmonary fibrosis: functional correlations and comparison with changes in visual CT scores. Eur Radiol. 2018;28:1318–27.

36. Jacob J, Bartholmai BJ, Rajagopalan S, Moorsel CHMv, Es HWv, Beek FTv, et al: Predicting Outcomes in Idiopathic Pulmonary Fibrosis Using Automated CT Analysis. Am J Res Crit Care Med 2018, 0:null. https://doi.org/10.1164/rccm.201711-2174OC

37. Lee HY, Lee KS, Jeong YJ, Hwang JH, Kim HJ, Chung MP, et al. High-resolution CT findings in fibrotic idiopathic interstitial pneumonias with little honeycombing: serial changes and prognostic implications. Am J Roentgenol. 2012;199:982–9.

38. Edey AJ, Devaraj AA, Barker RP, Nicholson AG, Wells AU, Hansell DM. Fibrotic idiopathic interstitial pneumonias: HRCT findings that predict mortality. Eur Radiol. 2011;21:1586–93.

39. Piciucchi S, Tomassetti S, Ravaglia C, Gurioli C, Gurioli C, Dubini A, et al. From "traction bronchiectasis" to honeycombing in idiopathic pulmonary fibrosis: a spectrum of bronchiolar remodeling also in radiology? BMC Pulm Med. 2016;16:87.

40. Sumikawa H, Johkoh T, Colby TV, Ichikado K, Suga M, Taniguchi H, et al. Computed tomography findings in pathological usual interstitial pneumonia. Am J Respir Crit Care Med. 2008;177:433–9.

41. Walsh SLF, Wells AU, Sverzellati N, Devaraj A, von der Thüsen J, Yousem SA, et al. Relationship between fibroblastic foci profusion and high resolution CT morphology in fibrotic lung disease. BMC Med. 2015;13:241.

42. Kim EJ, Elicker BM, Maldonado F, Webb WR, Ryu JH, Van Uden JH, et al. Usual interstitial pneumonia in rheumatoid arthritis-associated interstitial lung disease. Eur Respir J. 2010;35:1322–8.

43. Walsh SLF, Sverzellati N, Devaraj A, Keir GJ, Wells AU, Hansell DM. Connective tissue disease related fibrotic lung disease: high resolution computed tomographic and pulmonary function indices as prognostic determinants. Thorax. 2014;69:216–22.

44. Raghu G, Wells AU, Nicholson AG, Richeldi L, Flaherty KR, Le Maulf F, et al. Effect of Nintedanib in subgroups of idiopathic pulmonary fibrosis by diagnostic criteria. Am J Respir Crit Care Med. 2017;195:78–85.

45. Kondoh Y, Taniguchi H, Ogura T, Johkoh T, Fujimoto K, Sumikawa H, et al. Disease progression in idiopathic pulmonary fibrosis without pulmonary function impairment. Respirology. 2013;18:820–6.

46. Yamauchi H, Bando M, Baba T, Kataoka K, Yamada Y, Yamamoto H, et al. Clinical course and changes in high-resolution computed tomography findings in patients with idiopathic pulmonary fibrosis without honeycombing. PLoS One. 2016;11:e0166168.

47. Hansell DM, Goldin JG, King TE Jr, Lynch DA, Richeldi L, Wells AU. CT staging and monitoring of fibrotic interstitial lung diseases in clinical practice and treatment trials: a position paper from the Fleischner society. Lancet Respir Med. 2015;3:483–96.

48. Wu X, Kim GH, Salisbury ML, Barber D, Bartholmai BJ, Brown KK, et al: Computed Tomographic Biomarkers in Idiopathic Pulmonary Fibrosis: The Future of Quantitative Analysis. Am J Res Crit Care Med 2018, 0:null. https://doi.org/10.1164/rccm.201803-0444PP

49. Park HJ, Lee SM, Song JW, Lee SM, Oh SY, Kim N, et al. Texture-based automated quantitative assessment of regional patterns on initial CT in patients with idiopathic pulmonary fibrosis: relationship to decline in forced vital capacity. AJR Am J Roentgenol. 2016;207:976–83.

Permissions

The contributors of this book come from diverse backgrounds, making this book a truly international effort. This book will bring forth new frontiers with its revolutionizing research information and detailed analysis of the nascent developments around the world.

We would like to thank all the contributing authors for lending their expertise to make the book truly unique. They have played a crucial role in the development of this book. Without their invaluable contributions this book wouldn't have been possible. They have made vital efforts to compile up to date information on the varied aspects of this subject to make this book a valuable addition to the collection of many professionals and students.

This book was conceptualized with the vision of imparting up-to-date information and advanced data in this field. To ensure the same, a matchless editorial board was set up. Every individual on the board went through rigorous rounds of assessment to prove their worth. After which they invested a large part of their time researching and compiling the most relevant data for our readers.

The editorial board has been involved in producing this book since its inception. They have spent rigorous hours researching and exploring the diverse topics which have resulted in the successful publishing of this book. They have passed on their knowledge of decades through this book. To expedite this challenging task, the publisher supported the team at every step. A small team of assistant editors was also appointed to further simplify the editing procedure and attain best results for the readers.

Apart from the editorial board, the designing team has also invested a significant amount of their time in understanding the subject and creating the most relevant covers. They scrutinized every image to scout for the most suitable representation of the subject and create an appropriate cover for the book.

The publishing team has been an ardent support to the editorial, designing and production team. Their endless efforts to recruit the best for this project, has resulted in the accomplishment of this book. They are a veteran in the field of academics and their pool of knowledge is as vast as their experience in printing. Their expertise and guidance has proved useful at every step. Their uncompromising quality standards have made this book an exceptional effort. Their encouragement from time to time has been an inspiration for everyone.

The publisher and the editorial board hope that this book will prove to be a valuable piece of knowledge for researchers, students, practitioners and scholars across the globe.

List of Contributors

Masato Watanabe, Keitaro Nakamoto, Toshiya Inui, Mitsuru Sada, Kojiro Honda, Masaki Tamura, Yukari Ogawa, Takuma Yokoyama, Takeshi Saraya, Daisuke Kurai, Haruyuki Ishii and Hajime Takizawa
Department of Respiratory Medicine, Kyorin University School of Medicine, 6-20-3 Sinkawa, Mitaka-city, Tokyo 181-8612, Japan

Gyong Hwa Hong, Bo-Ram Bang, Sang-Yeob Kim, Chan-Gi Pack and Keun-Ai Moon
Asan Institute for Life Science, Seoul, Korea

Gyong Hwa Hong, Hyouk-Soo Kwon, Bo-Ram Bang, Keun-Ai Moon, Tae-Bum Kim, Hee-Bom Moon and You Sook Cho
Department of Internal Medicine, Division of Allergy and Clinical Immunology, Asan Medical Center, University of Ulsan College of Medicine, 88 Olympic-ro 43-gil, Songpa-gu, Seoul 138-736, Korea

So-Young Park
Department of Internal medicine, Division of Allergy and Respiratory Medicine, Konkuk University Medical Center, Seoul, Korea

Jaechun Lee
Department of Internal Medicine, Jeju National University School of Medicine, Jeju, Korea

Sang-Yeob Kim and Chan-Gi Pack
Department of Convergence Medicine, University of Ulsan, Seoul, Korea

Soohyun Kim
Laboratory of Cytokine Immunology, Institute of Biomedical Science and Technology, College of Medicine, Konkuk University, Seoul, Korea

Ann C. Gregory and Matthew B. Sullivan
Department of Microbiology, The Ohio State University, Columbus, OH 43210, USA

Matthew B. Sullivan
Department of Civil, Environmental and Geodetic Engineering, The Ohio State University, Columbus, OH 43210, USA

Leopoldo N. Segal
Division of Pulmonary, Critical Care and Sleep Medicine, New York University School of Medicine, New York, NY 10016, USA

Brian C. Keller
Division of Pulmonary, Critical Care and Sleep Medicine, The Ohio State University College of Medicine, 201 Davis Heart and Lung Research Institute, 473 West 12th Avenue, Columbus, OH 43210, USA

Christer Janson
Department of Medical Sciences: Respiratory, Allergy and Sleep Research, Uppsala University, Akademiska sjukhuset, 75185 Uppsala, Sweden

Gunnar Johansson, Björn Ställberg and Karin Lisspers
Department of Public Health and Caring Sciences, Family Medicine and Preventive Medicine, Uppsala University, Uppsala, Sweden

Petter Olsson
Novartis Sverige AB, Täby, Sweden

Dorothy L. Keininger and Florian S. Gutzwiller
Novartis, Basel, Switzerland

Milica Uhde
IQVIA, Stockholm, Sweden

Leif Jörgensen
IQVIA, Copenhagen, Denmark

Kjell Larsson
Karolinska Institutet, Solna, Sweden

Shuren Guo and Ming Liang
Department of Clinical Laboratory, The First Affiliated Hospital of Zhengzhou University, East Jianshe Road #1, Zhengzhou, Henan 450002, People's Republic of China
Key Clinical Laboratory of Henan province, Zhengzhou, Henan, People's Republic of China

Xiaohuan Mao
Department of Clinical Laboratory, Henan Provincial People's Hospital, Henan Province, Zhengzhou 450003, People's Republic of China

Bo He, Dan Han, Yuan-Ming Jiang, Zhen-Guang Zhang and Wei Zhao
Department of Medical Imaging, the First Affiliated Hospital of Kunming Medical University, No.295 Xichang Road, Kunming 650032, Yunnan, China

Wei Zhao
Department of Thoracic Surgery, the First Affiliated Hospital of Kunming Medical University, Kunming 650032, Yunnan, China

Jiang-Yuan Pi
Department of Pathology, Kunming Medical University, Kunming 650500, Yunnan, China

Lystra P. Hayden and Benjamin A. Raby
Division of Respiratory Diseases, Boston Children's Hospital, Boston, MA, USA

Lystra P. Hayden, Michael H. Cho, Benjamin A. Raby, Edwin K. Silverman and Craig P. Hersh
Channing Division of Network Medicine, Brigham and Women's Hospital, 181 Longwood Avenue, Boston, MA 02115, USA

Michael H. Cho Benjamin A. Raby, Edwin K. Silverman and Craig P. Hersh
Division of Pulmonary and Critical Care Medicine, Brigham and Women's Hospital, Boston, MA, USA

Terri H. Beaty
Bloomberg School of Public Health, Johns Hopkins University, Baltimore, MD, USA

Helena Crisford and Elizabeth Sapey
Institute of Inflammation and Ageing, University of Birmingham, Edgbaston, Birmingham B15 2GW, UK

Robert A. Stockley
University Hospital Birmingham NHS Foundation Trust, Edgbaston, Birmingham B15 2GW, UK

Helena Crisford
Institute of Inflammation and Ageing, College of Medical and Dental Sciences, Centre for Translational Inflammation Research, University of Birmingham Research Laboratories, Queen Elizabeth Hospital Birmingham, Mindelsohn Way, Birmingham B15 2WB, UK

Christian Domingo
Department of Medicine, Universitat Autònoma de Barcelona, Barcelona, Spain

Christian Domingo
Pulmonary Service, Corporació Sanitària Parc Taulí, Sabadell, Barcelona, Spain

Oscar Palomares
Department of Biochemistry and Molecular Biology, School of Chemistry, Complutense University of Madrid, Madrid, Spain

David A. Sandham
Novartis Institutes for Biomedical Research, Cambridge, MA, USA

Veit J. Erpenbeck
Novartis Pharma AG, Basel, Switzerland

Pablo Altman
Novartis Pharmaceuticals Corporation, One Health Plaza East Hanover, East Hanover, NJ 07936-1080, USA

Amelia Chiara Trombetta, Stefano Soldano, Veronica Tomatis, Barbara Ruaro, Sabrina Paolino, Renata Brizzolara, Paola Montagna, Alberto Sulli, Carmen Pizzorni and Maurizio Cutolo
Research Laboratory and Academic Division of Clinical Rheumatology, Department of Internal Medicine, University of Genova, Polyclinic San Martino Hospital, Genoa, Italy

Paola Contini
Clinical Immunology, Department of Internal Medicine, University of Genova, Genoa, Italy

Vanessa Smith
Department of Rheumatology, Ghent University Hospital, Ghent, Belgium
Department of Internal Medicine, Ghent University, Ghent, Belgium

Hye Jung Park, Min Kwang Byun and Hyung Jung Kim
Department of Internal Medicine, Gangnam Severance Hospital, Yonsei University College of Medicine, 211 Eonju-ro Gangnam-gu, Seoul 06273, Korea

Chin Kook Rhee and Kyungjoo Kim
Division of Pulmonary, Allergy and Critical Care Medicine, Department of Internal Medicine, Seoul St Mary's Hospital, College of Medicine, The Catholic University of Korea, Seoul, Korea

Kwang-Ha Yoo
Department of Internal Medicine, Konkuk University School of Medicine, Seoul, Korea

Joo Heung Yoon, Mehdi Nouraie, Xiaoping Chen, Richard H Zou, Jacobo Sellares, Kristen L Veraldi, Jared Chiarchiaro, Kathleen Lindell, David O Wilson, Kevin Gibson and Daniel J Kass
Dorothy P. and Richard P. Simmons Center for Interstitial Lung Disease and Division of Pulmonary, Allergy, and Critical Care Medicine, University of Pittsburgh, NW 628 UPMC Montefiore, 3459 Fifth Avenue Pittsburgh, Pittsburgh, PA 15213, USA

Jacobo Sellares
Interstitial Lung Diseases Program, Servei de Pneumologia, Institut Clinic Respiratori, Barcelona, Spain

Naftali Kaminski
Section of Pulmonary, Critical Care and Sleep Medicine, Yale University, New Haven, CT,USA

Timothy Burns
Division of Hematology and Oncology, University of Pittsburgh, Pittsburgh, PA, USA

Humberto Trejo Bittar and Samuel Yousem
Department of Pathology, University of Pittsburgh, Pittsburgh, PA, USA

Guangjie Liu and Jie Xu
Department of Respiratory Medicine, Beijing Tongren Hospital, CapitalMedical University, Beijing 100730, China

Peng Hao, Liming Wang, Yuchuan Wang, Ruifang Han, Ming Ying and Xuan Li
Tianjin Eye Hospital, Tianjin Eye Institute, Tianjin Key Lab of Ophthalmology and Visual Science, Tianjin 300020, China

Peng Hao, Liming Wang, Yuchuan Wang, Ruifang Han, Ming Ying, Shuangshuang Sui and Jinghua Liu
Clinical College of Ophthalmology, Tianjin Medical University, Tianjin 300020, China

Peng Hao, Liming Wang, Yuchuan Wang, Ruifang Han and Ming Ying
Nankai University Affiliated Eye Hospital, Tianjin 300020, China

Jing Yang, Jian Luo, Ling Yang, Dan Yang, Dan Wang, Bicui Liu, Tingxuan Huang, Xiaohu Wang, Binmiao Liang and Chuntao Liu
Department of Respiratory and Critical Care Medicine, West China School of Medicine and West China Hospital, Sichuan University, No.37, Guoxue Alley, Chengdu 610041, China

Jing Yang
Department of Respiratory Medicine, Mianyang Central Hospital, Mianyang 621099, China

Zhiheng Xu, Yimin Li, Jianmeng Zhou, Xi Li, Yongbo Huang, Xiaoqing Liu and Haibo Zhang
State Key Laboratory of Respiratory Diseases, National Clinical Research Center for Respiratory Disease, Guangzhou Institute for Respiratory Health, Guangzhou, China

Zhiheng Xu, Yimin Li, Jianmeng Zhou, Xi Li, Yongbo Huang and Haibo Zhang
Department of Critical Care Medicine, The First Affiliated Hospital of Guangzhou Medical University, Guangzhou, China

Karen E. A. Burns and Haibo Zhangs
Interdepartmental Division of Critical Care Medicine, University of Toronto, Toronto, ON, Canada
The Keenan Research Centre for Biomedical Science and the Li Ka Shing Knowledge Institute of St. Michael's Hospital, Toronto, ON M5B1W8, Canada
Departments of Anesthesia and Physiology, University of Toronto, Toronto, ON, Canada

Lukas Fischer, Nicola Benjamin, Benjamin Egenlauf, Satenik Harutyunova, Maria Koegler, Alberto M. Marra, Christian Nagel, Panagiota Xanthouli and Ekkehard Grünig
Centre for Pulmonary Hypertension, Thoraxklinik at Heidelberg University Hospital,Röntgenstrasse 1, D-69126 Heidelberg, Germany

Nicola Benjamin, Benjamin Egenlauf, Satenik Harutyunova, Alberto M. Marra, Christian Nagel, Panagiota Xanthouli and Ekkehard Grünig
Translational Lung Research Center Heidelberg (TLRC), Member of the German Center for Lung Research (DZL), Heidelberg, Germany

Norbert Blank and Hanns-Martin Lorenz
Department of Rheumatology, University Hospital Heidelberg, Heidelberg, Germany

Christine Fischer
Institute of HumanGenetics, University of Heidelberg, Heidelberg, Germany

Alberto M. Marra
IRCCS SDN Research Institute, Naples, Italy

Christian Nagel
Lung Centre, Klinikum Mittelbaden, Baden-Baden Balg, Baden-Baden, German

Eduardo Bossone
Heart Department, Cardiology Division, "Cava de' Tirreni and Amalfi Coast" Hospital, University of Salerno, Salerno, Italy

Line Verckist, Isabel Pintelon, Jean-Pierre Timmermans, Inge Brouns and Dirk Adriaensen
Laboratory of Cell Biology and Histology, Department of Veterinary Sciences, University of Antwerp, Universiteitsplein 1, 2610 Wilrijk, Antwerpen, Belgium

Lihui Zou, Junhua Zhang, Jingli Han, Wenqing Li and Fei Xiao
The MOH Key Laboratory of Geriatrics, Beijing Hospital, National Center of Gerontology, Beijing 100730, People's Republic of China

Fei Su
Department of Pathology, Beijing Hospital, National Center of Gerontology, Beijing 100730, People's Republic of China

Xiaomao Xu
Department of Respiratory and Critical Care Medicine, Beijing Hospital, National Center of Gerontology, Beijing 100730, People's Republic of China

Zhenguo Zhai
Department of Respiratory and Critical Care Medicine, China-Japan Friendship Hospital, Beijing 100029, People's Republic of China

Ian P. Naya, Hana Muellerova, Christopher Compton and Paul W. Jones
Respiratory Medicine, GSK, Brentford, Middlesex, UK

Lee Tombs
Precise Approach Ltd, Contingent worker on assignment at GSK, Uxbridge, Middlesex, UK

Toby C. Lewis, Ediri E. Metitiri, Ashley R. Carpenter, Adam M. Goldsmith, Kyra E. Wicklund, Breanna N. Eder, Adam T. Comstock, Jeannette M. Ricci, Sean R. Brennan, Ginger L. Washington, Kendall B. Owens and Marc B. Hershenson
Departments of Pediatrics and Communicable Diseases, University of Michigan Medical School, 1150 W. Medical Center Dr., Building MSRB2, Room 3570B, Ann Arbor, MI 48109-5688, USA

Marc B. Hershenson
Molecular and Integrative Physiology, University of Michigan Medical School, Ann Arbor, USA

Bhramar Mukherjee
Departments of Biostatistics, University of Michigan School of Public Health, University of Michigan, Ann Arbor, MI 48109, USA

Toby C. Lewis, Xiaodan Ren, Thomas G. Robins and Stuart A. Batterman
Environmental Health Sciences, University of Michigan School of Public Health, University of Michigan, Ann Arbor, MI 48109, USA

Kyra E. Wicklund
Epidemiology, University of Michigan School of Public Health, University of Michigan, Ann Arbor, MI 48109, USA

Toby C. Lewis, Ediri E. Metitiri and Graciela B. Mentz
Health Behavior/Health Education, University of Michigan School of Public Health, University of Michigan, Ann Arbor, MI 48109, USA

J. Clukers, W. De Backer and J. De Backer
Faculty of Medicine and Health Sciences, University of Antwerp (UAntwerpen), Universiteitsplein 1, 2610 Antwerpen, Belgium

M. Lanclus, B. Mignot, C. Van Holsbeke, J. Roseman, W. De Backer and J. De Backer
FluidDA nv, Groeningenlei 132, 2550 Kontich, Belgium

S. Porter, E. Gorina, E. Kouchakji and K. E. Lipson
FibroGen Inc., 409 Illinois Street, San Francisco, CA 94158, USA

Index